Challenging Bias in Forensic Psychological Assessment and Testing

Challenging Bias in Forensic Psychological Assessment and Testing is a groundbreaking work that addresses the biases and inequalities within the field of forensic psychology. It gives valuable insights into individual practices and wider criminal justice approaches at an international level, while providing tangible solutions to tackle the disparities.

This book constructively critiques current forensic practice and psychological assessment approaches through a variety of diverse voices from pioneering researchers around the world who offer their expertise on these challenges and assist the reader to consider their potential contribution to pushing forward the frontiers of Forensic Psychology. The authors also locate the origin of these biases in order to further dismantle them, and improve the outcomes for the forensic client base – especially specific diverse populations. They emphasise the need to be creative and evolve not just in line with the real-world changes of today, but also to prevent the issues of tomorrow before they become the next news headline.

This is a must read for professionals working in criminal justice, forensic psychology, legal psychology, and related fields. It is also a compelling resource for students and researchers of forensic psychology with particular interest in social diversity and inclusion.

Glenda C. Liell is a Forensic Psychologist with 24 years' experience in roles across criminal justice including high security prisons, regional psychology, headquarters, and probation. She is the current Chair of the BPS Committee on Test Standards and has represented the Division of Forensic Psychology on other BPS Committees. She has also guest lectured at various universities.

Martin J. Fisher is a Forensic Psychologist and has worked in the criminal justice field for over 33 years in England and Wales. He has honorary appointments within NHS Secure Services and Academia. He is also a past Chair of the BPS Committee on Test Standards, past member of the BPS Ethics Committee, and a member of the BPS Research Board.

Lawrence F. Jones, a Consultant Clinical and Forensic Psychologist, is the head of the psychology services at Rampton high secure hospital. He is an honorary clinical associate professor at Nottingham University and is a former chair of the Division of Forensic psychology. He has authored work on trauma, case formulation, and pragmatic risk assessment.

Issues in Forensic Psychology

Series Editors: Richard Shuker and Geraldine Akerman

The views expressed by the authors/editors may not necessarily be those held by the Series Editors or HMPPS.

Supervision for Forensic Practitioners
Edited by Jason Davies

Transforming Environments and Rehabilitation
A Guide for Practitioners in Forensic Settings and Criminal Justice
Edited by Geraldine Akerman, Adrian Needs, and Claire Bainbridge

The Psychology of Criminal Investigation
From Theory to Practice
Edited by Andy Griffiths and Rebecca Milne

Assessing and Managing Problematic Sexual Interests
A Practitioner's Guide
Edited by Geraldine Akerman, Derek Perkins, and Ross Bartels

Global Perspectives on Interventions in Forensic Therapeutic Communities
A Practitioner's Guide
Edited by Geraldine Akerman and Richard Shuker

Trauma-Informed Forensic Practice
Edited by Phil Wilmot and Lawrence Jones

Working with Autistic People in the Criminal Justice and Forensic Mental Health Systems
A Handbook for Practitioners
Edited by Nichola Tyler and Anne Sheeran

Challenging Bias in Forensic Psychological Assessment and Testing
Theoretical and Practical Approaches to Working with Diverse Populations
Edited by Glenda C. Liell, Martin J. Fisher, and Lawrence F. Jones

For more information about this series, please visit: www.routledge.com/Issues-in-Forensic-Psychology/book-series/IFP

Challenging Bias in Forensic Psychological Assessment and Testing

Theoretical and Practical Approaches to Working with Diverse Populations

Edited by Glenda C. Liell, Martin J. Fisher, and Lawrence F. Jones

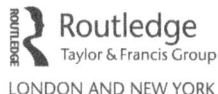
Routledge
Taylor & Francis Group

LONDON AND NEW YORK

Cover image: Getty

First published 2023
by Routledge
4 Park Square, Milton Park, Abingdon, Oxon OX14 4RN

and by Routledge
605 Third Avenue, New York, NY 10158

Routledge is an imprint of the Taylor & Francis Group, an informa business

British Library Cataloguing-in-Publication Data
A catalogue record for this book is available from the British Library

Library of Congress Cataloging-in-Publication Data
Names: Liell, Glenda C., editor. | Jones, Lawrence F. (Lawrence Francis), editor. | Fisher, Martin J., 1967- editor.
Title: Challenging bias in forensic psychological assessment and testing : theoretical and practical approaches to working with diverse populations / edited by edited by Glenda C. Liell, Martin J. Fisher, and Lawrence F. Jones.
Description: Abingdon, Oxon ; New York, NY : Routledge, 2023. | Series: Issues in forensic psychology | Includes bibliographical references and index.
Identifiers: LCCN 2022015244 (print) | LCCN 2022015245 (ebook) | ISBN 9781032138282 (paperback) | ISBN 9781032138299 (hardback) | ISBN 9781003230977 (ebook)
Subjects: LCSH: Forensic psychology. | Forensic psychology--Moral and ethical aspects. | Forensic psychology--Practice.
Classification: LCC RA1148 .C43 2023 (print) | LCC RA1148 (ebook) | DDC 614/.15--dc23/eng/20220505
LC record available at https://lccn.loc.gov/2022015244
LC ebook record available at https://lccn.loc.gov/2022015245

ISBN: 978-1-032-13829-9 (hbk)
ISBN: 978-1-032-13828-2 (pbk)
ISBN: 978-1-003-23097-7 (ebk)

DOI: 10.4324/9781003230977

Typeset in Baskerville
by MPS Limited, Dehradun

MF – "for Dexter, Oscar, Jake and Lucas and what the future holds".

GL – "For my husband Jim – thank you for believing in me, and for your love and support, & for my mum Elisa – I'm so glad you could see me do this".

LJ – "for my family for their forbearance".

ALL – "For all our colleagues working in forensic contexts around the world. We can, and will, strive to do better".

Contents

Future Directions

Glossary

(Chapter designation where acronym first appears.)

Chapter 1

DACES	Detection and Conviction Evasion Skills
CJS	Criminal Justice System
BPS	The British Psychological Society
D&I	Diversity and Inclusion
PAM	Predictive Agency Model
CAMCB	Cultural Agency-Model of Criminal Behaviour
RTO	Return to Offending
VR	Virtual Reality
HCPC	Health & Care Professions Council (UK)
PTMF	Power Threat Meaning Framework
PCP	Personal Construct Psychology
CJJI	UK Criminal Justice Joint Inspectorate
NDD	Neuro-Developmental Disorder
ADHD	Attention Deficit Hyperactivity Disorder
PCL-R	Psychopathy Checklist (Revised)
LGBTQIA	Lesbian, Gay, Bisexual, Transgender, Transsexual, Two- spirit, Queer, Questioning, Intersex, Asexual, Ally, A-gender, Bi-gender, Gender Queer, Pansexual, Pangender, and Gender Variant.

Chapter 2

EDI	Equality, Diversity and Inclusion
HCA	Health Care Assistant
AP	Assistant Psychologist

Chapter 3

RNR	Risk-Need-Responsivity (Model)
GPCSL	General Personality and Cognitive Social Learning
CBT	Cognitive-Behavioural Theory
PAM	The Predictive Agency Model
RCM	Risk-Causality Method

DRF   Dynamic Risk Factors
GLM   Good Lives Model

Chapter 4

CAMCB   Cultural Agency-Model of Criminal Behaviour

Chapter 5

IQ   Intellectual Quotient
DES   Detection Evasion Skills/Strategies
MAPPA   Multi Agency Public Protection Arrangements
DNA   DeoxyriboNucleic Acid
LOS   Levels of Surveillance
CES   Conviction Evasion Skills

Chapter 6

LSI-R   Level of Service Inventory – Revised

Chapter 7

CTT   Classical Test Theory
RAMAS   Risk Assessment Management and Audit System
ICD10   International Classification of Diseases – v10
WHO   World Health Organisation
PD   Personality Disorder
IRT   Item Response Theory
ICC   Item Characteristic Curve

Chapter 8

VR   Virtual Reality
VE   Virtual Environment
GPS   Global Positioning Satellite
SOCs   Sexual Offenders against Children
EMA   Ecological Momentary Assessments
VRAPT   VR Aggression Prevention Training
MEPS   Mobile-Enhanced Prevention Support
STD   Sexually Transmitted Disease

Chapter 9

CBT   Cognitive Behavioural Therapy
STI   Sexually Transmitted Illness

Chapter 10

PSYPACT   Psychology Interjurisdictional Compact
FMHA   Forensic Mental Health Assessments
HIPAA   Health Insurance Portability and Accessibility Act
GDPR   General Data Protection Regulations

Chapter 11
Chapter 12

PTMF Power Threat Meaning Framework
IPP Imprisonment for Public Protection

Chapter 13
Chapter 14

CFI Cultural Formulation Interview

Chapter 15

PCP Personal Construct Psychology
PCT Personal Construct Theory
PCA Principal Components Analysis

Chapter 16

ESI Electronically Stored Information
MSO Mental State at the Time of Offense

Chapter 17

PTSD Post Traumatic Stress Disorder
LSI Level of Service Inventory
SPJ Structured Professional Judgement
FAM Female Additional Manual (to the HCR-20 V2 & V3)

Chapter 18

GNC Gender Non-Conforming
WATHP World Association of Transgender Health Professionals

Chapter 19

LDDs Learning Difficulties and Disabilities
DCD Developmental Coordination Disorder
ADHD Attention Deficit Hyperactivity Disorder
ASC Autism Spectrum Conditions
DLD Developmental Language Disorder
ABI Acquired Brain Injury
PDA Pathological Demand Avoidance
TBI Traumatic Brain Injury
GEM Global Ethnic Majority
SEN Special Educational Needs

Chapter 20

LD Learning Disability
DRAMS Dynamic Risk Appraisal and Management System
CuRV Current Risk of Violence
SDRS Short Dynamic Risk Scale

Chapter 20
Chapter 22

BSL   British Sign Language
PHU   Units for Partially Hearing children
LDS   Language Deprivation Syndrome
VIQ   Verbal Intellectual Quotient
PIQ   Performance Intellectual Quotient

Chapter 23

EMDR   Eye Movement Desensitisation and Reprocessing

Chapter 24

P/CVE Prevent/Countering Violent Extremism
ERG   Extremism Risk Guide
VERA   Violence and Extremism Risk Assessment
MLG   Multi Level Guidelines

Chapter 25

CAPP   Comprehensive Assessment of Psychopathic Personality

Chapter 26

PPG   Penile Plethysmograph
ACE   Adverse Childhood Experience
ITSO   Integrated Theory of Sexual Offending
EISIP Explicit and Implicit Sexual Interest Profile

Chapter 27

Contributors

Natalie M. Anumba, Ph.D., is assistant professor of Psychiatry at UMass Chan Medical School, where she serves as Co-Director of the Law & Psychiatry Division in the Department of Psychiatry. She conducts forensic mental health evaluations; has co-authored articles and book chapters; and presents at local, national, and international conferences.

Dr. Palwinder Athwal-Kooner is a BPS Chartered and HCPC Registered Forensic Psychologist. She started her career working in forensic practice, predominantly forensic mental health services. She moved into academia in 2013. She is currently a Principal Lecturer at Nottingham Trent University since 2016. She is a member of the DFP committee and the EDI subcommittee.

Tanya Banfield leads in the Occupational Development Team of Genius Within CIC, a forensic and Autism Specialist qualified in psychometric testing, person-centred psychotherapy, coaching and disability inclusion. Currently completing a Professional Doctorate in Health: A Quantitative Study Within the Criminal Justice System: A Critical Evaluation of the Rehabilitation of Autistic Offenders in Prison.

Ashley B. Batastini is an assistant professor at the University of Memphis in the Department of Counselling, Educational Psychology, & Research. Her professional interests include development of and research on mental health interventions for criminal justice-involved populations and best practices in forensic mental health assessment.

Kerry Beckley is a Consultant Clinical Forensic Psychologist and Trainer/ Supervisor in Schema Therapy. She previously worked in NHS secure hospital and community forensic settings in the United Kingdom and is now in independent practice, primarily conducting risk assessments. Kerry also continues to provide schema therapy training and supervision for forensic practitioners.

Dr Nicholas Blagden is a co-founder and trustee of the charity Safer Living Foundation, Associate Professor in Forensic Psychology, Chartered Psychologist and Head of the Sexual Offences Crime and Misconduct

Research Unit at Nottingham Trent University. He has worked and researched within criminal justice and prison settings for 15 years. Dr Blagden has a track record of high quality research, has led programme evaluations and has disseminated his work in high ranking international journals and conferences.

Rachel N. Bomysoad is a doctoral student in clinical psychology at Montclair State University. Her research interests are in the area of forensic psychology and include eyewitness interviewing, forensic mental health assessment, substance misuse, dishonesty, juvenile justice, and opportunities for technological innovations.

Luke Butcher has spent over 15 years working in senior levels within government and non-government organisations in regional, rural, and remote Australia. His research interests include service user involvement in health and human service delivery, engagement of cultural knowledge holders in service design, and place-based models of care.

Mark Callender is a Principle Forensic Psychologist working within the National High Secure Learning Disability and Autism Service. For 20 years he has worked across high, medium, and low secure settings. He specialises in engaging individuals with intellectual and developmental difficulties that present behaviours that challenge and low motivation.

Ana Clara DaSilva is a BPS DFP in-training representative helping to bring awareness to the lack of ethnic diversity in the field. Ana contributed to numerous events regarding her trainee journey and is the force behind the DFP Network of Black and Asian Forensic Psychologists. Has worked in mental health, secure and community settings.

Jason Davies is a chartered (BPS) and registered (HCPC) clinical and forensic psychologist, BPS Fellow and AdvanceHE Senior Fellow. He has worked as a clinician in secure inpatient and community based forensic mental health services. His current research includes forensic assessment and formulation; treatment impact, and staff support, performance and well-being.

Andrew Day is a Professor in the discipline of Criminology in the School for Social and Political Sciences. A clinical and forensic psychologist by training, his research interests have generally been in the area of correctional psychology and rehabilitation.

Christopher Dean is a chartered and registered forensic psychologist, director of Identify Psychological Services Ltd, senior fellow at the Global Center on Cooperative Security and a Parole Board member. For the past 13 years he has provided specialist psychological services and consultancy to prevent terrorism and violent extremism.

Mats Dernevik is a Clinical and Forensic Psychologist from Sweden. He did his PhD on mentally disordered offenders at the Karolinska Institute in Stockholm. He works as Consultant Psychologist with Deaf people in the private healthcare sector and is a visiting research fellow at University of Lincoln.

Dr Nancy Doyle is an Occupational Psychologist specialising in disability inclusion, founder of the non-profit company Genius Within. Genius Within provides career and occupational inclusion consulting in prisons, unemployed communities, businesses, and corporates. Nancy is the Co-Director of the Centre for Neurodiversity Research at Work, at Birkbeck, University of London.

Jean-Louis van Gelder is Director of the MPI for the Study of Crime, Law and Security, and Full Professor at the Institute of Education and Child Studies, University of Leiden. Research interests include emotions and personality, novel technologies such as virtual reality, and the relation between short-term mindsets and crime.

Kenny Gonzalez, MA, is a clinical psychology PhD student at Montclair State University. He is also an adjunct instructor at John Jay College in New York City. His research interests include violence risk assessment, psychopathy, police and public safety psychology, and cross-cultural considerations in forensic assessment.

Lauren Grove, MA, is a doctoral candidate in the clinical psychology PhD programme at Montclair State University. She earned her BA in psychology from Temple University and her MA in clinical psychology from Towson University. Her research interests include adolescent decision making and treatment and assessment of justice-involved youth.

Michelle Guyton is a licensed psychologist board-certified in forensic psychology. She is co-owner and training director at Northwest Forensic Institute, a private practice forensic evaluation practice, in Portland, Oregon. Before entering full-time practice, Dr Guyton taught at Pacific University Graduate School of Psychology.

Sean Hammond is retired from the School of Applied Psychology, University College Cork where he served as Statutory Lecturer, Director of the Forensic Psychology Postgraduate Programme and Head of School. Prior to this, he was the Head of the Clinical Decision Making Support Unit at Broadmoor Hospital and Senior Lecturer at the University of Surrey. He has an expertise in Forensic Psychometrics and multivariate data analysis.

R. Karl Hanson co-developed several widely used risk tools, including Static-99R and STABLE-2007 when working for Public Safety Canada (1991–2017). Currently, he is an Adjunct Research Professor in the Psychology Department of Carleton University, and President of the Society for the Advancement of Actuarial Risk Need Assessment (SAARNA).

Roxanne Heffernan has published numerous academic papers on the relationship between dynamic risk factors and crime and developed explanations of offending based in human agency, her recent book is Heffernan and Ward (2020) *Dynamic Risk in Sexual Offending: Causal Considerations.* Springer.

Sören Henrich is a lecturer in Forensic Psychology at the University of Central Lancashire and Research Associate working for secure forensic settings across the Merseycare NHS Foundation Trust. He leads research establishing non-pathologising guidance for trans care and is part of national and international work groups and forums on this topic.

Rachel Hicks is an Assistant Psychologist and Forensic Psychologist in Training for the National High Secure Learning Disability and Autism Service.

Todd E. Hogue is a Registered Forensic and Clinical Psychologist, Professor of Forensic Psychology at the University of Lincoln. Having worked in prison, community and secure mental health settings with individuals who have personality disorder and sexual or violent offending histories he currently researches the impact of attitudes and individual factors on professional judgements.

Lorraine Hough is a Chartered Occupational and Forensic Psychologist, with over 30 years applied experience, within Employment Service, Disability Service; RNIB and RNID, (Rehabilitation). An Assessor for Division of Occupational Psychology, she is currently Senior Forensic Verifier for the BPS, serving on the Committee on Test Standards and the Verifier Group.

Elizabeth Kimber is a research assistant at Greater Manchester Mental Health NHS Foundation Trust. Lizzie has a clinical psychology research masters and experience of working in Deaf services as an assistant psychologist. Lizzie intends to pursue a career in clinical psychology and holds a special interest in Deaf mental health.

Christopher M. King, JD, PhD, is a member of the psychology faculty at Montclair State University. He teaches and conducts research related to forensic psychology, correctional psychology, police and public safety psychology, and mental health law. He also works as an independent contracting psychologist in private practice.

Daryl G. Kroner, PhD, is a professor in the School of Justice and Public Safety at Southern Illinois University Carbondale. Prior to this position, he was employed as a correctional psychologist from 1986 to 2008. His current research interests include risk assessment, measurement and mechanisms of change, and criminal desistance.

Monica Lloyd is a chartered and registered forensic psychologist who worked in HMPPS and HMI Prisons before joining the University of Birmingham. Following dedicated work with terrorist offenders in custody she continues to research and publish in extremist violence, and to provide consultancy to the European Radicalisation Awareness Network.

Emma Longfellow is a Consultant Forensic Psychologist and Psychology Lead for the National High Secure Learning Disability and Autism Service. She has over 20 years' experience of working with Intellectual and Developmental difficulties across the National Health Service and Her Majesty's Prison and Probation Service.

Madison Lord earned her master's from Georgia State University and is a current Counselling Psychology doctoral student at the University of Memphis. As a member of the Correctional and Forensic Psychology Research Lab, her interests include bias in forensic assessment and the use of social media evidence across psycholegal contexts.

Dr Brendan Monteiro is a Consultant Psychiatrist in Deaf Mental Health Care. He has led the development and delivery of Mental Health services for Deaf people. He is Honorary Professor of Health & Society, University of Salford. He has extensive experience worldwide of lecturing on Mental Health and Deafness.

Adrian Needs did extensive work in HM Prison Service which encompassed high security and training services, the latter leading to a prominent role with the BPS in developing national standards for professional qualification in forensic psychology. This led to university-based work, including recent research with veterans, trauma, personal change and related intersubjective and systemic processes.

Margaret O'Rourke is a Chartered Forensic Clinical Psychologist and Researcher with over 25 years experience in NHS services in mental health, addiction, and forensic services. Dr O'Rourke has held a number of national roles, including risk management advisor Department of Health, National Strategy for Healthy Doctors, Ireland, Clinical Governance Panel British Psychological Society, President of Psychological Society Ireland, Clinical Director of SafeNOW USA and Chair of BPS Forensic Clinical Psychology Group.

Meera Patel is a third-year Counselling Psychology Doctoral Student at the University of Memphis. Her ongoing clinical research interests include jury decision making, re-entry programmes, criminality in minority populations, and personality disorders.

Derek Perkins, PhD, is a Registered Clinical and Forensic Psychologist, Professor of Forensic Psychology at Royal Holloway University of London and Co-Director of online PROTECT research group. He has published on sexual offending, online child sexual abuse and sexual homicide, and is an expert witness in Family and Criminal Court proceedings.

Ignazio Puzzo, PhD, is a Senior Lecturer in Psychology at Brunel University London. His current research focuses on understanding the interplay between affective, neurocognitive, and social factors contributing to the development of aggressive and antisocial behaviour in children and adolescents as well as in adults mentally disordered offenders.

Jo Ramsden is the clinical lead for Leeds Personality Disorder Services and works as a consultant clinical psychologist for the cluster of services in the Yorkshire region commissioned under the Offender Personality Disorder strategy. Jo regularly teaches for UCLAN on the Knowledge and Understanding Framework MSc and is a certified MBT therapist and supervisor.

Martine Ratcliffe has worked in the Criminal Justice System for 21 years. She has worked with Young Adults facilitating and managing Offending Behaviour Programmes, as well as offering a Crisis Intervention Service. She has also worked with male and female life sentenced prisoners for over 10 years. Her roles have included the supervision of Trainee Forensic Psychologists. Martine is now Diversity and Inclusion National Lead for a Psychology Services Group in a large UK Public Sector Organisation.

Job van der Schalk is an assistant professor at the Institute of Education and Child Studies, University of Leiden. He previously was an assistant professor at Cardiff University and was associate editor of the British journal of Social Psychology. His research interests include social psychology, emotion, and decision making.

Stefanie Schmidt is a postdoctoral researcher at the faculty of Psychology at FernUniversität in Hagen. Her research focuses on understanding how cultural socialisation shapes the development of offending behaviour and on how to adapt risk assessment and offender rehabilitation accordingly. She trains forensic practitioners on risk assessment and intercultural competence.

Jacob Seaward has worked for HMPPS for 20 years. He currently works across several different prisons in Hampshire, Wiltshire, and the Thames Valley. He has maintained an interest in the assessment of personality and psychopathy in a forensic context throughout his career, including its ethics.

Aniek Siezenga is a doctoral student at Leiden University in the Netherlands and the MPI for the Study of Crime, Law and Security in Germany. She studies the interaction between technology, such as virtual reality and smartphone applications, and human behaviour.

Jenny Tew has worked for HMPPS for over 20 years. She is the head of Psychology at HMP Long Lartin and previously worked in the Chromis and Psychopathy team within Interventions Services. Her PhD is in the Assessment and treatment of those with high levels of psychopathic traits.

Karen Thorne is a Chartered and Registered Forensic Psychologist, with over 26 years' experience of working in forensic settings. She has extensive experience in the assessment and treatment of people with convictions and her research interests include traumatic brain injury and sexual offending.

Loumarie Vasquez is a master's student in clinical psychology at Montclair State University, currently completing an externship at a community mental health centre. She also works as an allied human services professional. Her professional interests include evidence-based mental healthcare and social justice.

Michael Vitacco is a board-certified forensic psychologist who is a Professor in the Institute of Public and Preventive Health and in the Department of Psychiatry and Health Behaviour at Augusta University in Augusta, Georgia. His primary area of research is in the forensic psychological assessment including violence risk assessment, malingering, and the use of social media to improve forensic decision making.

Vivienne de Vogel PhD is professor of Forensic Mental Health Care at Maastricht University and at the University of Applied Sciences Utrecht. Furthermore, she works as researcher at the Van der Hoeven Kliniek, a forensic psychiatric centre in Utrecht. Her research focuses on gender differences in forensic care, violence risk assessment and management, resilience, and inpatient violence.

Tony Ward, DipClinPsyc, PhD has over 460 research publications and his current research focuses on the development of explanatory models in psychopathology and forensic psychology. His recent publications include "Why Theoretical Literacy is Essential for Forensic Research and Practice" in *Criminal Behaviour and Mental Health* (2020) and "Practice Frameworks in Correctional Psychology: Translating Causal Theories and Normative Assumptions Into Practice" in *Aggression and Violent Behavior* (2021).

Phil Willmot is a Consultant Forensic and Clinical Psychologist and Joint Lead Psychologist for the Men's Personality Disorder Service at Rampton Hospital. He is also a Senior Lecturer in Forensic Psychology at the University of Lincoln, United Kingdom.

Yilma Woldgabreal is a Senior Rehabilitation Psychologist with more than 20 years' experience working for both community corrections and prisons. During this time, he has held various positions, including his role as a parole officer, researcher, team leader, and manager. His research focuses on assessment and rehabilitation programmes, with particular interest in the application of positive psychology interventions with individuals who have committed offences.

Dr Rachel Worthington is a Forensic Psychologist and Associate Fellow of the Division of Forensic Psychology. She is a Senior Lecturer and works in private practice. She has published a range of peer reviewed articles and has presented both nationally and internationally on working positively with people with complex needs.

Foreword

With the historic social turbulence caused by Brexit, the COVID-19 lockdown, #MeToo, BLM, the deadly attempted coup at the US Capitol Building, and the Russian invasion of Ukraine, the past few years have seen seismic shifts across many walks of life. Remarkably, the world of forensic psychology has to date largely avoided an existential re-examination of our place in this challenging new environment. After all, working with some of the most vulnerable individuals in the most extreme circumstances of state control, we work on what might be considered the "frontlines" of the social politics of trauma, race, class, gender, and social justice. This remarkable volume, then, represents an overdue but incredibly rich opening of this conversation with contributions from many of the leading lights of the field.

We are told that the genesis of this edited volume arose from the tragic killing of George Floyd by officer Derek Chauvin in the United States in the summer of 2020. That incredibly graphic footage, broadcast all over the world, has instigated a pointed, global debate around policing, criminal justice and (remarkably) the value of Black lives. The fact that it also triggered this brave, thoughtful collection of essays clustering around the issue of bias in forensic assessment and testing is highly reassuring for those of us in the field. Moreover, although the authors started with questions around the challenges of racial diversity in psychological practice, they do not stop there. Contributions expand this discussion to wider issues of culture, diversity, and social justice across forensic psychology domains.

The relevance of the killing of George Floyd to risk assessment practices or personality testing may not be initially obvious to the outsider. Yet, anyone who has worked in a prison environment in any capacity watched that infamous footage with a painful sense of recognition, immediately familiar with Chauvin's self-righteous violence, toxic masculinity and racist dehumanisation.

The killing of George Floyd graphically reminded us that justice work is practiced by humans – all of us with the same frailties and, yes, biases that can be found in the subjects of our psychological research and practice. As actors in the justice system, forensic psychologists have tremendous power. We may not carry deadly weapons like police officers or have the power to sentence people to prison like judges, but we have enormous power over human lives, nonetheless.

As such, we are obligated to scrutinise our own biases and explore the ways that our practices can exacerbate inequalities, re-traumatise the victimised, or set up self-fulfilling prophecies of doom.

Indeed, in re-watching the infamous George Floyd footage, the most painful recognition for forensic psychologists may not be Chauvin's murderous violence, but rather the culpable passivity of the more junior police officers who ignored the pleas of onlookers and did nothing as Chauvin took Floyd's life. Like those officers, forensic psychologists have too long been passive observers of the enormous social inequalities built into the criminal justice system and the violence of incarceration. As experts in mental health and well-being, we simply know too much to plea innocence at this stage. Precisely because of our scientific training, because we strive to be evidence-based and objective, we are compelled to act as forensic psychologists, to acknowledge the stark injustices of a system that claims the word justice.

To that end, this book provides an essential, if at times uncomfortable lens on forensic psychology that fits the turbulent times we are living through. Far from the last word, I hope this work at the very least opens up a wider conversation for our field.

Professor Shadd Maruna
Queen's University Belfast

Preface

The genesis of this edited volume arose from one of the editors (GL) reflecting on the events which transpired in the late spring period of 2020. This wasn't the developing COVID-19 pandemic, but rather the death of George Floyd in the United States. This event has prompted many responses as we have all seen, across the world, and this volume, grew from a desire to try and make a difference in Forensic Psychology.

As is often the case in the field of Forensic Practice, we reflect on thoughts that we have about the world around us, and in this case, those conversations between the editors, all of us having lengthy and significant involvement with the area of psychological assessment and testing, led to our jointly acknowledging that aspects of Forensic Psychology, especially in the fields of assessment and testing (which we would all wish to profess expertise in), seemed to fall somewhat short of the aspiration in the field.

Sharing our thinking with colleagues internationally and in the United Kingdom, it quickly became apparent that others had similar views and spent a good deal of time working on the issues presenting and moreover progressed shared concerns towards solutions.

Our endeavour then in this volume is to share and develop how the field of forensic assessment and testing can be responsive to the challenges of diversity and culture in all their forms, and start to rethink and question the assumptions that many practitioners will have held in the doctrine that has been followed historically.

Our service users are amongst the most vulnerable in the face of professional expertise: as editors and authors here recognise, and articulate – those vulnerabilities are exacerbated and intensified when individuals aren't in the "universal normal" that is often the premise of or assessment and testing approaches.

Growing from an initial review of assessment and testing with people of colour, we have sought to also include thinking about the diversity of diversity, and what we as forensic psychologists and practitioners can do to make a difference in the way that we work with our service users, whatever their heritage, culture, faith, or the way that they experience the world in which we all live.

Glenda, Martin and Lawrence
January 2022

Acknowledgements

It has been an absolute pleasure working with all our contributors. Thank you so much for all your hard work and for sticking with it – we really appreciated it.

Editors Note: The Editors have made every effort to ensure that the language and terminology used in this text by ourselves and our contributors is both inclusive and in keeping with current perspectives at the time the manuscript was being prepared. Use of language continues to evolve, and we hope that no part of this book will cause offence to any body or group.

Part I

Present Day Issues in Forensic Psychological Assessment

1 Forensic Context Assessment: Some Current Challenges

Glenda Liell, Martin Fisher, and Lawrence Jones

With Lorraine Hough

Introduction

Everyone has a part to play in addressing bias and a lack of inclusivity in society, and one of the ways professionals can help is by committing to their ongoing learning and development. All those working in forensic contexts need to consider the ways that they and/or their working environments have contributed to this longstanding problem. This book is intended to encourage both reflection and action, and so the editors have sought to consider the accessibility of the material for students of forensic psychology, experienced practitioners, and academic researchers alike.

All contributors were encouraged to write from the perspective of how either concepts, theories, or practices within their areas of interest and expertise, can offer a path towards developing greater equality across forensic contexts. All the chapters offer suggestions for either; applied practice, a different perspective which can foster inclusion, or recommend where further research is needed to enable further progress. The content is deliberately wide-ranging in an effort to appeal to as large a cross section of the forensic profession as possible.

Whilst a challenge to group the chapters due to the naturally overlapping themes within them, there are, overall, three broad themes which capture the content of the book:

- Biases arising from the way risk is measured, and the methods used in the development of assessments which also reflect broader societal issues and encourage bias
- Biases arising from professionals themselves, and their management of the assessment or treatment process
- Biases which arise from working with the diversity that *is* the forensic population

This introductory chapter begins with some historical context setting in relation to discrimination in forensic testing and the development of forensic testing more

DOI: 10.4324/9781003230977-2

generally – highlighting the legal requirement for forensic psychologists to present reliable evidence. The chapters in Part I: Present Day Issues in Forensic Psychological Assessment have been grouped into distinct areas to facilitate describing them here. They are as follows:

- Issues of culture, and developments in thinking around dynamic risk factors
- Challenges to the actuarial approach, risk classification, and the impact of detection and conviction evasion skills (DACES) on assessment
- The positive contribution of technology in improving parity and inclusivity

Latter parts then reflect parts II and III of the book. Whilst these largely present descriptions of the content, context is described where possible, and links to chapters. The purpose is to offer a real flavour of what readers can expect to find in the main body of the book. Contributor names and chapter headings/topics are in bold to offer a quick point of reference.

The editors asked all contributors to offer tangible suggestions for developing thinking or practice which readers could act on immediately. As such all readers will find something to assist them with their own professional development.

Discriminating as a Result of Psychological Testing

Whilst the history of psychological testing is beyond the scope of this chapter, suffice to say it has enabled difference in human variation to be measured, and for decisions to be reached about normative (typical) and what has been considered non-normative (atypical) behaviours or outcomes. It supports individuals being compared with each other, facilitating measurement of difficult to observe psychological characteristics, traits or concepts to be operationalised and quantified. It allows for comparison of an individual within a specified population and for decisions to be made on the basis of such comparisons, allowing cohorts to be differentiated in a relatively quick and systematised manner, in what has been considered a scientific manner.

There has long been a recognition, however, of the limitations of psychological testing, and its discrimination towards certain groups or individuals (e.g., recruitment). High-profile legal test cases concerning the misuse of occupational tests have been followed by financial penalties, highlighting both the direct and indirect discriminatory practices in the recruitment and selection field. In the United Kingdom, changes were subsequently made to legislation which included the Sex Discrimination Act 1975 (UK Public General Acts, 1975, c. 65), the Race Relations Act 1976 (UK Public Relations Acts, 1976, c.74), and the Disability Discrimination Act 1995 (UK Public General Acts, 1995, c. 50). Unfortunately, one could argue that the misuse of testing has not been sporadic or infrequent. Indeed, as Vermeren (2013) notes:

> Typologies are as old as the road to Rome. In ancient times, Hippocrates and Galenus divided people into types according to the mixture of 'the four bodily fluids': the sanguine temperament (warm blooded), the choleric temperament (hottempered, due to too much yellow bile), the melancholic temperament (due to too much blackbile), and the phlegmatic temperament (due to too much phlegm). (p. 2)

As such, in the forensic context, practitioners must be wary of the temptation to typify and categorise.

Psychometric Test Use in the Forensic Context

In the relatively recent past, forensic assessment has experienced considerable growth, with the nature and variety of forensic context assessment tools increasing also, alongside the range of applications of such tools. These tools inform anything from committal, sentencing, or diversion decisions in the Criminal Justice System context. They support release decisions made by the Parole Board or Mental Health Tribunals, and support Civil Court decisions such as in the Family Courts. Police methods are underpinned by psychological approaches to witness interviewing and advocacy considerations. Forensic assessment informs sentence progression decisions as well as treatment or intervention requirements.

Forensic psychologists, when presenting evidence as expert witnesses are minded to consider Frye v United States (Cir. 1923) which "states that an expert opinion is admissible if the scientific technique on which the opinion is based is "generally accepted as reliable in the relevant scientific community" (Cappellino, 2021). However, in the case of the Daubert ruling (*Daubert v. Merrell Dow Pharmaceuticals, Inc.*, 1993), the court emphasised the importance of a trial judge's "gatekeeping responsibility". The case resulted in a list of factors requiring consideration:

> - Whether the expert's technique or theory can be tested and assessed for reliability
> - Whether the technique or theory has been subject to peer review and publication
> - The known or potential rate of error of the technique or theory
> - The existence and maintenance of standards and controls
> - Whether the technique or theory has been generally accepted in the scientific community
>
> (Cappellino, 2021)

These rulings established the need for theoretically and psychometrically adequate data-gathering instruments. The abstraction of conclusions from these must be grounded in empirically validated theories, requiring the weighing up and qualifying of testimony on the basis of theory and empirical research, with the psychologist being prepared to describe their decision-making rationale and the status of any data-gathering instrument.

Developments in Forensic Risk Assessment

During the 1990s, forensic risk assessment moved from unstructured clinical assessments (first generation), towards actuarial instruments (second generation), to more recently, evidence-based assessment (third generation), with fourth generation risk assessment now incorporating risk management planning. Structured professional judgement tools (SPJs) focus the practitioners' attention on criminogenic needs, incorporating the research into dynamic risk factors, as well as a wider consideration of risk, need, and responsivity principles, alongside protective factors. There have been recent developments in thinking around the notion of risk factors and their utility.

Structured assessments were a starting point for addressing concerns around the validity of unstructured judgement in terms of subjectivity and unconscious bias in clinical interviewing (Grove, 2005; Grove & Meehl, 1996). The shared terminology of these tools, whilst placing importance on inter-rater reliability and the consideration of dynamic factors, did not necessarily ensure effective consideration of what is the expected "normal". That is, incorporating within their design the appropriate inclusion and representation of protected characteristics, the consideration of language and cognitive developmental factors, and the very real notions of privilege and social inequality. That is notwithstanding whether these assessments have cultural applicability, are able to include as opposed to exclude, and do not contribute to some individuals experiencing worse outcomes than others. The fourth generation of risk assessment incorporates the notion of integrated case management, places a greater focus on responsivity, and the wider availability of appropriate tools facilitates a broader case formulation process. There is also the corresponding opportunity to consider protective factors, the need for active risk management, the "best-fit" intervention, as well as the monitoring of progress and change (Andrews et al., 2006).

Reliability and Validity

When we consider issues that arise in the application of psychological tests and instruments to forensic populations (with their inherent diversity in profile), we should be clear about the definitions being applied here:

- *Reliability* is concerned with the accuracy and precision of a score on a test. All measures have some degree of variance, and the reliability of a test is a measure of its accuracy. In individual assessments, accuracy is crucial given the potential outcomes which could result from their use. In a forensic context, individual assessments are at the centre of practice, and therefore reliability is a key issue.

- *Validity* is concerned with what the test score actually measures. Assertions of the validity of a measure must be supported by research that demonstrates an outcome (score) is in and of itself a meaningful measure of the quality or qualities intended. In a forensic context, ensuring that the measure has relevance and is meaning for the individual in question is critical. Unless there is certainty that a measure has meaning when applied to a given individual, the assessment project falls.

Validity is contextual. A test can be valid for one application but completely irrelevant for another (BPS, 2017). Assessors in the forensic context then need to be certain that the approach being used is relevant for the individual being assessed, and that the outcome has meaning in terms of *what* is being assessed. For example, rating the risk of future violence has little meaning unless the practitioner understands that risk rating is relative to the degree to which the rating might be deemed to be reliable. The *scoring* of tests taken by a subject in the pursuit of assessment must not be conflated with the *rating* of a subject in a framework of professional judgements. The two are distinct and different.

With certain types of assessment, the stakes for the public, and indeed the impacts and outcomes for the individuals themselves, are both higher and far reaching. Where the context itself appears adversarial, this impacts the individual's presentation. Indeed, the reliability of self-report and the validity of assessments about risk of future re-offending have been evidenced as being greater when not for risk assessment purposes (Mann et al., 2011). Working collaboratively and minimising the perspective of an adversarial approach can help decrease forensic clients' need to present in a less than genuine way in an effort to steer the outcome of the assessment in their favour. The validity of an assessment can thus be increased with a more genuine presentation.

Part I: Present Day Issues in Forensic Psychological Assessment

Issues of Culture and Developments in Thinking around Dynamic Risk Factors

Research on both cognitive assessment (Rock & Price, 2019) and risk assessment of indigenous Australian Aboriginal communities (Shepherd et al., 2014) indicates that there are qualitative differences in terms of the nature of risk factors for First Nations groups; with a need to consider the implications of this in terms of the use of violence and the normalising of it within certain cultural groups.

This includes the development of attitudes, values, and social norms, as well as the specific contexts linked to individual or group-based beliefs, values, or attitudes. There are now a variety of tools which aim to address such considerations. These include, for example, the Multi-Level Guidelines (MLG; Cook et al., 2013) for exploring group-based violence such as within organised crime. Arguably, newer tools must be subject to further validation research, and more attention should be given to the relevance and appropriateness of norms. Some measures tend to be validated only on US or Canadian populations, which raises questions about (cultural) generalisability, although some tools have corresponding UK norms (such as the Hare Psychopathy Checklist-Revised; Cooke et al., 2005), and questions of transferability and generalisability of norms in relation to Correctional Facility vs Secure Hospital and/or Psychiatric vs Prison Populations.

White privilege (McIntosh, 1989) has long been recognised as having major implications in terms of its socio-economic and cultural impact on all forms of psychological testing, with most measures reflecting white, westernised language, experience, and cultural values. There are also known limitations of equality of access in terms of educational opportunity for some justice-involved people, with recognition in the literature of disenfranchisement with societal norms, and different life experiences well documented in developmental and life-course of-fending literature (i.e., Farrington, 2005; Sampson & Laub, 1993). Furthermore, developments in approaches to formulation have arguably encouraged a much broader perspective to include other important individual factors such as absence of parenting skills, exposure to early childhood experiences (ACEs), socio-economic and cultural deprivation, early exposure to substances, and the absence of positive role models or secure attachments – all of which can impact cognitive development. Risk assessment tools in forensic contexts must therefore consider cultural, developmental, and a wider social narrative to be fully meaningful. The interpretation of outcomes for the use of any assessment tool should be within the context of an individual's "normative" experience and cultural milieu.

As much as it is important to consider the issues of culture in relation to the forensic population a further consideration is the impact of our own past experiences and how it has shaped us as professionals. Chapter 2 offers **the lived experience perspective** of three female colleagues from black, Asian, and minority ethnic backgrounds working in our profession. **Palwinder Athwal-Kooner, Martine Ratcliffe, and Ana Da Silva** share what have been the common themes from their personal experiences growing up, and from their journeys into and within this profession. They have described the experience of writing their chapter as "fearful and exposing". Having been asked to "represent all minorities" and how exposing it is to ask people of colour to share their lived experience (when others are not expected to) is something requiring further consideration by all. And to think that the fear of "getting it wrong" is a barrier stopping some from speaking up! Their message is clear – it starts with "you" – which really does mean *everyone*. They present some helpful tips for developing your "lens" which everyone would benefit from trying. This all highlights the importance of taking a more considered approach to how workplaces can be-come safer, more equal, and foster a spirit that encourages people to work at their best, and be the best version of themselves.

Two chapters by Stefanie Schimidt, Roxanne Hefferman, and Tony Ward pick up some particular issues in relation to culture in assessment and treatment. In Chapter 3, **Roxanne Hefferman and Tony Ward – *The Role of Dynamic Risk Factors in Forensic Assessment and Treatment Planning*** sets the scene for Chapter 4 lead by **Stefanie Schmidt**. Chapter 3 describes the theoretical problems with conceptualising risk factors and explains how the current way of thinking can restrict their contribution to our under-standing of offending behaviour and subsequent treatment planning. Due to formulations being commonly guided by a cognitive-behavioural or social-learning approach, the outcomes can appear fairly similar as practitioners seek to make sense of them by fitting them into a well-established set of risk factors. The authors argue that the underlying assumption (and problem) in this process is that dynamic risk factors are theoretically coherent constructs, and can be considered causes of offending behaviour. Their proposal is that alternative case formulation approaches, which can explain offending in terms of agency and motivation, provide a way forward, and go on to describe the predictive agency model (PAM) – developed by these same authors. The description of this model lays the foundations for their second chapter.

Chapter 4 considers the effect of bias during the risk assessment process, how it risks invalidating the outcome, and how cultural bias in particular has multiple impacts on minority groups. *Why dynamic risk factors cannot be applied universally* argues the importance of establishing equivalence when applying risk assessment measures cross-culturally, and suggests how it may be possible to mitigate biases in cross-cultural risk assessment settings. The authors describe the development of the Cultural Agency-Model of Criminal Behaviour (CAMCB) to facilitate a culturally sensitive approach to identifying the causes of offending. They state that cultural sensitivity requires that researchers and practitioners are well-aware of the relevant cultural context(s) and understand how particular cultural traits influence per-ception, cognition, and behaviour.

Challenges to the Actuarial Approach, Risk Classification, and the Impact of "DACES" on Assessment

The roots of the actuarial approach to risk assessment in the early part of the 20th century concerned an interest in ascertaining the likelihood of an individual being successful on parole. This lead to the notion of risk factors (identified as variables such as nature of offence, previous arrests, and age). Developments in this area were grounded in a desire to assist the Parole Board in its decision making around who to release, and involved the use of data to describe those variables. In the years that have followed the focus has shifted to an interest in the severity of offending with a view to ranking the seriousness of offences for the purposes of informing sentencing policy. Readers are directed to, for example, Taxman et al. (2006) for further detail.

Subsequently more statistically based, formalised assessment instruments which employed the use of the commonly termed static or historical items were developed. The promise of the actuarial approach included the replication of test scores by different raters thereby limiting the problem of subjectivity, but importantly the ability to predict (potential) outcomes and the likelihood of these in a given population within a defined period. Tools were designed to provide indicative levels of risk via the use of relative classifications such as low, medium, or high. This was then used to support decisions about intensity of treatment or required intervention, as compared to others in that population. The scale items in an assessment tool are empirical, and typically weighted or combined using specific algorithms.

The editorial team, in Chapter 5, consider **False Convictions** and *Detection and Conviction Evasion Skills (DACES)* present a third challenge to assessment which explores how clinical judgement may be predicting re-offending whereas actuarial assessment predicts reconviction (a smaller subset of those re-offending). Reconviction is considered a problematic measure of re-offending due to the fact that a significant amount of offending goes unreported, undetected, or un-convicted. This is further confounded by the fact that re-conviction is considered a measure of a return to offending (RTO), and that biases in the CJS are determining both re-conviction and conviction rates. Privilege and prejudice have a role to play as do biases in terms who gets investigated and then caught – and who doesn't. To this end the factors that may determine being detected and convicted arguably rival the weight traditionally placed on individual risk factors and assessments of risk by actuarial measures. We explain how social and interpersonal dynamics together with the skills and propensities of the individual contribute to either good or poor detection and evasion skills. One of the implications of this concerns how best to make use of actuarial assessments. What is presented are the beginnings of a new model for incorporating DACES into clinical formulation, and how it may be possible to incorporate this perspective into clinical decision making. The complication with this lies in its challenge to standard policy around how re-offending is understood and risk measured, but arguably the evidence should not be ignored.

There are inherent dangers in categorising individuals by their risk outcomes due to the increased likelihood of this being incorrect if test takers/evaluees are from a minority group in particular. Assessment outcomes can lead to significant impacts for individuals, and it is the problem of mis-categorising which is the topic of Chapter 6 in which **Daryl Kroner and R. Karl Hanson** look at *standardised risk levels for criminal recidivism risk*. Their argument is that whilst there is evidence to support the notion of biased classification, the situation is not helped by the lack of a common language for describing and communicating risk of recidivism.

The authors describe the development of a standardising risk classification and communication system, named the 5-Level System advanced by the Justice

Center of the US Council of State Governments (Hanson et al., 2017). The underlying assumption in its development is the presence of a general latent construct of criminal risk, which most risk assessment instruments tap into this construct (antisociality). The process involved integrating features of criminal risk such as percentile ranks and recidivism rates, with the overall outcome being a set of risk levels with explicit definitions which assists decision makers with coming to more just conclusions. The authors explain how those from minorities groups often come to be assessed as being higher risk than their white counterparts when risk assessment tools are used, and how prediction is difficult when greater criminal justice involvement inflates the outcomes. They argue, for example, that if minorities are more policed then criminal history is arguably less of a reliable measure of antisociality for non-whites. Furthermore, they describe how by standardising risk levels it is possible to arrive at more reliable conclusions regarding the extent of racial bias.

The idea that we might be able to reliably *predict* the likelihood of an individual causing harm is both fundamental and deeply ingrained in the forensic psychological approach. There are however inherent issues in an approach which relies on actuarial measures. These issues are not new, and are helpfully summarised in Chapter 7 by **Sean Hammond and Margaret O'Rourke –*The Cumulative Modelling of Risk***. They describe the process of how risk factor checklists are generated (and subsequently used to rate their presence or not in an individual), and produce either a weighted or unweighted outcome. The issue with the outcome is that normative data from an apparently representative sample is then used to assess risk in a single individual case. In the case of minority groups, the authors suggest that using a cumulative model can identify "elevated misfits" – highlighting that a bias may be present. This chapter offers of way of identifying when further caution should be exercised when interpreting test scores – in other words how to include a potential safeguard.

The Positive Contribution of Technology in Improving Parity and Inclusivity

Arguably many, if not most people around the world with the means and opportunity to access technology during the COVID-19 pandemic, did so, and probably benefited from it in a positive way. Many organisations delivering a variety of services found themselves needing to make adjustments to their usual ways of working, which may have included increasing their use of technology. The health professions responded to the need to adapt, equally, and a rise in the use of technology for remote assessment and treatment was observed. Research has been undertaken in areas such as videoconferencing-based services telepsychiatry, and telepsychology (e.g., Johnson et al., 2021). Three chapters exemplify and demonstrate the potential utility of employing technological solutions as part of the response to addressing bias, promoting inclusivity, and improving service delivery to disadvantaged groups coming into contact with criminal justice systems.

In Chapter 8, the findings of an extensive review into the use of state-of-the-art VR and apps in forensic contexts, and the opportunities these could present for risk assessment, rehabilitation, and reintegration are reviewed. **Aniek Siezenga and colleagues – *What Works in the Digital Age? VR and Smartphone Applications for Forensic Psychology*** – provide a useful resource for those looking to incorporate such technologies in the development of their services, in particular, virtual reality (VR) and smartphone apps. They discuss how VR enables objective data gathering and standardised treatment, resulting in less biased and more individualised assessment, and how role play exercises set up in VR can be created to be more culturally relatable to minority groups.

In Chapter 9, **Christopher King and colleagues** in their chapter ***Assessment and Intervention Technologies in Juvenile Justice*** describe some of the challenges faced by justice-involved youth who tend to come from multiculturally diverse and socioeconomically disadvantaged backgrounds, namely the barriers preventing access to interventions services. They note that technology-facilitated services have potential benefits where responsivity issues are concerned, and may "speak" to youth's generally high rates of technology usage. However, they also highlight that those from disadvantaged communities may not have access to the technology that could facilitate them attaining those much-needed e-mental health services. The need for further research is emphasised along with a caution that arguably no type of e-mental health can be said to have been fully validated for this population.

On the theme of using technology to assist disadvantages groups, in Chapter 10, ***Conducting Remote Evaluations in Underserved and Marginalised Communities***, Ashley Batastini and colleagues highlight the racial and economic imbalances in forensic assessment faced by pre-trial individuals in economically disadvantaged areas. Some of the challenges to offering these services to remote communities include: long wait-times; the use of incentives to drop charges or offer quick plea deals that may infringe on a defendant's rights; and the use of practitioners lacking in specific forensic mental health training. Recommendations are made for how to improve such services, whilst also drawing attention to practice and policy issues in relation to undertaking remote assessments using this approach.

Part II: Forensic Practice and Working with Biases

Whilst engaging in supervision is a *requirement* under the Health & Care Professions Council (HCPC) in the United Kingdom, it is arguably an *ongoing personal commitment* to this as well as a willingness to both challenge and be challenged which will encourage the broader development of the profession. On this theme of personal development the chapters below in the second section encourage a range of approaches practitioners may find helpful when trying to mitigate against bias. Supervision and reflection have a key role to play in ensuring that inclusive working environments are created which foster excellence, as well as helping to mitigate against the biases presenting themselves in the professional-client relationship. The first two chapters here pick up on these issues.

In Chapter 11, **Supervising Assessment Practice, Jason Davies** reviews models of supervision and in particular, how to use supervision effectively – with attention being given to the possible "deaf, dumb, and blind spots" within assessment practice. He highlights how powerful – yet hidden bias can be, and how it's an acceptance of our susceptibility to being influenced which can pave the way for engaging with supervision effectively. Furthermore, by remaining curious about ourselves, our practice, and others, this can assist with exploring bias and truly embracing diversity.

As well as having an awareness of biases and taking responsibility for managing them, practitioners have a choice as to which construct(s) or framework(s) will help make sense of an individual's presentation, and from which they'll then draw conclusions as to the risk of harm to self or others.

One such framework is the **Power Threat Meaning Framework** (PTMF; Johnstone et al., 2018). In Chapter 12, **Jo Ramsden and Kerry Beckley** present its potential utility within the CJS by way of a case examples. These examples helpfully explain how the CJS can fail to account for trauma and context when considering those who have offended, and how people are shaped by their circumstances to respond to the world in destructive and dangerous ways. The authors explore how the CJS system itself can induce threat responses and hence exacerbate risk. A key thread in their discussion is how risk assessment approaches fail to take into account individual's lived experiences, and as part of this biased assumptions are made in day-to-day practice. Three key recommendations are made for integrating the PTMF into practice: reframe offending as a threat response, talk explicitly about power, and use it to help a traumatised system.

With supervision remaining a key theme, in Chapter 13 **Todd Hogue and Mats Dernevik** in **Individual Bias** in **Forensic Practice** specifically explore the implicit bias process and how this influences judgements and behaviour without individuals having a conscious awareness of this. It cannot be assumed that judgements made by forensic practitioners do not carry any influence from the persons themselves, although the precise impact of implicit bias on forensic judgements is yet to be determined. Research into bias present in forensic decision making is presented, and they argue that Dror's (2020) model, developed from forensic science research, offers a framework which could be applied to psychological/psychiatric expertise in forensic practice.

Attention is drawn to the issue of **Cultural Bias in Forensic Assessment** in Chapter 14. This has not necessarily been at the forefront of discussions about practice, until perhaps, more recently. **Andrew Day and colleagues** offer an exposé of this area, drawing on Canadian Court cases which highlighted how the identity of the service user and the cultural context of the assessment can influence both the quality and admissibility of the findings. Importantly, they explain some of the reasons why contemporary forensic assessments have largely remained anglophonic in their orientation and development, and challenge the view that one can become competent in another's culture. The benefits of increased service user involvement as well as the use of "cultural consultants" are some of the ways the authors suggest that preparations prior to undertaking assessments could be enhanced.

A whole-system perspective of the CJS using the PTMF would go some way to further contextualising individuals' behaviour within that system, and offer a different interpretation – and hence response – which could usefully avoid inflicting further trauma on that individual. However, the practitioner must also consider which approach to take during that direct interaction during assessment. Whether it is possible to arrive at a *true* understanding of someone else's thinking and behaviour, which is not impacted by personal bias or the context, cannot be debated here. In Chapter 15, an approach underpinned by **Personal Construct Psychology (PCP;** Kelly, 1955) **– the use of Repertory Grids** – may assist in the practitioners' aspiration to arrive at such a position. **Nicolas Blagden and Adrian Needs'** chapter discusses PCP and the value of employing repertory grids in forensic psychological assessment. A clear benefit of the PCP lies in its wholly collaborative approach, and the idea of making sense "with" during the process of encouraging clients to reveal their ways of making sense of things. Importantly, the authors highlight how repertory grids "privilege the individual's own culture, meanings and experiences, attempting proactively to understand the individual's world", and as an open-ended method can be tailored to the concerns, culture, and context of the individual in a way that a standardised assessment tool cannot.

The rapid growth in social media in the last 20 years have challenged different aspects of the CJS and impacted on psychology practice. Arguably, with ongoing evolution it is necessary for practice to keep pace. A central component of assessment is the use of wide-ranging sources of information. The final chapter (Chapter 16) in this section by **Ashley Batastini and colleagues** explores the use of **Social Media Data in Forensic Evaluations**. It offers an alternative to the bias that exists in the perception of its perceived utility. The authors argue that social media data could offer important insights about the timing of behaviours, patterns of functioning, communication style, or contextual factors that may be less apparent from other sources. The question raised is whether the lack of guidance around how best to utilise this information allows for the introduction of bias in how it is construed and interpreted. Whilst the limitations of this data are presented, so too is the argument for its utility as another source of potentially valuable collateral information for assessment.

Part III: Diversity and Forensic Populations: Theoretical and Practical Approaches

Whilst practitioners will rightly consider the need to identify an assessment designed with their client's characteristics and the assessment's aims in mind, the forensic population is arguably so diverse that it is unrealistic to expect to find the right tool for all clients and populations. There are a number of chapters in this book which highlight some of the very particular issues in respect of assessing certain groups. These are outlined below, and whilst it's working with that population which is the subject of those chapters, there are also clear reflections on how certain views and attitudes in society have also impacted those areas.

Chapter 17 addresses **Gender-Sensitive Violence Risk Assessment**, and the wider societal issues which impact how practitioners approach working with their clients. **Vivienne de Vogel** highlights how gender bias is still considered to be a detectable and powerful factor in psychological practice which may lead to the inappropriate use and overuse of certain diagnoses in women, like borderline personality disorder. The clinical presentation of women can also be characterised by internalising disorders and self-injury behaviours, as well as a more complex trauma history, especially sexual abuse – hence she suggests that the assessment approach should be directed by this. There is also now more awareness of transgenerational trauma, and she calls for the voice of black women with lived experience to work in partnership with practitioners in order to educate and support staff working in these settings.

Gender Identity Assessments with Trans and Gender Non-Binary Individuals are covered within chapter 18 which highlights the challenges being experienced by trans and gender non-binary individuals. **Soren Henrich** explains the role of medicalisation and criminalisation, as well as colonialism in the creation of the binary gender system, and offers a contemporary criticism of several approaches in trans care, including gender identity assessment. He highlights how the assessment of trans individuals' gender identities, often a central requirement to access any form of support, is not adhering to any agreed guidelines, or sound empirical evidence base, and presents a newly developed non-pathologising assessment approach for use with this client group.

A recent UK Criminal Justice Joint Inspectorate Neurodiversity Review (CJJI, 2021) considered "neurodivergence" an umbrella term referring to the group of conditions falling under the category of neurodevelopmental disorders (NDDs). There are three chapters which address key issues in relation to disorders captured by this umbrella. Neurodivergence and assessment issues are addressed in 3 chapters. Chapter 19: **Neurodiversity by Nancy Doyle and colleagues** introduce the umbrella term of "neurodivergence" which encapsulates a range of disorders, the relative prevalences of which are also presented. Socio-historic influences which have impacted this area are discussed, as are, importantly, the implications for the assessment of this client group. The authors highlight how the very nuances of the testing context and administration practice can impact reliability and validity. They also emphasise the importance of the practitioners' skills in being able to employ a range of strategies to, for example, promote effective communication. In Chapter 20, **Emma Longfellow and colleagues** consider the issues around **Risk Assessment in Learning Disability Populations**, highlighting the heterogeneity of this group, and the limitations of the assessments currently available. They identify the need for further research which considers the socio-cultural difference and the potential implications for assessing both risk and protective factors. In Chapter 21, **Rachel Worthington** considers the issues around challenging bias in the **assessment and treatment of people with Attention Deficit Hyperactivity Disorder (ADHD)**. She highlights the presence of racial disparities in the diagnosis of ADHD, and the increased vulnerability for ADHD of those classed as "immigrants", or those who have had to flee their home country due to war or conflict. She discusses where biases appear for those living with ADHD, and makes recommendations for both assessment and treatment.

Chapter 22 is about **Deaf People in Forensic Contexts**. Mats Dernevik and colleagues present a detailed exposition of the challenges faced by deaf people as a result of a lack of understanding of deafness and communication on the part of those working in the criminal justice system. The availability of experts with the required expertise can be limited, and there is a lack of valid assessment and treatment methods. Models for understanding deafness are presented, and it is explained how being deaf can be understood as being part of a cultural and linguistic minority, parallel to other minority groups. Some important considerations for practitioners are presented such as how to work with interpreters, as well as some of the issues around mental health and risk assessment.

In Chapter 23, Phil Willmot considers our approaches to offending behaviour and treatment through a discussion of **Criminally Diverse Offending**. Those with multiple convictions tend not to specialise in a particular type of offence, and whilst many programmes are designed with the most serious offender in mind, their complexity and diversity is not necessarily recognised as they are placed into overarching categories of, for example, that "violent" or "sexual". Phil argues that these terms serve to obscure further underlying causal processes or treatment needs, whilst also masking other personal, social, and cultural factors which should be addressed on an individual formulation-led basis. The treatment model used in the Men's Personality Disorder Service at Rampton Hospital which aims to work with these complexities is discussed, and particular links drawn between developmental adversity and criminal diversity.

Issues about societal impact could not be more applicable than when working with those convicted of extremist offences. **Christopher Dean and Monica Lloyd** in their chapter on **Challenging Bias in the Assessment of Extremist Offending** (24) explain how working with this group encompasses a susceptibility to bias, and specifically issues associated with race and privilege. They explain how bias can influence the assessment process through terminology and the use of language, through the level of risk aversion created by large-scale terrorist attacks, by overlooking the role of context, and through subtle biases that demonise and homogenise this group. They point out that whilst assessment frameworks have been developed to assist in the task of making basic risk discriminations, they are only as good as the skills and mindset of the assessor. The authors offer their perspective on how practitioners can strive to mitigate against biases when working with this group.

In the case of the PCL-R v.2 (Hare, 2003), there is good research on cultural differences in the exposition of the construct (e.g., see Cooke et al., 2005). **Jenny Tew and Jacob Seaward** in chapter 25 address the Assessment of Psychopathy, which aims to provide an overview of the key considerations in the assessment of psychopathy, with a focus on diversity factors such as cognitive functioning, gender, culture, and ethnicity. They highlight the importance of considering the individual and their context when choosing and applying an assessment for psychopathy and making use of findings in practice. This is a key area of assessment which has experienced much development, and has continued to be the subject of research in recent years.

Picking up on the theme of individualised and accurate formulation when working with individuals who have committed sexual offences, **Derek Perkins and Ignacio Puzzo** in Chapter 26 discuss recent advances in this area in Technological Assessment Methods which can assist with removing the biases commonly present in the development of psychometric measures – the key example being a lack of diversity in norm groups. A range of different methods are discussed which the practitioner could introduce into their assessment repertoire which, if further developed, could assist with minimising biases during the assessment process.

Some Final Comments

There is clearly more work to be done around specific cohorts of the forensic population, for example improving the ways we work with those with the full range of neurodivergent conditions, and the LGBTQIA+ community for whom CJS needs to be better prepared to care for. With all populations, the challenge lies in how to assess in a reliable and valid way, taking into account some of the issues around measurement, categorisation, and representation in any norm group. The question to keep asking, however, is who are we *not* talking about now? We are arguably in a less than ideal situation, with several pressing issues around assessment for which there are no clear answers right now. However, we are in an evolving field, and so this is to be expected.

Some of the issues around measurement appear to be pointing us towards the need for a more single idiographic approach to formulation, with minimal use of tests, in which the task is to truly understand *all* the possible factors which may have contributed to that individual coming into contact with a CJS. In the fullest sense, that means an appreciation of broader societal factors and the impact that structural social factors have on criminalisation. Where suitability for re-integration is concerned, a culturally informed approach to the barriers to practicing any skills learned in treatment back in the "home" environment is needed. The goal is to enable people to live a life that has meaning to *them* and which fulfils their basic human needs in *their* environment.

It is not the editors' intention to conclude this introduction with our position on the "what next"? Instead, **Yilma Woldgabreal** was invited to write the concluding chapter (Chapter 27) for this book **Summary Perspectives** in which he offers his perspective on the key messages and future direction for this area of work. We are very grateful to him for this.

There is much we are responsible for as practitioners such a willingness to reflect and an openness to personal challenge. In our own workplaces there is much we can do and try to influence. There is more scope for international collaboration as we work through how to integrate a cultural perspective into our work – video call anyone? Where there is a need for policy change, the profession is uniquely placed to help policy colleagues make sense of the available evidence, and facilitate the generating of tangible – if interim – solutions to some of the bigger problems.

The editors were not able to incorporate as much as would have been preferable around the developments in the use of technology in forensic contexts. This area does, however, provide much opportunity for both improving accessibility to much needed services, and for assisting with addressing bias. It has arguably been a challenge for research to keep up. The editors would encourage all those practitioners with new ideas in this area to collaborate with academic colleagues who can assist in the development of evaluation programmes to help ensure that further progress in this area is both safe and the evidence base sound.

References

Andrews, D. A., Bonta, J., & Wormwith, J. S. (2006). The recent past and near future of risk and/or needs assessment. *Crime & Delinquency, 52*(1), 7–27.

BPS. (2017). Psychological testing: A test user's guide. Retrieved December 28, 2021, from https://ptc.bps.org.uk/sites/ptc.bps.org.uk/files/guidance_documents/ptc02_test_users_guide_2017_web.pdf

Cappellino, J. D. (2021). Daubert vs. Frye: Navigating the standards of admissibility for expert testimony. *Expert Institute*, 7th September. https://:Daubert vs. Frye: Standards of Admissibility for Expert Testimony (expertinstitute.com).

CJJI. (2021). *Neurodiversity in the criminal justice system: A review of evidence.* Retrieved from https://www.justiceinspectorates.gov.uk/cjji/wp-content/uploads/sites/2/2021/07/Neurodiversity-evidence-review-web-2021.pdf

Cook, A. N., Hart, S. D., & Kropp, P. R. (2013). *Multi-level guidelines for the assessment and management of group-based violence.* Burnaby, Canada: Mental Health, Law, & Policy Institute, Simon Fraser University.

Cooke, D. J., Michie, C., Hart, S. D., & Clark, D. (2005). Assessing psychopathy in the UK: Concerns about cross-cultural generalisability. *British Journal of Psychiatry, 186*(4), 335–341. 10.1192/bjp.186.4.335

Daubert v. Merrell Dow Pharmaceuticals, Inc., 509 U.S. 579 (1993).

Dror, I. E. (2020). Cognitive and human factors in expert decision making: Six fallacies and the eight sources of bias. *Analytical Chemistry, 92*(12), 7998–8004. 10.1021/acs.analchem.0c00704

Farrington, D. P. (2005). *Integrated developmental and life-course theories of offending: Advances in criminological theory* (Vol. 14). New York: Routledge. ISBN9780203788431.

Frye v United States 293 F. 1013 (D.C. Cir. 1923)

Grove, W. M. (2005). Clinical versus statistical prediction: The contribution of Paul E. Meehl. *Journal of Clinical Psychology, 61*(10), 1233–1243.

Grove, W. M., & Meehl, P. E. (1996). Comparative efficiency of informal (subjective, impressionistic) and formal (mechanical, algorithmic) prediction procedures: the clinical-statistical controversy. *Psychology, Public Policy and Law*, 2(2), 293–323.

Hanson, R. K., Bourgon, G., McGrath, R. J., Kroner, D. G., D'Amora, D. A., Thomas, S. S., & Tavarez, L. P. (2017). A five-level risk and needs system: Maximizing assessment results in corrections through the development of a common language. U.S. Department of Justice, Bureau of Justice Assistance: The Council of State Governments Justice Center.

Hare, R. D. (2003). *Hare psychopathy checklist-revised (PCL-R)* (2nd ed.). Canada, Toronto: Multi-Health Systems Inc.

Johnson, L., Gutridge, K., Parkes, J., Roy, A., & Plugge, E. (2021). Scoping review of mental health in prisons through the COVID-19 pandemic. *BMJ Open*, *11*, e046547. 110.1136/bmjopen-2020-046547

Johnstone, L., Boyle, M., Cromby, J., Dillon, J., Harper, D., Kinderman, P., Longden, E., Pilgrim, D., & Read, J. (2018). *The power threat meaning framework: Towards the identification of patterns in emotional distress, unusual experiences and troubled or troubling behaviour, as an alternative to functional psychiatric diagnosis*. Leicester: British Psychological Society.

Kelly, G. A. (1955). *The psychology of personal constructs* (Vols. 1 & 2). New York: W.W.Norton.

Mann, R. E., Ware, J., & Fernandez, Y. M. (2011). Managing sexual offender treatment programmes. In Douglas P. Boer, Reinhard Eher, Leam A. Craig, Michael H. Miner, & Friedemann, Pfäfflin (Eds.). *International perspectives on the assessment and treatment of sexual offenders: Theory, practice, and research* (pp. 331–353). Chichester, UK: Wiley-Blackwell.

McIntosh, P. (1989). White privilege: Unpacking the invisible knapsack. *Peace & Freedom*. July/August.

Rock, D., & Price, I. R. (2019). Identifying culturally acceptable cognitive tests for use in remote Northern Australia. *BMC Psychology*, *7*, 62. 10.1186/s40359-019-0335-7

Sampson, R. J., & Laub, J. H. (1993). *Crime in the making: Pathways and turning points through life*. Cambridge, MA: Harvard University Press.

Shepherd, S. M., Adams, Y., McEntyre, E., & Walker, R. (2014). Violence risk assessment in Australian aboriginal offender populations: A review of the literature. *Psychology, Public Policy and Law*, April 20, Vol. 3. 10.1037/law0000017

Taxman, F. S., Thanner, M., & Weisburd, D. (2006). Risk, need, and responsivity (RNR): It *all* depends. *Crime Delinquency*, *52*(1), 28–51. 10.1177/0011128705281754

UK Public General Acts. (1975). *Sex Discrimination Act*, c.65.

UK Public General Acts. (1995). *Disability Discrimination Act*, c. 50.

UK Public Relations Acts. (1976). *Race Relations Act*, c.74.

Vermeren, P. (2013). The undesired popularity of typologies and other 'Jung'. (translation). *Gedrag & Gezondheid (Behaviour and Organisations)*. Retrieved December 27, 2021, from https://www.researchgate.net/publication/275945722_The_Undesired_Popularity_of_Typologies_and_other_%27Jung%27_translation

2 Challenging Bias in the Forensic Context: Lived Experiences

Palwinder Athwal-Kooner, Martine Ratcliffe, and Ana Da Silva

Introduction

There has been a focus on Equality, Diversity and Inclusion (EDI) within the criminal justice system, for example, the Lammy Review (2017). High profile reports such as these have put inequality, particularly race, in the spotlight for individuals, organisations, and the wider public. These recommendations have been influential in developing the EDI agenda in various contexts. A vital part of this agenda is reflecting on our practice and challenging biases. This is very much the focus of this chapter; by sharing our lived experience, we hope to prompt thinking about bias and support reflective thinking for those supporting the EDI agenda.

It is essential to acknowledge that the service user lived experience is missing from our discussions, which we hope to address in future work. However, we hope that the Black, Asian, and Minority Ethnic staff perspectives shared in this chapter are helpful, as we are also part of the same system that our service users belong to or have faced some similar barriers to them. It is hoped that by sharing our experiences, we can prompt awareness and understanding of what it could be like for our service users experiencing this.

This chapter outlines the lived experience of three females from a Black Asian and Minority Ethnic background working different roles within forensic psychology. This provides breadth and depth in experience and perspective. We will each reflect on some key topics relating to EDI, drawing from our lived experience. Based on this, we will suggest some potential next steps for progressing this work in the future. It was also deliberately written in a non-traditional academic tone. It is intentionally a reflective and narrative piece, again demonstrating that knowledge, experience, and voice can be presented differently.

Journey within Forensic Psychology

Martine: When thinking about my career journey for this chapter, I realised that how I would navigate my career journey was shaped by my early life experiences, well before I even knew what psychology and the psychology profession was. From as young as primary school, I was

DOI: 10.4324/9781003230977-3

very aware of my ethnicity (mixed race; white British and black Caribbean), being one of the very few children of colour in a predominantly white working-class school. I recall hearing parents talking in the playground about my mixed-race heritage. I recollect the lack of anyone who looked like me on TV, in the newspapers, magazines, and toys I played with. I remember the racist name-calling and the less overt, insidious comments made by adults and children alike. The comments took different forms and used different words, but all placed race at the centre of the abuse. Then there were the defensive denials of the credibility of my lived experience if I "complained" about a racist comment, with the rebuttal often being "it was just a joke, can't you take a joke" and "I'm not racist, I have Black friends".

As I grew older, I felt that society moved into a space of "colour blindness", which led to comments such as "when I look at you I don't see a colour" and "there is one race, and that's the human race". Attitudes such as this led me to feel like my identity and experience were being denied and not important. "Otherising"[1] treatment that I experienced led me to often feel alone, less than, different and that I always had to think about what I said or did to not draw attention to, or live up to the stereotypes placed upon me.

On the one hand, my experiences gave me the impetus and motivation to work hard, to do well and prove to people that I was worthy. However, the negative narrative was frequently louder, drowning out the positivity I had tried to turn it into. My lived experience of the influence bias and negative perceptions can have, played a role in shaping how I approached my career. I still feel the impact of those biases and negative perceptions, which continue to thrive at times in the form of imposter syndrome.

My early childhood experiences shaped my interest in human behaviour, so when I embarked on my A-Levels, I became interested in psychology. By the time I got to university, I knew I wanted to be a psychologist. However, becoming a psychologist felt like a dream. I was the first in my immediate family to go to university. I was from a working-class background. My experiences growing up had led me to believe some of the biases that others had held about me, my ethnicity, and my class. My socio-economic status also impacted my financial capacity. It felt like deciding to try and access the profession was a huge gamble. There was no second chance. If I got into debt for this, I couldn't just chalk this down to experience; a lot was riding on my decision. Financial security (individual or familial) affords more freedom around decisions and the risks you can take, which can impact career possibilities. Organisations need to consider this when considering career pipelines which may disadvantage some people to consider psychology as a profession.

I graduated with my psychology degree, and I applied to work for a large UK public sector employer. This was decades ago when there were psychology assistant roles and funding for MSc's (a pre-requisite to becoming a Forensic Psychologist in Training). This enabled me to take the risk of moving forward with a career in psychology. I remember feeling that the organisation welcomed people who could not afford to pay for the qualifications themselves; it felt inclusive. After I joined the organisation, some years later, the entry requirements to apply to be a Forensic Psychologist in Training changed to require people to have an MSc. I remember the change happening and how that made me feel. Whilst I know that organisations are businesses, I subconsciously heard this change's message was not one of "welcome". It made me feel like our profession was more about who can afford to fund themselves to gain the necessary qualifications and was less about who has the talent and ability. Therefore, organisations need to consider via Equality Impact Assessments what a change to recruitment, such as the one I have aforementioned, impacts minorities and social mobility. Organisations should ask themselves what message it sends to current and future staff from minority and marginalised backgrounds.

I recently met with several teenagers who wanted to know about the psychology profession as a possible career. They were from a diverse community with a similar socio-economic background to my own growing up. One of the things that came out of this was a surprise at seeing a woman of colour in the profession and that being a psychologist was the sole domain of "posh" people. This reinforced to me the impact on the perceptions of the psychology profession and on who fits into that world and will be welcomed into it. Therefore organisations wishing to attract a diverse range of people into the profession need to consider engaging with children from a young age about what the profession is like and why it may be for them. As a psychology profession, we also need to consider why we may be perceived as "posh", what this means for people accessing the profession and how this impacts engagement with service users.

Ana: I felt "lucky" to have started my new job as a Health Care Assistant (HCA) the Monday after my last day at university, although I had no idea of the journey I had ahead of me.

The foundation of support that I received within this role allowed me to learn and appreciate the real-life implications of having mental health difficulties, following learning about it for the last three years. After working as an HCA for two years, I finally bagged my first paid assistant psychologist (AP) position. This role was physically and mentally strenuous, but it was also very frustrating as I spent most of the time working at an HCA capacity rather than the advertised AP role due to "staff shortages". I am sure I am not the only one to have experienced this, a daunting reality for many. After many rejections and a minor "breakdown", I decided to apply for a lower band role, allowing me to get into the forensic world. Six months into the post, I applied for and was offered my first forensic AP role, where I was supported more than ever before.

I would like to kindly point out that the above paragraph does not even begin to touch on the emotional and physical ride that it was! From colleagues to patients and numerous incidents, it was most definitely a rollercoaster of a journey that contributed to the person and clinician I am today.

The forensic AP role involved a considerable amount of lone working, and I spent much time by myself, reading through the documentation, composing audits, and virtually assessing patients due to the nature of the post. I remember feeling like I might be losing my people skills, as I spent many days jumping from one office to another and often not saying more than "hello" to other office frequenters. On the other hand, I had been blessed with two brilliant supervisors. These individuals often surprised me with how much potential they saw in me than I could see in myself. They asked about my mental health and wondered how well I was coping, as I would often spend a significant amount of time reading through what I can only describe as disturbing information and not having someone readily available to discuss it with – which was at times challenging. However, they reminded me, they were only a phone call or text away, which I ever so appreciated. Eventually, I became comfortable. I had my routine, was aware of my triggers, and was more than happy to discuss anything during supervision. I was also offered further opportunities to partake in other work that the probation office provided, which I readily accepted. One day, one of my supervisors asked me when I would be providing her "with something to read as application season was due soon". I was utterly lost, and it took me what felt like minutes to realise she was talking about me applying for the forensic doctorate courses. I told her the truth. I said I was not thinking of applying so soon because I did not believe I had acquired enough experience, and most significantly, I did not think I could afford the fees. She disagreed and quickly did the maths and clarified that it would have been exactly one year that I had been in the role by the time I applied. She encouraged me, reassuring me that if anything, it would give me insight into what the application process is like and added, "you never know, you might prove yourself wrong and get accepted the first time … ".

I was invited for an interview for both courses. The first interview was a shambles; the nerves got the best of me! The second, which took place a week after, was weirdly okay. I was nervous but just kept reminding myself, "if anything, I am gaining experience". Whilst sitting in the classroom waiting for the group interview to start, I took a glance around and just sighed and thought to myself, "I have no chance, being the only black person here", but still vowed to do my best. At my solo interview, I quickly bonded with the interviewers who seemed genuinely intrigued by my "years of experience" and asked me, "why not sooner?" I explained that the student loan would be why, without it, I would not be considering taking that step and that it was also new information to me as it was my supervisor who had told me about it. Upon saying that, they exchanged a "look" with each other. I was sure of it and wondered why. They must have noticed I saw it, and one of them broke the sudden silence to clarify that the loan did not cover the total fees and asked me if I was aware. I nervously replied "yes" and explained to them my proposed plan: I would apply for advertised posts and use them as placements to fund my living and save up to top up my fees. They seemed convinced, and I thought I was too…

A week later, I received an email congratulating me on being accepted to the course.

Telling my parents was such a bittersweet moment. They seemed proud that their daughter was on the path to achieving her dream of becoming a forensic psychologist. It was a relief to see all of those years of hard work, hardship, tears, and rejection finally leading to an excellent resolution. On the other hand, it also meant that they would have to become financially independent from me, something they were no longer used to; they still rebuffed the incoming hurdle and celebrated my achievement. My first-generation African immigrant parents were proud of me. It was also a mini celebration at work, coupled with a few "I told you so". I was eternally grateful to my supervisors and felt ready to embark on this new journey ahead of me. Little did I know how much my life was about to change …

I had days I wanted to tell everyone and days where self-doubt crept in and tried to paralyse me. I thought that if I surrounded myself with other black trainees, I would be fine, as long as I had people alongside me on this journey. I quickly scoured through the internet to find a network of black forensic psychology trainees, but I could not find anything after searching for days. Whilst looking, I came across on social media an event that was due to occur in the following months about black professionals in psychology and psychiatry. I emailed the organisers offering to support the day's facilitation as a ticket inspector or seat usher. I was desperate to do anything to increase my network of black individuals in the field. However, I was instead invited to participate as a speaker to my biggest surprise, which I readily accepted.

The event was a success, and I was astounded by its reception afterwards. Many reached out asking "how I had done it" or "whom I knew", something that saddened me, but I completely understood. On that day, I was surrounded by qualified and aspiring black psychologists, something I had been so eager and excited about. However, I knew it did not look like that in various workplaces, and it certainly did not look like it in the classroom. So I understood. I, too, questioned whether it would be possible for someone who looked like me and had a journey similar to mine to become a forensic psychologist in a world everyone calls "so small". I had wondered if it was, in fact, too small for people like us to be allowed to enter. Or whether it meant it could indeed expand with our presence and improve. Though I leaned more towards the former, I vouched to do my best, succeed, and bring everyone else along with me. Even if "everyone else" was just one person.

When the first day of lectures arrived, it still felt too good to be true. I was in a new town, away from my loved ones and all that I knew, and the "newness" most definitely continued. In a cohort of about 15 individuals, I was the only black student, something I had not experienced since my early childhood in Lisbon, Portugal. It was weird and somewhat uncomfortable; I automatically put myself in a "do not belong here" box. Being naturally shy, I spent the first few days just smiling and nodding away, but I ultimately found my bearings; slowly but surely (as some of my classmates and lecturers would confirm), my confidence found its voice.

Pally: Whenever I'm asked "why did you become a forensic psychologist", my response is, "I want to help people, especially those less fortunate, the 'underdog' so to speak, and I want to make a difference in the world". I've realised that this isn't that "far" away from my experience through engaging in reflective practice. This realisation starts when I think about my experiences at primary school, being the only Indian child in the class (to my knowledge) and struggling to make friends because I'm different. So, I made friends with the black girl in the class, as we are both different and understand what this feels like.

Reflecting on this experience has made me realise that this is still how I feel now in my career as a forensic psychologist. Whenever I go somewhere new and unfamiliar, whether it is a meeting, conference, or social situation, I feel nervous and anxious about whom I will sit with. In this type of situation, I automatically gravitate towards the other individuals from a minority group, as it feels comfortable. However, by interacting in this way, am I perpetuating these "lines"? When I became conscious that this is my pattern, I decided that I would try to consciously go against my natural response to go to my "in-group" (Tajfel, 1974) as a commitment to work on these issues. Upon reflection, perhaps others feel like this as well when it comes to these types of situations, and this may well be the case. But for me, it is certainly a challenge: It relates to me feeling different and wanting to be accepted, which I believe is related to not being part of the ingroup in these situations.

I've also reflected on how this could be the case for our minority service users. When they go to an unfamiliar situation, whether it's a new treatment group, an assessment session, or a decision-making meeting such as a tribunal or panel, they perhaps have the same worry and concern about being different, judged, and accepted for their background, etc. This is in addition to the individual and contextual factors relating to their status as service users. Interestingly service users have said to me in clinical work that I don't know what it's like for them, that I must have had an easy life being a psychologist. I don't address their assumptions directly but ponder that it hasn't been as easy as they may think.

So, being from a second-generation immigrant family and the first person in the family to go to university, navigating the education system wasn't easy. Indeed, coming to university was a privilege being from a single-parent family where employment was centred on low paid manual labour. I was lucky to have this opportunity as the family migrated to the United Kingdom to gain a better life. There wasn't a template for being a university student, but also what would happen after university, so becoming an educated professional. This was a personal and familial goal, but no one knew what this would look like, as being educated wasn't something we were used to. To me, being professional meant you are clever, had knowledge, a good vocabulary, are articulate, cultured, and come from wealth, privilege and power. This wasn't something I was, as I'm not clever and articulate, I now know this to be imposter syndrome, and I have to remind myself, I have made it to this point, so I have some worth.

I have been in situations where I don't understand the words and phrases that have been used, as I don't know all the cultural inferences and expressions, as I wouldn't have grown up being exposed to these. So in these instances, I have secretly googled these phrases, as I felt embarrassed that I didn't know what they meant, which triggered "I'm not good enough" to be in these "circles" and I "don't belong". In more recent times, as my confidence has grown. I have felt confident enough to ask for clarification or mention to the individual that I don't understand the reference, so gently reminding them to think about the cultural inferences they have used and to explain what they mean. It isn't easy to do this as it triggers vulnerability to admit this. However, I've realised that if we don't give this feedback, how will others reflect and learn about the cultural inferences being used and to challenge these biases? Again, I have reflected on what this must be like for our service users. Not to make assumptions and recognising individuality, but I now have some privilege. I've been able to gain an education and a career as a forensic psychologist following this, which has given me some status and power, but they have little privilege. They may not have the confidence to say, "I don't understand what you mean". Instead, they may communicate this in perhaps unhelpful ways.

When thinking about my postgraduate training in forensic psychology, I don't recall there being a strong focus on EDI, which is probably how things were at that time. This is really at the forefront of my mind, especially working in an academic setting. I have wondered about what it must be like being a minority student at university. When I was in university as an undergraduate, 9/11 happened. It was difficult being from an Indian background then; the feeling of "I don't belong" and "don't fit in" was prevalent. I remember going to the supermarket in my traditional Indian clothing and feeling "stared at", which made me feel so uncomfortable that I learnt to avoid wearing my traditional Indian clothes in public. This may be my subjective experience, but I feel that I am responded to differently according to whether I wear my Indian clothes or what I call my "English" clothes. So, I have learnt to fit in by suppressing my Indianness and perhaps this has helped me get to the position I have now?

Whilst these reflections don't directly relate to my route into forensic psychology, these experiences have underpinned my journey to becoming a forensic psychologist. In terms of wanting to become a forensic psychologist to make a difference and make a better life for myself and the next generation. This is why there were mixed emotions upon completing my postgraduate training. On the one hand, graduation was recognition that we (my family were just as invested) had made it; maybe I am good enough and could belong in this world. However, I now have a responsibility to do something with this privilege I have been given.

Experience of EDI Agenda

Martine: I am passionate about diversity and inclusion (D&I). It allows me to amplify the voices of others, provide a "critical friend" regarding projects, policies, and conversations to ensure that D&I is embedded into all we do and that it is the "golden thread" within our forensic practice. However, there are several challenges to the work, and I think engaging in D&I work as a woman of colour has been a complex one.

One of the complexities is that the work feels like it brings an unconscious expectation for me to represent "all minorities", which can weigh heavy when trying to convey a point or a message. Besides the weight, I cannot speak for all minorities, and no white colleagues would ever be expected to articulate the lived experience of all white people. Organisations need to reflect on this and take a more individualised approach. Within the psychology profession, who are used to and have a focus on being responsive, we need to translate this into the treatment of minority groups. All individuals within those groups also have nuanced needs requiring individualised responses.

Another challenge comes with disclosure of lived experience. To raise awareness of issues faced by less represented groups, other individuals from those less represented groups and I are often asked to share their experiences. This can be very exposing, sharing and showing a level of vulnerability that others usually do not share or wish to share at work. Nevertheless, experiences are shared, and it's my observation from sharing and through speaking to others, that this can be triggering and traumatising without aftercare provision, beyond a possible check-in. The individuals who hear the experience often then feel a sense of guilt, shame and sometimes anger and talk about wishing to do better/do more/offer support etc. Those feelings can then become the focus of the discussions, with the meaning of the original message getting lost or consumed in the feeling of the guilt expressed.

I think disclosure of lived experience can be helpful, but it has to be handled with care and needs to be a safe and positive experience for all parties. I share when I feel other colleagues who do not feel represented get a moment of community or validation. I share when I feel that it will provoke thought and conversation. I share when I feel that the sharing will lead to positive action and change. I share if I feel it will dispel myths and where I think it will help in fostering diversity and inclusion. However, it's been disappointing to share when I get a sense of inaction, and this can take varying forms, such as when I am used as the first port of call without any action on the part of the person making contact or when people freeze in their guilt and shame and do not put that into the internal work of "doing better". That's when sharing can feel painful and that you have been leaned on for plans, ideas, work without it being reciprocal. I am fortunate that I conduct a lot of the sharing as part of my full-time role where I am immersed in D&I. However, some colleagues often conduct D&I work on top of their day to day jobs (where D&I is one thing they may lead on for their region along with many other roles). This can come with a heavy emotional price tag and this must be understood, empathised with and considered by colleagues and leaders. It's important for organisations to remember that D&I work and the sharing of trauma (because that is what it is) can be onerous. It is also difficult to explain and educate colleagues on the impact of systemic discrimination. This is why leaders and managers should consider their asks of marginalised peoples and what the ask means for them in terms of the task and the emotional labour; what are the implications beyond the "can you just".

Ana: In early 2020, not only was the world "shutting down" due to COVID-19, but another critical event that affected me more than I could imagine was the killing of George Floyd. Watching the death of George Floyd on numerous news outlets, continuously revisiting the horrific event and how the world reacted to it, did something to my being. I remember discussing it with a close black friend who is also in their journey to becoming a psychologist, how I felt like I was grieving for someone I knew and how the worlds' reaction just made me want to shut away. I was grateful for how we could support each other, attended free online support events, and learned how we were not alone in feeling that way. At that time, I could also see how different divisions of psychology in the United Kingdom were rolling out statements about the events and signposting supportive services. However, there had been nothing from the division I thought I wanted to belong to. I was already involved with the division of forensic psychology and wondered whether I should say something. Still, I was concerned about being blacklisted for life or ignored and wondered how that would affect me personally and my current journey towards qualifying. My friend so kindly listened as I battled with what to do. She then proposed that I needed to think about whether I would be okay with identifying myself as part of a team that did not acknowledge what I and other black aspiring, trainees and qualified forensic psychologists, as well as clients and patients and colleagues, might also be feeling at that time.

"I've done it", I said and let out a concerned sigh of relief as I sent a two-page email explaining my disappointment and suggesting what and how we could learn from the whole situation: the murder and their lack of reaction.

That email was the beginning of a new thing for me and what I hope will be a new thing for others. The courage came from a change that I want to see and that I might also have to be – and become. Apologetic emails began flooding my inbox about the failure to recognise and acknowledge the impact the death of George Floyd had on black aspiring trainees and qualified forensic psychologists. I was then invited to present at my first division of forensic psychology conference and brought along fellow trainees. Together we presented and discussed our experiences as black trainees and the challenges of pursuing careers in forensic psychology.

I have since had the chance to meet and be introduced to people in the field whom I admire or whom I have read or heard about. They look like me, have had similarly complex journeys, and crave seeing a different psychology world. I have been blessed with the honour of being involved in unique projects, have written articles, contributed to talks and much more; currently, I am being entrusted and supported with birthing the support network I once looked for.

Pally: I sense that there is some recognition that EDI is an important issue, but there can be a "stuckness" of what can we do to address this and/ or its "someone else's responsibility". EDI is everyone's "business". Sometimes I experience an internal conflict between speaking about this and voicing it, as it's important to address it in terms of my values. But then there is the concern about being viewed as the Indian person talking about race again. But then, if I don't say anything, am I being complicit? So, what do I do? This can be tiring to have to navigate.

EDI should be embedded in our values and approach. We should be open and curious to listening and reflecting, even if we aren't always clear about what to do, and we may not always get it right or say the right thing. I have tried to promote practices supportive of EDI in my work with postgraduate students. For example, when thinking about EDI in forensic practice, I've asked students to reflect on what lens they see the world through based on their past experiences. I role-modelled this myself by speaking about how my past experiences got me into forensic psychology and how I have a strong multi-cultural aspect to my lens. Specifically, I have encouraged students to read the work of Bashe et al. (2007) and reflect upon their values, how this relates to EDI, and how this impacts on them working within and/or becoming forensic psychologists. Students have found this to be a very valuable exercise.

Thinking further about the training route using an EDI lens, how might this be experienced by an individual whose first language may not be English? How might the tasks of risk assessment and formulation writing be experienced? The individual is trying to learn these tasks conceptually and communicate their understanding in their non-native language. I've encouraged students to focus on understanding the skill and story conceptually rather than writing competence, as fears about writing competence can be a barrier. Whilst the argument might be that written communication is a crucial employability skill within forensic psychology, this can be developed over time and shouldn't be a barrier to joining and progressing in the field. Building confidence in this way will be vital if we want to develop a more diverse and inclusive workforce.

Overall, we all have a responsibility to take ownership of the EDI agenda. However, the barrier to this can be the fear of saying and doing the wrong thing. I have this concern myself at times of offending others. But the consequence of this concern could be that we don't do anything, and we don't ask any questions – because we don't know what the right ones are. Perhaps in these instances, we can ask others, curiously and inquisitively, what the right question is? What the correct term is that they would prefer? By taking that "leap" and asking these types of questions, we are connecting, modelling, working towards being inclusive, and moving towards making change a reality.

Leadership

Martine: Being in a minority in the workplace can have a significant impact with far-reaching consequences. It has impacted how I have acculturated into the profession and the level of authenticity I have felt able to show. I spent a lot of time early on in my career, trying to morph into what I thought a "psychologist" should be – which included buying a suit and slicking my hair back. I subconsciously worried about feeding into any stereotypes and worried that colleagues may hold or could call into question whether I was "suitable" for the profession based on the biases I already knew people had the capacity for. This was "stuff" I was carrying from my past, but I would suggest that several people from less represented backgrounds would have an affinity with this experience. I think seeing diversity within senior roles would have helped make me feel part of the profession and broader organisation and provide me with a frame of reference to orientate me into the profession and workplace, giving me confidence that I, too, could form a career as a psychologist.

Being a mixed-race woman and a minority in society, as well as in forensic psychology and my job role, has also impacted how I engage with and encounter leadership spaces. In my career, I am very used to seeing people look like me in non-leadership roles and being over-represented in the custodial setting. So when in leadership spaces, particularly now that I am a senior manager, I am very aware of the lack of representation of anyone that looks like me. This creates pressure to maximise the impact I have in meetings to make up for the lack of representation. I try to speak up consistently as I am aware others may not get the chance to be in the space I am. It's my view that minority leaders can feel a heavy sense of responsibility and weight to represent other minorities and make the most of being afforded the opportunity of being in a leadership position. Diversity in leadership and senior management would help ease the pressure felt by the less represented and increase the feeling of more diversity of thinking when making decisions and generating ideas and solutions in the leadership space.

Pally: Gaining a promotion into management in my current context has made me really reflect on EDI and leadership. I've thought about what kind of leader I want to be and what kind of leader I should be. This journey of becoming a leader has brought the difference between my eastern and western roots to the forefront. In particular, being from a culture where perhaps females haven't always had such a strong voice or much opportunity to express it. To now be in a leadership position where I am expected to have a voice, which I should express.

It has been difficult for me to find my voice transitioning into a leadership position and have the confidence to express it. I've had to push myself outside of my comfort zone. When you have been part of a marginalised group that hasn't traditionally had a voice, it's hard to use it. Sometimes from an EDI perspective, it feels that the solution is to give the person the opportunity to express their voice, in my case, in a management position. However, that doesn't mean that the person who is "given" the opportunity and "voice" knows how to use this or that they have the personal resources (i.e., confidence) to engage with this. There is a lot of emotional labour in putting yourself out there in this way and dealing with any potential consequences of doing so. How I express myself and my voice may be different due to cultural differences, and I've had to reflect on how my voice will "land" and be "viewed". Will I get caught out as an imposter, and as not really knowing what I'm talking about? Could I be upsetting the "status quo" by speaking out, and what will be the consequences of this? So my leadership position is encouraging me to be brave and speak up, as I now have a responsibility to do this. This comes back to my values about doing the right thing. In this context, the challenge of coming from a marginalised group and struggling to have a voice can be encouraged by others inviting you to express your voice and reminding you how valuable it is. This can be really supportive in terms of good practice.

In summary, I have had to work on developing my leadership identity as a minority female. I don't have any role models in similar leadership positions that I could relate to inside and outside of a work context to help me on this journey. I've realised that what I want to do in my leadership position is make a difference and live authentically within my values. And to do this, I just need to be me.

"What Now?"

Martine: I have talked about some of the complexities of D&I work and the challenges faced when conducting this work as a person of colour, but I often get asked how the most represented with structural enabled advantages in a workplace and organisation can support D&I work.

I would say that D&I is a collective responsibility; it is everyone's business! Only YOU are in that therapeutic space at that moment and can make a difference to whether a service user feels seen, heard and validated. YOU are the only one who can take responsibility for your actions in a meeting or conversation with a colleague. Maybe ask yourself these questions:

• How do you play your role in making all your colleagues feel included, especially those you feel you do not necessarily "click" with?

• Do you create a safe space or perpetuate fear and silence?

• Do you let your discomfort centre itself and dictate how you deal with a situation?

• Do you let it silence you or freeze you into no action at all?

Do you let your inner voice eat away at your confidence and lead you not to do the internal work required to be genuinely pro-inclusion and anti-discriminatory – and instead seek the work from others to provide you with the answers to your discomfort?

At this juncture, I want to focus on two things as take-home messages. Firstly it is a focus on YOU. This is, I think, one of the most important messages I would like to get across about D&I progress within the profession; D&I is more likely to embed and flourish if you are doing the work on yourself, and it's in your practice and behaviour. Reflective practice is a crucial part of our work, and part of this has to be the internal work to understand what our lived experiences mean for our practice. We must understand our biases and blind spots to understand what we need to work on professionally and what may be areas of introspection we may shy away from because it's a challenge for us. Finding ways to achieve this is the start of understanding ourselves better and what this means for our practice and cultural competence. If we can't do this or make the time for such work when we ask so much of our service users, we are not practising what we expect from them.

The second focus I want to highlight is discomfort. In my experience, this seems to place a huge role in the "what next" bit. Colleagues, friends, and family have often talked about being faced with a situation whereby inequality requires challenge. The theme that arises is that this has led to their discomfort and the individual letting that become the focus of the situation rather than the inequality. In other examples, the discomfort has led to feeling overwhelmed and inaction. Therefore, I take this opportunity to urge people to take ownership of and hold on to this discomfort whilst not letting it own you. Do the internal work to understand the discomfort, read, research, do your bit – and if the discomfort begins to take control, remind yourself that there are lots of people who do not have the embedded advantages to avoid the discomfort; they have to live and navigate it every day.

Lastly, in this chapter, I wanted to note the importance of allyship/solidarity and the value of having courageous practitioners around you. This has been invaluable to me in my career. During my route to qualification and forensic practice, I have had supervisors, some line managers, and colleagues who have been at the forefront of challenging inequality, have done the internal work to unpick their biases so that they can approach their work and me with cultural humility, and are very clear in the part they play in D&I. They have worked to strive towards doing and being better in terms of anti-discriminatory practice.

Individuals such as these around me during my career means I have breathed a little easier. The burden has been lighter, and I feel I have grown in my confidence and ability to be authentic in my work and the profession. That is the difference that collective responsibility and internal work can achieve.

Ana: It is a tiny start, but it is a start nonetheless. Despite many other factors that have impacted my journey (too many to list here), I appreciate the ups and downs and the journey it has started. Do not be fooled; imposter syndrome is real, but I believe dreams and aspirations are even more real. I hope that encouraging and helping others in the field will be something that will continue for me. I also hope to see changes in curriculums, workplaces and even policies and guidelines that will challenge and educate people and lead to a better understanding rather than ostracising Black, Asian and other Ethnic Minorities and encouraging all different types of disproportionalities. I genuinely hope to see a day where greater accessibility and affordability, increased support and guidance, and a visual representation of ethnic diversity is found and experienced in forensic psychology.

Table 2.1 Themes and questions to aid reflection about bias

Theme	Questions
Lens	What is my lens to view the world?
	What impact has my past experiences had on my lens?
	How have my values impacted on my lens?
	What impact might this lens have on me? On my choice to select the profession of forensic psychology?
	What impact does my lens have on my practice?
	What is the lens of the person I'm supporting and working with? How do they view the world?
Power and privilege	What is my power and privilege?
	How am I using this?
	How do I experience inequality?
	How do I experience others' experience of inequality?
	How do I respond to this?
Assumptions	What assumptions am I making about this person?
	What might be influencing me to make such assumptions?
	What questions can I ask that make me question my assumptions?
Inferences	What cultural inferences and behaviours am I promoting in my language and my behaviour?
	How may others experience this?
	How might this impact on inclusivity in my context?
	What can I do to work on this?
Developing my lens	It may be hard to change your lens, but you can be aware of the impact of it in the different situations we have to be within. It can perhaps be adapted over time with experience and reflection. Some questions to consider:
	How open am I to this?
	What might impact on my openness to adapt my lens? (fears, barriers)
	How can I work with this?
	Who is my "critical friend" that can help me reflect about my lens?

Pally: As mentioned, reflective practice is one way of reflecting on the ideas discussed in this chapter. In particular, the ethics autobiography (Bashe et al., 2007) is a tool that can be used to aid reflective practice. Relatedly, presented in Table 2.1 are some themes and questions that could be useful to think about your "lens". I hope that by sharing this I/we can promote discussion and reflection. My ultimate goal is to promote connection, belonging and acceptance (Brown, 2012). I'm still trying to figure out the ways to get there or if this is even realistic, but I hope the discussions in this chapter are certainly a starting point.

Conclusion

The writing of this chapter was a fearful and exposing process. It made us feel vulnerable to criticism and judgement as we put ourselves out there. We don't have the usual anchor of references and science. We want to celebrate and acknowledge difference; isn't this what diversity is? But there's a tension between acknowledging difference and not be accepted; there is a lot of shame associated with this. Fundamentally, as Brown (2012) suggested, we want connection, belonging, and acceptance. Through us writing this, we hope that we have supported the development of connection and made this discussion feel safe and comfortable, and if one person reads this and feels less lonely in this world, then in our view, that has made a difference.

Departing comment: "Change will not come if we wait for some other person or some other time. We are the ones we've been waiting for. We are the change that we seek" – Barack Obama.

Note

1 View or treat (a person or group of people) as intrinsically different from and alien to oneself.

References

Bashe, A., Anderson, S. K., Handelsman, M. M., & Klevansky, R. (2007). An acculturation model for ethics training: The ethics autobiography and beyond. *Professional Psychology: Research and Practice, 38*(1), 60–67.

Brown, B. (2012). *Daring greatly: How the courage to be vulnerable transforms the way we live, love, parent, and lead.* London: Penguin Books Ltd.

Lammy, D. (2017). *The Lammy review: An independent review into the treatment of, and outcomes for, black, Asian and minority ethnic individuals in the criminal justice system.* London: Lammy Review.

Tajfel, H. (1974). Social identity and intergroup behaviour. *Social Science Information, 13*(2), 65–93.

3 The Role of Dynamic Risk Factors in Forensic Assessment and Treatment Planning

Roxanne Heffernan and Tony Ward

Introduction: Forensic Assessment and Treatment Planning

Assessment and treatment planning are an important initial step in any forensic intervention, they help a practitioner gain an understanding of the person they are working with, their needs, and how best to work with them to reduce the likelihood that they will commit further offences. Assessment generally includes a thorough file review, a clinical interview (sometimes supplemented with collateral interviews), use of psychometrics and/or risk-need assessment tools, a case formulation, and a treatment plan (Sturmey et al., 2019; Ward et al., 2016). The first three steps are aimed at gathering information about the persons' history, their characteristics and capacities, and the problems they experience which relate to their offending. Thus, in psychological assessment, clinicians attempt to systematically collect data that enable them to identify a client's difficulties and their causes. The result of this process is a conceptual model representing the client's various complaints, their causes, and their interrelationships; what is termed a *case formulation*. A case formulation ideally represents a coherent explanation describing the development of personal characteristics and situations which are relevant to the offence and other problematic behaviours, and then makes predictions about the most useful intervention.

The treatment plan sets out the goals and tasks for the intervention in terms of what capacities need to be developed or strengthened to obtain important individual goals and prevent reoffending. While there is no standard approach to forensic assessment, it should be systematic, comprehensive, and relevant (Day, 2019). It typically involves an in-depth analysis of events (both internal and external) before and after offending and the practitioner makes judgements about what is relevant to the particular case; it has been likened to putting together a puzzle (Day, 2019).

One component of forensic assessment, *risk-need assessment*, is widely used to classify individuals in terms of their level of *risk* and thus *need* for intervention (Day, 2019). This is in line with the risk and need principles of the widely utilised Risk-Need-Responsivity (RNR) model (Bonta & Andrews, 2017). The RNR model assumes a linear relationship between risk and need and proposes that the

DOI: 10.4324/9781003230977-4

factors which are statistically associated with recidivism are the most appropriate targets for intervention. Risk-need assessment typically relies on standardised tools containing items related to domains of risk or aspects of the person's functioning and lifestyle which correlate with crime. This standardised approach ensures that "risky" characteristics are considered in terms of their presence and severity, rather than simply relying on professional judgement in determining risk level and thus need for intervention. While risk-need assessment may provide information about level of risk and factors which contribute to this prediction, it does not *explain* the development (i.e., causes), function, and maintenance of harmful patterns of behaviour for the individual. In contrast to risk-need assessment, which is largely based on aggregate information and predictors at the population level, a case formulation is highly individualised (Sturmey et al., 2019).

When completing a risk-need assessment, background information is gathered, which will also contribute to the case formulation. This includes early development and life domains associated with offending in general (e.g., family, peers, substance use, relationships, education, employment) and past offending (i.e., patterns in offending, thoughts about offending). It is important to note that the information gathered for the risk-need assessment only forms part of the picture; further information is required to complete a comprehensive case formulation. While a case formulation should account for the whole person, a specific problem formulation may inform this (Sturmey et al., 2019). In the forensic field these focus on recent past offences and patterns of offending, and they provide a reference point to understand the proximal influences on offending (Sturmey et al., 2019). Importantly, formulating an offence provides meaning and reasons for why and how the behaviour has developed, contextual influences, and maintaining factors, rather than simply describing the behaviour. Key features of the offence formulation include how historical events/influences have shaped certain reactions (e.g., sensitisation, learned behaviours, reinforcement), schema which have developed due to past experiences, interpersonal problems, proximal triggers, cognition and emotion, patterns of behaviour (e.g., avoidance, aggression), and its function (e.g., self-protection, control). Functional analysis is most often used and involves identifying the purpose of the behaviour, the factors which cause and maintain it, and alternative behaviours which perform a similar function for the individual (Day, 2019). Practitioners may also consider offence paralleling behaviours (OPB) when formulating offending. OPB is a method of formulation which looks at similar recurring behaviours which can be observed (i.e., in prison, in treatment) and more readily explored with the individual (Sturmey et al., 2019). Thus, OPB provides opportunities to observe behaviour and monitor change, alternative behaviours can be reinforced throughout the intervention, and test hypothesised mechanisms and processes thought to influence past offending and identify whether they are still present.

As a formulation is essentially an individualised theory of behaviour, generating hypotheses about its causes (and potential solutions) must rely on some theory of human functioning. In general, case formulation can be based on any theory available to the practitioner. However, it is suggested that offence-related information must be interpreted in line with a "generally accepted theory" (McMurran & Bruford, 2015) or an empirically supported theory (Sturmey et al., 2019). In the forensic field, cognitive-behavioural theories tend to be most widely used (Sturmey et al., 2019), within a General Personality and Cognitive Social Learning (GPCSL) approach (Bonta & Andrews, 2017). According to this theory the causes of criminal behaviour, or "criminogenic needs", include seven of the central eight (most predictive) risk factors: antisocial attitudes, associates, personality pattern, family and marital problems, education, employment, leisure, and substance use. These factors then become the targets of intervention.

Despite its importance in guiding intervention, until recently, forensic case formulation has received relatively little attention in the literature (Sturmey & McMurran, 2011). Relatedly, there is little to no agreement about what exactly a good case formulation looks like, and the methods and theories used vary across practitioners (Day, 2019). Various researchers have put forward suggestions for what a case formulation should contain and how one may evaluate these. For example, according to Sturmey (2010) case formulations should pick out the *relevant* parts of the presenting issue, be able to *explain* the onset and maintenance of the behaviour, and inform an *individualised* intervention plan. Case formulations should also be iterative, with each stage being tested and refined in accordance with new information (Davies et al., 2013). Sturmey (2010) acknowledges that while case formulations have these common elements, they vary in terms of the emphasis placed on specific factors (e.g., personal characteristics, the environment/situation, relationships, historical events) and how much attention is given to identifying opportunities for change. Despite potential inconsistencies in practitioner approach and the subjectivity of these judgements, what all good case formulations have in common is that they aim to pick out the *causes* of offending and reoffending.

The Role of Dynamic Risk Factors in Assessment and Formulation

As discussed, risk factors are central to risk-need assessment, subsequent decisions about programme placement (i.e., treatment intensity), and areas of need to be targeted (Sturmey et al., 2019). The tools used in these assessments tend to converge on well supported correlates of reoffending which can be divided into those which are static (i.e., unchanging, historical) and those which are dynamic. Dynamic risk factors are important because risk assessment has moved from merely being concerned with prediction to being concerned with intervention. Static factors are good predictors but, as they cannot be changed, they have little utility in treatment planning and monitoring progress (Olver & Wong, 2019). Dynamic risk factors can be defined as features of the individual, their lifestyle, and environment, which are statistically associated with recidivism and are changeable. Examples include seven of the central eight (listed above) for general offending and additional risk factors for specific types of offending, for example, intimacy deficits and sexual deviance for sexual offending (Mann et al., 2010).

These factors originate from risk prediction, as they are correlated with re-cidivism at the population level, they can be used to predict likelihood of re-offending. These factors were then transported into the arena of treatment and are the most common targets of change for interventions designed to reduce recidivism (i.e., the need principle). The underlying assumption is that correlates of reoffending must be targeted or changed to prevent crime. While we do not dispute the utility of dynamic risk factors in *prediction*, their role as treatment targets requires the existence of causal links with offending behaviour.

Unlike clinical case formulations which typically draw from a range of etio-logical theories, forensic or offence-based formulations tend to centre around or at least refer to dynamic risk factors. Typically, formulation is based upon the widely accepted "propensity model" of risk, where long-term vulnerabilities (i.e., dynamic risk factors) interact with environmental triggers and opportunities to influence behaviour (Beech & Ward, 2004). As above, case formulation is gen-erally guided by practitioners' training in cognitive-behavioural theory (CBT; Beck, 1970) and a General Personality and Cognitive Social Learning (GPCSL; Bonta & Andrews, 2017) perspective of persons. There is an emphasis on faulty thinking, offence-supportive core beliefs, antisocial traits, and learned behaviour. This approach can result in case formulations which look incredibly similar across individuals, as practitioners attempt to fit individuals' experiences within a well-established set of factors (Ward & Fortune, 2016a). In the sense that it links risk factors with behaviour, a formulation aims to bridge the gap between pre-diction and explanation. It guides practice via the integration of empirical knowledge and theoretical understanding of the factors which are strongly linked with offending. Therefore, theories of risk factors and offending are a crucial foundation; they guide the process of inference from descriptions of thoughts and behaviours to explanations of their possible causes and targets for intervention. The problem currently facing practitioners is that existing case formulation ap-proaches assume that dynamic risk factors are theoretically coherent constructs and therefore can be viewed as causes of offending behaviour. However, as we will now argue, this assumption is incorrect.

Conceptual Problems with the Reliance on Dynamic Risk Factors

There has been increasing critical attention towards dynamic risk factors over the last five to ten years, both in terms of their predictive and construct validity, and their conceptualisation and ability to explain crime. In this section we will focus only on the conceptual problems with these factors which reduce their utility in case formulation and treatment planning. Following this, we will describe a re-cent approach aimed at overcoming these problems and discuss its utility in informing case formulation.

There are four key conceptual problems which undermine the potential causal status of dynamic risk factors and thus their utility in formulation and treatment (see Ward & Fortune, 2016a). The first is that they lack *coherence*; they contain

several types of variables (e.g., mental states, contexts, underlying causal processes) and therefore are composite rather than coherent concepts (Ward &
Fortune, 2016a). It is likely these categories contain multiple potential causal
strands, but in their current form also include contextual/environmental (e.g.,
employment), behavioural (e.g., aggression), and psychological state (e.g., attitudes and emotions) aspects. A second issue is that due to their many possible
causal elements, they *lack specificity*. In other words, it is unclear which of the
potential causes embedded within each risk factor are relevant for explaining
certain phenomena in any particular case. A third issue is that dynamic risk
factors suffer from the *grain problem*, meaning there is no consensus about which
level of abstraction is most appropriate for conceptualising them. For example,
they can be described as umbrella categories (e.g., antisocial personality pattern,
relationship problems) or more fine-grained categories composed of specific
features (e.g., impulsivity, aggression). Finally, they are not "scientific kinds"
(Ward, 2016) and thus *lack factualness* or objectivity. They are (at least partially)
normative constructs; they exist due to their relationship with behaviours deemed
harmful and/or unlawful (i.e., crime) rather than being real things that exist
independently of normative practices.

To illustrate these issues, we will explore the example of "emotional congruence with children". This risk category has strong empirical support for its
association with sexual reoffending against children and has been described as:

> relationships with children are more emotionally satisfying … may find
> children easier to relate to than adults, may feel he is still like a child himself,
> and may believe that children understand him better than adults do. He
> often feels himself to be "in love" with his child victims.
>
> (Mann et al., 2010, p. 201)

This factor is judged present based on the way the person talks about their
offending and their relationship with the (child) victim. Thus, it is possible that
rather than representing an enduring propensity or affiliation with children in
general, it may simply reflect the individual's attempt at justifying their behaviour
in the moment or be specific to certain victims. It is also possible that indicators
of emotional congruence with children could be symptoms of problems in other
risk domains, such as sexual deviance, attachment problems, social skill or
cognitive deficits, and offence supportive attitudes such as "children can enjoy
sex" (Mann et al., 2010). Thus, it is unclear what underlying mechanism(s) the
category refers to and how it might increase risk at the individual level (i.e., it
lacks specificity). In addition, it is, in part at least, a normative category in the
sense that emotional congruence with others, including children, varies across
the population and is only deemed dysfunctional when it occurs in the context of
sexual offending. In other words, having some level of emotional congruence
(i.e., empathy and care) for children is healthy and can be protective, however,
when paired with inaccurate beliefs about the nature and capacities of children
and sexual motivations, it can be harmful.

To illustrate the remaining two problems, lack of coherence and the grain problem, we will explore the composite nature of emotional congruence with children. The processes which hang together across explanatory levels and grains of analysis (i.e., from general categories to specific) to cause or constitute this factor may include (but are not limited to):

- *Cultural/contextual level*: Norms and laws specifying the types of relationships that are appropriate and what these should involve (i.e., age of consent, boundaries); gender norms; ideal sources and amount of emotional congruence; and contextual opportunities (i.e., social roles)
- *Interpersonal/social level*: Interpersonal skills (e.g., communication); social learning; social roles; social isolation or rejection from adults; expectations and responsibilities in adult relationships
- *Phenomenological/psychological level*: Emotional connection/congruence; love; empathy; sexual preferences; beliefs about relationships (i.e., self and others); cognitive capacity; perspective-taking; and attachment style
- *Neuropsychological level*: Brain regions and neurotransmitters such as oxytocin; vasopressin; pre-frontal cortex; brain injury; and hormones that underpin psychological problems and experiences indicative of intimacy and congruence
- *Biological level*: Sexual arousal; physical health; and physical attributes (i.e., size, attractiveness)

Each level of analysis draws from various kinds of evidence and research, and varies in its type of explanation, for example, from biological to socio-cultural. In addition, this category varies in its level of abstraction depending on the task at hand, this is known as the grain problem. For example, emotional congruence with children can be thought of as an overarching category which contains more specific problems such as emotional (e.g., congruence, safety, love) and cognitive (e.g., beliefs about children and relationships, attributions of behaviour) processes at lower levels. No level can provide a comprehensive explanation of emotional congruence with children; unique properties and processes exist at each level. We hope these examples illustrate the range of influences and potential processes which exist in just one risk category, and that they highlight the overlap between different categories (e.g., cognition, emotion, and interpersonal factors). This should clarify how the composite nature of dynamic risk factors creates incoherence and conceptual confusion and provide support for the assertion that they are ill suited for the purposes of explanation and formulation. They are useful for prediction, but if they are to be useful in case formulation or treatment, arguably they need to be reworked.

The key difficulty with using dynamic risk factors in formulation is that it is assumed that they are coherent constructs which are causally linked with crime (e.g., Hart et al., 2011; Sturmey & McMurran, 2011). In our opinion this is not currently the case; dynamic risk factors are best thought of as red flags which signal the presence of problems (i.e., interpersonal, skill deficits) but fail to account for their development and maintenance. The focus in formulation on empirically established lists of risk factors within a GPCSL approach (Andrews & Bonta, 2010; Bonta & Andrews, 2017) falls short of causal explanation (see Ward & Fortune, 2016a) and thus is limited in its ability to guide interventions.

Further, it is argued that "the theoretical legitimacy of incorporating dynamic risk factors into the domain of treatment depends on their causal status" (Ward & Fortune, 2016a, p. 80). A counter argument is that as changes to dynamic risk factors are predictive and correspond to changes in behaviour (i.e., reduced recidivism), their causal status is not important. However, empirical findings concerning the links between improvement on areas of risk and subsequent changes in offending are currently mixed (Klepfisz et al., 2016; Duwe & Rocque, 2016; Serin et al., 2013), there are concerns about construct validity (Cording et al., 2016; Polaschek, 2016), and there is little understanding of the mechanisms underlying the change process. While researchers often acknowledge that dynamic risk factors are (or at least point to) *potential* causes, practitioners are effectively treating them as causes when they make them the focus of treatment. If we hope to change behaviour, then the best way to do this is to alter its causes, there is little point targeting a correlate to change an outcome.

Alternative Case Formulation Models

Recently there have been calls for a shift in focus, from a preoccupation with correlates to instead grounding our understanding of offending within psychological theories of human agency. It is beyond the scope of this chapter to outline the theories which have recently been developed to explain offending in terms of agency and motivation (e.g., Heffernan & Ward, 2015; Schmidt et al., 2021; Serin et al., 2016; Strauss-Hughes et al., 2019; Thornton, 2016; Thornton et al., 2017; Ward, 2017; Ward & Carter, 2019). Here we will briefly describe one model and one methodological framework, and then make some suggestions about how these may overcome some of the limitations with basing case formulation on dynamic risk factors.

The Predictive Agency Model (PAM; Heffernan & Ward, 2017, see Figure 3.1) is based on the assumption that persons are goal-directed (Ward, 2002) and future focussed (Seligman et al., 2016; Ward, 2017). Human beings' selective advantage lies in their capacity to mentally represent their environment and make informed predictions about the future responses of the self and others in any given situation (Heffernan & Ward, 2017). According to this approach, humans have evolved to be dynamic learners whose ability to adapt depends on their constructing *general models* that accurately predict other peoples' mental states, behaviour, and events. The capacity to construct, test, and revise general models enables persons to evaluate the outcomes of their actions and give meaning to their experiences. Through a lifetime of experience and social/cultural learning individuals develop these capacities and general models. Persons are essentially forward-looking and predisposed to construct plans and predictions to guide their behaviour. Adaptive functioning requires internal and external capacities and resources to achieve valued outcomes and avoid potential harm.

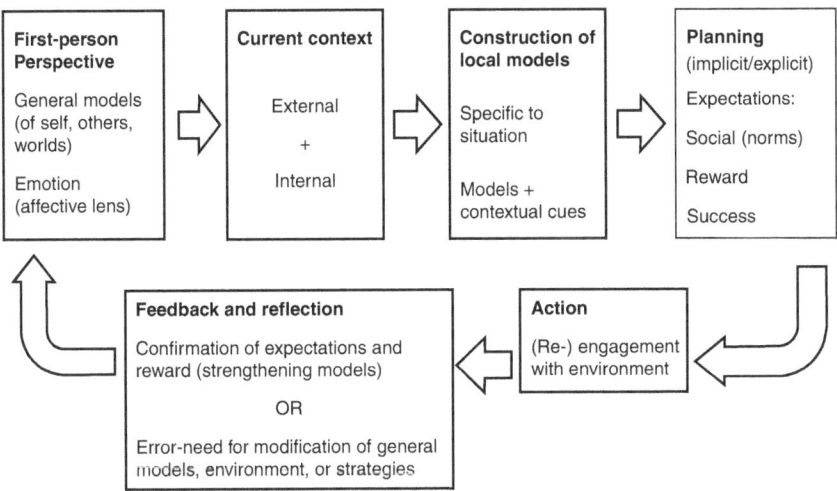

Figure 3.1 Predictive agency model.

Source: Adapted from R. Heffernan & T. Ward (2017). A comprehensive theory of dynamic risk and protective factors. *Aggression and Violent Behavior, 37,* 137.

In the PAM, a *first-person perspective* is comprised of general models (of the self, others, world) and an affective lens through which the person experiences the world. This allows a person to create predictions or simulations, which are crucial for long-term thinking and decision making. The person must project the self into the future and link these possibilities with authentic emotion (i.e., feel what that future situation would be like). Seligman et al. (2013) call these "if-then conditionals"; general models develop from past experiences where the individual learned what to expect from different situations and behaviours. Particular situations, environments, and mental states (i.e., the *current context*) prompt the person to access relevant general models, which inform situation specific *local models* (i.e., a mental representation of present opportunities, threats, options to act). However, constraints on cognitive resources can affect the capacity to generate accurate local models, as well as subsequent phases (Seligman et al., 2013), possibly explaining why some people only offend when experiencing distress or intoxication. *Planning* (implicitly or explicitly) involves identifying possible actions and predicting likely outcomes, emotion helps to evaluate these options (i.e., they are affectively tagged based on experience). This part of the model is based on the theory of reasoned action (Fishbein & Ajzen, 2010), which proposes that decision making relies on expectations of reward, success, and others' perception. Many actions will have the possibility of both positive and negative outcomes, linked with an individual's values and priorities (i.e., emotions track value). There may be deficits in the capacity to generate multiple options or evaluate possible outcomes. After an action has occurred, *feedback and reflection* help make sense of behaviour and its outcomes. Reflection draws on values, emotion, and general models. For example, an individual may experience aversive outcomes/feedback (e.g., arrest and/or feeling guilt) and modify general models or the costs of behaviour can be compensated for through justifications or minimisations, avoiding the need to adjust general models. Within the PAM, dynamic risk factors are conceptualised as problems in the capacities (including internal and external components) and processes which underpin agency.

The *Risk-Causality Method* (RCM; Heffernan et al., 2019) conceptual framework (see Figure 3.2) capitalises on the strengths of previous suggested research methods (e.g., Ward & Fortune, 2016b) by analysing dynamic risk factors through three phases: deconstruction, analysis, and reintegration. While this method was developed as a framework to generate further research into the composition and function of dynamic risk factors, it can also be applied to the exploration of areas of risk in case formulation.

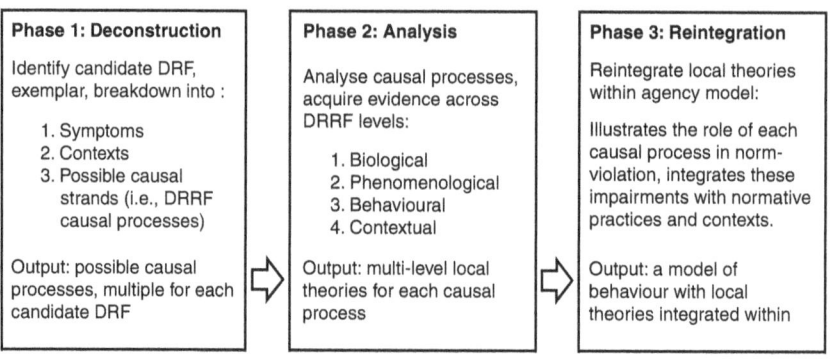

Figure 3.2 The risk-causality method.

Source: Adapted from R. Heffernan, T. Ward, S. Vandevelde, & L. Van Damme (2019). Dynamic risk factors and explanation: The risk-causality method. *Aggression and Violent Behavior, 44,* 53.

Phase one views dynamic risk factors as useful markers of (or red flags for) crime related problems. Thus, their key function is to indicate potential causal processes, contextual features, and behavioural and mental state variables (i.e., symptoms). Once a dynamic risk factor is selected, researchers should develop an exemplar (i.e., a typical description) of this risk domain which will anchor the first phase. The next step is to describe its behavioural or mental state (i.e., symptom-like) aspects, the contexts in which these aspects are observed, and identify the *potential causal processes* underpinning these. Breaking dynamic risk factors down in this way overcomes their composite nature and the grain problem. It also allows researchers and practitioners to isolate the potential causal strands within these categories, consider how these have developed and been shaped by the environment, and how they might interact with each other. To provide structure to the identification of these causal processes, researchers should consider a range of psychological systems, for example, negative and positive affective, cognitive, interpersonal, self-regulatory, and intrapersonal (see Ward & Fortune, 2016b).

Phase two begins with the list of possible causal processes, each of which should be explored across several levels of analysis to discern their possible influences and the evidence for these. This phase draws from research and theory (e.g., psychological, social, biological, and neuroscientific) to identify potential causal mechanisms. This phase has the potential to be complicated and laborious, but it is an important task which requires sufficient attention to provide comprehensive multi-level accounts of areas of risk. Ultimately, in the realm of research, phase two will provide mini theories of each potential causal process for all risk categories identified in phase one. These will explain how a particular system should work and thus help to identify whether there is dysfunction. In *phase three* these mini theories should be integrated within a model of human agency (e.g., the PAM) to understand their interactions how they influence action – no system on its own can explain offending. This final phase aims to explain the cumulative role of various causal processes in offending, essentially reintegrating information concerning the causal elements of dynamic risk factors with the sorts of tasks and environments in which they play out (e.g., intimacy seeking, emotion-regulation, resource attainment). This phase helps to address the normative nature of risk categories, as it links them with the goals, behaviours, capacities, and social contexts within which they are observed.

Because case formulation should be inferential rather than merely descriptive, the development of mechanistic explanations is directly relevant to forensic practice, both in helping to locate the source (i.e., underlying cause) of impairments and understanding how these problems have developed over time. Etiological explanations typically refer to events or features which temporally precede and generate an offence (i.e., potential causes). For example, loneliness and intoxication may lead to a sexual offence. *Compositional* explanations on the other hand refer to the structure of phenomena across multiple levels of analysis. For example, the functioning of the brain while a person is experiencing loneliness constitutes the emotion, rather than causing it (perhaps it is partially caused by an external event and/or a previous thought). Case formulations typically provide an etiological explanation in the sense that they contain proposed distal and proximal influences upon behaviour, and support predictions about the sorts of triggers and contexts which are likely to precede any future offences. We suggest that these explanations will be more useful if they are supplemented by compositional explanations concerning the phenomena implicated within these narratives. In other words, both types of explanation are necessary for developing comprehensive explanations. In case formulation practitioners can use the three phases of the RCM to structure their reasoning about the composition of relevant areas of risk for the individual and the underpinning mechanisms which can be altered through treatment.

In terms of intervention, the above approach aligns with strength-based frameworks such as the Good Lives Model (GLM; Ward, 2002; Ward & Stewart, 2003), which aim to support healthy agency (i.e., needs attainment). The PAM and RCM can add depth to the GLM by pointing to more specific areas where weakness (or strength) may be present. Simply relying on existing case formulation models or etiological theories that assume that risk factors (as currently stated in the literature) are possible causes is likely to result in overly general, poorly integrated formulations (i.e., everyone looks the same or possible hypotheses are overlooked). We suggest that in case formulation dynamic risk factors should only be used to indicate *general problem areas* and be regarded as summaries of possible causes, contextual factors, behavioural, and mental state variables. By the processes of deconstruction, analysis, and reintegration practitioners can put dynamic risk factors to work in ways that can provide a deeper understanding of why and how individuals act in ways that harm other people.

In order to do this, it is important for practitioners to consider the levels of explanation most appropriate for the task at hand. For example, the mechanisms underpinning offending are comprised of genetic, neurobiological, psychological, social/cultural, and ecological systems (Weerasekera, 1996). Persons are comprised of hierarchical systems, with unique properties emerging at each level. This means that explanations pitched at just one level and ignoring others will be impoverished; all will form a piece of the explanatory picture. For example, when explaining an offence it would be a mistake to overlook the importance of the physical and social environment (e.g., laws, norms, opportunities), the psychological features (e.g., emotion, cognition), or the biological and neurological influences upon cognition and behaviour. While one level may not be reduced to another (e.g., anger cannot be fully explained by physiological arousal) a certain level of analysis could be more suited to a particular task. Certain levels are influenced by others in a process of upward (e.g., biological influences on mood) and downward (e.g., environmental stressors influencing thoughts) causation, reflecting both horizontal and vertical interactions (i.e., between mechanisms and across levels of analysis).

We suggest that, generally speaking, first person, intentional (psychological level) explanations are privileged for the purposes of case formulation, and these should focus on descriptions of behaviour – what people do or fail to do, and why. While biological and social levels are also important, we ultimately need to understand why the person acted in ways that harmed others. This means that useful explanations of offending and its potential causes must refer to mechanisms and offer an explanation which differentiates adaptive or optimum functioning from dysfunction in particular contexts (Ward & Fortune, 2016a). Further, these explanations must be able to account for the interaction of mechanisms (within various risk categories) which result in offending; it is not enough to specify the various mechanism components without a satisfactory account of their causal trajectories. A framework such as the RCM has the potential to both guide the development of compositional explanations within individual case formulations (i.e., via local models) and describe how various mechanisms are linked with each other and behaviour through their integration within a model of agency (i.e., the PAM).

To make these implications more concrete, we will now make some preliminary suggestions concerning how case formulations can be responsive to the problems with and reconceptualisation of dynamic risk factors described throughout this chapter. Firstly, risk-need assessments may provide guidance on problem areas to be explored in the formulation. However, it is important not to jump to conclusions about the causes of behaviour, or to rely solely on identified risk factors to guide case formulations. Rather, practitioners can use these ratings as one source of information (i.e., as potential barriers to prosocial agency or red flags to explore), and later check whether they are likely to be linked with or addressed within their case formulation. The most important source of information for constructing the formulation will be the individual's account of their behaviour, including the motivations and values underpinning it and the context in which it occurred.

The practitioner should conduct an exploratory, collaborative, and semi-structured interview to draw out the different elements of the offence. This conversation may be guided by the PAM or a similar model. For example, considering the person's background, culture, early experiences, and how these have shaped their identity and world view. They will explore the individual's priorities, how they conceptualise a good life and how they have in the past strived to reach this, which may relate in different ways to offending (i.e., function of behaviour). Thus, there is a dual focus on well-being and risk. The practitioner will consider emotional functioning, the role of emotion in motivating behaviour within certain contexts and how their general affect influences their perceptions of the world. They will then look at the situation in which the offence occurred, including external conditions and internal states, and explore local models or situation specific representations of the offending context. It is important here to explore the role of the context and cultural norms (i.e., others present) in shaping their response. This will lead into a discussion of the planning phase, considering the expectations which (implicitly or explicitly) influenced their choice of behaviour. The individual can then describe the behaviour and its consequences, including responses from others and themselves. This will help to understand how the behaviour aligns with their existing general models and priorities/values, for example, whether and how the behaviour was rewarding (i.e., was it successful in meeting needs?), and if it was congruent with expectations. The impact of feedback/outcomes on general models can be explored in terms of any learning or sense-making.

This whole conversation can be used to develop a narrative (or visual depiction) of the distal and proximal influences on offending behaviour. Depth can then be added through using the RCM phases to explore the possible mechanisms underpinning areas of risk or deficits in the agency process (this can also draw from the risk-need assessment). Practitioners can locate potential sources of problems and then draw from existing psychological theories to increase specificity and understanding. This step may involve additional levels of explanation – including social, contextual, and behavioural, as well as sub-personal mechanisms (i.e., neurological and biological processes). In saying this, in the interests of collaboration and case formulation usability, it is important that the explanation makes sense to the individual. This might mean that certain levels of explanation are included in a more implicit way, or they are not discussed with the individual. The case formulation should represent a bridge between scientific method and the individual's common-sense explanation of their own behaviour. The individual may provide their own theories about the causes of their behaviour and what they need to change. The first-person perspective is invaluable because it is gives insight into their own understanding and provides cultural nuances which may not be picked up by the practitioner. It also facilitates ownership of their own case formulation and buys in for the goals which emerge from it and creates a sense of balance in the therapeutic relationship.

When it comes to setting goals and delivering interventions, practitioners can use this formulation to develop goals based on the specific causes identified (i.e., hypothesised areas of vulnerability) and the individual's priorities. Of course, this is easier in settings with more flexibility to deliver individualised interventions, rather than "one size fits all" programmes. The strategies for developing strengths or resources will vary. For example, vulnerabilities in the planning stage may be addressed by increasing options for action selection, and problems with general models may be addressed by shifting these to more healthy, adaptive, or prosocial alternatives. These alternative models and options must be feasible to the individual and congruent with their culture and environment. According to the PAM, behaviour will change when expectations change, and expectations change via feedback signals. Therefore, rehabilitation should aim to provide learning opportunities or situations where error signals (i.e., unexpected outcomes) are experienced to alter expectations for future scenarios. For this to happen individuals must possess the capacities required to learn from these situations, and so this process (i.e., feedback and reflection) may need to be guided and supported by therapists. We suggest that, with support, capacities can be built which allow the individual to explicitly identify and implement alternative strategies, and that with practice (and reward) these may become part of their behavioural repertoire.

This approach is intended to be complementary to widely used frameworks such as the GLM and the RNR model but adds depth concerning the mechanisms underpinning criminal behaviour (i.e., the need principle) and integrates these within a model of human agency which can guide individualised (i.e., responsive) treatment. In this approach dynamic risk factors are viewed as predictive devices which may indicate areas for further inquiry, and they are likely to demonstrate changes following effective treatment. However, treatment is more broadly focused on strengthening the internal and external resources required to meet needs in prosocial and healthy ways. This approach overcomes the issues listed earlier; it is more individualised and accounts for parts of the person which are not necessarily statistically related to offending at the population level. A related strength of this approach is that it can account for diversity; the individual is viewed within their socio-cultural context rather than being reduced to a list of risk factors.

Conclusion and Future Directions

The analysis provided throughout this chapter has questioned the utility of relying on dynamic risk factors as explanations for offending and targets of interventions.

The domains of functioning and arenas of life reflected within risk categories are most likely in "need" of prosocial change and when this occurs, we should see changes in behaviour (i.e., they are symptoms of antisocial life orientation). However, without an in-depth understanding of what specifically needs to change and how we might facilitate this for individuals, practitioners are unable to effectively formulate, plan, and deliver treatment or monitor its success. Comprehensive and individualised formulation requires practitioners to identify the most likely causes of the problems reflected within patterns of offending. In addition, we must consider the possibility that the factors which reduce crime vary from those which have been shown to correlate with offending (Kroner et al., 2017; Polaschek, 2016; Serin & Lloyd, 2009). Even if we can identify the range of potential causes of offending, practitioners should also consider the causes of desistance to understand and influence the change process. A potential way to do this is to adopt a more holistic view of persons as goal-directed agents.

It makes little sense to construct formulations and intervention plans without a reasonable understanding of what the possible causes of crime and related phenomena are. Relying on dynamic risk factors as treatment targets is a mistake as they do not reliably identify underlying causes at all; they are in effect *summary labels* for possible causes, contextual features, behaviours, and mental state variables. Strictly speaking, they do not exist for the purposes of treatment, and there is little point targeting symptom-like summaries and assuming this will alter the mechanisms generating them. Further theoretical work is needed, however, from a pragmatic viewpoint the PAM and RCM can play valuable roles in structuring clinical inquiry and, in conjunction with knowledge of etiological theories, risk assessment, and classification models, can assist practitioners to arrive at a working explanation of an individual's crime-related problems. It can bridge the gap between risk assessment and intervention and ensure that practitioners carefully consider the explanatory possibilities offered by dynamic risk factors and avoid the trap of assuming they directly pick out causal factors. An advantage of structuring assessment and subsequent treatment in this way is that it confers a degree of epistemic scepticism on practitioners' conceptualisations of clients and reminds them that they critically depend on theoretical and methodological assumptions.

References

Andrews, D. A., & Bonta, J. (2010). *The psychology of criminal conduct* (5th ed.). New Providence, NJ: LexisNexis.

Beck, A. T. (1970). Cognitive therapy: Nature and relation to behavior therapy. *Behavior therapy*, *1*(2), 184–200.

Beech, A. R., & Ward, T. (2004). The integration of etiology and risk in sexual offenders: A theoretical framework. *Aggression and Violent Behavior*, *10*(1), 31–63. 10.1016/j.avb. 2003.08.002

Bonta, J., & Andrews, D. A. (2017). *The psychology of criminal conduct* (6th ed.). New York, NY: Routledge.

Cording, J. R., Beggs Christofferson, S. M., & Grace, R. C. (2016). Challenges for the theory and application of dynamic risk factors. *Psychology, Crime & Law, 22*(1–2), 84–103. 10.1080/1068316x.2015.1111367

Davies, J., Black, S., Bentley, N., & Nagi, C. (2013). Forensic case formulation: Theoretical, ethical and practical issues. *Criminal Behaviour and Mental Health, 23*(4), 304–314. 10.1002/cbm.1882

Day, A. (2019). *Psychological assessment in the correctional setting.* The Wiley International Handbook of Correctional Psychology, pp. 488–497. NJ: USA, & Chichester, UK-both listed in original text: https://onlinelibrary.wiley.com/doi/pdf/10.1002/9781119139980.fmatter

Duwe, G., & Rocque, M. (2016). A jack of all trades but a master of none? Evaluating the performance of the Level of Service Inventory–Revised (LSI-R) in the assessment of risk and need. *Corrections, 1*(2), 81–106. 10.1080/23774657.2015.1111743

Fishbein, M., & Ajzen, I. (2010). *Predicting and changing behavior: The reasoned action approach.* New York, NY: Psychology Press (Taylor & Francis).

Hart, S., Sturmey, P., Logan, C., & McMurran, M. (2011). Forensic case formulation. *International Journal of Forensic Mental Health, 10*(2), 118–126.

Heffernan, R., & Ward, T. (2015). The conceptualization of dynamic risk factors in child sex offenders: An agency model. *Aggression and Violent Behavior, 24*, 250–260. 10.1016/j.avb.2015.07.001

Heffernan, R., & Ward, T. (2017). A comprehensive theory of dynamic risk and protective factors. *Aggression and Violent Behavior, 37*, 129–141. 10.1016/j.avb.2017.10.003

Heffernan, R., Ward, T., Vandevelde, S., & Van Damme, L. (2019). Dynamic risk factors and constructing explanations of offending: The risk-causality method. *Aggression and Violent Behavior, 44*, 47–56. 10.1016/j.avb.2018.11.009

Klepfisz, G., Daffern, M., & Day, A. (2016). Understanding dynamic risk factors for violence. *Psychology, Crime & Law, 22*(1–2), 124–137. 10.1080/1068316X.2015.1109091

Kroner, D. G., Polaschek, D. L., Serin, R. C., & Skeem, J. L. (2017). An exploration of the symmetry between crime-causing and crime-reducing factors: Implications for delivery of offender services. *Psychological Services, 16*(2), 329–339. 10.1037/ser0000199

Mann, R. E., Hanson, R. K., & Thornton, D. (2010). Assessing risk for sexual recidivism: Some proposals on the nature of psychologically meaningful risk factors. *Sex Abuse, 22*(2), 191–217. 10.1177/1079063210366039

McMurran, M., & Bruford, S. (2015). Case formulation quality checklist: A revision based upon clinicians' views. *Journal of Forensic Practice, 18*(1), 31–38. 10.1108/JFP-05-2015-0027

Olver, M. E., & Wong, S. C. (2019). *Offender risk and need assessment: Theory, research, and applications* (pp. 461–475). The Wiley International Handbook of Correctional Psychology. NJ: USA, & Chichester, UK - both listed in original text: https://onlinelibrary.wiley.com/doi/pdf/10.1002/9781119139980.fmatter

Polaschek, D. L. (2016). Desistance and dynamic risk factors belong together. *Psychology, Crime & Law, 22*(1–2), 171–189. 10.1080/1068316X.2015.1114114

Schmidt, S., Heffernan, R., & Ward, T. (2021). The cultural agency-model of criminal behavior. *Aggression and Violent Behavior, 58*, 101554.

Seligman, M. E., Railton, P., Baumeister, R. F., & Sripada, C. (2013). Navigating into the future or driven by the past. *Perspectives on Psychological Science, 8*(2), 119–141. 10.1177/1745691612474317

Seligman, M. E. P., Railton, P., Baumeister, R. R., & Sripada, C. (2016). *Homo prospectus.* New York, NY: Oxford University Press.

Serin, R. C., Chadwick, N., & Lloyd, C. D. (2016). Dynamic risk and protective factors. *Psychology, Crime & Law*, *22*(1–2), 151–170. 10.1080/1068316X.2015.1112013

Serin, R. C., & Lloyd, C. D. (2009). Examining the process of offender change: The transition to crime desistance. *Psychology, Crime & Law*, *15*(4), 347–364. 10.1080/106831 60802261078

Serin, R. C., Lloyd, C. D., Helmus, L., Derkzen, D. M., & Luong, D. (2013). Does intra-individual change predict offender recidivism? Searching for the holy grail in assessing offender change. *Aggression and Violent Behavior*, *18*(1), 32–53. 10.1016/j.avb.2012.09.002

Strauss-Hughes, A., Heffernan, R., & Ward, T. (2019). A cultural–ecological perspective on agency and offending behavior. *Psychiatry, Psychology and Law*, 10.1080/13218719. 2019.1644250

Sturmey, P. (2010). Case formulation in forensic psychology. In M. Daffern, L. Jones, & J. Shine (Eds.). *Offence paralleling behaviour: A case formulation approach to offender assessment and intervention* (pp. 25–51). Chichester: Wiley.

Sturmey, P., & McMurran, M. (Eds.). (2011). *Forensic case formulation* (Vol. 49). Chichester, UK: John Wiley & Sons.

Sturmey, P., McMurran, M., & Daffern, M. (2019). *Case formulation and treatment planning*. The Wiley International Handbook of Correctional Psychology. NJ:USA, & Chichester, UK, pp. 476–487. both listed in original text: https://onlinelibrary.wiley.com/doi/pdf/10. 1002/9781119139980.fmatter

Thornton, D. (2016). Developing a theory of dynamic risk. *Psychology, Crime & Law*, *22*(1–2), 138–150. 10.1080/1068316x.2015.1109092

Thornton, D., Kelley, S. M., & Nelligan, K. E. (2017). Protective factors and mental illness in men with a history of sexual offending. *Aggression and Violent Behavior*, *32*, 29–36. 10.1016/j.avb.2016.12.003

Ward, T. (2002). Good lives and the rehabilitation of sexual offenders: Promises and problems. *Aggression and Violent Behavior*, *7*, 513–528. 10.1016/S1359-1789(01)00076-3

Ward, T. (2016). Dynamic risk factors: Scientific kinds or predictive constructs. *Psychology, Crime & Law*, *22*(1–2), 2–16.

Ward, T. (2017). Prediction and agency: The role of protective factors in correctional rehabilitation and desistance. *Aggression and Violent Behavior*, *32*, 19–28. 10.1016/j.avb. 2016.11.012

Ward, T., & Carter, E. (2019). The classification of offending and crime related problems: A functional perspective. *Psychology, Crime, & Law*, *25*(6), 542–560. 10.1080/1068316X.2018. 1557182

Ward, T., Clack, S., & Haig, B. (2016). The abductive theory of method: Scientific inquiry and clinical practice. *Behaviour Change*, *33*, 212–231.

Ward, T., & Fortune, C.-A. (2016a). The role of dynamic risk factors in the explanation of offending. *Aggression and Violent Behavior*, *29*, 79–88. 10.1016/j.avb.2016.06.007

Ward, T., & Fortune, C.-A. (2016b). From dynamic risk factors to causal processes: A methodological framework. *Psychology, Crime & Law*, *22*(1-2), 190–202. 10.1080/1068316x. 2015.1117080

Ward, T., & Stewart, C. A. (2003). The treatment of sex offenders: Risk management and good lives. *Professional Psychology: Research and Practice*, *34*, 353–360. 10.1037/0735-7028. 34.4.353

Weerasekera, P. (1996). *Multiperspective case formulation: A step towards treatment integration*. Malabar, FL: Krieger Publishing Company.

4 Why Dynamic Risk Factors Cannot Be Applied Universally: Their Normative Nature and the Importance of Cultural Awareness in Risk Assessment and Intervention

Stefanie Schmidt, Roxanne Heffernan, and Tony Ward

Introduction

Risk assessment and intervention in forensic psychology are largely based on the prominent Risk-Need-Responsivity (RNR) principle developed by Andrews and Bonta (2010). In accordance with these principles, intervention should be delivered proportionate to *risk* level; targets of intervention should address criminogenic *needs* (i.e., dynamic risk factors); and treatment should be *responsive* to evidence-based types of intervention as well as individual needs of participants (e.g., intellectual abilities; for more detail see Heffernan and Ward in Chapter 3). As a consequence, differences in dynamic risk factors across various (cultural) groups directly affect assessment and intervention. For example, Indigenous people are more frequently classified as high risk and so receive more supervision and intervention due to a higher exposure to common risk factors (Martel et al., 2011).

Although currently considered best practice, the RNR model contains a number of assumptions that need to be validated: That differences in risk level are meaningful rather than artefacts of measurement tools; that dynamic risk factors explain why some people offend and others do not; and that the causes of offending and their various indicators are similar for Indigenous people and people from North America (Shepherd & Lewis-Fernandez, 2016). As most risk assessment tools and theories in forensic psychology were developed within a Euro-American context, these (largely implicit) assumptions need to be evaluated (Reisig et al., 2006).

In this chapter, we will first argue for the importance of establishing equivalence when applying risk assessment measures cross-culturally. We will point to potential biases that can threaten equivalence and suggest how we can (in principle) mitigate biases in cross-cultural risk assessment settings. We will argue that the construct of dynamic risk factors (DRF), in their current conceptualisation, impede researcher's and practitioners' ability to be culturally aware, and illustrate this via several examples. As a way forward, we will present

DOI: 10.4324/9781003230977-5

a stepwise approach to culturally sensitive identification of potential causes of crime using a framework called the Cultural Agency-Model of Criminal Behaviour (Schmidt et al., 2021).

Importance of Equivalence in Forensic Psychology

Risk assessment tools and intervention programmes, which were mainly developed in Euro-American countries, are routinely applied within various cultural contexts (Pusch & Holtfreter, 2018). This practice is common despite scarce knowledge about their cross-cultural transferability (Hart, 2016; Jones et al., 2002; Martel et al., 2011; Shepherd & Lewis-Fernandez, 2016). Practitioners need to be aware that the accuracy of risk prediction depends upon the representativeness of samples on which the tools were developed and validated (Gottfredson & Moriarty, 2006). However, most samples predominantly comprise Euro-American males (Douglas et al., 2017; Jones et al., 2002; Shepherd & Lewis-Fernandez, 2016). Several cross-cultural analyses have shown that the predictive validity of common (violence) risk assessment tools is higher if the samples comprise mainly white Euro-Americans (Edens et al., 2007; Gendreau et al., 1996; Leistico et al., 2008; Onifade et al., 2009; Schlager & Simourd, 2007; Schmidt et al., 2018; Shepherd et al., 2015; Wilson & Gutierrez, 2014; for a meta-analytical review see Singh et al., 2011).

Biases affect actuarial risk assessment procedures and other associated tasks. For example, individual case formulations are based on well-known theories of the potential causes of crime (i.e., criminogenic needs) and as such often refer to DRF (Heffernan & Ward in Chapter 3). If there is scarce literature about the cross-cultural validity of DRF and the role of other culture-specific or migration related stressors in the development of criminal conduct (Schmidt et al., 2019), practitioners must make these judgements themselves based on their own opinions and experiences. They can either ignore potential differences and additional factors, resulting in ethnocentricity at the risk of invalid and unfair assessment and treatment. Or, they can try to adapt common measures, theories, and procedures in accordance to the specific individual and cultural context. To adapt as one thinks is best may lack both theoretical and empirical frames of reference that would make such judgements transparent (Schmidt & Ward, 2020). This procedure is also highly prone to stereotyping and biased judgements which might result in even less valid and more unfair results compared to no adaptation (Shepherd & Spivak, 2021).

Thus, cultural bias may not only result in institutional discrimination (e.g., by placing people falsely considered high risk into high security placement or intensive intervention) but also influence case management, treatment decisions, and decisions around preparedness to release on a more subtle and implicit level (e.g., stereotypes affecting the explanation of individual offending behaviour; Minhas & Walsh, 2018). This may have a cumulative negative effect for people from minority groups who are evaluated and treated by such methods, as they likely already suffer from marginalisation and disadvantage (Shepherd, 2015a).

This issue not only applies to racial or ethnic minorities, but many other dimensions of diversity as well (e.g., gender, sexual orientation, beliefs; Berry et al., 2011).[1] To be fair and valid in cross-cultural settings is not just an ethical requirement relating to the person being assessed (American Psychological Association [APA], 2017). It is crucial in forensic psychology (Haag et al., 2016), because every decision and intervention that is based on such evaluations also affects the public as a whole and the wider aims of the justice system. Therefore, it is mandatory to strive for equivalence of actuarial risk assessment conscientiously and to be sure that biases are mitigated – an issue that has rarely been addressed in forensic psychology (Cooke et al., 2005b; Veen et al., 2011).

Potential Bias and Ways to Mitigate It

Cross-cultural equivalence is only achieved when biases are absent. Although these two concepts, briefly explained in Table 4.1, are defined differently (He & van de Vijver, 2012), we will elaborate on them together in the following sections. We will then provide examples and recommend ways to (in principle) ensure equivalence and mitigate biases in forensic risk assessment. For more details see Schmidt et al. (2020).

Construct Equivalence Threatened by Construct Bias

If a theoretical construct (e.g., procriminal attitudes) has exactly the same meaning across cultures then *construct equivalence* is achieved (He & van de Vijver, 2012; van de Vijver & Leung, 2011; van de Vijver & Tanzer, 2004). *Construct bias* can be detected by comparing the definition and indicators of a construct across

Table 4.1 Bias and equivalence taxonomies

Term	Description
Equivalence	Level of comparability of measurement outcomes
Construct	Constructs have the same meaning across groups
Structural and functional	Instrument measures the same construct across groups
Measurement unit	Measurement scales have the same measurement units but different origins
Scalar or full score	Measurement scales have the same measurement units and the same origin
Bias	Factors which threaten the comparability of scores
Construct bias	Conceptualisation of the construct is not identical across groups
Method bias	Nuisance resulting from sampling, instrument characteristics, or administration
Item bias	Nuisance at the item level

Note: Table taken from Schmidt et al. (2020) originally adapted from van de Vijver and Rothmann (2004) and van de Vijver and Leung (2011).

cultures (van de Vijver & Tanzer, 2004). For example, at least one aspect of procriminal attitudes in Western cultures, denial of responsibility (Bonta & Andrews, 2017), is considered an appropriate response in many other cultures and not a sign of maladaptive behaviour (Kitayama et al., 2009; Maddux et al., 2011). This cross-cultural difference suggests that denial of responsibility is not suitable for a definition of procriminal attitudes across cultures. Thus, a construct bias is very likely for this DRF.

To mitigate construct bias, it is necessary to (a) reduce the definition to universal aspects (which may or may not be possible), or (b) clearly differentiate between universal and culturally variable aspects. Either way, researchers might start with a qualitative approach (e.g., interviewing) to test the suitability of construct definitions and related instruments informally before using the construct in new cultural contexts (He & van de Vijver, 2012). For example, Kreis and Cooke (2011) ran a prototypical analysis via a lexical approach to examine the definition of the construct "psychopathy" across gender and found many similarities as well as differences. Thus, it is necessary to ask people within each culture of interest what, for example, "procriminal attitudes" are, how they are expressed, and how they can be characterised and measured, before using this dynamic risk factor in assessment and treatment planning.

Structural Equivalence Threatened by Construct or Item Bias

Structural and functional equivalence are achieved when all underlying dimensions are identical (i.e., factor structure, e.g., arrogant and deceitful interpersonal style, deficient emotional experience, and impulsive and irresponsible behavioural style as factors of psychopathy; Cooke & Michie, 2001) and nomological networks are similar (patterns of convergent and discriminant relationships with other constructs, e.g., relations of psychopathy with offending) across groups (van de Vijver & Leung, 2011).

Researchers may evaluate structural equivalence by running exploratory or confirmatory factor analysis (van de Vijver & Tanzer, 2004). For example, Shariat et al. (2010) examined the three-factor structure of the psychopathy checklist: Screening Version (PCL:SV; Hart et al., 1995) within an Iranian sample compared to the Canadian and American standardisation sample. Although the three-factor-solution showed a good fit for both samples, the model fit differently in the two samples, indicating structural differences. Further analysis of potential item bias (i.e., items are inappropriate indicators of a construct because they do not have the same meaning across cultures) revealed that in particular a superficial and deceitful style could not effectively differentiate the Iranian people who scored above the cut off for psychopathy from those who did not (Shariat et al., 2010). That is, being superficial and deceitful can be considered less problematic and can be viewed as an adaptive behaviour in a collectivistic and hierarchical society to maintain harmony and honour.

Measurement Equivalence Threatened by Method or Item Bias

Measurement equivalence refers to whether an instrument measures the construct similarly across cultures (He & van de Vijver, 2012). Method biases (i.e., related to the application and assessment of a construct) that threaten measurement equivalence may be present when conditions vary between different cultural groups. For example, a lack of information about past criminal offending for people who have recently migrated may jeopardise the assessment of criminal history (Schmidt et al., 2018) – one of the most important risk factors in risk assessment. Furthermore, varying language abilities or culturally influenced communication styles (e.g., discomfort in rapid direct questioning, fear/mistrust of authority) may result in differences in the quantity and quality of information gathered in interviews that inform risk assessment (Shepherd & Lewis-Fernandez, 2016).

Researchers and practitioners can detect and control for method biases of this kind when they ensure comparable assessment conditions (e.g., by consulting interpreters, cultural training) or when they systematically take potential subjective and contextual variables into account (van de Vijver & Tanzer, 2004).

Along with method biases, differential item functioning (i.e., indicating item bias) may threaten measurement equivalence. This might be the case if one item is related differently to the construct across cultures. For example, compliance with treatment, as one indicator of procriminal attitudes (Bonta & Andrews, 2017), may differ because people from different cultures may have different experiences and thus expectations of treatment (Sue & Sue, 2013) rather than signalling a lack of motivation to change or attitudes supportive of continued offending. For example, Loya et al. (2010) illustrated that the use of counselling services for mental health problems is associated with greater reluctance and less favourable attitudes among South Asians compared to Caucasians in the United States.

Full Score Equivalence Threatened by Method or Item Bias

Finally, full score or scalar equivalence is achieved if absolute scores have exactly the same meaning without additional influences of sample characteristics (van de Vijver & Tanzer, 2004). Only when this is the case is it feasible to make cross-cultural comparisons and to justify decisions about supervision levels and treatment targets and methods cross-culturally.

When differences between samples (e.g., age, socio-economic status) are present that affect scores, method bias is present. Forensic practitioners must keep in mind that minorities (due to processes such as colonisation and/or marginalisation) often have higher rates of family disruption, problems in education, and unemployment (Schmidt et al., 2018; Shepherd, 2015b; Shepherd & Lewis-Fernandez, 2016), which are likely to influence their scores.

Along with method bias, item bias also threatens full score equivalence. Applying differential item as well as test function analysis, Cooke et al. (2005a) found cross-cultural differences between North-American and UK samples when using the Psychopathy Checklist-Revised (PCL-R; Hare, 2003). As a consequence, North-American cut-offs cannot be used in European populations as they do not represent the same level of psychopathy.

All potential biases must be appropriately taken into account (He & van de Vijver, 2012). Researchers and practitioners must put in a lot of effort into ensuring full equivalence and be very careful before applying risk assessment tools and related intervention planning methods universally. This task is made even more challenging due to the problems with their underlying constructs, DRF.

Why Dynamic Risk Factors Cannot Be Assessed in a Culturally Sensitive Manner

All of these potential ways to ensure equivalence and mitigate bias (illustrated above) presuppose that the underlying concept of interest is defined appropriately. A proper definition involves precisely formulated (inclusion and exclusion) criteria that describe the construct of interest. Such definitions are characterised by coherence (i.e., every aspect is clearly related to all other aspects in a logical order), specificity (i.e., narrowness of the range of meaning), and factualness (i.e., being real and thus falsifiable). A clear definition is also the basis for sophisticated development of an assessment tool. An instrument has favourable psychometric properties if it measures the construct of interest precisely (e.g., internal consistency, test-retest-consistency, inter-rater-consistency) and accurately (e.g., construct validity, predictive validity; Cohen et al., 2018). Thus, the evaluation of psychometric properties of a test is highly dependent upon the conceptualisation of the constructs (Gottfredson & Moriarty, 2006).

Unfortunately, the contemporary conceptualisation of DRF in general and commonly used DRF in particular (e.g., intimacy problems) do not meet the requirements mentioned above. DRF in general suffer from four key conceptual problems that are illustrated in more detail by Heffernan and Ward in Chapter 3.

First, DRF are *composite constructs* containing a number of variables from different conceptual categories (i.e., mental states, enduring vulnerabilities, contextual variables, behaviours) and, thus, they lack coherence (Ward & Fortune, 2016). For example, the DRF antisocial personality pattern is defined by: impulsiveness, adventurous pleasure-seeking, generalised trouble (multiple victims, multiple settings), restless aggression, and callous disregard for others (Bonta & Andrews, 2017). These variables may be indicative of different, possibly even contradicting, pathways to criminal behaviour (Ward & Fortune, 2016). This becomes even more likely in cross-cultural settings. For example, Bonta and Andrews (2017) "hypothesise that families that promote prosocial norms and are characterised by warm emotional attachments would have the lowest rates of delinquency" (p. 151). Thereby, Bonta and Andrews conflate two different concepts (i.e., prosocial norms and attachments) within one DRF (i.e., family problems), without clarifying the logic behind it. Cross-cultural research shows that among people with a Turkish or Arab migration background who have offended, emotional attachment between family members is strongly pronounced while delinquency of family members is also highly prevalent, compared to native Germans (Schmidt et al., 2018). However, researchers and practitioners cannot differentiate clearly between the different ways in which family dynamics may influence offending because of the composite nature of DRF. This also influences the psychometric properties of instruments measuring DRF. Because DRF are not unidimensional but heterogeneous (Hanson et al., 2013), many sophisticated (statistical) methods (e.g., differential item functioning analysis; see also Hammond in Chapter 7) simply cannot be applied in order to detect (item) biases.

Secondly, DRF *lack specificity*. Because of their composite nature (Via et al., 2016), it is not possible to define clear inclusion and exclusion criteria and determine which features point to causal mechanisms and are thus a necessary condition for the existence of the phenomenon. This lack of specificity calls for additional reasoning about the potential causal mechanisms which are relevant for explaining the relationship between DRF and offending (Ward & Fortune, 2016). Returning to the example of antisocial personality pattern, it is not specified whether aggressive behaviour, a parasitical lifestyle, or problems in delaying immediate gratification is the main causal aspect which links this category with offending. Consequently, we cannot evaluate whether different scores of antisocial personality pattern in fact point to cross-cultural differences in the DRF-crime relationship (e.g., problems in delaying immediate gratification are less causal in a diverse culture) or if they only pertain to secondary contextual aspects (e.g., a parasitical lifestyle is defined, expressed, and observed differently across cultures).

Given this lack of specificity, we cannot ascertain whether indicators of constructs are similarly appropriate (i.e., to detect item bias) across cultures. When we do not know how indicators (i.e., items of risk assessment tools) relate to the latent constructs of DRF (Ward, 2016) in general, we cannot examine if this also applies in other cultural contexts.

Third, DRF are formulated at *multiple levels of abstraction* ranging from more general terms to more concrete ones (Ward & Fortune, 2016). Thereby, broad terms often include several lower-level categories within them (Haynes, 1992). For example, they can be formulated as general categories (e.g., personality pattern, attitudes) and more specific factors within these categories (i.e., empathy problems, impulsivity). In addition, they can be explained at various levels of analysis, for example, via behavioural, social-contextual, psychological, neurological, and biological processes. Because unique properties and processes exist at each level of explanation, we do not know what exactly to refer to when we want to examine them cross-culturally (e.g., to ensure construct equivalence).

Fourth, DRF are *normative by nature*, they lack factualness because they only exist in relation to crime or judgements about what is antisocial versus prosocial. In many cases, DRF are even prefaced with terms like "procriminal", "poor", or "problematic" (Ward & Heffernan, 2017). However, these judgements necessitate the existence of norms concerning what is right/wrong and desirable/undesirable; these are based on a particular legal system which is in itself highly culture-dependent (Friedman, 1990). For example, in honour-cultures violent reactions to threats are considered appropriate or even desirable, while being against the law in dignity cultures (Arsovska & Verduyn, 2007). This illustrates that "risk item content often reflects the practices, perceptions, norms, belief systems, and behavioural expectations of Western culture" (Shepherd & Lewis-Fernandez, 2016, p. 429). Many theories about the causes of offending, risk assessment tools, and treatment programmes were developed in Euro-American contexts. This fact requires a thorough differentiation between potential universal and culture-specific aspects of crime-related concepts (i.e., DRF) in order to undertake risk assessment and intervention in a culturally sensitive manner (Hart, 2016; Jones et al., 2002; Martel et al., 2011; Shepherd & Lewis-Fernandez, 2016).

A Framework for Culturally Sensitive Identification of the Causes of Crime

A possible way forward towards culturally informed risk assessment and intervention planning is an explicit reference to agency as described in the Predictive Agency-Model (PAM; Heffernan & Ward, 2017; see also Heffernan and Ward in Chapter 3). Building on the premises of the PAM; the Cultural Agency-Model of Criminal Behaviour (CAMCB; Schmidt et al., 2021) was specifically designed to assist in culturally sensitive identification of the possible causal processes underpinning DRF and crime (Schmidt et al., 2021). The CAMCB can be used by researchers and practitioners as a framework to formulate context-specific (individual) theories of crime, such as those developed in case formulation and treatment planning. The CAMCB draws attention to the underlying psychological mechanisms of (criminal) behaviour and thereby allows for differentiation between universal processes and culturally bound manifestations of these processes. In order to achieve maximum flexibility (given the diversity of potential cultural influences) and to be transparent at the same time (which is necessary for a fair and valid decision-making process) we propose a stepwise approach:

1   Define the universal aspects and mechanisms of behaviour (e.g., motivational process and planning) which are inherited predispositions evident in all humans (Del Giudice, 2018) and use them to structure the explanation.
2   Identify core cultural traits (i.e., mindsets like interdependency as being broad knowledge networks; Oyserman, 2011) which vary across cultures and influence perception and behaviour deeply and systematically. Then, work through all universal aspects and mechanisms by specifying how they are shaped by the relevant cultural trait (e.g., interdependency).
3   Evaluate a particular behavioural outcome (e.g., specific offending) and its components according to functionality (i.e., if the underlying agency-process is impaired in any way), adaptivity (i.e., if it is appropriate with respect to the cultural context), and normativity (i.e., if it meets normative standards).

We will illustrate this process with a brief example utilising the three steps above. First, we outline the universal planning process (Crick & Dodge, 1994) which involves goal identification (Custers & Aarts, 2005; Danner et al., 2008; Kruglanski et al., 2002; Moskowitz et al., 2004) and decision-making about which action to take to meet a goal (Crick & Dodge, 1994; Fishbein & Ajzen, 2010; Heffernan & Ward, 2017). Secondly, we refer to an interdependent style of processing (compared to an independent style) as a key cultural trait that influences the universal process of planning in various ways. Markus and Kitayama (1991, 1998, 2010) introduced this trait to explain cross-cultural differences between Asian (interdependent) and Euro-American (independent) people. Broadly, independent people experience themselves as separate from others and feel a need to highlight their uniqueness. Independency is associated with autonomy, individually oriented achievement, affiliation, exhibition, and power. In contrast, interdependent people experience themselves as closely connected to others within the social context and feel the need to fulfil obligations and maintain harmony. Interdependency is associated with subordination, socially oriented achievement, patience, and nurturance. Applying these explanations to individual behaviour, differences in independence/interdependence affects universal aspects and mechanisms of behaviour (e.g., planning; Markus, 2016).

In terms of the third step, this can result in the identification of different causes of (sometimes the very same) behaviour. As Table 4.2 illustrates, offending behaviour must be explained in different ways due to cultural differences. While someone who is influenced by an independent style of processing might use criminal conduct to achieve personal goals (e.g., violence towards an associate to seek status), someone who is influenced by an interdependent style of processing might use criminal conduct as means to fulfil perceived role expectations (e.g., violence towards an associate to protect others or as a response to a threat to a group's cohesion or harmony). This suggests that it might be more useful to look at personal attitudes and personality traits for causes of crime when an independent style of processing is present, but to look more closely at social and contextual factors when an interdependent style of processing is prevalent (Dwairy, 2002).

Implications for Practice

To move from an ethnocentric approach to risk assessment and intervention in forensic psychology to a culturally-sensitive approach which mitigates biases, researchers and practitioners need to undertake a systematic process. Cultural sensitivity requires that researchers and practitioners are well-aware of the relevant cultural context(s) and that they understand how particular cultural traits influence perception, cognition, and behaviour. We suggest that *cultural competence training* might help to build up this awareness, transmit knowledge, and train competency in intercultural contexts (Sue & Sue, 2013). In order to be effective and avoid producing unwanted side effects (e.g., further discrimination), such training must also involve reflection on the role of stereotypes and potential bias in risk assessment (Shepherd & Spivak, 2021).

Table 4.2 Varying causes of crime depending on different cultural traits

Universal aspect (planning)	Cultural trait	Culturally shaped style of processing	Potential causes of crime
Goals	IND	Personal goals, desires, and approach goals	Self-centred goals (e.g., "I will benefit by dominating") in order to defend the self, cultivate desired images, or get desired outcomes to the self
	INT	Shared social goals, social demands and expectations, and avoidance goals	Social-centred goals favouring the in-group (e.g., "My group will benefit by dominating") in order to defend status as in-group member, positive group-evaluation, the reputation of the group, or gain desired outcomes to important others
Evaluating means	IND	Focus on the self and emotional consequences	Highly accessible scripts that include crime-promoting aspects, a limited alternative behavioural repertoire, positive evaluation of these responses and their outcome as benefiting the self
	INT	Focus on (important) others, social norms, and relational consequences	Highly accessible scripts that include crime-promoting aspects, social norms that limit an alternative behavioural repertoire, the positive evaluation of these responses, and the expectation of rewarding outcomes as benefitting important others

Note: Excerpt of Table 4.2 from Schmidt et al. (2021); IND = Independency; INT = Interdependency; Eid und Diener (2009), Kitayama et al. (2006), Tsai et al. (2006).

If researchers and practitioners want to acknowledge culture they need to first identify *relevant cultural traits*. The question that needs to be answered is: Which cultural trait(s) might be relevant to this behaviour? Thereby, is necessary to differentiate between a highly probable activation of a cultural trait (e.g., someone living a cultural community favouring family-orientation) and the actual activation of that trait through situational cues (e.g., collectivist family orientation during a family meeting). In multi-cultural environments the specific context in which a particular behaviour is enacted plays an even more important role. Different cultural traits might interact (Vignoles et al., 2016) and also form new hybrid identities combining cultural traits of host country and county of origin (Foroutan, 2013). When identifying cultural traits, we also have to be aware of and transparent about our limited knowledge of diverse cultural traits and the fact that any observation made is also influenced by central cultural traits of the observer himself/herself.

When there is a strong awareness of relevant cultural traits, the CAMCB can be used to *systematically identify the relevant causes of an offence* for a particular individual. For example, case formulations should be grounded in generally accepted (McMurran & Bruford, 2016) or empirically supported theories (Sturmey & McMurran, 2011), but they also need to be adapted to the relevant cultural context. Cultural adaptation is often hindered by the lack of coherence and specificity of the foundational concepts (i.e., DRF) of risk assessment tools and common theories of crime (Ward, 2016). The CAMCB, however, can provide practitioners with a template to assist culturally sensitive case formulation due to the explicit differentiation between universal processes and their culturally shaped individual realisations.

The task of *predicting further offending* can also benefit from case formulations that are built on the CAMCB. Once the culturally shaped potential causal factors are identified for the individual, they can be evaluated with respect to their stability over time and context. Thereby, the prediction of behaviour for people favouring an independent style of processing can be compared to people favouring an interdependent style, and the key differences observed can inform future practice. For example, interdependency is associated with high context-sensitivity, which is why practitioners need to clearly specify all relevant context variables when formulating predictions (Schmidt & Ward, 2020).

Having identified the potential causes of an individual's behaviour in a culturally sensitive manner (e.g., via the CAMCB), *treatment programmes* can then be directed towards these hypothesised causes. Referring to our earlier example, it may be more useful to apply programmes which focus on changing individual cognition, emotion, and behaviour when an independent style of processing is the prevalent mindset, while a more systemic (e.g., family focussed) approach could be more useful when an interdependent style of processing is preferred (Schmidt & Ward, 2020). Integrating indigenous models of behaviour, change, and treatment might also be very effective in multi-cultural settings (Strauss-Hughes et al., 2019). Using the CAMCB aligns with a strength-based resource-building approach in treatment (e.g., Good Lives

Model [GLM]; Ward & Stewart, 2003), due to the focus on the functioning of universal psychological mechanisms that are not dependent upon social norms. This positive approach in correctional services is especially important for this group of already highly stigmatised people; those who have committed offences and belong to marginalised cultures (Jones et al., 2002; Shepherd & Lewis-Fernandez, 2016).

Conclusion

In sum, the contemporary conceptualisation of DRF impedes researchers' and practitioners' ability to be culturally aware when undertaking and evaluating risk assessment practices. Due to significant theoretical problems in the way DRF are conceptualised and, and taking into account their normative nature, researchers and practitioners cannot ensure equivalent measurement in cross-cultural settings even if they would like to. As a consequence, commonly accepted DRF should not be routinely used for risk assessment and intervention planning in intercultural contexts. To do so is likely to result in flawed explanations of offending, incorrect prediction, impoverished classification systems, unjust outcomes, and ultimately poor practice.

Note

1 We will mainly focus on culture in a more narrow sense in this chapter, following the ongoing discussion in the forensic scientific community (Haag et al., 2016; Hart, 2016; Shepherd & Spivak, 2021).

References

American Psychological Association (Ed.) (2017). *Ethical principles of psychologists and code of conduct*. http://www.apa.org/ethics/code/

Andrews, D. A., & Bonta, J. (2010). *The psychology of criminal conduct*. NY, USA: Anderson Publishing.

Arsovska, J., & Verduyn, P. (2007). Globalization, conduct norms and 'culture conflict': Perceptions of violence and crime in an ethnic Albanian context. *British Journal of Criminology*, *48*(2), 226–246. 10.1093/bjc/azm068

Berry, J. W., Poortinga, Y. H., Breugelmans, S. M., Chasiotis, A., & Sam, D. L. (2011). *Cross-cultural psychology: research and applications* (3rd ed.). Cambrideg, UK: Cambridge University Press.

Bonta, J., & Andrews, D. A. (2017). *The psychology of criminal conduct* (6th ed.). NY, USA: Routledge Taylor & Francis Group.

Cohen, L., Manion, L., & Morrison, K. (2018). *Research methods in education* (8th ed.). London, UK: Routledge.

Cooke, D. J., & Michie, C. (2001). Refining the construct of psychopathy: Towards a hierarchical model. *Psychological Assessment*, *13*(2), 171–188. 10.1037/1040-3590.13.2.171

Cooke, D. J., Michie, C., Hart, S. D., & Clark, D. (2005a). Assessing psychopathy in the UK: Concerns about cross-cultural generalisability. *The British Journal of Psychiatry*, *186*, 335–341. 10.1192/bjp.186.4.335

Cooke, D. J., Michie, C., Hart, S. D., & Clark, D. (2005b). Assessing psychopathy in the UK: Concerns about cross-cultural generalisability. *The British Journal of Psychiatry, 186*(4), 335–341.

Crick, N. R., & Dodge, K. A. (1994). A review and reformulation of social information-processing mechanisms in children's social adjustment. *Psychological Bulletin, 115*(1), 74–101.

Custers, R., & Aarts, H. (2005). Positive affect as implicit motivator: On the nonconscious operation of behavioral goals. *Journal of Personality and Social Psychology, 89*(2), 129–142. 10.1037/0022-3514.89.2.129

Danner, U. N., Aarts, H., & Vries, N. K. de (2008). Habit vs. intention in the prediction of future behaviour: The role of frequency, context stability and mental accessibility of past behaviour. *British Journal of Social Psychology, 47*(Pt 2), 245–265. 10.1348/0144 66607X230876

Del Giudice, M. (2018). *Evolutionary psychopathology: A unified approach.* Oxford, UK: Oxford University Press.

Douglas, T., Pugh, J., Singh, I., Savulescu, J., & Fazel, S. (2017). Risk assessment tools in criminal justice and forensic psychiatry: The need for better data. *European Psychiatry: The Journal of the Association of European Psychiatrists, 42*, 134–137. 10.1016/j.eurpsy.2016. 12.009

Dwairy, M. (2002). Foundations of psychosocial dynamic personality theory of collective people. *Clinical Psychology Review, 22*(3), 343–360. 10.1016/S0272-7358(01)00100-3

Edens, J. F., Campbell, J. S., & Weir, J. M. (2007). Youth psychopathy and criminal recidivism: A meta-analysis of the psychopathy checklist measures. *Law and Human Behavior, 31*(1), 53–75. 10.1007/s10979-006-9019-y

Eid, M., & Diener, E. (2009). Norms for experiencing emotions in different cultures: inter- and intranational differences. Michalos, A.C., & Diener, E. *Social indicators research series. Culture and well-being, 38*, pp. 169–202. 10.1037//0022-3514.81.5.869. Netherlands: Springer.

Fishbein, M., & Ajzen, I. (2010). *Predicting and changing behavior: The reasoned action approach.* US: Psychology Press.

Foroutan, N. (2013). Hybride identitäten. In H. U. Brinkmann & H.-H. Uslucan (Eds.). *Dabeisein und Dazugehören* (pp. 85–99). Germany: Springer Fachmedien Wiesbaden. 10. 1007/978-3-531-19010-5_5

Friedman, L. M. (1990). *The republic of choice: Law, authority, and culture.* NY: Harvard University Press.

Gendreau, P., Little, T., & Goggin, C. (1996). A meta-analysis of the predictors of adult offender recidivism: What works! *Criminology, 34*(4), 575–596. 10.1111/j.1745-9125. 1996.tb01220.x

Gottfredson, S. D., & Moriarty, L. J. (2006). Statistical risk assessment: Old problems and new applications. *Crime & Delinquency, 52*(1), 178–200. 10.1177/0011128705281748

Haag, A. M., Boyes, A., Cheng, J., MacNeil, A., & Wirove, R. (2016). An introduction to the issues of cross-cultural assessment inspired by Ewert v. Canada. *Journal of Threat Assessment and Management, 3*(2), 65–75. 10.1037/tam0000067

Hanson, R. K., Babchishin, K. M., Helmus, L., & Thornton, D. (2013). Quantifying the relative risk of sex offenders: Risk ratios for Static-99R. *Sexual Abuse: A Journal of Research and Treatment, 25*(5), 482–515. 10.1177/1079063212469060

Hare, R. D. (2003). *The Hare Psychopathy Checklist-Revised.* Toronto, ON, Canada: Multi-Health Systems.

Hart, S. D. (2016). Culture and violence risk assessment: The case of Ewert v. Canada. *Journal of Threat Assessment and Management, 3*(2), 76–96. 10.1037/tam0000068

Hart, S. D., Cox, D. N., & Hare, R. D. (1995). Manual for the Hare Psychopathy Checklist: Screening Version (PCL:SV). Toronto, ON, Canada: Multi-Health Systems.

Haynes, S. N. (1992). *Models of causality in psychopathology: Toward dynamic, synthetic and nonlinear models of behavior disorders. Pergamon general psychology series: Vol. 168.* Macmillan; Maxwell Macmillan Canada.

He, J., & van de Vijver, F. (2012). Bias and equivalence in cross-cultural research. *Online Readings in Psychology and Culture, 2*(2). 10.9707/2307-0919.1111

Heffernan, R., & Ward, T. (2017). A comprehensive theory of dynamic risk and protective factors. *Aggression and Violent Behavior, 37,* 129–141. 10.1016/j.avb.2017.10.003

Jones, R., Masters, M., Griffiths, A., & Moulday, N. (2002). Culturally relevant assessment of indigenous offenders: A literature review. *Australian Psychologist, 37*(3), 187–197. 10.1080/00050060210001706866

Kitayama, S., Mesquita, B., & Karasawa, M. (2006). Cultural affordances and emotional experience: Socially engaging and disengaging emotions in Japan and the United States. *Journal of Personality and Social Psychology, 91*(5), 890–903. 10.1037/0022-3514.91.5.890

Kitayama, S., Park, H., Sevincer, A. T., Karasawa, M., & Uskul, A. K. (2009). A cultural task analysis of implicit independence: Comparing North America, Western Europe, and East Asia. *Journal of Personality and Social Psychology, 97*(2), 236–255. 10.1037/a0015999

Kreis, M. K. F., & Cooke, D. J. (2011). Capturing the psychopathic female: A prototypicality analysis of the comprehensive assessment of psychopathic personality (CAPP) across gender. *Behavioral Sciences & the Law, 29*(5), 634–648. 10.1002/bsl.1003

Kruglanski, A. W., Shah, J. Y., Fishbach, A., Friedman, R., Chun, W. Y., & Sleeth-Keppler, D. (2002). A theory of goal systems. In *Advances in experimental social psychology* (Vol. 34, pp. 331–378). Cambridge MA, US: Elsevier. 10.1016/S0065-2601(02)80008-9

Leistico, A.-M. R., Salekin, R. T., DeCoster, J., & Rogers, R. (2008). A large-scale meta-analysis relating the hare measures of psychopathy to antisocial conduct. *Law and Human Behavior, 32*(1), 28–45. 10.1007/s10979-007-9096-6

Loya, F., Reddy, R., & Hinshaw, S. P. (2010). Mental illness stigma as a mediator of differences in Caucasian and South Asian college students' attitudes toward psychological counseling. *Journal of Counseling Psychology, 57*(4), 484–490. 10.1037/a0021113

Maddux, W., Martin, A., Sinaceur, M., & Kitayama, S. (2011). *In the middle between east and west: Implicit cultural orientations in Saudi Arabia.* Paper Presented at the 24rd Annual International Association of Conflict Management Conference Istanbul, Turkey. July 3 –6, 2011.

Markus, H. R. (2016). What moves people to action? Culture and motivation. *Current Opinion in Psychology, 8,* 161–166. 10.1016/j.copsyc.2015.10.028

Markus, H. R., & Kitayama, S. (1991). Culture and the self: Implications for cognition, emotion, and motivation. *Psychological Review, 98*(2), 224–253.

Markus, H. R., & Kitayama, S. (1998). The cultural psychology of personality. *Journal of Cross-Cultural Psychology, 29*(1), 63–87. 10.1177/0022022198291004

Markus, H. R., & Kitayama, S. (2010). Cultures and selves: A cycle of mutual constitution. *Perspectives on Psychological Science: A Journal of the Association for Psychological Science, 5*(4), 420–430. 10.1177/1745691610375557

Martel, J., Brassard, R., & Jaccoud, M. (2011). When two worlds collide: Aboriginal risk management in Canadian corrections. *British Journal of Criminology, 51*(2), 235–255. 10.1093/bjc/azr003

McMurran, M., & Bruford, S. (2016). Case formulation quality checklist: A revision based upon clinicians' views. *The Journal of Forensic Practice, 18*(1), 31–38. 10.1108/JFP-05-2015-0027

Minhas, R., & Walsh, D. (2018). Influence of racial stereotypes on investigative decision-making in criminal investigations: A qualitative comparative analysis. *Cogent Social Sciences*, *4*(1), 1538588. 10.1080/23311886.2018.1538588

Moskowitz, G. B., Li, P., & Kirk, E. R. (2004). The implicit volition model: On the pre-conscious regulation of temporarily adopted goals. In *Advances in experimental social psychology* (Vol. 36, pp. 317–413). Cambriudge MA, US: Elsevier. 10.1016/S0065-2601(04)36006-5

Onifade, E., Davidson, W., & Campbell, C. (2009). Risk assessment: The predictive validity of the youth level of service case management inventory with African Americans and girls. *Journal of Ethnicity in Criminal Justice*, *7*(3), 205–221. 10.1080/15377930903143544

Oyserman, D. (2011). Culture as situated cognition: Cultural mindsets, cultural fluency, and meaning making. *European Review of Social Psychology*, *22*(1), 164–214. 10.1080/10463283.2011.627187

Pusch, N., & Holtfreter, K. (2018). Gender and risk assessment in juvenile offenders: A meta-analysis. *Criminal Justice and Behavior*, *45*(1), 56–81. 10.1177/0093854817721720

Reisig, M. D., Holtfreter, K., & Morash, M. (2006). Assessing recidivism risk across female pathways to crime. *Justice Quarterly*, *23*(3), 384–405. 10.1080/07418820600869152

Schlager, M. D., & Simourd, D. J. (2007). Validity of the Level of Service Inventory-Revised (LSI-R) among African American and Hispanic male offenders. *Criminal Justice and Behavior*, *34*(4), 545–554. 10.1177/0093854806296039

Schmidt, S., Bliesener, T., & van der Meer, E. (2019). Risk and protective factors of delinquency that are sensitive to migration and culture. *Psychology, Crime & Law*, *18*(2), 1–27. 10.1080/1068316X.2019.1597088

Schmidt, S., Heffernan, R., & Ward, T. (2020). Why we cannot explain cross-cultural differences in risk assessment. *Aggression and Violent Behavior*, *50*, 101346. 10.1016/j.avb.2019.101346

Schmidt, S., Heffernan, R., & Ward, T. (2021). The cultural agency-model of criminal behavior. *Aggression and Violent Behavior*, *58*(1), 101554. 10.1016/j.avb.2021.101554

Schmidt, S., van der Meer, E., Tydecks, S., & Bliesener, T. (2018). How culture and migration affect risk assessment. *The European Journal of Psychology Applied to Legal Context*, 1–14. 10.5093/ejpalc2018a7

Schmidt, S., & Ward, T. (2020). Delinquenz kultursensibel erklären – ein theoretisches Rahmenmodell. *Forensische Psychiatrie, Psychologie, Kriminologie*, *30*, 47. 10.1007/s11757-020-00638-5

Shariat, S. V., Assadi, S. M., Noroozian, M., Pakravannejad, M., Yahyazadeh, O., Aghayan, S., Michie, C., & Cooke, D. (2010). Psychopathy in Iran: A cross-cultural study. *Journal of Personality Disorders*, *24*(5), 676–691. 10.1521/pedi.2010.24.5.676

Shepherd, S. M. (2015a). Criminal engagement and Australian culturally and linguisti-cally diverse populations: Challenges and implications for forensic risk assessment. *Psychiatry, Psychology and Law*, 1–19. 10.1080/13218719.2015.1053164

Shepherd, S. M. (2015b). Finding color in conformity: A commentary on culturally specific risk factors for violence in Australia. *International Journal of Offender Therapy and Comparative Criminology*, *59*(12), 1297–1307. 10.1177/0306624X14540492

Shepherd, S. M., & Lewis-Fernandez, R. (2016). Forensic risk assessment and cultural diversity: Contemporary challenges and future directions. *Psychology, Public Policy, and Law*, *22*(4), 427–438. 10.1037/law0000102

Shepherd, S. M., Singh, J. P., & Fullam, R. (2015). Does the youth level of service/case management inventory generalize across ethnicity? *International Journal of Forensic Mental Health*, *14*(3), 193–204. 10.1080/14999013.2015.1086450

Shepherd, S. M., & Spivak, B. L. (2021). Finding colour in conformity part II – reflections on structured professional judgement and cross-cultural risk assessment. *International Journal of Offender Therapy and Comparative Criminology*, *65*(1), 92–99. 10.1177/0306624X20928025

Singh, J. P., Grann, M., & Fazel, S. (2011). A comparative study of violence risk assessment tools: A systematic review and metaregression analysis of 68 studies involving 25,980 participants. *Clinical Psychology Review*, *31*(3), 499–513. 10.1016/j.cpr.2010.11.009

Strauss-Hughes, A., Heffernan, R., & Ward, T. (2019). A cultural–ecological perspective on agency and offending behaviour. *Psychiatry, Psychology and Law*, *39*(2), 1–21. 10.1080/13218719.2019.1644250

Sturmey, P., & McMurran, M. (Eds.) (2011). *Wiley series in forensic clinical psychology. Forensic case formulation*. Chichester, UK: Wiley-Blackwell. http://public.eblib.com/choice/publicfullrecord.aspx?p=819263

Sue, D. W., & Sue, D. (2013). *Counseling the culturally diverse: Theory and practice* (6th ed.). Chichester, UK: Wiley.

Tsai, J. L., Knutson, B., & Fung, H. H. (2006). Cultural variation in affect valuation. *Journal of Personality and Social Psychology*, *90*(2), 288–307. 10.1037/0022-3514.90.2.288.

van de Vijver, F., & Leung, K. (2011). Equivalence and bias: A review of concepts, models, and data analytic procedures. In D. R. Matsumoto & Fons J. R. van de Vijver (Eds.). *Culture and psychology. Cross-cultural research methods in psychology* (pp. 17–45). Cambridge, UK: Cambridge University Press.

van de Vijver, F., & Rothmann, S. (2004). Assessment in multicultural groups: The South African case. *SA Journal of Industrial Psychology*, *30*(4). 10.4102/sajip.v30i4.169

van de Vijver, F., & Tanzer, N. K. (2004). Bias and equivalence in cross-cultural assessment: An overview. *Revue Européenne De Psychologie Appliquée/European Review of Applied Psychology*, *54*(2), 119–135. 10.1016/j.erap.2003.12.004

Veen, V. C., Stevens, G. W. J. M., Andershed, H., Raaijmakers, Q. A. W., Doreleijers, T. A. H., & Vollebergh, W. A. M. (2011). Cross-ethnic generalizability of the three-factor model of psychopathy: The youth psychopathic traits inventory in an incarcerated sample of native Dutch and Moroccan immigrant boys. *International Journal of Law and Psychiatry*, *34*(2), 127–130. 10.1016/j.ijlp.2011.02.007

Via, B., Dezember, A., & Taxman, F. S. (2016). Exploring how to measure crimenogenic needs: Five instruments and no real answers. In F. S. Taxman (Ed.). *The ASC division on corrections & sentencing handbook series. Handbook on risk and need assessment: Theory and practice* (pp. 312–330). Australia: Taylor and Francis.

Vignoles, V. L., Owe, E., Becker, M., Smith, P. B., Easterbrook, M. J., Brown, R., González, R., Didier, N., Carrasco, D., Cadena, M. P., Lay, S., Schwartz, S. J., Des Rosiers, S. E., Villamar, J. A., Gavreliuc, A., Zinkeng, M., Kreuzbauer, R., Baguma, P., Martin, M., …, Bond, M. H. (2016). Beyond the 'east-west' dichotomy: Global variation in cultural models of selfhood. *Journal of Experimental Psychology. General*, *145*(8), 966–1000. 10.1037/xge0000175

Ward, T. (2016). Dynamic risk factors: Scientific kinds or predictive constructs. *Psychology, Crime & Law*, *22*(1–2), 2–16. 10.1080/1068316X.2015.1109094

Ward, T., & Fortune, C.-A. (2016). From dynamic risk factors to causal processes: A methodological framework. *Psychology, Crime & Law*, *22*(1–2), 190–202. 10.1080/1068316X.2015.1117080

Ward, T., & Heffernan, R. (2017). The role of values in forensic and correctional rehabilitation. *Aggression and Violent Behavior*, *37*, 42–51. 10.1016/j.avb.2017.09.002

Ward, T., & Stewart, C. A. (2003). The treatment of sex offenders: Risk management and good lives. *Professional Psychology: Research and Practice, 34*(4), 353–360. 10.1037/0735-7028. 34.4.353

Wilson, H. A., & Gutierrez, L. (2014). Does one size fit all? A meta-analysis examining the predictive ability of the Level of Service Inventory (LSI) with aboriginal offenders. *Criminal Justice and Behavior, 41*(2), 196–219. 10.1177/0093854813500958

5   The Validity of Reconviction as a Proxy Measure for Re-offending: Interpreting Risk Measures and Research in the Light of False Convictions and Detection and Conviction Evasion Skills (DACES) and Processes

Lawrence Jones, Glenda Liell, and Martin Fisher

Introduction

Jacobs and Wallach (2021) wrote: "Researchers and practitioners are often inclined to conflate constructs and their operationalisations – i.e., to collapse the distinction between them … . collapsing these distinctions elides the space in which fairness-related harms are most often introduced" (p. 10); this chapter is an attempt to try and explore some of the issues raised by this observation. The whole project of risk assessment and treatment evaluation pivots on the assumption of reconviction and conviction being a valid measure of return-to-offending (RTO). Any bias in this as a measure of RTO inevitably influences the inferences we can make about the constructs used to evaluate reconviction or conviction. Understanding the processes linked with detection and conviction evasion skills and processes, DACES (see Figure 5.1), helps us to better interpret findings that are based on reconviction as an operationalisation of RTO. A number of consequences of this bias linked to reconviction and conviction will be outlined. In particular, the possibility that risk assessments will be systematically biased by racism and white privilege will also be considered.

The construct validity of the concept of risk as measured by conviction histories will be explored. The work of Monahan et al. (2001) has examined this issue in the context of forensic psychiatric patients, but here we argue that in terms of how we assess for future risk, the issues are far wider. We are referring to the issue of bias here in the context that Jensen (1980) describes as predictive test bias. That is within the groups to which the test/assessment is being applied, there is a difference in the regression equation between the test and its criterion. Simply arguing that differing cultures, standardisation samples or egalitarianism bias tests is fallacious; it is the validity of the measure in the first place that is the problem, not the diversity in the test takers (Kline, 2000).

DOI: 10.4324/9781003230977-6

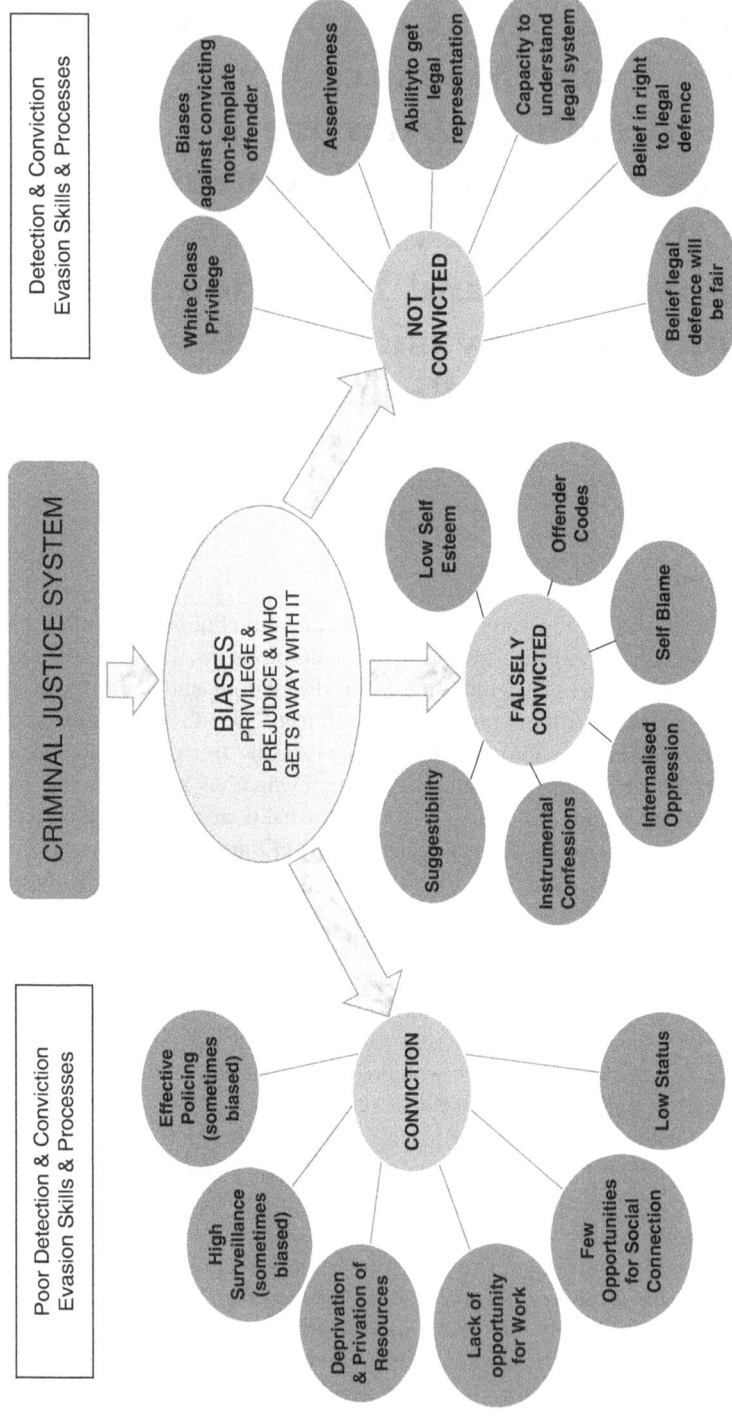

Figure 5.1 Diagram illustrating the interface between the criminal justice system, biases and Detection and Conviction Evasion Skills (DACES).

This chapter starts with an exploration of the nature of detection and conviction vulnerability, evasion skills, and contextual influences on these. In other words, how has the person we are working with ended up here? A more nuanced understanding of what reconviction actually means will be suggested by describing the different ways in which offending does not result in a conviction, and *not* offending can result in a false conviction, i.e., developing a measurement model (Jacobs & Wllach, 2021). This will be explained by considering: reporting rates, recording rates by the police, charging rates, and conviction rates. We will also explore the role of systemic social and interpersonal dynamics, as well as the skills and propensities of the individual in relation to the false positives/negatives and true positives/negatives of convictions.

We conclude with an examination of the practical implications of this for clinical practice, assessing dynamic risk and safety issues, and making sense of research that has used reconviction as a measure of reoffending. A new model for conceptualising individual and social detection and conviction evasion, and the various kinds of bias influencing whether or not a crime committed results in a conviction will also be outlined, as well as suggestions for future research and development.

The Nature of Detection and Conviction Vulnerability, Evasion Skills, and Contextual Influences on These

Construct Validity and the Concept of Risk

Messick (1995) highlighted the importance of looking at the consequences of decisions based on the use of a particular approach to measuring a construct as a central aspect of assessing construct validity. We argue that reconviction as a measure, is an underspecification of the construct of RTO. Many people who offend do not get convicted, and conversely, some people who get convicted have not offended. Moreover, as Mayson (2019) and Woldgabreal et al. (2020) point out there are systemic/structural processes that bias who actually gets caught for offending and who doesn't. Table 5.1 illustrates the true positives and negatives for offending or not offending, highlighting the biases attached to these.

Table 5.1 Type 1 and type 2 errors noted

	Detected and convicted	*Not detected or convicted*
Offended	Correctly convicted (true positive); biased in terms of who gets investigated and caught and who doesn't, e.g., privilege and prejudice	Got away with it, false acquittal (false negative); DACES Privilege and prejudice at play in who manages to "get away with" offending.
Didn't offend	Falsely convicted (false positive); lack of self advocacy skills and systemic and structural processes impacting on false convictions – shaped by privilege and prejudice	Didn't do it and correctly not convicted (true negative)

Each of the cells in Table 5.2 can be explored in terms of both the individual's skills and inclinations as well as the systemic/structural factors that contributed to the outcome – following Monohans et al. (2001) recommendation that we follow an interactional approach to risk. Analysed in this way, there are eight different types of causal pathway to an outcome of "has re-offended or not" each with a range of sources of bias demonstrated in Table 5.2.

It is important to emphasise that what we are looking at here is the construct validity of reconviction as a measure of re-offending. Not to include contextual interaction factors would amount to construct underspecification. Clinically what we are interested in is identifying what factors, if left unchanged, can contribute to the chances of an individual returning to offending.

Understanding the causal processes of each of the pathways in each of the cells in Table 5.2 is critical to interpreting any measurement that uses reconviction as an outcome. Dynamic risk factors, that correlate with reconviction, can be theoretically associated with any of these. For example, impulsivity would likely be linked to poor conviction avoidance skills.

The potential harm brought about by neglecting to consider systemic/structural factors and DACESs when interpreting the use of reconviction as a measure of RTO, will be examined within the framework offered by Messick (as suggested by Sizmur, 2008) for evaluating construct validity. Messick argues that validity should considered both in terms of the impact on the psychometric properties (reliability/validity etc.), and what the consequences and meaning could be of using a particular measure, in this case thinking about the impact of DACES. The consequences are shown in Table 5.3 in terms of both score interpretation and score usage.

What are the consequences of being judged to be a "high risk" as opposed to a "low risk" if one is not either of these in reality – if DACES and systemic biases had been accounted for? Or, perhaps more pertinently if the degree of certainty (in terms of relative outcomes or empirical bases) we can offer to support the judgement is unclear.

The importance of assessing systemic/structural bias and DACES when using measures based on reconviction as a measure of RTO is a natural consequence of this.

Bias in Identification of True Positives

Systemic: Social and Interpersonal Dynamics

If an individual is released into a context where there is a higher than average level of either statutory or societal surveillance/monitoring (e.g., the mandated registration of those convicted of sexual offences in Engand and Wales), then it might be expected that the clear up rate in that context would be higher than that obtained in the context where the risk assessment instrument was developed. Higher levels of surveillance can be linked with a range of factors.

Table 5.2 Examples of possible biases underpinning type 1 and type 2 errors

	True positive	False positive	True negative	False negative
Contextual/systemic social and interpersonal dynamics	High surveillance (potentially biased in different ways), effective policing (but possibly focussing more on one specific group than another), deprivation and privation of key resources, opportunity for work, social connection, status	Racism, sexism, homophobia, coercive policing obtaining false confessions, ineffective policing	Effective policing (potentially applied unevenly to different groups), availability of evidence	White and class privilege, biases against charging and convicting people who don't manage to resemble "template" of being "an offender" (Larcombe, 2012)
Intrapersonal, e.g., skills and propensities of individual	Willingness to admit and confess poor detection and conviction avoidance skills	Suggestiblity, self-blaming, instrumental "confessions", internalised oppression, low self-esteem offender codes (taking the blame for others)	Assertiveness, ability to get legal representation, capacity to understand legal system (i.e., neurodiversity impact) and use it effectively to prevent false positives, belief in the right to a legal defence and that the legal system will be fair	Detection and conviction evasion skills, values, and propensities (e.g., scripts and implicit theories)

Table 5.3 Interactions between evidential and consequential outcomes

	Score interpretation	*Score use*
Evidential basis	Construct validity	Construct validity + relevance/utility
Consequential basis	Value implications	Social consequences

Source: Adapted by Sizmur, 2008 from Messick, 1989, p. 20.

Note: The term "score" has been substituted for "test" in this adaptation.

This is critically important in the analysis of re-offending studies using re-conviction as an outcome. If following, or in association with, an intervention addressing offending behaviour a systemic change is brought in that impacts on levels of surveillance, or levels of intelligence in relation to a particular category of offender, then we might expect some change in reconviction rates that are not due to the intervention. An example of this has been the introduction of the sex offender register and the use of multi-agency public protection arrangements (MAPPAs) panels for people who have offended sexually. If intelligence and consultation between police and workers with access to an understanding of risk assessments are introduced, then the level of surveillance for that offender will be increased and this would lead to a higher rate of conviction. This could look as if it was the intervention that caused an apparent deterioration but in fact it is the individual becoming more detectable as a consequence of a change in practice compared to when the registers and MAPPA panels were not in existence (for a review see Vess et al., 2014).

Simply having been convicted before should theoretically mean that the individual is "on the police radar" and therefore more susceptible to being detected if they offend again. They are perhaps less likely to be in the majority group of undetected offences and more likely to be in the minority group of detected offences. Whilst in theory the more prolific an offender is the more likely they are to be detected, differing levels of resource are allocated to different types of offence, which may also be subject to regional variation. Detection rates in the United Kingdom are referred to as "cleared up" crimes by the police – that is they are either sanction or non-sanction detections. Sanction detection involves a formal sanction. The detection rates in 2009/10, for example were highest for drugs offences, which can be explained by the ability to issue a warning for possession without a visit to a police station (Ogunbur & Taylor, 2010).

Biases in the allocation of resources to detection and conviction will also be relevant to this. If the police only stop and search people of colour then there will be an over-representation of people of colour in the criminal justice system, not because people of colour are more risky but because they have been singled out for detection (Mayson, 2019). Privilege is then at play in risk assessments where low scores can be due to people not having been detected because they haven't been sought out as much by the police at the time the data set used to validate the risk assessment was obtained. This bias cannot be offset by using different groups to establish norms because it is "baked in" to the outcome measure (see Mayson, 2019).

True positives, if conceptualised as having a systemic component, should also be thought of as being impacted on by contextual deprivation and privation of resources. That is, the context is criminogenic. Releasing an individual into a context where they are exposed to racism, homophobia, poverty, stigma, social ostracism, unemployment, lack of opportunity for social connection (Social Exclusion Unit Report, 2002) or any other kinds of resource deprivation will increase the risk of offending as a way of meeting basic needs (Jones, 2022). To attribute the eventual re-offending, if it happens, to the individual alone would be to miss-construe or underspecify the causal factors driving the behaviour. There is a danger of over valourising or reifying psychological processes in specifying a valid causal model, at the expense of social structural factors when considering risk. Arguably, risk assessment processes currently do not necessarily consider the aforementioned systemic components – much like some years ago we did not consider protective factors as part of formulation.

Risk factors then cannot be conceptualised without conceptualising, at the same time, the contexts in which the propensity is likely to be activated. If a person of colour is released into an abusive and racist context where there are few resources to support them, and little opportunity for social connection, or police are stopping and searching them in a disproportionate manner, then risk factors such as antisocial attitudes or mixing with antisocial peers could become more salient.

Intrapersonal: Skills and Propensities of the Individual

Not being able or willing to use detection and conviction evasion skills is an example of an intrapersonal factor that could contribute to an individual being convicted. If it is hard to detect who has committed an offence of a particular kind, or if it is hard to obtain a conviction if an offence that has been committed, then not having detection and conviction evasion skills could well lead to an individual having a greater likelihood of being caught and convicted for crimes they have committed.

In some ways this is not a problem, in that we generally want people who have committed offences to be caught for them. However, when it comes to inter-preting reconviction as a measure of re-offending it becomes problematic in that reconviction is not measuring all offending, it is only measuring offending by people who don't have detection evasion skills, low IQ, values that are congruent with disclosing, and maybe also suggestible people. Young age and low IQ are associated with poor DACES (Jones, 2013); Hanson and Wallace-Carpetta (2000) write:

> The … similarity of risk predictors for male batterers and general offenders … could be attributed to a common outcome criterion (arrest). … risk factors, such as young age and low verbal IQ, could be substantially related to the probability of getting caught and processed by the criminal justice system. (p. 75)

How are these factors linked to getting caught?

> Young age could be related to lack of experience of the criminal justice system (CJS) and thus absence of DES [Detection Evasion Skills]. Young age could be related to a reduced detection evasion context; that is, younger people may be exposed to higher levels of supervision and older people to more opportunities to offend without being detected.
>
> (Jones, 2010, p. 75)

Similar processes could also be at play with Low IQ.

Gudjohnson (e.g., 2017) has identified suggestibility as being associated with false confessions, but this is may also be associated with an increased tendency to make true confessions, and hence the increased likelihood of being convicted for offences committed. Levels of suggestibility and the likelihood of a false or true confession are likely linked to cognitive capacity or neurodiverse presentations (e.g., Trowbridge, 2003), particularly in the context of coercive interrogations (Chapman, 2013). Whilst not necessarily common, it is possible to have people with particularly strong religious beliefs being opposed to *not* telling the truth (Stavrova & Siegers, 2014), or people who have feelings of guilt and want to be punished. Whilst previous research has failed to conclude that guilty people wish to suffer or be punished (Baumeister et al., 1994), there may be a link between guilt and self-harm (Inbar et al., 2013). Individuals who believe strongly in the need to be truthful or feel they should be punished may therefore have a greater chance of being detected and convicted as a consequence of their actions or decisions around this. Should we consider the risk of these individuals in the same way as the rest of the validation sample for the risk assessment instrument? Or should we think about their uniqueness.

Bias in Identification of False Negatives

The "Dark Figure"

Crime survey data suggests that the majority of offending does not get reported. Typically in crime surveys a random sample of people are contacted by telephone and interviewed about their experience of crime over a specified period. The "dark figure of crime" refers to the difference in criminal acts as measured by criminal justice system records and offenders' self-reported acts (Biderman & Reiss, 1967) or estimates of the true rate of offending from sources such as crime surveys.

Figure 5.2 illustrates the various stages at which an offence that has been committed can drop out of the process whereby it gets recorded and convicted as an offence (Figure 5.3).

In looking at the Crime Survey for England and Wales data it is almost always estimated that about 40% of crime gets reported to the police in some way and

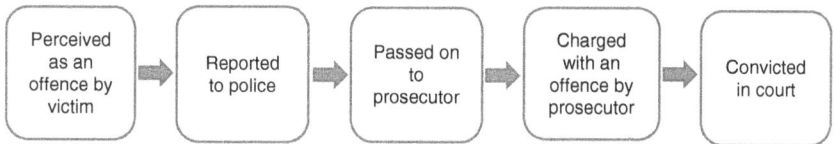

Figure 5.2 Crime survey data information flows.

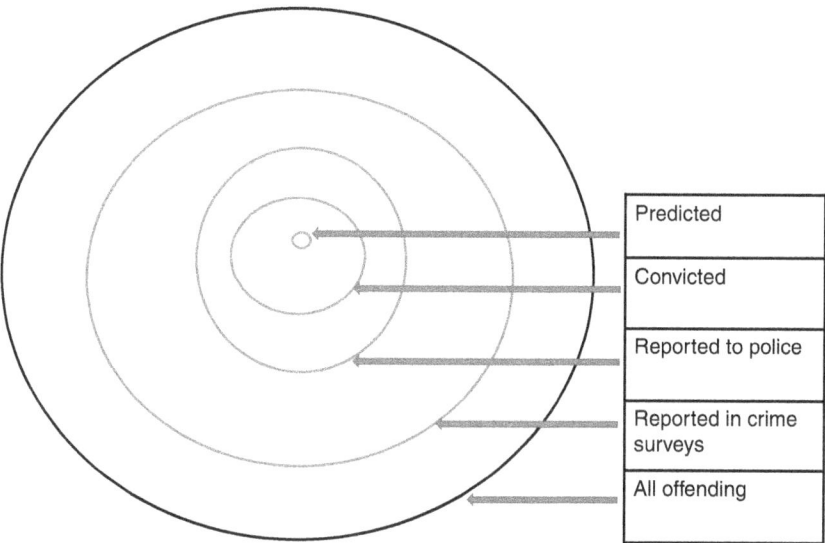

Figure 5.3 Diagram illustrating difference between operationalisation of crime by using reconviction and actual offending.

that the "dark figure" is about 60%. Some offences, for example, burglaries and car thefts are reported more often (Table 5.4), and are more likely therefore to constitute a greater proportion of recorded crime. The "dark figure" of crime also varies between crime types (Gove et al., 1985; Tarling & Morris, 2010).

Buil-Gil et al. (2020) in a review of the evidence for factors leading to crime being reported found that:

> … rates are larger for female victims than males, and elderly citizens are more likely to report crimes than young people … Victims from suburban areasreport crimes less frequently than urban and rural residents and the neighbourhoods' economic disadvantage, concentration of immigrants andsocial cohesion affect crime reporting rates … (p. 365)

Table 5.4 Contextual factors impacting on DACESs

Victim perception of offending

An offence needs to be recognised and seen as an offence in order to be reported to the police. Arguably, his requires a number of things.

1 Noticing that the offence has taken place.
2 Believing that the activity encountered was "wrong" in some way.
3 Recognising the severity of the activity.
4 Wanting the perpetrator to be punished. Understanding or agreeing with the idea that reporting the offence is important as a deterrent/preventative measure against future offending against them or against others.

Victim not disclosing to the police

If a victim recognises that they have been offended against then the next step is for them to disclose to the police. A number of factors can lead to non-disclosure:

1 Fear of reprisals or revenge from perpetrator or the perpetrators social network can lead to victims not disclosing.
2 If the victim event occurred in the context of the victim breaking the law then the victim may fear self-incrimination if they disclose.
3 Victims believe that the authority will take little if any action as their beliefs in the ability of the police to act is undermined.

Other factors also impact on victim's willingness to report offences (Posick & Singleton, 2014), for example,

1 Lower rates of reporting by youth and minorities – they have previously experienced what they perceive to be unfair police enforcement activities, leading them to distrust the police.
2 Police are more likely to be called when the injuries are serious.
3 More intense responses of emotional distress are linked to calling the Police – but these victims are less likely to be satisfied with the Police's response. Levels of satisfaction increase however when confidence in the police was already high.

Police not prosecuting effectively

This process may be independent of the individual person who has offended. Gould et al. (2021) hypothesise and review a set of processes that can result in failure to prosecute or "falsely acquit":

1 Flawed police investigations
2 Forensic error
3 Official misconduct
4 Errors in charging
5 Prosecutor biases
6 Competence of prosecutors victim/witness
7 Cooperation victim/witness
8 Credibility

Gould et al. (2021) point out that many of the processes that result in false convictions also result in false acquittals. Whether the biases are the same is not clear however.

Level of Surveillance

People who have previously offended are likely to be monitored and suspected, and therefore charged and convicted, more often than those who haven't. Therefore, a proportion of the variance in the number of previous convictions which contribute to the prediction of reconviction is attributable to systemic factors.

It is, for example, conceivable that one of the reasons that people who are "low risk" become "worse" (e.g., Lowenkamp & Latessa, 2004) if engaging in therapy is that they are subjected to a higher level – quantitatively or qualitatively – of surveillance and are therefore detected and convicted more often than those who are not.

Taylor (1999) points out that burglary is a good predictor of reconviction partly because the police target people with previous convictions. This is likely to be the case for other kinds of offending too. Indeed Sizmur (2008) suggests that the lack of specificity of many risk assessment instruments (e.g., Coid et al., 2013, who found that many of risk assessments seem to be as good at predicting offending generally as they are at predicting specific offences), could reflect this process whereby predictive factors are putative measures of the extent to which the individual is on the police's radar, not of specific propensities to offend in particular ways.

An illustrative example of this in interpreting studies of treatment efficacy using reconviction as an outcome measure is that a possible explanation for interventions apparently making people worse is that the mere act of engaging in a therapeutic intervention can mean that the system, and more specifically the police, is/are more knowledgeable about the areas of risk presented by the individual. The introduction of MAPPA panels in the United Kingdom has meant that for "high risk" offenders surveillance and monitoring of post release behaviour has been more informed and focussed in a manner that is influenced by knowledge of the individual gained in the context of therapy.

Innocent People Wrongly Convicted: False Positives

Burnham (2017), in the United States, reviewed the data on false convictions for rape which emerged after the introduction of DNA testing that allowed convicted individuals to contest their convictions in the United States, and highlighted the disproportionate representation of people of colour in the wrongful convictions population. For homicides and sexual assaults, in 5% of the cases DNA evidence didn't support the conviction. She goes on to point out that "whereas in 2011 black men were about 40–50% of the prison population, they were about 70% of the exonerated population"(Smith & Hattery, 2011). She also highlights the bias in those wrongfully convicted of rape where 84% of exonerated men were people of colour charged with rape or murder of a white woman (Smith & Hattery, 2011).

It is estimated that 30–35% of the incarcerated population of people who have committed sexual offences deny that they have committed an offence (e.g., Hood et al., 2002; Kennedy & Grubin, 1992). If we use the DNA data as a very rough estimate of false positives (5%) this suggests that 1 in 6 or 7 of people who deny their offence (assuming that all innocent offenders deny the offences they have been convicted for) are actually telling the truth – at least prior to the introduction of DNA testing in the investigative process.

The main reasons for the miscarriage of justice in these cases were identified by Burnham (2017) as being cross-racial misidentifications, false confessions "and ingrained racial attitudes of decision-makers, both white and black (Kang et al., 2012; Smith et al., 2015), from the police to the appellate court judges [that] predispose them to find the accused culpable" (p. 397).

Interpreting Research into Interventions Using Reconviction Rates as a Measure of Efficacy

A key challenge to the argument that the difference in reconviction rates between a control or comparison group and an intervention group is that the intervention has resulted in an increase or decrease in conviction rates that is not due to a change in offending. The individual may move into the group of individuals who offend but do not get convicted, or do not offend and do get convicted as a consequence of changes in DACES or changes in contextual processes such as surveillance linked with the intervention.

Jones (2013) asked an audience of forensic psychologists how likely it is that: learning to be less impulsive, avoiding contact with other offenders, problem solving skills, good lives planning, hearing accounts of others offending, emotional regulation, victim "mentalizing" skills (all putative treatment targets) could increase DACES? The response from the audience confirmed that each of these intervention strategies, according to the practitioners in the audience, could, in theory, significantly impact on increasing DACES.

In exploring the problem of reconviction as a measure of RTO Jones (2004) wrote:

> It is possible to have interventions resulting in an apparent reduction in offending behaviour (with the treated group being reconvicted far lesscompared to either what was expected from the actuarially assessed probability of being reconvicted or to the untreated group), but which in reality have not changed offending behaviour at all. An example might be a thinking skills intervention. If the treated individualbecame more adept at thinking about creative detection evasion strategies or effective prosecution evasion strategiesand developed the self-restraint not to offend in an impulsive way, the reconviction rates might plummet whereas the actual offending could remain unchanged or even increase. Alternatively, an intervention could have the effect of increasing reconviction rates and this being a desirable outcome if the treatment graduates go on to hand themselves in to the police more readily, perhaps as a self-regulatory relapse prevention strategy to prevent an escalation in offending. Or perhapsthe intervention fostered honesty and a genuine concern about being lawful which lead to disclosure to police of offences that the individual previously would not have disclosed. (p. 36)

In order to attribute changes in reconviction rates, for the better or for worse, to the impact of an intervention on RTO it is important to establish the following:

1 The difference in reconviction rates between the comparison group and the intervention group is not due to intervention impacting on

   a The individuals willingness or unwillingness to conceal their offending in the context of detection and conviction processes
   b The individuals detection and conviction evasion skills being improved or depleted by the intervention

2 The difference in reconviction rates between the comparison group and the intervention group is not due to a change of surveillance – or some other significant systemic process – brought about by increased knowledge of the individual deriving from the intervention, then informing police resulting in an increased chance of conviction.

Potential Impact of Therapeutic Interventions on DACES

Some people, in the authors' clinical experience, have deliberately either handed themselves in to the police for an offence they had committed, or committed another lesser offence (e.g., putting a brick through a window) in order to get themselves into a situation – custody – where they could not offend in a serious way (and indeed where they felt safe). These individuals wanted to stop themselves from seriously offending after having worked on the ways they had previously harmed others, and building up a commitment to stop hurting people. This illustrates the way in which treatment can potentially increase reconviction rates but this still being a desirable outcome.

Some interventions shape up the skill of confessing and taking responsibility – e.g., in a therapeutic community where the peer group encourage owning responsibility and being able to reflect on the processes leading up to problematic or harmful behaviour. If these interventions had been evaluated using reconviction for any offence as an outcome – and had been effective – it would probably look as if the individual had been made worse by the therapy, when in fact the therapy had had a potentially positive impact (see also Jones, 2004). We should also consider therefore, the potential for "thinking skills" developed in treatment being used in decisions to re-offend – but perhaps in a different way and with different consequences (which could include less harm caused).

Cultures That Prevent or Inhibit Offence Disclosure

"Turning a blind eye" to offending behaviour is a significant feature of social responses to crime. The assumption that crime gets reported to the police is flawed. Crime surveys, as discussed earlier, typically indicated that a significant amount of offending isn't taken to the police. Indeed a significant amount could not be reported to crime survey researchers also. This kind of social response is more common in cultures where "grassing" or "snitching" are seen as antisocial and frowned on for many types of offending.

Prison cultures are an example of this kind of culture. They are described as "universities of crime" (Tremblay et al., 2018) because often individuals learn from each other ways in which they can commit offences more effectively without getting caught. Some of this learning is direct, and some is through seeing and hearing others offending or hearing about offences that others have committed (Jones, 2007).

There are also cultures where culpability is seen differently; where there is a reluctance to report crime and consequently people do not build up a criminal record if they offend. Examples of this are mental health settings, some kinds of response to female offending – where they are seen through a distorting stereotype of women as not offending – and some kinds of response to people with intellectual disabilities or neurodiversity, where the offending is seen as "part of the condition" and not something they should be held accountable for. Following Larcome's model (2012) this is an example of people not fitting the "template" of an offender.

Comparing Clinical Judgement with Actuarial Modelling Is Comparing Apples and Oranges

We have so far argued that what is being predicted by actuarial risk assessment is different from what is being predicted by clinical judgement. If clinical assessment is assessing propensity to offend and actuarial assessment is predicting reconviction, and much offending doesn't result in a conviction, then it is likely that clinicians will make predictions of re-offending when algorithms would not predict reconviction. The assumption here would be that re-offending rates are much higher than reconviction rates.

Clinical judgement should consistently obtain a high number of apparent "false positives" when using conviction as an outcome; because it should formulate and therefore predict RTO, not reconviction. If RTO rates are substantially higher than reconviction rates, then the predicted rate arrived at through case formulation and clinical judgement will be higher than the obtained reconviction rate. When comparisons are made between clinical judgement and actuarial modelling this is indeed what is found; typically comparisons between clinical judgement and actuarial predictions identify clinical judgement as resulting in a higher number of "false positives" (e.g., Hood et al., 2002; Mossman, 1994).

It is important to highlight however that this is *not* a reason not to be using actuarial measures; it is simply an important factor for practitioners to think about when they are conducting and interpreting risk assessments. This is not a criticism of the Meehlian finding that actuarial prediction is superior to clinical prediction, it is simply pointing out that in the two contexts fundamentally different things are being predicted; for the clinician propensity to re-offend is predicted, for the statistical prediction reconviction is predicted.

Mossman's (1994) meta-analysis suggests false positive rate of 44% for "pure" clinical judgements of dangerousness. Some of these, we have argued, could be undetected offenders and therefore true positives however.

Beginnings of a Model for Incorporating DACES into Risk Assesment and Formulation

Any variable substantially related to the probability of getting caught and processed by the criminal justice system needs to be considered when understanding what is being measured by reconviction or re-arrest as an outcome. (Re)conviction is correlated with exposure to the CJS in two ways: Increases in knowledge of DACES through exposure to systems, procedures and other offenders, but it also increases levels of future police surveillance. Biases such as racism and white privilege will impact also on levels of police surveillance. Low IQ and young age can be linked with absence of effective DACES; however, they are also associated with higher levels of diversion from the CJS. Anecdotally, high numbers of people with learning difficulties do not get convicted for offences that they commit (Jon Taylor personal communication), and police services explicitly have a policy to divert people with learning difficulties – and indeed people with psychological problems – from the CJS (e.g., Jacobson, 2008).

Contextual levels of surveillance (LOS) are critical to understanding conviction. If an individual moves to a non-urban context, where surveillance might be low then there may be a lesser chance of them getting caught and offending if norms were developed from people in a context where supervision is higher – in some urban settings for example. In custody, surveillance levels are higher than in community, so capacity to predict getting caught actuarially should be better. High surveillance contexts can (a) increase detection rates and (b) increase context specific DACES. Contexts where there are high levels of punishment will lead to the development of DACES; Hollin (2002) argues that the impact of punishment is not to reduce offending but to increase motivation and skills to hide offending and evade detection.

All statistically identified risk factors can be conceptualised as factors that facilitate getting caught, as well as factors associated with risk of reoffending. How then, theoretically, are other risk factors possibly linked with getting caught? Gendreau et al. (1996) highlighted that the persistent offender tends to be young, have unstable employment, abuse alcohol and drugs, hold pro-criminal attitudes, and associates with other criminals. Are these factors that facilitate getting caught rather than – or as well as – specifically predicting offending? Number of previous convictions (one of the most robust predictors of reconviction) could be a

Table 5.5 Risk/need factors and their impact in getting caught

Major risk/need factor	Processes linking factor with risk of getting caught
Antisocial personality pattern	Impulsivity and reduced self-management skills leading to reduced use of DACES.
Procriminal attitudes	Associate with people who are offending, present as "fitting the template" (Larcombe, 2012) of a "criminal". Easily suspected of offending. Individual comes into contact with police more often, and when they do their presentation may lead to an escalation in problematic behaviour due to problems with people in "authority".
Social supports for crime	Criminal friends and isolation from prosocial others result in increased probability that police suspect an individual of committing offences – when compared with individual who doesn't have "criminal friends".
Substance abuse	Reduced capacity to implement DACES due to substance misuse linked with increased impulsivity, and reduced capacity to think effectively and use consequential thinking in relation to getting caught and avoiding conviction.
Family/marital relationships	Poor family relationships linked with increased surveillance from social services, and lack of support for implementing DACES and gaining resources to facilitate avoiding conviction.
School/work	Unemployment linked with lifestyle that results increased visibility to police.
Prosocial recreational activities	Lack of prosocial recreational activity resulting in increased levels of offending that then result in increased visibility and "being on the police's radar".

measure of the extent to which an individual is subjected to forensic surveillance; the police look first of all for people with a history of offending in a particular way. Table 5.5 outlines some risk/need factors and how they might impact individuals getting caught.

When building up an understanding of non-detection in relation to measures using reconviction as an outcome it is important to recognise that many of the offences that are not detected or convicted may be committed by people who have already been caught. Abel et al. (1987) found that adults who committed sexual offences were guaranteed anonymity disclosed having committed an average of 533 sex offenses over a 12-year period before being detected (Abel et al., 1987; Abel et al., 1988). The researchers concluded that "arrest records of paraphiliacs do not provide a reliable indication of the true scope of paraphilic acts" and that "most paraphilic acts are not reported".

In another study, it was found that people who had committed rape, assured that their responses would stay anonymous, described having six times as many victims as could be identified from official records, and each of the people who had offended sexually against children in the study reported having hundreds of previously unknown sexual contacts with children (Weinrott & Saylor, 1991). People who had offended sexually taking polygraph tests (e.g., Ahlmeyer et al., 2000) offenders who were known to have an average of two victims at the time of their arrest subsequently reported having an average of 184 victims after taking polygraph tests while in treatment (see also Emerick & Dutton, 1993). Underwood, Patch, Cappelletty, and Wolfe, (1999) found that individuals who have sexually molested children eventually report, while in treatment, having committed an average of 88 crimes each. Other researchers have reported that the number of sex offences reported by those who had committed sexual offences in treatment increased by three to four times (Emerick & Dutton, 1993).

If antisocial orientation/lifestyle instability is the best predictor of both sexual and general recidivism in those convicted of sexual offences it is doubtful that it is predicting the probability of reoffending rather than only the probability of being arrested and convicted for subsequent offending.

Clinical Implications

Risk Assessment Considerations

Risk assessments need to take into account the limitations identified in this chapter. If an individual is assessed using a risk assessment instrument and the outcome identifies characteristics also identified in the research as representing a cohort of people who had a high level of reconviction, then this needs to be considered in terms of the following questions. *Has this person evidenced or not evidenced this risk factor because they don't have good detection and conviction evasion skills, or they do have good detection and conviction evasion skills?*

Broadening Your Clinical Risk Formulation: Assessing DACES

When considering how DACES might be assessed it would be useful to consider detection evasion strategies (DES). The literature highlights a range of strategies that individuals use in order to evade detection (e.g., Beauregard & Bouchard, 2010; Chopin et al., 2019; Chopin et al., 2021; Nee, 2015; Nee & Meenaghan, 2006; Nee & Taylor, 2000; Nee & Ward, 2015) as outlined in Table 5.6.

Table 5.6 Detection evasion strategies

Literature suggests the following as detection evasion strategies

 1 Planning offending and resisting offending impulsively
 2 Offending sober and not under influence of drugs
 3 Thinking about ways of not getting caught
 4 Anticipating police strategies for catching them (e.g., fingerprints, DNA, surveillance)
 5 Using gloves and masks to prevent recognition
 6 Selecting victims that are less likely to disclose or, if they do, that are less likely to be deemed "credible" in legal context
 7 Concealing physical, contextual and memorial aspects of the offence that could contribute to detection
 8 Learning about what not to do from hearing about others offending and getting caught
 9 Offending whilst sober or not using drugs in order to avoid making mistakes
10 Hiding skills (self and evidence)
11 Deception and fraud skills
12 Lying to those close to them
13 Persuading the victim that what is happening is not an offence
14 Persuading the victim that the activity isn't wrong, even if it is seen as an offence by the law
15 Persuading the victim that the activity isn't significant or impactful even if they acknowledge that it is "wrong" and illegal
16 Offending in social and cultural contexts where reporting things to the police is actively discouraged, e.g., cultures where it is seen as "grassing" and disloyalty, or where retributive justice is accepted and going to the police seen as a subcultural crime or evidence of weakness
17 Supporting this kind of culture by engaging in retributive responses to others reporting offences to the police
18 Using weapons to threaten victim of adverse consequences of disclosure
19 Threatening the victim with revenge, loss of love or friendship or other negative consequences
20 Using vulnerabilities in the victim to make disclosure to the police un-attractive
   a Building emotional or material dependency on them so that disclosure is associated with the fear of losing these resources
   b Offending against relatives or cultural peers where disclosure will result in family or peers ostracising the individual
   c Shaping fear of stigma in the victim "if you tell anyone then your parents will hate you"
   d Shaping misattribution of blame/guilt "it was your fault because … you left your window open, you were wearing provocative clothing, you provoked me …".
   e Shaping beliefs about being believed in people who haven't been believed in the past. A significant component of this facet of DACES is involved in what has been called in the literature "grooming" in sexual offending. It isn't however limited to sexual offending.

Second to DES is a consideration of the individual's conviction evasion skills (CES). Once an individual has been apprehended for an offence a different set of skills come into play aimed at avoiding conviction. See Table 5.7.

Table 5.7 Conviction evasion skills

1 Skills and knowledge about accessing a good lawyer
2 Knowing people who can help with either advice or money
3 Utilising knowledge about legal rights to limit police activity and scope
4 Knowledge about and skills in relation to what to say and what not to say in police interviews
5 Deception skills
6 Skills at performing effectively and "credibly" in court
7 Skills at deflecting or pointing blame at others
8 Skills in offering mitigating circumstances
9 Knowledge of most effective defence strategies; knowledge and skills in relation to appealing against convictions

The following is a checklist of both static and dynamic factors to consider as part of a DACES assessment:

Static factors: Fitting a "template" of what an offender of this kind looks like (Larcombe, 2012):
• Being a person of colour (increasing chances of allegation and conviction) as opposed to being white (decreasing chances of allegation and conviction due to white privilege)
• Being a person with a lower SES (increasing chances of allegation and conviction) as opposed to coming from "higher" SES (decreasing chances of allegation and conviction)
• Being a person who is not well integrated and lacking in social connections
• Being a person who is more likely to be monitored
• Being a person who is socially identified due to factors such as their sexuality
• Being a person who is likely suggestible and may wrongly confess

Skills factors: Not having a good repertoire of DACES (see list above):
• If the individual is assessed as having good DACES then the estimate needs to be seen as an under estimate. It isn't, however, clear by how much.
• If they are assessed as having poor DACES then the estimate might be seen as an under estimate of their chances of returning to offending.
• If they are assessed as having criminogenic factors which could explain their lack of DACES and hence their conviction.

If they are assessed as not having the skills abilities to fully navigate the legal system or access the required support available, i.e., legal aid.

If an individual is claiming that they are innocent of an offence, it needs to be acknowledged that a proportion of those who have a conviction are people who have not committed an offence. The possibility that the individual is actually innocent needs to be acknowledged and work needs to be undertaken that allows for both these possibilities. The overrepresentation of people with intellectual difficulties or from black and ethnic backgrounds needs to be considered.

If a clinician is convinced that an individual is innocent then they need to have a strategy for dealing with this in their setting. Feeding back reasons for this kind of judgement needs to have a place in clinical practice. It isn't the job of a forensic psychologist to make judgements about innocence or guilt, this is a legal judgement and needs to be done through the appropriate legal means. It is the job of the psychologist to contextualise risk, develop a full understanding of the potential factors that lead to imprisonment, and hypothesise about their relative impacts on the likelihood of being RTO. The focus will likely shift as the client nears release, and one considers the release context more closely alongside the environmental, individual, and contextual factors impacting on a person's likelihood of living a fulfilling life.

Carrying Out a DACES Assessment

When considering how best to explore DACES within the context of a formulation, the following (see Table 5.8) may form a useful starting point:

Table 5.8 DACES assessment

Considerations within a DACES assessment
• Explore and individual's offending history from the perspective of having been charged but not convicted.
• Whilst challenging, ask about undetected offences (whilst being clear about the responsibility to report).
• Ask the individual to describe their DACES, and the ways in which these were not effective in the context of their current offence.
• A sequence of offences can be analysed to identify what has been learned in the context of one offence that has been part of a subsequent offence, i.e., the skills learned to avoid detection. A form of formulation called Multiple Sequential Functional Analysis (Dawson & Gresswell, 2010) could be used.
• Looking at offence paralleling behaviour and DACES in the current setting can be useful in thinking about DACES in the past.
• Whilst relationally problematic and intrusive, clinical use of polygraphy can be useful for exploring offending activities including DACES.

Monitoring impact of surveillance and sanctions on covertisation of offending can also be useful. Covertisation is the process whereby an individual increasingly conceals offending behaviour in custodial settings each time it is responded to through punishment and surveillance. High surveillance and punishment result in an increase in covert activity. Custodial contexts shape up fantasy or imaginative rehearsal of offending behaviour that can later be acted on. The important point is that the behaviour and the motivation for it doesn't necessarily "go away", the individual simply founds more and more effective ways of hiding it.

Figure 5.4 shows now the impacts of the CJS and DACES on formulation can be conceptualised diagrammatically.

Implications for Research and the Future Development of DACES

How forensic practitioners engage with accounting for the differences between reported crime, reconviction and returning to offending requires access to a

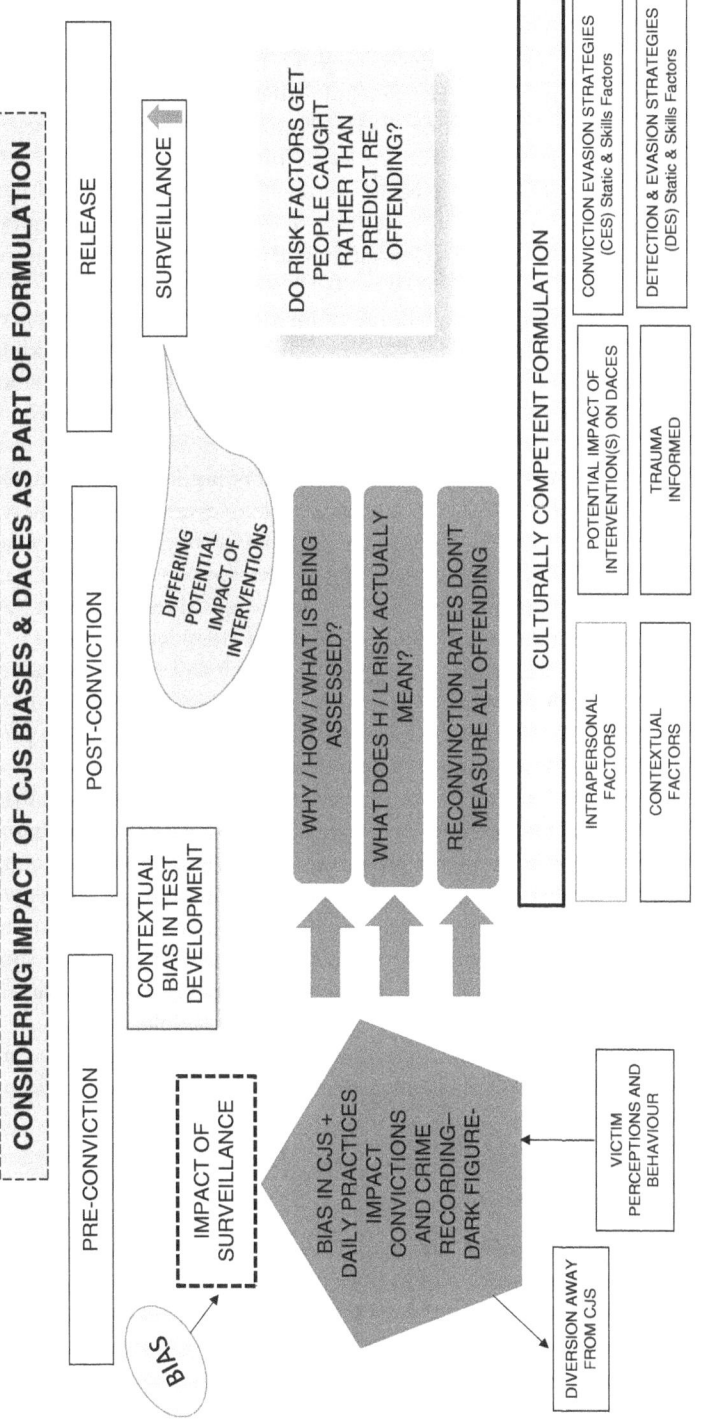

Figure 5.4 Impacts of of CJS and DACES on bias in formulation.

broader evidence base than what is available for, or is a constituent of, the the forensic psychology field per se. Jacques (2019) describes the role of criminological research in examining the knowledge base in respect of crime and where the optimal data arises. He concludes that in order to best understand the context and detail of offending, then accessing data sources with the most information is an optimal approach. As such, forensic practitioners, in seeking to better understand DACES, need to consider the data arising and conclusions drawn from wider fields of study and expertise such as victimology, criminology, and wider social research initiatives that are less exclusive in terms of participants.

Nee (2015) and with other collaborators for example has undertaken work, albeit indirectly in the field of DACES, which helps us to see methodologies that might enhance our ability to apply findings and better understand the basis of the assessments that are completed with those individuals who have been convicted.

As noted at the start of this chapter, practitioners need to be cautious about being drawn into fallacious conclusions when making assumptions about testing and assessment (Kline, 2000). Understanding what it is that we are seeking to measure is critical, as we have argued, and in terms of research activity methodologies which draw upon ecological approaches (e.g., Tremblay et al., 2018), will enable the examination of people per se rather than "criminals".

There is a need for theory driven support for making links between changes in therapy and changes in conviction which involves linking process variables with outcome variables in a more sophisticated manner. This is likely to prove a significant challenge. Furthermore, whilst treatment should necessarily seek to examine an individual's life and its trajectories, it is after that is achieved that one should consider what has been the criminal behaviour. On a more fundamental level, the relative impacts of interventions must be more clearly understood, and consideration given to what the consequences would be if an improvement in DES was the primary outcome? Equally, what if it could be further demonstrated that treatment resulted in more self-regulatory offending? How should such individuals be processed through the CJS, and whether this would merit an adjustment of the punishment is a debate that is yet to take place.

Clearly, there is a need for practitioners and researchers to begin incorporating DACES into their work so that further development of the model and can be undertaken.

Concluding Comments

It was not within the scope of this chapter to present all the statistics or arguments supporting the presence of bias both in the creation and analysis of crime statistics. However, what has been presented is arguably sufficient to support its presence. We have sought to present the relative impacts of these biases on the different pathways which can lead individuals to being imprisoned – with contextual and intrapersonal factors impacting on this also.

Whilst in its infancy, there are the beginnings of a model for enhancing formulations and adding a further trajectory incorporating DACES. The forensic psychology profession embraced the Good Lives Model (Ward, 2010) and subsequently protective factors (De Vries Robbé et al., 2012), as they were introduced to encourage a more balanced approach to our understanding of our clients and to address construct underspecification. The forensic psychology profession continues to evolve, as we currently seek to do our part to address bias and misrepresentation, through the ongoing development of our practice, clarifying construct underspecification and the confusion between a construct and its operationalisation is a process that requires further work. Whilst this introduces a degree of uncertainty into risk assessment, coping with, communicating about and being transparent in relation to uncertainty should be a key skill in risk assessment – particularly when under organisational pressures to make predictions.

References

Abel, G. G., Becker, J. V., Cunningham-Rathner, N., Rouleau, J. L., & Murphy, W. D. (1987). Self-reported sex crimes of non-incarcerated paraphiliacs. *Journal of Interpersonal Violence*, *2*, 3–25.

Abel, G. G., Mittelman, M., Becker, J. V., Rathner, J., & Rouleau, J. (1988). Predicting child molesters' response to treatment. In R. A. Prentky & V. L. Quinsey (Eds.). *Human sexual aggression: Current perspectives* (pp. 223–234). New York: New York Academy of Science.

Ahlmeyer, S., Heil, P., McKee, B., & English, K. (2000). The impact of polygraphy on admissions of victims and offenses in adult sexual offenders. *Sexual Abuse: Journal of Research & Treatment*, *12*(2), 123–138.

Baumeister, R. F., Stillwell, A. M., & Heatherton, T. F. (1994). Guilt: An interpersonal approach. *Psychological Bulletin*, 115, 243–267. 10.1037/0033-2909.115.2.243

Beauregard, E., & Bouchard, M. (2010). Cleaning up your act: Forensic awareness as a detection avoidance strategy. *Journal of Criminal Justice*, *38*(10), 1160–1166. 10.1016/j. jcrimjus.2010.09.004

Biderman, A. D., & Reiss, A. J. (1967). On exploring the "dark figure" of crime. *The ANNALS of the American Academy of Political and Social Science*, *374*(1), 1–15. 10.1177/0002 71626737400102

Buil-Gil, D., Medina, J., & Shlomo, N. (2020). Measuring the dark figure of crime in geographic areas. Small area estimation from the Crime Survey for England and Wales. *The British Journal of Criminology*, *0*, [azaa067]. 10.1093/bjc/azaa067

Burnham, M. (2017). Retrospective justice in the age of innocence: The hard case of rape executions. In D. S. Medwed (Ed.). *Wrongful convictions and the DNA revolution twenty-five years of freeing the innocent* (pp. 291–313). Cambridge: Cambridge University Press.

Chapman, F. E. (2013). Coerced internalized false confessions and police interrogations: The power of coercion. *Law Psychology Review*, *37*, 159–209.

Chopin, J., Beauregard, E., Bitzer, S., & Reale, K. (2019). Rapists' behaviors to avoid police detection. *Journal of Criminal Justice*, *61*, 81–89. 10.1016/j.jcrimjus.2019.04.001

Chopin, J., Paquette, S., & Beauregard, E. (2021). Is there an "expert" stranger rapist? *Sexual Abuse*. Advance online publication. 10.1177/1079063221993478

Coid, J. W., Ullrich, S., & Kallis, C. (2013). Predicting future violence among individuals with psychopathy. *The British Journal of Psychiatry*, *203*(5), 387–388.

Dawson, D. L., & Gresswell, D. M. (2010). Offence paralleling behaviour and multiple sequential functional analysis. In M. Daffern, L. F. Jones, & J. Shine (Eds.). *Offence paralleling behaviour: A case formulation approach to offender assessment and intervention* (pp. 89–104). Chichester: John Wiley & Sons. ISBN 9780470744475, 9780470744482, 9780470970270

De Vries Robbé, M., De Vogel, V., & Stam, J. (2012). Protective factors for violence risk: The value for clinical practice. *Psychology*, *13*(12a), 1259–1263.

Emerick, R. L., & Dutton, W. A. (1993). The effect of polygraphy on the self report of adolescent sex offenders: Implications for risk assessment. *Annals of Sex Research*, *6*(2), 83–103. 10.1007/BF00849301

Gendreau, P., Little, T., & Goggin, C. (1996). A meta-analysis of the predictors of adult offender recidivism: What works!. *Criminology*, *34*, 575–607.

Gould, J. B., Smiegocki, V. M., & Leo, R. A. (2021, February 1). Theorizing failed prosecutions. *Journal of Criminal Law and Criminology*. Forthcoming, American University School of Public Affairs Research Paper Forthcoming, SMU Dedman School of Law Legal Studies Research Paper No. 509, Univ. of San Francisco Law Research Paper No. 2021-10, Available at SSRN: https://ssrn.com/abstract=3792518

Gove, W. R., Hughes, M., & Geerken, M. (1985). Are uniform crime reports a valid indicator of the index crimes? An affirmative answer with some minor modifications. *Criminology*, *23*, 451–501.

Gudjonsson, G. H. (2017). False confessions and suggestibility. In P. Basant & I. Treasaden (Eds.). *Forensic psychiatry: Fundamentals and clinical practice*. Boca Raton: Imprint CRC Press. 10.1201/9781315380797

Hanson, K., & Wallace-Carpetta, S. (2000). *Predicting recidivism among male batterers 2000-06*. Department of the Solicitor General Canada. Public Works and Government Services Canada Cat. No.: JS42-91/2000 ISBN: 0-662-65222-3.

Hollin, C. R. (2002). Does punishment motivate offenders to change? In M. McMurran (Ed.). *Motivating offenders to change. A guide to enhancing engagement in therapy* (pp. 235–246). West Sussex: Wiley Series in forensic clinical psychology. 10.1002/9780470713471.ch14

Hood, R., Shute, S., Feilzer, M., & Wilcox, A. (2002). Sex offenders emerging from long-term imprisonment. A study of their long-term reconviction rates and of parole board members' judgements of their risk. *British Journal of Criminology*, *42*(2), 371–394.

Inbar, Y., Pizarro, D. A., Gilovich, T., & Ariely, D. (2013). Moral masochism: On the connection between guilt and self-punishment. *Emotion*, *13*(1), 14–18.

Jacobs, A. Z., & Wallach, H. (2021). Measurement and fairness. In Conference on Fairness, Accountability, and Transparency (FAccT '21), March 3–10, 2021, Virtual Event, Canada. ACM, New York, 11 pages. 10.1145/3442188.3445901

Jacobson, J. (2008). *No one knows police responses to suspects, learning disabilities and learning difficulties: A review of policy and practice*. London: Prison Reform Trust.

Jacques, S. (2019). Which source possesses the best data on the empirical aspects of criminal events? A theory of opportunity and necessary conditions. *Deviant Behavior*, *40*(12), 1543–1552. 10.1080/01639625.2018.1559635

Jensen, A. (1980). *Bias in mental testing*. New York: Free Press.

Jones, L. (2004). Offence paralleling behavior (OPB) as a framework for assessment and interventions with offenders. In A. Needs & G. J. Towl (Eds.). *Applying psychology to forensic practice* (pp. 34–63). Oxford: British Psychological Society Blackwell.

Jones, L. F. (2007). Iatrogenic interventions with personality disordered offenders. *Psychology Crime and Law*, *13*(1), 69–79. 10.1080/10683160600869809

Jones, L. F. (2010). History of the offence paralleling behaviour construct and related concepts. In M. Daffern, L. Jones, & J. Shine (Eds.). *Offence paralleling behaviour: A case formulation approach to offender assessment and intervention* (pp. 1–23). West Sussex, UK: John Wiley & Sons.

Jones, L. F. (2013). Detection and conviction evasion skills. *Presentation at the Lincoln University Sex Offender Research*. Lincoln University Sex Offender Research Program.

Jones, L. F. (2022). Trauma informed risk assessment and intervention: Understanding the role of triggering contexts and offence related altered states of consciousness (ORASC). In P. Willmot & L. F. Jones (Eds.). *Trauma informed care in forensic practice*. London: Routledge.

Kang, J., Bennett, M. W., Carbado, D. W., Casey, P., Dasgupta, N., Faigman, D., & Mnookin, J. (2012). Implicit bias in the courtroom. *UCLA Law Review, 59*, 1124–1186.

Kennedy, H., & Grubin, D. (1992). Patterns of denial in sex offenders. *Psychological Medicine, 22*, 191–196.

Kline, P. (2000). *The handbook of psychcological testing* (2nd ed.). Oxford, UK: Routledge.

Larcombe, W. (2012). Sex offender risk assessment: The need to place recidivism research in the context of attrition in the criminal justice system. *Violence Against Women, 18*, 482–501. 10.1177/1077801212452249

Lowenkamp, C. T., & Latessa, E. J. (2004). Understanding the risk principle: How and why correctional interventions can harm low-risk offenders [Technical report]. *Topics in community corrections* (pp. 3–8). Washington, DC: U.S. Department of Justice, National Institute of Corrections.

Mayson, S. G. (2019). Bias in, bias out. *Yale Law Journal, 128*(8), 2122–2473.

Messick, S. (1989). Validity. In Linn, R. L. (Ed.), *Educational measurement*. 3rd ed. 13–103. New York: American Council on Education/Macmillan.

Messick, S. (1995). Validity of psychological assessment: Validation of inferences from persons' responses and performances as scientific inquiry into score meaning. *American Psychologist, 50*(9), 741–749. https://doi.org/10.1037/0003-066X.50.9.741

Monahan, J., Steadman, H. J., Silver, E., Appelbaum, P. S., Robbins, P. C., Mulvey, E. P., Roth, L. H., Grisso, T., & Banks, S. (2001). *Rethinking Risk Assessment: The MacArthur Study of Mental Disorder and Violence*. Oxford: Oxford University Press.

Mossman, D. (1994). Assessing predictions of violence: Being accurate about accuracy. *Journal of Consulting and Clinical Psychology, 62*, 783–792.

Nee, C. (2015). Understanding expertise in burglars: From pre-conscious scanning to action and beyond. *Aggression and Violent Behavior, 20*, 53–61. 10.1016/j.avb.2014.12.006

Nee, C., & Meenaghan, A. (2006). Expert decision making in burglars. *British Journal of Criminology, 46*(5), 935–949. 10.1093/bjc/azl013

Nee, C., & Taylor, M. (2000). Examining burglars' target selection: Interview, experiment or ethnomethodology? *Psychology, Crime & Law, 6*(1), 45–59. 10.1080/10683160008410831

Nee, C., & Ward, T. (2015). Review of expertise and its general implications for correctional psychology and criminology. *Aggression and Violent Behavior, 20*, 1–9. 10.1016/j.avb.2014.12.002

Ogunbur, I., & Taylor, P. (2010). Detection of crime. In J. Flatley, C. Kershaw, K. Smith, R. Chaplin, & D. Moon (Eds.). Crime in England and Wales 2009/10. Findings from the British Crime Survey and police recorded crime. *Home Office Statistical Bulletin*. July 2010. London: Home Office.

Posick, C., & Singleton, M. (2014). Why crimes aren't reported: The role of emotional distress and perceptions of police response. *The Journalist's Resource, Scholar's Strategy Network*. May 13.

Sizmur, S. (2008, July). Construct validity and risk assessment for serious offending. Paper presented at the 8th International Association of Forensic Mental Health Services, Vienna.

Smith, E., & Hattery, A. J. (2011). Race, wrongful conviction and exoneration. *Journal of African American Studies*, *15*, 74–94. 10.1007/s12111-010-9130-5

Smith, R. J., Levinson, J. D., & Robinson, Z. (2015). Implicit white favoritism in the criminal justice system. 66 Alabama Law Review 871.

Social Exclusion Unit Report. (2002, July) *Reducing re-offending by ex-prisoners.* https://publications.parliament.uk/pa/cm200405/cmselect/cmhaff/193/19306.htm

Stavrova, O., & Siegers, P. (2014). Religious prosociality and morality across cultures: How social enforcement of religion shapes the effects of personal religiosity on prosocial and moral attitudes and behaviors. *Personality and Social Psychology Bulletin*, *40*, 315–333. 10.1177/0146167213510951

Tarling, R., & Morris, K. (2010). Reporting crime to the police. *The British Journal of Criminology*, *50*(3), 474–490. 10.1093/bjc/azq011

Taylor, R. (1999). Predicting reconvictions for sexual and violent offences using the revised Offender Group Reconviction Scale. *Research Findings 104*. Home Office.

Tremblay, R. E., Vitaro, F., & Côté, S. M. (2018). Developmental origins of chronic physical aggression: A bio-psycho-social model for the next generation of preventive interventions. *Annual Review of Psychology*, *69*, 383–407. 10.1146/annurev-psych-010416-044030

Trowbridge, B. C. (2003). Suggestibility and confessions. *American Journal of Forensic Psychology*, *21*, 5–23.

Underwood, R. C., Patch, P. C., Cappelletty, G. G., & Wolfe, R. W. (1999). Do Sexual Offenders Molest When Other Persons Are Present? A Preliminary Investigation. *Sexual Abuse: A Journal of Research and Treatment*, *11*(3), 243–247. 10.1023/a:1021316525940

Vess, J., Day, A., Powell, M., & Graffam, J. (2014). International sex offender registration laws: Research and evaluation issues based on a review of current scientific literature. *Police Practice & Research*, *15*(4), 322–335. 10.1080/15614263.2011.646744

Ward, T. (2010). The good lives model of offender rehabilitation: Basic assumptions, etiological commitments, and practice implications. In F. McNeill, P. Raynor, & C. Trotter (Eds.). *Offender supervision: New directions in theory, research and practice*. Cullompton: Willan Publishing.

Weinrott, M., & Saylor, M. (1991). Self-report of crimes committed by sex offenders. *Journal of Interpersonal Violence*, *6*(3), 286–300.

Woldgabreal, Y., Day, A., & Tamatea, A. (2020). Do risk assessments play a role in the enduring 'color line'? *Advancing Corrections*, *10*, 18–28.

6 Measuring What Matters: Standardised Risk Levels for Criminal Recidivism Risk

Daryl G. Kroner and R. Karl Hanson

Introduction

Risk assessments have a profound impact on individuals in criminal justice and forensic mental health systems, guiding supervision, classification, and release decisions. They also influence the treatment and services provided, particularly in settings that aspire to the Risk/Need/Responsivity (RNR) rehabilitation model (Andrews et al., 1990). One perennial concern is whether these classifications are correct. This is a particular concern given the overrepresentation of historically disadvantaged groups in criminal justice systems, who often are rated "high" on risk assessment tools. Debates about biased classification, however, have been hindered by the ambiguity in the meaning of the risk levels. If we are going to work towards effective, fair, and equitable risk classifications, we need a common language for describing and communicating the risk for criminal recidivism.

In this chapter we discuss one approach to standardising risk classification and communication, specifically, the 5-Level System advanced by the Justice Center of the US Council of State Governments (Hanson et al., 2017). This system integrates diverse features of recidivism risk, including statistical indicators (e.g., percentile ranks, recidivism rates), the density of criminogenic needs, strengths, and antecedents, along with recommended correctional responses and expected outcomes. By providing explicit meanings to risk levels, the 5-Level system helps decision-makers, evaluators, and the individuals assessed determine the extent to which classification decision are accurate and just (Council of State Governments Justice Center, 2014).

Statement of Problem

There has been an explosion of risk tools in corrections and forensic mental health, with hundreds of different measures currently available. Each comes with its own risk categories. Often individuals are assessed on multiple tools. For example, an individual in the criminal justice system might be assessed on one instrument for bail release, another for sentencing, another for prison placement, and yet another for community supervision. As well, individuals can also be assessed for specific types of criminal outcomes, such as intimate partner

DOI: 10.4324/9781003230977-7

violence, or sexual offending. In high stakes evaluations, evaluators typically use multiple instruments. When each of these measures has different risk categories, expect confusion.

Research on risk category consistency finds, instead, inconsistency. Jung and colleagues (2013), for example, found that the percentage agreement among four sexual recidivism risk assessment instruments varied from a low of 23.2% to a high of 71.4%. Barbaree et al. (2006) found that approximately half of their sample of individuals with a sexual offending history was identified as high risk by one of the five risk assessment instruments; however, only 3% were placed in the high-risk category by all five instruments.

Such inconsistency should not be surprising given that the meaning of risk levels is rarely defined (Hanson et al., 2017). Apart from a general expectation that individuals with higher scores are more likely to reoffend than individuals with lower scores, it is unclear what other inferences should be made from risk level placement. Should the recidivism rates per category be the same across samples and settings? What about relative risk? Treatment needs?

A related concern is that the target population of risk tools is often unknown. If an individual has a relatively high score, evaluators must ask "relative to what?" A lack of consistency can occur because of (a) differences in sample base rates, (b) differences in mean scores and distribution characteristics, and (c) differences in the endorsed content within the categories. Consider, for example, a comparison between the Canadian samples of the Youth Level of Service/Case Management Inventory (YLS/CMI) and the application to young persons convicted of an offence in Japan (Takahashi et al., 2013). In the Japanese sample, only 3.1% of the sample was placed into the "high" and "very high" categories. This under-representation in the top two categories occurred even though the relative risk statistic ($r = .34$) was the same as in Canadian studies (random effects $r = .34$, Table 12, Olver et al., 2014).

Consistent interpretation of risk categories has multiple benefits. First, risk level placement would not depend on the instrument used; instead, all (equally valid) risk tools would say the same thing. As well, consistent interpretations would support theory testing of crime-related etiologies (Krauss et al., 2000). Consistent placement into risk categories would also inform optimal levels of supervision or interventions. Furthermore, consistency increases the confidence in the results. As noted by Heilbrun et al. (2007), "[c]onsistency across sources makes it more likely that the agreed-upon information is accurate" (p. 53). Finally, theoretically coherent, consistent risk categories can do much to reduce ethnic and cultural biases in recidivism risk assessments.

Solution – The Justice Center's 5-Level System

One attempt to increase consistency in risk categories is the five-level risk as-sessment system developed by the Justice Center of the US Council of State Governments (Hanson et al., 2017). Applied to a client, the 5-Level system starts with the individual's risk score on a specific tool (e.g., 10 out of 30) and then uses a set of decision rules to determine which one of five standardised risk levels the individual most closely resembles. The decision rules are based upon previous research that identifies the risk-relevant characteristics typically observed for individuals with these scores on this measure. Instead of the original risk levels asserted by the test developers, the obtained risk score is interpreted according to the standardised 5-Level System, which *mean the same thing* regardless of the risk tool used.

Between 2014 and 2016, the Justice Center hosted a series of meetings of criminal justice researchers, managers, and practitioners aimed at developing generalised risk levels. The first meeting involved risk assessment researchers. The initial proposals had a range of 2–11 risk categories, with 3, 4, and 5 categories receiving serious consideration (CSG Justice Center, 2014). Another consultation involved correctional administrators and managers (i.e., system directors, deputy directors), who considered the systems' potential application of a common risk category system. A subsequent consultation involved assessment practitioners (i.e., probation officers, supervisors), who considered scoring and translational issues. Finally, the synthesised information from the previous meetings guided discussions of the initial group of researchers, accompanied by a broader group of 20 risk assessment researchers representing universities, correctional systems, and nonprofit criminal justice agencies. This group examined conceptual issues and potential research in the implementation of the 5-Level System.

The 5-Level System integrates the most significant features of risk level placements into a framework aligned with the RNR model of correctional rehabilitation. Not only do the levels inform the likelihood of recidivism, they also present a psychological profile of the typical individuals at each level, indicate recommended correctional responses, and describe expected outcomes. In the language of psychological assessment, the 5-Level system aspires to *construct validity*, that is, a theoretically coherent set of inferences associated with each risk level (Cronbach & Meehl's, 1955, *nomological nets*).

Level I is the lowest risk level, describing individuals who are similar to non-criminal justice involved persons, that is, individuals with no criminal record in a typical Western-based criminal justice system. The recidivism rate for Level I is around 3% after two years, with the upper limit of 5%. Level II indicates a temporary offending profile with strong prosocial tendencies. Level II individuals are higher risk than the general population, but lower than the average for those involved in the typical criminal justice system. The recidivism rate for Level II is about 19% with a range from 5% to 29%. Level III describes individuals in the middle of the risk distribution of the entire correctional population. The average recidivism rate for Level III is around 40%, with a range from 30% to 49%. Level IV describes individuals with chronic and lengthy criminal involvement, with expected recidivism rates of approximately 65% (50–84%). The highest-risk level, Level V, describes individuals with entrenched criminal profiles who are nearly certain to reoffend (average $\approx$ 90%, lower limit of 85% within two years).

Percentile rank norms, relative risk, and recidivism rates can be used to derive the five risk levels from existing criminal recidivism risk tools (Hanson et al., 2017). More specifically, the three steps involve calculating (a) the median score for the risk instrument, (b) odds ratios, and (c) recidivism rates estimates associated with scores (Babchishin et al., 2017). As in traditional inferential statistics, the 5-Level System is based on the population median, not the sample median. In other words, the reference population would be the entire criminal justice and forensic population to which the measure could potentially (ever) be used. Practically, the median and other statistics are derived from samples (not populations). Next, the boundary scores between Level II and Level III, and between Level III and Level IV are determined by an odds ratio of .70/1.43 from the median value. An odds ratio of this size was selected because it corresponds to the recidivism reduction that occurs with the typical published treatment intervention (i.e., $r = .10$, $d = .20$; e.g., Bonta & Andrews, 2016; Hanson et al., 2009). The boundary score between Level I and Level II (5%) and between Level IV and Level V (85%) are based on two-year recidivism rates estimated by logistic regression (Hanson, 2022, Chapter 11; Helmus & Hanson, 2011).

Almost any criminal recidivism risk assessment scale can be converted into the 5-Level System, given the necessary data: (a) two-year recidivism study with a sample size of 500, at least 100 recidivists, (b) a score range of 15 points (or percentage points), and (c) at least moderate predictive accuracy (AUC of .66 or higher). Note that the different statistics can be derived from different samples. For example, the median value could be based on large, representative samples whereas the relative risk statistics could be based on smaller, more diverse samples.

Core Assumptions

The 5-Level System is predicated on the assumption that there is general latent construct of criminal risk, and that most risk assessment instruments tap into this construct (antisociality). This construct is considered a dimension whose core feature is the propensity for rule violation. Associated features include all those characteristics that we find on recidivism risk tools, which have been well summarised by Bonta and Andrews (2016) as the Central Eight (history of antisocial behavior, antisocial personality pattern, antisocial cognition, antisocial associates, and problems with family/marital circumstances, school/work, leisure/recreation, and substance abuse). A general latent construct of criminal risk is supported by a study that found that a risk tool created from randomly selected items from other risk tools predicted recidivism as well as any of the original tools (Kroner et al., 2005).

A second major assumption is that estimates of the likelihood of criminal recidivism can, and should, be based on placement on this latent dimension. Individuals at each of the risk levels are expected to systematically differ on indicators of psychological and community adjustment, and these individual differences are associated with recidivism risk. One implication of this assumption is that the reverse is also true: valid assessments of recidivism risk (however conducted) are also valid indicators of the density of risk-relevant propensities.

Individuals with elevated procriminal attitudes are likely to reoffend, and individuals who are likely to reoffend have elevated procriminal attitudes.

A related assumption is that data from samples of similar individuals should inform decisions about both risk-relevant propensities and the likelihood of recidivism of individuals. As Mossman (2015) states, risk estimates for individuals "flow naturally and obviously from information about groups of outcomes" (p. 94; see also Imrey & Dawid, 2015).

Another important assumption is that the 5-Level System is a broadly applicable, not jurisdiction specific. Most individuals within most criminal justice systems in Westernised democracies can be reasonably fit into one of the five risk levels, although the proportion at each level will depend on local criminal justice policies. For instance, in the consultations leading to the development of the 5-Level System, representatives from one jurisdiction stated that there are almost no Level I cases in their correctional system because they diverted such cases at the point when police decide whether or not to lay charges. Similarly, if we apply the 5-Level System to a sample of lower risk probationers, we would expect to have few or no cases in Level IV and Level V. This is, in fact, what happens. In a study of probationers administered the LSI-R ($N = 24,936$), there were no cases in Level V; in contrast, Level V cases were found in a higher-risk parole community sample ($N = 36,303$; Kroner et al., 2020). Even through the 5-Level System has five levels, the actual number of discernable levels will vary across settings.

Benefits of the 5-Level System

The 5-Level System is a principled approach to establishing risk levels. It has credible, explicit procedures, which were derived from both norm-referenced and criterion-referenced assessment models. Instead of the cacophony produced by unharmonised risk levels, the 5-Level System aspires to improve both case-specific risk communication, and advance research on effective interventions in corrections and forensic mental health. Other benefits include increasing the consistency in risk-level placements, clear implications for action, improved risk communication, practical advantages for corrections administrators, and reduced racial/ethnic biases. Each of these benefits will be elaborated below.

Increasing Consistency in Risk-Level Placements

The 5-Level System can increase the consistency of risk-level placement in routine corrections. In one of our studies (Kroner & Derrick, 2020), we compared a normative percentile method of creating risk categories with the 5-Level System. The comparisons used the LSI-R and two "made-up" risk instruments derived from administrative data. Both derived tools had a limited range of total scores, which was a less than optimal condition for creating risk categories. Penalising the created risk scales in this way allowed for a stronger conclusion about the effectiveness of the 5-Level System. One derived instrument maximised the relationship between the administrative items and outcome, and the other derived instrument maximised the relationship between the administrative items and LSI-R total score. The agreement among the LSI-R and the two derived instruments was higher when the 5-Level System was used to create the risk categories compared to using the percentile norm approach. The increase in agreement was approximately 5%. This per cent may not seem large, but when applied to an overall correctional system, it would increase the consistency of placements for a substantial number of individuals.

Clear Implications for Action

Associated with each of the risk levels are guidelines for correctional intervention dosage, the level of supervision, and expected results of intervention. Congruent with the risk principle in the RNR model, as the risk levels increase, so do the required number of criminogenic need areas that need to be addressed. At Level I, there are none or few; at Level II, there are few needs, mostly mild and transitory; at Level III, there are multiple needs, some severe; at Level IV, there are multiple needs, with some chronic and severe; and at Level V, there are multiple needs that are severe, chronic, and entrenched.

It should be noted that how the intervention addresses these needs makes a difference. It is assumed that interventions are based on valid principles of change. If not, the impact of addressing more criminogenic need areas is mute. For example, for interventions for higher-risk persons involved in the criminal justice system, having substance abuse intervention only in an educational format may reduce the overall effectiveness of the intervention (Polaschek, 2011). The intended use of risk assessment instruments to identify and address individuals' needs is often poorly implemented (Viljoen et al., 2018), which could be partially attributed to a lack of clear direction on which risk levels require what amounts of intervention. The explicit recommendations built into the 5-Level System may increase the concordance between treatment needs and treatment received.

The dose-response rehabilitation research continues to evolve. There is consensus that as the number of criminogenic need areas increase, so does the recommended dose of correctional interventions; however, without standardised risk levels, it is difficult to interpret dose-response studies. Not that long ago, 100–200 hours was considered intensive intervention for higher-risk groups (Cortoni et al., 2006). Now, for higher-risk groups approximately 250 hours would be considered appropriate (Lester et al., 2020; Makarios et al., 2014), with approximately 300 hours of intervention for the highest-risk persons involved in the criminal justice system (Polaschek, 2011). Based on these and similar studies, the 5-Level System recommends 100–200 hours at Level III, 200–300 hours at Level IV, and even more for Level V. In contrast, the limited concerns of individuals at Level II can be effective addressed with supportive counselling and case management. For Level I, no psychological intervention is indicated, and could even be counterproductive.

Similarly, the intensity of supervision should increase as risk levels increase. For example, correctional policy could stipulate no or bi-weekly contact for the lowest-risk levels, weekly or bi-weekly contact for mid-risk range, and contact every 48 hours for nearly all the high-risk cases (Luong & Wormith, 2011). Although explicit policy is helpful, officer adherence to risk/supervision dosage will also increase when officers receive risk assessment training (Ricks et al., 2016).

At Level V, it is unrealistic to expect significant reductions in recidivism risk in the short term. Meaningful change may take decades. Polaschek (2011) found only slight recidivism reductions with persons who were very high risk. Consequently, rather than directly addressing specific criminogenic needs, it may be more effective to focus on preparing for future change, and for future participation in interventions (Polaschek & Yesberg, 2015). Developing the skills to maintain treatment engagement may also be an appropriate target for individuals at Level V (Lester et al., 2020).

Although slavish adherence to specific dose levels can be counterproductive (Simourd & Olver, 2019), the recommendations of the 5-Level System provide useful guidance for planning service delivery in corrections and forensic mental health. When individual routine receives substantially more, or substantially less, than that recommended by the five levels, administrators need to carefully consider the rationale for the prevailing practices. When treatment is financed by the state, administrators would be expected to welcome reductions in service implied by the 5-Level Model. In contrast, Hogan and Sribney (2019) have suggested that administrators may have little enthusiasm for the 5-Level System should it imply the need to increase the amount of treatment provided.

Improved Risk Communication

There are four general ways that evaluators can speak about an individual's propensity for a future negative event: percentile ranks, absolute likelihoods, relative risk, and risk category labels (Davies et al., 2020; Hanson et al., 2017). Each method has advantages and disadvantages. One of the benefits of the 5-Level Systems is that it informs each of these four types of risk communication. The five levels are named categories, and can be used as such (i.e., evaluators can simply report the risk level and be done with it); however, placement in any of the five levels allows evaluators and decision-makers to infer likelihoods, percentile ranks, and relative risk.

Percentile ranks are the most common method of communicating assessment results in psychology (Crawford & Garthwaite, 2009; Crawford et al., 2009). Although helpful, they only address whether the individual is more or less "risky" than other individuals. Percentiles say nothing about the likelihood of the outcome. The *absolute likelihood* approach assigns a probability to the outcome of interest (e.g., out of 100 individuals like Mr. Jones, 37 would be expected to be reconvicted for a violent offence within three years). One problem with absolute likelihoods is that they are difficult to estimate with precision. The base rate of the outcome changes based on follow-up time, the definition of the outcome, and other factors that may not be fully understood (Helmus et al., 2012). In contrast, relative risk, expressed as rate ratios or odds ratios, are a much more stable feature of prediction schemes (Helmus et al., 2012; Matheny et al., 2005). Relative risk, however, is difficult to interpret without some notion of the base rate. If the risk score indicates that the individual is four times as likely to re-offend as the average individual, the next obvious question should be "What is the average recidivism rate?", which returns us to the absolute likelihoods.

Evaluators and decision-makers have a near universal preference for named risk levels over any form of numeric risk communication (Heilbrun et al., 2016). A benefit of nominal labels for risk levels is that they indicated proscriptive plans of action. Without a label, decision-makers may not know how to respond to an evaluation that concludes that the individuals has a 22% likelihood of sexual recidivism within five years. It would be much easier to respond if this likelihood was described as unusually high.

When developing the 5-Level System, we quickly concluded that the levels must be names (e.g., Level III), not numbers (42%). We were also keenly aware, however, that without grounding in statistical indicators, the meaning of risk levels would vary across risk tools. Through a multi-stage process, the 5-Level System integrates percentiles, absolute risk, and relative risk into named levels. The importance of using all four approaches is supported by research indicating that noise in risk level placement can be reduced when diverse, case-specific statistical indicators are considered (Mills, 2017), and risk information is presented in multiple formats (Davies et al., 2020; Harris et al., 2015). When the five-level development group was deciding on names, we avoided the traditional labels of "low", "medium", and "high" because they were already associated with multiple meanings that varied by context. During the consultation process, various labels were considered, including colours and animals (Fuzzy Bunnies to Rabid Hyenas), ultimately landing on ordered levels identified by Roman numerals.

Advantages for Corrections Administration

The 5-Level System offers two clear benefits for corrections administration: (a) improved resource allocation planning (i.e., number of staff supervisors, client intervention slots), and (b) reduced noise in risk level placements. With regard to resource allocation, knowing the number of clients at each risk level and the appropriate proscriptive efforts for each level allow correctional administrators to calculate, in advance, the resources necessary to manage and reduce risk. Furthermore, these system-wide calculations can be made independent of specific risk assessment instruments.

The misclassification of clients is costly for both systems and individuals. Even with the use of a valid risk assessment instrument, there are two situations that commonly add noise to risk level placements: (a) overrides, and (b) the administration of multiple risk tools to the same individual. Professional overrides of risk assessment instruments are far too common given that they degrade predictive accuracy (Cohen et al., 2020; Hanson & Morton-Bourgon, 2009; Schmidt et al., 2016). Of concern, overrides are not evenly split between upward and downward reclassifications. Instead, overrides in the criminal justice system are usually conservative (i.e., individuals are placed in higher-risk categories; 98.3%, Cohen et al., 2016; 100%, Schmidt et al., 2016). Furthermore, most overrides involved factors that were already accounted for in the risk tools used (Cohen et al., 2016).

Some evaluators may increase risk levels because the recidivism rate estimates associated with actuarial risk tools fail to account for undetected recidivism. This practice is problematic for several reasons. First, raising actuarial low-risk cases to moderate- or high-risk cases decreases the evaluator's ability to make meaningful distinctions between cases. The primary use of risk tools is to efficiently align rehabilitation and public protection measures with the risk and need profiles. Rarely does the referral question hinge on an absolute likelihood of recidivism – detected or not. Furthermore, upper level correlations are found between undetected and detected recidivism rates. Ranking individuals based on the likelihood of either type of recidivism will also rank order individuals on the latent propensity for rule violation, which most risk tools aspire to assess. Another problem is that evaluators who make decisions based on undetected recidivism rates distance themselves from evidence-based practice, as these rates, by definition, are unobservable events. Professional opinions gain scientific credentials by reference to empirical findings. Basing decisions on inherently unobservable events risks introduces personal biases and unfounded speculations into otherwise credible evaluations.

Overrides may occur because evaluators do not have a clear sense of what the risk levels mean. When this occurs, the inclination is to increase the risk level. The 5-Level System aims to improve this situation by providing clear descriptions of the criminogenic needs, prosocial strengths, and recommended correctional response at each of the levels. Evaluators should be able to match the case-at-hand to the risk level the individual most closely resembles. This should increase case managers' confidence in the risk level placements provided by the risk tool, and support their activities that addressing client criminal justice issues related to risk.

The second situation that can result in misclassification is the use of multiple risk assessment instruments on a single individual. This is common in court, and when individuals go from one part of a system to another (i.e., jail to prison, forensic hospital to community corrections). Just as most overrides increase risk, evaluators typically based their overall assessment on the highest category assigned when using two or more risk tools. This is likely to overestimate risk (Babchishin et al., 2012). The actual effect, however, is difficult to anticipate because the meaning of most risk levels is unknown. An individual classified as high risk on one instrument may be lower risk than an individual classified as moderate risk on a different risk tool (Bourgon et al., 2018). The 5-Level System decreases such apparent inconsistencies across risk tools. The standardised and sequential statistical methods for creating the levels becomes the defining qualities for the risk levels, resulting in unified risk levels. Consequently, evaluators are better able to identify when disagreements between risk tools are substantive, rather than artefacts of divergent definitions of risk level.

Risk Assessment Bias

Racial/ethnic differences are, regrettably, systemic to the criminal justice system. In the United States, minorities are more likely to be stopped by police (Gelman et al., 2007; Pierson et al., 2020) arrested (Wu, 2016), require high pretrial bonds (Wooldredge, 2012), receive harsher sentences for person crimes (Kutateladze et al., 2014), and be incarcerated (Bales & Piquero, 2012). These events impact the measurement of criminal history, which is included in nearly every risk assessment instrument tool, directly or indirectly. Consequently, racialised minorities involved in the criminal justice system receive higher risk assessment instrument scores than non-minority populations. These differences can be expected starting when the first risk assessment instrument is administered. It appears that this impact is greater for classification than prediction, as the predictive ability of risk assessment instruments can be similar between minority and non-minority populations (Lowder et al., 2019; Skeem & Lowenkamp, 2016). The prediction studies are difficult to interpret, however, because the increased criminal justice involvement for minority groups inflates both the prediction tools and the outcome. For a number of risk assessment instruments, minority and non-minority classification differences have been noted at the each risk category (Ostermann & Salerno, 2016; Perrault et al., 2017).

The 5-Level System could advance discussions of equity and fairness by focusing attention on what risk assessments should be assessing. If, fundamentally, criminal recidivism risk tools are assessing a latent dimension of antisociality, then it is reasonable to ask the extent to which this dimension varies across groups. It is also important to ask whether the same indicators mean the same thing for groups who are substantially different in terms of social status, targets of racism, and history of oppression. If minorities are overpoliced, then criminal history should be a less valid measure of antisociality among minorities than it is among whites. Similarly, negative attitudes towards police may be an effective indicator of antisociality among affluent, white youth, whereas such attitudes could simply be justified, true belief for minority males, particularly in this post-Floyd era. Evaluators and decision-makers need to consider the intent and purpose of risk assessments when deciding if its application to a particular individual is accurate and just. The 5-Level System provides a framework for such deliberations.

Another strength of the 5-Level Systems is that it allows for the identification of racial biases that is independent of a particular risk assessment instrument. Currently, the analysis of bias is based on thresholds unique to each risk tool. By standardising the risk levels, a clearer and a more robust conclusion can be made regarding the nature and extent of racial bias.

Another contribution of the 5-Level System is its ability to tailor proscriptive components according to minority concerns. Intervention dosage, criminogenic need areas, supervision recommendations, and expected results of intervention at each of the five levels could be tailored according to racial/ethnic concerns. Minority status can, and should, influence criminal justice interventions. Minority status is predictive of treatment dropouts (Olver et al., 2011), underlining the need for culturally informed programming.

Challenges

The difficulties and challenges of the 5-Level System can be placed into the two broad categories of (a) inputs (i.e., risk assessment instrument characteristics) and (b) outputs (i.e., inferences and recommendations). Although the system aspires to apply to almost all criminal risk tools, this may not be the case. Hogan (2020), for example, has questioned the feasibility of inferring criminogenic needs from risk tools that contain predominantly static, historical factors.

Although research has found a correspondence between the level of criminogenic needs and the five levels derived from static risk tools (Blais et al., 2021; Hanson et al., 2017), this is not always the case (Coulter, Lloyd, & Serin, 2021). Furthermore, the correspondence between static and dynamic risk factors is only approximate. In general, risk level placement should improve when evaluators consider more features of the 5-Level System (e.g., both static and dynamic risk factors, see Olver et al., 2020).

Most risk assessment instruments in the criminal justice system reflect a latent construct of antisociality. The model assumes that individuals vary on this relatively enduring propensities, such that relative placement on the construct can be inferred from past behaviours, and use to estimate the likelihood of future rule violations. However, if the risk assessment instrument is too far away from measuring this latent construct (it is measuring something else, such as poverty), the 5-Level System might not work. The 5-Level System has been successfully adapted for sexual recidivism risk tools (Hanson et al., 2017; Moore, 2018; Olver et al., 2018; Olver et al., 2020). Currently, there is ongoing debate about how it should be applied to risk tools designed to assess general violence (Davies et al., 2020) or intimate partner violence.

The 5-Level System assumes that the propensity for criminal recidivism is proportional to the density of criminogenic needs, that is, the psychological and community adjustment problems that figure on risk tools. Although this generalisation is well supported by research, it may not describe certain criminal subgroups. Drug dealers, for example, may live otherwise prosocial lives yet be high risk for recidivism. At the other end of the spectrum are older individuals who have desisted from crime many years ago, but who still retain certain antisocial features. These older individuals should be classed in Level I based on very low recidivism rates; however, they look quite different from the Justice Center's description of Level I as otherwise prosocial individuals who made an isolated mistake (Blais et al., 2021). Research has yet to determine how different a subgroup needs to be before the 5-Level System stops making sense.

Although a comprehensive survey is beyond the scope of the current paper, we are aware that the 5-Level System has so far been adopted in a few US states (e.g., Colorado), some Canadian jurisdictions (e.g., British Columbia, Correctional Service of Canada) and a few international settings (e.g., Singapore, Hong Kong).

Much broader use is needed before it can fulfil its potential as a common language for risk communication.

Directions for Future Research

The 5-Level System was developed to reduce what Kahneman and colleagues refer to as noise in human judgement (Kahneman et al., 2021). This is a testable hypothesis. For example, the variability in decision-makers' final judgements should be lower (reduced variance) when the results of different risk tools are presented in the language of the five levels instead of in the original categories of the risk tools. In applied practice, reduced noise would be indicated by fewer professional overrides.

One of the biggest evidence gaps concerns the five-level's recommendations for treatment dose. Although we believe these recommendations are reasonable, they are based on a limited number of studies (see Simourd & Olver, 2019 for a review). Significantly, none of these studies classified initial risk using the five levels. Consequently, there is a need for many more treatment outcome studies that vary the number of hours of credible interventions delivered to individuals classed into the 5-Level System.

How protective factors might work at each risk level is also unknown. Protective factors are considered to have a central role in intervention efficacy and in the desistance process. Knowing how these factors assist with risk reduction, and if they differ among the risk levels, would be helpful in assisting persons involved with the criminal justice system to be crime free.

Conclusion

The science and practice of recidivism risk assessment has advanced to the point that we can say more than the individual's risk is "low", "moderate", or "high". Nevertheless, poorly defined risk label persistent in applied practice. The Justice Center's 5-Level System provides an opportunity to decrease noise in risk level placement by standardising criminal recidivism risk levels in corrections and forensic mental health. Not only should this lead to more accurate placements, it also has the promise of reducing bias. A common understanding of the meaning of risk levels is a prerequisite for determining whether risk level placement is valid and just.

References

Andrews, D. A., Bonta, J., & Hoge, R. D. (1990). Classification for effective rehabilitation: Rediscovering psychology. *Criminal Justice and Behavior, 17*(1), 19–52. 10.1177/0093854 890017001004

Babchishin, K. M., Hanson, R. K., & Helmus, L. (2012). Communicating risk for sex offenders: Risk ratios for Static-2002R. *Sexual Offender Treatment, 7*(2), 1–12.

Babchishin, K. M., Kroner, D. G., & Hanson, R. K. (2017). Standardized risk/need levels for corrections. *Crime Scene*, *24*(1), 9–13.

Bales, W. D., & Piquero, A. R. (2012). Racial/ethnic differentials in sentencing to incarceration. *Justice Quarterly*, *29*, 742–773. 10.1080/07418825.2012.659674

Barbaree, H. E., Langton, C. M., & Peacock, E. J. (2006). Different actuarial risk measures produce different risk rankings for sexual offenders. *Sexual Abuse: A Journal of Research and Treatment*, *18*(4), 423–440. 10.1007/s11194-006-9029-9

Blais, J., Babchishin, K. M., & Hanson, R. K. (2021). Improving our risk communication: Standardized risk levels for the BARR-2002R. *Sexual Abuse*. 10.1177/1079063221047185

Bonta, J., & Andrews, D. A. (2016). *The psychology of criminal conduct* (6th ed.). New York, NY: Routledge.

Bourgon, G., Mugford, R., Hanson, R. K., & Coligado, M. (2018). Offender risk assessment practices vary across Canada. *Canadian Journal of Criminology and Criminal Justice*, *60*(2), 167–205. 10.3138/cjccj.2016-0024

Cohen, T. H., Lowenkamp, C. T., Bechtel, K., & Flores, A. W. (2020). Risk assessment overrides: Shuffling the risk deck without any improvements in prediction. *Criminal Justice and Behavior*, *47*(12), 1609–1629. 10.1177/0093854820953449

Cohen, T. H., Pendergast, B., & VanBenschoten, S. W. (2016). Examining overrides of risk classifications for offenders on federal supervision. *Federal Probation*, *80*(1), 12–21.

Cortoni, F., Nunes, K. L., & Latendresse, M. (2006). *An examination of the effectiveness of the violence prevention program* (2006 No R-178). Correctional Service Canada.

Coulter, D. J., Lloyd, C. D., & Serin, R. C. (2021, April). Combining static and dynamic recidivism risk information into the Five-Level Risk and Needs system: A New Zealand example. Manuscript under review.

Council of State Governments Justice Center. (2014). *A common language for risk assessment: Experts convene in Washington.* http://csgjusticecenter.org/a-common-languagefor-riskassessments-experts-convene-in-washington/

Crawford, J. R., & Garthwaite, P. H. (2009). Percentiles please: The case for expressing neuropsychological test scores and accompanying confidence limits as percentile ranks. *The Clinical Neuropsychologist*, *23*(2), 193–204. 10.1080/13854040801968450

Crawford, J. R., Garthwaite, P. H., & Slick, D. J. (2009). On percentile norms in neuropsychology: Proposed reporting standards and methods for quantifying the uncertainty over the percentile ranks of test scores. *The Clinical Neuropsychologist*, *23*(7), 1173–1195. 10.1080/13854040902795018

Cronbach, L. J., & Meehl, P. E. (1955). Construct validity in psychological tests. *Psychological Bulletin*, *52*(4), 281–302. 10.1037/h0040957

Davies, S. T., Helmus, L. M., & Quinsey, V. L. (2020). Improving risk communication: Developing risk ratios for the VRAG-R. *Journal of Interpersonal Violence*. Advance online publication. 10.1177/0886260520914555

Gelman, A., Fagan, J., & Kiss, A. (2007). An analysis of the New York City police department's "stop-and-frisk" policy in the context of claims of racial bias. *Journal of the American Statistical Association*, *102*, 813–823. 10.1198/016214506000001040

Hanson, R. K. (2022). *Prediction statistics for psychological assessment*. Washington: American Psychological Association. https://doi.org/10.1037/0000275-000

Hanson, R. K., Babchishin, K. M., Helmus, L. M., Thornton, D., & Phenix, A. (2017). Communicating the results of criterion referenced prediction measures: Risk categories for the Static-99R and Static-2002R sexual offender risk assessment tools. *Psychological Assessment*, *29*(5), 582–597. 10.1037/pas0000371

Hanson, R. K., Bourgon, G., Helmus, L., & Hodgson, S. (2009). The principles of effective correctional treatment also apply to sexual offenders: A meta-analysis. *Criminal Justice and Behavior, 36*(9), 865–891. 10.1177/0093854809338545

Hanson, R. K., Bourgon, G., McGrath, R. J., Kroner, D. G., D'Amora, D. A., Thomas, S. S., & Tavarez L. (2017). *A five-level risk and needs system: Maximizing assessment results in corrections through the development of a common language.* New York, NY: The Council of State Governments Justice Center.

Hanson, R. K., & Morton-Bourgon, K. E. (2009). The accuracy of recidivism risk assessments for sexual offenders: A meta-analysis of 118 prediction studies. *Psychological Assessment, 21*(1), 1–21. 10.1037/a0014421

Harris, G. T., Lowenkamp, C. T., & Hilton, N. Z. (2015). Evidence for risk estimate precision: Implications for individual risk communication. *Behavioral Sciences & the Law, 33*(1), 111–127. 10.1002/bsl.2158

Heilbrun, K., Marczyk, G., DeMatteo, D., & Mack-Allen, J. (2007). A principles-based approach to forensic mental health assessment: Utility and update. In A. M. Goldstein (Ed.). *Forensic psychology: Emerging topics and expanding roles* (pp. 45–72). Hoboken: John Wiley and Sons.

Heilbrun, K., Newsham, R., & Pietruszka, V. (2016). Risk communication: An international update. In J. P. Singh, S. Bjorkly, & S. Fazel (Eds.). *International perspectives on violence risk assessment* (pp. 150–165). Oxford: Oxford University Press.

Helmus, L., & Hanson, R. K. (2011). More fun with statistics! How to use logistic regression to predict criminal recidivism risk. *Crime Scene, 18*(2), 8–12.

Helmus, L., Hanson, R. K., Thornton, D., Babchishin, K. M., & Harris, A. J. R. (2012). Absolute recidivism rates predicted by Static-99R and Static-2002R sex offender risk assessment tools vary across samples: A meta-analysis. *Criminal Justice and Behavior, 39*(9), 1148–1171. 10.1177/0093854812443648

Hogan, N. R. (2020). Critical considerations in the development and interpretation of common risk language. *Psychiatry, Psychology and Law.* Advance online publication. 10.1080/13218719.2020.1767719

Hogan, N. R., & Sribney, C. (2019). *Combining Static-99R and STABLE-2007 risk categories: An evaluation of the five-level system for risk communication. Sexual Offender Treatment, 14.* http://www.sexual-offender-treatment.org/187.html

Imrey, P. B., & Dawid, A. P. (2015). A commentary on statistical assessment of violence recidivism risk. *Statistics and Public Policy, 2*(1), 1–18. 10.1080/2330443X.2015.1029338

Jung, S., Pham, A., & Ennis, L. (2013). Measuring the disparity of categorical risk among various sex offender risk assessment measures. *Journal of Forensic Psychiatry & Psychology, 24*(3), 353–370. 10.1080/14789949.2013.806567

Kahneman, D., Sibony, O., & Sustein, C. R. (2021). *Noise: A flaw in human judgment.* 1–384. Glasgow, Scotland: William Collins Publishers.

Krauss, D. A., Sales, B. D., Becker, J. V., & Figueredo, A. J. (2000). Beyond prediction to explanation in risk assessment research. *International Journal of Law and Psychiatry, 23*(2), 91–112. 10.1016/S0160-2527(99)00032-1

Kroner, D. G., & Derrick, B. (2020). The Council of State Governments Justice Center approach to increasing risk-level consistency in the application of risk assessment instruments: *Assessment.* Advance online publication. 10.1177/1073191120958066

Kroner, D. G., Mills, J. F., & Reddon, J. R. (2005). A coffee can, factor analysis, and prediction of antisocial behavior: The structure of criminal risk. *International Journal of Law and Psychiatry, 28*(4), 360–374. 10.1016/j.ijlp.2004.01.011

Kroner, D. G., Morrison, M. M., & Lowder, E. M. (2020). A principled approach to the construction of risk assessment categories: The Council of State Governments Justice Center Five-Level System. *International Journal of Offender Therapy and Comparative Criminology, 64*(10–11), 1074–1090. 10.1177/0306624X19870374

Kutateladze, B. L., Andiloro, N. R., Johnson, B. D., & Spohn, C. C. (2014). Cumulative disadvantage: Examining racial and ethnic disparity in prosecution and sentencing. *Criminology, 52*(3), 514–551. 10.1111/1745-9125.12047

Lester, M. E., Batastini, A. B., Davis, R., & Bourgon, G. (2020). Is risk-need-responsivity enough? Examining differences in treatment response among male incarcerated persons. *Criminal Justice and Behavior, 47*(7), 829–847. 10.1177/0093854820915740

Lowder, E. M., Morrison, M. M., Kroner, D. G., & Desmarais, S. L. (2019). Racial bias and LSI-R assessments in probation sentencing and outcomes. *Criminal Justice and Behavior, 46*(2), 210–233. 10.1177/0093854818789977

Luong, D., & Wormith, J. S. (2011). Applying risk/need assessment to probation practice and its impact on the recidivism of young offenders. *Criminal Justice and Behavior, 38*(12), 1177–1199. 10.1177/0093854811421596

Makarios, M., Sperber, K. G., & Latessa, E. J. (2014). Treatment dosage and the risk principle: A refinement and extension. *Journal of Offender Rehabilitation, 53*(5), 334–350. 10.1080/10509674.2014.922157

Matheny, M. E., Ohno-Machado, L., & Resnic, F. S. (2005). Discrimination and calibration of mortality risk prediction models in interventional cardiology. *Journal of Biomedical Informatics, 38*(5), 367–375. 10.1016/j.jbi.2005.02.007

Mills, J. F. (2017). Violence risk assessment: A brief review, current issues, and future directions. *Canadian Psychology/Psychologie Canadienne, 58*(1), 40–49. 10.1037/cap0000100

Moore, L. (2018). Static risk assessment of sexual offenders in New Zealand: Predictive accuracy, classification of risk, and the moderating effect of time offence-free in the community. Doctoral Dissertation, Psychology, University of Canterbury, Christchurch, NZ.

Mossman, D. (2015). From group data to useful probabilities: The relevance of actuarial risk assessment in individual instances. *Journal of the American Academy of Psychiatry and the Law Online, 43*(1), 93–102. 10.2139/ssrn.2372101

Olver, M. E., Kelley, S. M., Kingston, D. A., Beggs Christofferson, S. M., Thornton, D., & Wong, S. C. P. (2020). Incremental contributions of static and dynamic sexual violence risk assessment integrating Static-99R and VRS-SO common language risk levels. *Criminal Justice and Behavior*. Advance online publication. 10.1177/0093854820974400

Olver, M. E., Mundt, J. C., Thornton, D., Beggs Chrstofferson, S. M., Kingston, D. A., Sowden, J. N., Nicholaichuk, T. P., Gordon, A., & Wong, S. C. P. (2018). Using the Violence Risk Scale – sexual offense version in sexual violence risk assessments: Updated risk categories and recidivism estimates from a multisite sample of treated sexual offenders. *Psychological Assessment, 30*(7), 941–955. 10.1037/pas0000538

Olver, M. E., Stockdale, K. C., & Wormith, J. S. (2011). A meta-analysis of predictors of offender treatment attrition and its relationship to recidivism. *Journal of Consulting and Clinical Psychology, 79*(1), 6–21. 10.1037/a0022200

Olver, M. E., Stockdale, K. C., & Wormith, J. S. (2014). Thirty years of research on the Level of Service Scales: a meta-analytic examination of predictive accuracy and sources of variability. *Psychological Assessment, 26*(1), 156–176. 10.1037/a0035080

Ostermann, M., & Salerno, L. M. (2016). The validity of the Level of Service Inventory – revised at the intersection of race and gender. *The Prison Journal, 96*(4), 554–575. 10.11 77/0032885516650878

Perrault, R. T., Vincent, G. M., & Guy, L. S. (2017). Are risk assessments racially biased?: Field study of the SAVRY and YLS/CMI in probation. *Psychological Assessment, 29*, 664–678. http://dx.doi.org/10.1037/pas0000445.

Pierson, E., Simoiu, C., Overgoor, J., Corbett-Davies, S., Jenson, D., Shoemaker, A., Ramachandran, V., Barghouty, P., Phillips, C., Shroff, R., & Goel, S. (2020). A large-scale analysis of racial disparities in police stops across the United States. *Nature: Human Behaviour, 4*(July), 736–745. 10.1038/s41562-020-0858-1

Polaschek, D. L. L. (2011). High-intensity rehabilitation for violent offenders in New Zealand: Reconviction outcomes for high- and medium-risk prisoners. *Journal of Interpersonal Violence, 26*(4), 664–682. 10.1177/0886260510365854

Polaschek, D. L. L., & Yesberg, J. A. (2015). Desistance in high-risk prisoners: Pre-release self-reported desistance commitment and perceptions of change predict 12-month survival. *Practice: The New Zealand Corrections Journal, 3*(1), 24–29.

Ricks, E. P., Eno Louden, J., & Kennealy, P. J. (2016). Probation officer role emphases and use of risk assessment information before and after training. *Behavioral Sciences & the Law, 34*(2/3), 337–351. 10.1002/bsl.2219

Schmidt, F., Sinclair, S. M., & Thomasdóttir, S. (2016). Predictive Validity of the Youth Level of Service/Case Management Inventory with Youth who have Committed Sexual and Non-Sexual Offenses: The Utility of Professional Override. *Criminal Justice and Behavior, 43*(3), 413–430. 10.1177/0093854815603389.

Simourd, D. J., & Olver, M. (2019). Prescribed correctional treatment dosage: Cautions, commentary, and future directions. *Journal of Offender Rehabilitation, 58*(2), 75–91. 10.1 080/10509674.2018.1562503

Skeem, J. L., & Lowenkamp, C. T. (2016). Risk, race, and recidivism: Predictive bias and disparate impact. *Criminology, 54*(4), 680–712. 10.1111/1745-9125.12123

Takahashi, M., Mori, T., & Kroner, D. G. (2013). A cross-validation of the Youth Level of Service/Case Management Inventory (YLS/CMI) among Japanese juvenile offenders. *Law and Human Behavior, 37*(6), 389–400. 10.1037/lhb0000029

Viljoen, J. L., Cochrane, D. M., & Jonnson, M. R. (2018). Do risk assessment tools help manage and reduce risk of violence and reoffending? A systematic review. *Law and Human Behavior, 42*(3), 181–214. 10.1037/lhb0000280

Wooldredge, J. (2012). Distinguishing race effects on pre-trial release and sentencing decisions. *Justice Quarterly, 29*(1), 41–75. 10.1080/07418825.2011.559480

Wu, J. (2016). Racial/ethnic discrimination and prosecution: A meta-analysis. *Criminal Justice and Behavior, 43*(4), 437–458. 10.1177/0093854815628026

7 The Cumulative Modelling of Risk

Sean Hammond and M.M. O'Rourke

Introduction

Forensic Clinical Risk Assessment is an inherently risky enterprise. It has long been recognised that false negative judgements may lead to service users perpetrating damaging behaviour which can sometimes raise serious doubts about forensic clinical judgement (Reed, 1997; Richie et al., 1994). Perhaps less potentially spectacular are false positive judgements that may lead to users being labelled "dangerous" with a knock-on impact on their liberty (Beckett, 2008; Carson & Bain, 2008).

Leading into the 21st century, risk assessment was widely seen as a polarised exercise with pure clinical judgement at one end of the spectrum and the actuarial method at the other. There had been ample demonstration of the limitations of clinical judgement in making risk assessments (Dawes et al., 1989; Grove & Meehl, 1996) building on Paul Meehl's seminal work on clinical diagnosis (Meehl, 1954). Quinsey et al. (1998) in particular, argued that the use of actuarial instruments to inform decisions would hugely mitigate the subjectivism of clinical judgements in a context where accuracy in risk judgements is vitally important.

The actuarial approach involves an identification of those characteristics that predict damaging behaviours and then a quantification of the cumulative effect of those characteristics as they apply to the patient being assessed. It is an essentially two-stage process. First, the predictors are identified using a large normative sample usually carried out by some form of general linear procedure. Second, informed by this information, some form of aggregation is applied to produce an individual risk "score".

In its simplest and most common form, the predictors are identified and then a checklist is drawn up for each service-user indicating the presence or absence of that predictor. Aggregation is often carried out by a simple or weighted summation. Sometimes the predictors are weighted in some manner but more often the summation is unweighted. The important point to be made here is that we are using normative data to judge the potential risk that a single individual poses.

There is a lot of merit in the actuarial approach. It focuses upon empirical evidence drawn from large sample data – it provides a clear and objective outcome and the process by which the score is arrived at is transparent and

DOI: 10.4324/9781003230977-8

replicable. There are now in excess of 200 forensic tools for assessing the risk of violence for example (Singh et al., 2014).

Unfortunately, the literature on actuarial risk assessment reveals a host of difficulties which have militated against the practical application of much of the interesting research (Douglas et al., 2017). There appear to be five main difficulties:

1 The construct of risk is not easily defined in mental health settings (Appelbaum, 2005).
2 The outcomes by which risk assessments may be validated are often unclear and unreliable (Coid et al., 2015; Siontis et al., 2015).
3 There would appear to be biases with regard to diversity irrespective of the purported objectivity of actuarial instruments (Shepard & Lewis-Fernandez, 2016).
4 A full understanding of the interaction between risk indicators is a perennial challenge in prediction analysis especially when trying to justify the subsequent use of a summative score (Keating & Boster, 2019).
5 The essentially normative focus of much risk assessment research does not always map onto the essentially idiographic task of assessing an individual patient (DeMateo et al., 2010).

The great caveat of the actuarial approach is that individuals do not always conform to normative behaviour, especially in people with extreme behaviours or people whose behaviour is largely characterised by unpredictability and impulse.

This chapter attempts to address the latter three issues but in doing so, may throw some light on the other two. The focus of the chapter is on the psychometric modelling of risk in which the emphasis is one of measurement rather than prediction. As such it proposes that a fundamental part of the actuarial approach to risk assessment is to properly address the measurement properties of the tools being used. When done in a detailed manner this should have the effect of clarifying the construct being measured and also provide the basis for an idiographic input into the decision-making process.

Psychometrics and Risk Assessment

Typically, in the risk assessment literature the measurement properties of checklists is dealt with in a cursory and naive manner in which Classical Test Theory (CTT) is utilised and alpha coefficients are routinely applied to infer psychometric quality. The primary drawbacks with this approach are that the total score is the sole unit of analysis, the standard error of measurement is a property of the test score and not the individual being assessed and there is no inherent model binding the risk indicators together.

It has long been known in the psychometric testing tradition that respondents may obtain the same total score but may have earned that score by responding to the items in entirely different ways. Exactly the same situation applies in forensic clinical assessment and risk assessment checklists are no exception. This issue is

Table 7.1 Illustration of two cases on an ICD-10 dissocial PD checklist

Symptom	Person A	Person B
Blames others	1	0
Callous unconcern	1	0
Relationship failures	1	0
Frustration	0	1
Feels no guilt	0	1
Irresponsibility	0	1
Total score	3	3

largely skirted over in traditional psychometric texts where the CTT focus is on the total score. However, anyone with any pretensions towards psychometric expertise is now fully aware of the limitations of CCT and the important role that Item Response Theory has in the development and appraisal of psychological measures (Embretson & Hershberger, 1999; McDonald, 1999).

For illustration, let us suppose that we have a six-item checklist that purports to measure dissocial personality disorder. Each of the items is drawn from the ICD10 criteria (WHO, 1993). We have two people who have been referred for assessment and we find that each person meets three of the six criteria. In Table 7.1, the symptom profiles for each person are displayed in which 1 represents the presence of that symptom and 0 represents its absence.

Since the ICD-10 classification for dissocial PD requires three symptoms to be present and the fact that each person demonstrates three of the six criteria leads us to conclude that both patients may be classified as dissocial personality disordered. The problem emerges when we compare the profiles of each person. Although they receive an identical classification it is clear that persons A and B have no symptoms in common.

Thus, the simple summation of symptoms to obtain a total score has offered up something of a quandary, for while it is mathematically perfectly acceptable to add up numbers in this way, it does not sit well in measurement terms where the focus is upon discriminating between objects. In this case, two people have an identical score but are entirely dissimilar. Consider the distinct clinical or therapeutic issues that each person poses, despite the fact that they apparently share the same diagnosis.

While, we have used the, largely superseded, ICD10 criteria here for illustration, it should be borne in mind that all such additive classification systems carry the same risk. For example, the ICD-11 dissocial PD construct proposed by Carnoval et al. (2020) contains 12 items but summation still remains the method of scoring.

In order to legitimately sum item responses, we must assume that the items describe a unidimensional structure, and this specifies a particular pattern of relationships between the items known as a simplex pattern. The most effective way of ascertaining unidimensionality is to examine the cumulative structure of the items.

The Cumulative Scale

The issue of inconsistent profiles was addressed very early on in the development of the discipline of psychometrics (Guttman, 1944; Mokken, 1971; Rasch, 1960; Walker, 1931), where it became clear that the valid use of simple summation implied a cumulative structure to the items being used. For illustration, let us digress briefly to consider the case of a short, four-item test of numerical ability used on a sample of six 5-year-old children.

Figure 7.1 shows the unfolded relationship between the children and the items in the test. Here we see that Lenny has not mastered the concept of multiplication yet and has not been able to correctly answer any of the items and scores 0. Dirk, on the other hand, has succeeded in getting all the items correct and so has a score of 4.

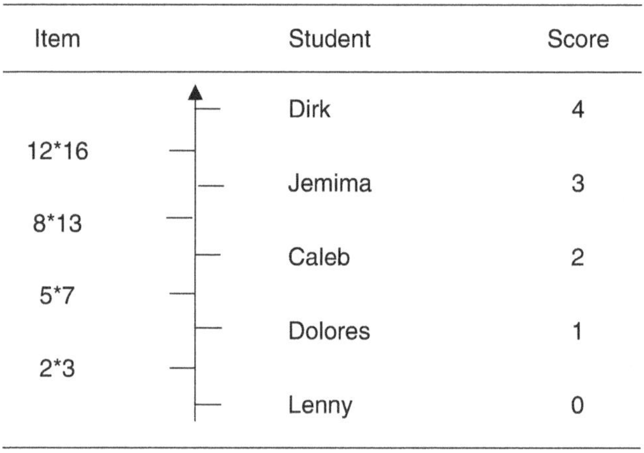

Item		Student	Score
		Dirk	4
12*16			
		Jemima	3
8*13			
		Caleb	2
5*7			
		Dolores	1
2*3			
		Lenny	0

Figure 7.1 An illustration of a unidimensional cumulative scale for four multiplication items and five children.

If we consider Jemima, we see that she has scored 3, which means she got one item incorrect. It makes sense to suppose that the item she could not answer is the most difficult. Equally, Caleb obtained a score of 2 and we may suppose that this means he was able to correctly answer the two easiest items while Dolores obtained a score of 1, which indicates she got the easiest item correct.

This joint ordering of item difficulty and responder ability is the root feature of a cumulative scale. The model that underpins a cumulative scale states that the total score that a person obtains allows the researcher to accurately reproduce that person's profile of item responses. However, in the real world such a model is unlikely to reflect everyone. With four items, it is possible to have 2^4, or 16 distinct profiles of answers while only five fit the model expectations. In Table 7.2, we show all possible profiles for the items ordered by difficulty (1 indicates a correct answer and 0 indicates an incorrect answer). According to the model, five profiles are legitimate and 11 are illegitimate.

Table 7.2 All profiles obtainable from a four-item checklist, where items are ordered from high frequency (common) to low frequency (rare)

Legitimate profile	Illegitimate profiles					Total score
0000						0
1000	0100	0010	0001			1
1100	0110	0101	0011	1010	1001	2
1110	0111	1011	1101			3
1111						4

It is, of course, a legitimate question to ask, how does this advance the practice of risk assessment? If we extrapolate this rather simplistic example to risk assessment checklists, we have to assume that we can order our risk indicators in terms of their commonality. Thus, in a risk assessment for violent assault the risk indicator "past trouble with the law" is probably more common than, "impulse control disorder" which is more common than "routinely carries firearms". Thus, if an individual is assessed on this three-item checklist and obtains a score of 1 we could assume it is the most common feature that applies. But this only applies if we can assume that the checklist items conform to a cumulative scale.

In order to test for the presence of a cumulative scale there are essentially three avenues of investigation. The earliest approach was pioneered by Louis Guttman (1944) and is widely known as Guttman Scaling or Scalogram Analysis (Dunn-Rankin, 2004). This was largely replaced by the more statistically sophisticated Rasch Model (Fischer & Molenaar, 1995; Rasch, 1960). A further non-parametric approach was developed by Mokken (1971) and is commonly known as Mokken Scaling (van Schuur, 2003; Bedford et al., 2009; van der Ark, 2012).

The Scalogram

Using the scalogram technique the items are ordered according to their frequency and each profile is examined to identify whether it conforms to the model. Deviations from the model expectations are taken as errors and these are aggregated. An index of reproducibility can then be obtained:

Formula 1

$$R = \frac{E}{n * m} \tag{7.1}$$

where E is the aggregation of errors, n is the number of cases, and m is the number of items. Guttman argued that when R exceeds 0.9, it is safe to proceed on the assumption that the items conform to a cumulative scale. Summation is therefore psychometrically valid. There have been a number of developments in evaluating scalograms (Goodenough, 1944; Green, 1956; Coombs, Coombs & Lingoes, 1978) and it is often now integrated into a more general set of procedures under the general name latent structure analysis (Goodman, 1975; Proctor, 1970).

The major limitation of the scalogram approach is the fact that it reflects a deterministic model. That is, all profiles are simply categorised as legitimate or illegitimate. In real-world data random fluctuations occur all the time due to a wide range of factors. As a result, it is often very hard to fit the scalogram model, especially if a large number of items are required.

The Rasch Model

A breakthrough emerged with the work of Georg Rasch (1960) who pioneered a probabilistic cumulative model, known widely as the Rasch model, which specified that the probability of a particular item response is directly dependent on the strength of a person's score through the following probabilistic function:

Formula 2

$$p_{ij} = \frac{1}{1 + \exp^{(\theta_i - \delta_j)}} \tag{7.2}$$

In which θ_I is the location of person i on the joint cumulative scale and δ_j is the location of item j on the same scale. Although θ is not the same as the total score of the person and δ is not the same as the frequency of the item, they have the same order as each other. The process of a Rasch analysis identifies the θ and δ parameters in such a way that the data fits as well as possible to a cumulative scale. Because these parameters can be estimated pretty robustly, usually to a maximum likelihood, the whole model can be tested as a goodness of fit problem.

Once we obtain the θ and δ parameters we can generate a standardised residual for every response for each person:

Formula 3

$$z_{ij} = \frac{x_{ij} - p_{ij}}{\sqrt{p_{ij}(1 - p_{ij})}} \tag{7.3}$$

Summing these residuals across people gives us an item misfit statistic with $n - 1$ degrees of freedom:

Formula 4

$$\chi_j^2 = \sum_{i=1}^{n} z_{ij} \tag{7.4}$$

Summing across items gives a person misfit statistic with $m - 1$ degrees of freedom:

Formula 5

$$\chi_i^2 = \sum_{j=1}^{m} z_{ij} \tag{7.5}$$

This is a fairly crude method of assessing fit, in fact there are many more sophisticated procedures available (see, e.g., Debelak, 2019; Glas & Verhelst, 1995), but it serves here for a simple illustration of the logic.

The Rasch model has a number of very attractive features. For example, it provides standard errors of estimate for each person and each item separately which leads to a feature known as specific objectivity (Rasch, 1977). This makes the model particularly useful for examining change and also measuring bias between groups (Fischer, 1985). This is an important feature in the risk assessment domain, when one is checking that a particular assessment tool is valid for a small subgroup of service-users.

It is beyond the scope of this chapter to delve further into the many psychometric advantages (and limitations) of the Rasch model but a comprehensive pedagogical text may be found in Bond et al. (2020) and, for more mathematical detail, Fischer and Molenaar (1995).

Mokken Scaling

One of the potential drawbacks of Rasch modelling is that it presupposes a logistic relationship between each item and the test scores. This relationship can be demonstrated for two items in Figure 7.2. Essentially it is a plot of the probability function given in equation 2, where θ ranges between $-\alpha$ and $+\alpha$.

The Rasch model specifies the shape of the relationship and assumes the trace lines to be parallel (i.e., they can never intersect with each other). This is a defining aspect of the cumulative model.

Mokken suggested a scaling approach that would relax the assumption that the item characteristic curves (ICCs) have a common shape. In fact, he suggested two

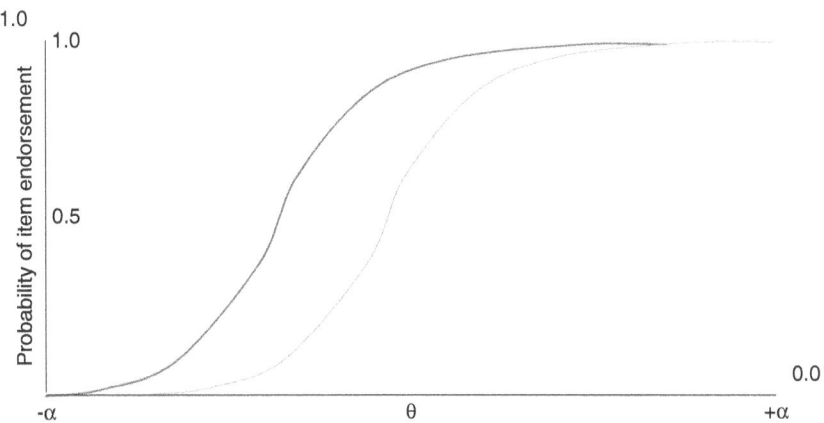

Figure 7.2 Item characteristic curves (ICCs) for two items showing the identical shape of the function.

distinct models, the second of which builds upon the first. The first model, widely known as the Monotone Homogeneity (MH) model simply asserts that the ICCs start low down on the left and then rise monotonically to the top right as the ability (or level of risk) increases. There is no assumption that the ICCs do not intersect and so this model does not imply a cumulative scale. In Figure 7.3, we see an example of two such items.

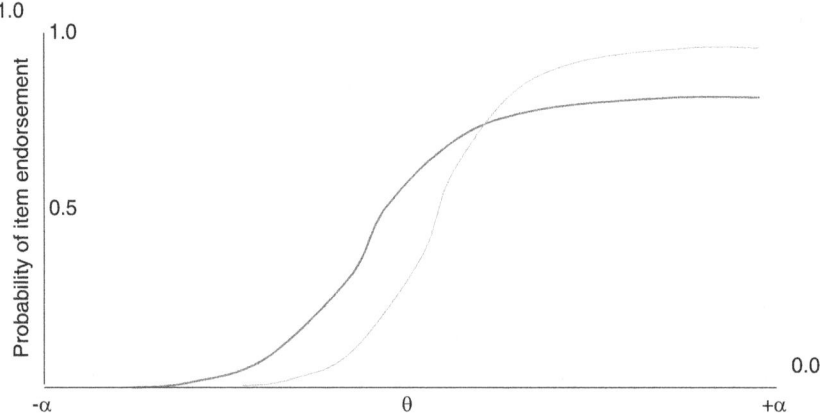

Figure 7.3 Item characteristic curves (ICCs) for two non-parallel items showing the monotonic trend for each.

Traditionally, the MH model is tested by generating a homogeneity coefficient H. The homogeneity coefficient for each item is found using the following formula:

Formula 6

$$H_i = \frac{\sum_{j<>i}^{m} (1 p_{ij} - p_i p_j)}{\sum_{j>i}^{m} (p_i - p_i p_j) + \sum_{j<i}^{m} (p_j - p_i p_j)} \tag{7.6}$$

where p_i is the proportion of times item i occurs and p_{ij} is the proportion of times item i occurs and item j does not. An exactly equivalent procedure exists to identify the person fit in which the data file is turned on its side so that the nxm file becomes mxn and using the same formula:

Formula 7

$$H_i = \frac{\sum_{j<>i}^{n} (p_{ij} - p_i p_j)}{\sum_{j>i}^{n} (p_i - p_i p_j) + \sum_{j<i}^{n} (p_j - p_i p_j)} \tag{7.7}$$

The total fit is found by:

Formula 8

$$H = \frac{\sum_{i=1}^{m-1} \sum_{j=i+1}^{m} (p_{ij} - p_i p_j)}{\sum_{i=1}^{m-1} \sum_{j=i+1}^{m} p_i (1 - p_j)} \tag{7.8}$$

H is not, itself, a statistic and Mokken recommends that a value of 0.3 is required before it can be claimed that the MH model describes the data. Mokken argues that 0.3–0.4 represents a weak fit and a strong fit requires that the H exceeds 0.5.

The second of Mokken's models is known as the Double Monotonicity (DM) model and this model assumes that the MH fits the data but also that the ICCs do not intersect. In order to test the DM model a number of rather convoluted, but relatively straight forward techniques are employed (see Sijtsma & Molenaar, 2002). However, one simple strategy worth mentioning here is to generate person fit coefficients. Simply put, if both the item and person H coefficients reveal a reasonable fit, then we can assume that the joint scale is indicated and so a cumulative structure exists (Sijtsma & Meijer, 1992).

Idiographic Caution Indices

Once it is established that a risk assessment checklist conforms to a cumulative scale, we may have confidence that an additive accumulation of the risk indicators to obtain a risk score is appropriate and psychometrically justified. However, this does not remove the issue of inconsistent profiles. Modelling the scale using normative data defines the normal or expected patterns of response, but it also allows us to identify deviations from these patterns that may be of clinical or forensic interest.

A wide range of approaches for identifying aberrant response profiles have been derived (Karabatsos, 2003; Tatsuoka, 1984) mostly within the educational context where concerns about cheating or guessing in educational tests was the prime motivator. These methods usually involve the use of misfit coefficients in which individual response profiles are evaluated against a particular psychometric model. Such coefficients are widely termed "caution indices" to reflect the fact that confidence in the total score should be dependent on the degree of idiosyncrasy in the manner it was arrived at.

In the context of testing in risk assessment spurious profiles may emerge because there may be insufficient information to make a concise judgement, the rater may make a careless mistake or the rater may have a biased view of the individual being assessed. Of course, these issues are mitigated if the risk assessment is part of a full case conference with multiple agency participation. However, even when these procedural artefacts are removed, there will be service-users who present an unusual profile, and the nature and extent of "unusual" can only be viewed against the backdrop of norm-based modelling.

Karabatsos (2003) identified 36 well-used person-fit coefficients many of which are specific to the particular psychometric model being used. In this chapter, we describe a general index for any of the three cumulative models described above. The Sato Caution Index, proposed by Sato (1980) and modified by Tatsuoka and Linn (1983), is calculated as:

Formula 9

$$SCI_i = \frac{\sum_{j=1}^{s} (1 - x_j) c_j - \sum_{j=s+1}^{m} x_j c_j}{\sum_{j=1}^{s} c_j - \sum_{j=m+1-s}^{m} c_j}$$ (7.9)

where x_j is the person's score for item j (1 = present, 0 = absent), c_j is the item total count for item j and s is the person's total score.

The SCI ranges between 0 and 1 and Sato suggests that a value of 0.5 indicates substantial deviation from expectation.

Application of Cumulative Modelling in Risk Assessment

The account above has been necessarily theoretical, we can finally turn to consider the applications of cumulative modelling within a risk assessment context. For most readers who are new to these ideas it may at first appear daunting to apply cumulative modelling to their data. Some will have been using a preferred risk assessment instrument quite happily but may feel it needs a psychometric review, while others may be contemplating development of a new bespoke tool for their service.

Evaluating an Existing Risk Assessment Instrument

Let us suppose that we have been using a risk assessment checklist for some time and we have gathered a large data set from our service users. We now wish to carry out a psychometric appraisal and, in particular, we hypothesise that it conforms to a cumulative model such that a simple summation is all that is required to generate a risk score. We decide to test this hypothesis by applying the Rasch model so we subject the data file to the requisite analysis (we give a brief description of freely available software below). Perhaps we find one or two checklist items do not fit the model but when we remove them we find a very good cumulative structure. Providing the remaining items can be shown to describe the domain in question, we can have confidence in our scale.

Developing Our Own Bespoke Risk Assessment Instrument

Developing one's own instrument may be time consuming and usually involves the following four steps:

1   Identify the risk indicators that will comprise the checklist. This is a largely qualitative process in which a deep understanding of the risk domain is assumed.

2   Generate a checklist using these indicators and gather a large sample that represents the client group.
3   Perform an actuarial analysis (often some form of regression analysis) to demonstrate the checklist's ability to predict a chosen outcome.
4   Form a final version of the checklist and subject it to a cumulative modelling analysis.

This may prove to be an iterative process in which the checklist is refined over a number of years. However, finally we find a measure we can be confident in.

Using Our Cumulative Risk Assessment Instrument

The typical application of a risk assessment checklist is to aggregate responses to each item to form a total score. As we mentioned above, this is usually done by simple summation. Once we can demonstrate that our checklist conforms to a cumulative scale, this way of generating the score is fully justified. Once we have an individual service-user's score we can place that person either along some risk continuum or, more commonly, into a usable risk category (e.g., high – medium – low) based upon an a priori normative based classifier.

However, a cumulative model also allows us to generate a caution score for each service user assessed. This provides an index of the degree of person-fit and is an indicator of how confident we can be in ascribing the risk score to that individual. If the misfit is high, we must conclude that the degree of risk of that individual cannot be confidently asserted without further investigation.

Misfit as an Index of Predictability

There are a number of possible reasons for an individual's misfit, but one in particular may be that they manifest very few low-level risk indicators but many more high-risk indicators. Because of regression to the mean, their score may place them in a medium risk category but once this is flagged by a high caution index the assessor can revisit the profile to discover that greater concern may be indicated. Essentially then, a high degree of misfit may signify unpredictability, which may moderate the risk assessors decision. Of course, not all misfit will lead to cause for concern but in signalling closer inspection of the case they can serve as aids for the decision making process.

Misfit as an Index of Model Adequacy in the Face of Diversity

The model parameters should have been built by using a large representative sample of service users. This implies that a diverse range of individuals comprise the normative sample. However, by definition, some minority groups may be under-represented in the normative data. Thus, when members of that minority group are assessed, it may be found that they manifest elevated misfit. This may be an indication of bias and suggests that the checklist has limited applicability to these cases.

In fact, the Rasch model is particularly well equipped to identify these biases due to the fact that it is based upon the principle of specific objectivity (Fischer,

1985). It may be that the risk assessor has a sample of people from the minority group in which case a Differential Item Functioning (DIF) analysis (Hagquist & Andrich, 2017) may be carried out to explore the item level differences between the normative and the minority groups. This may help in disentangling the differential meaning of the measure in the two groups (Hammond, 1995).

However, if such an analysis is not possible, the misfit score may be seen as an indicator of bias in the case of a minority service-user and may suggest a further refinement of the risk model being applied.

Example

We will now turn to an example in an attempt to clarify some of the issues discussed. The Risk Assessment Management and Audit System (RAMAS) was developed as a multiagency risk management system (O'Rourke et al., 1996) in community forensic settings. Part of this system is a risk checklist comprising 66 risk indicators for three areas of risk, Dangerousness (risk of harm to others), Self-Harm (risk of self-harm/suicide), and Mental Instability (risk of mental health crisis). The scores on the three risk facets are used to inform decisions regarding risk management. In developing the checklist, the cumulative structure of each facet was tested using the Mokken Scaling approach. This was followed up some time later using Rasch modelling. For illustration, we will consider the self-harm subscale which consists of nine risk indicators or items although initially ten items were used.

In Table 7.3, the Rasch analysis of the original ten-item self-harm scale is summarised. This was carried out on a sample of 621 service users from community forensic and probation services. There was a pretty good fit to this scale although one item, *Refuses Treatment*, manifested a substantial degree of misfit. In fact, that this item was subsequently excluded from the self-harm scale. When this is done the scale manifests a good fit to the cumulative Rasch model.

Table 7.3 Fitting self-harm to the Rasch model

Item	Item count	δ	S.E.	Fit
24. Risk to self	366	−1.455	0.229	−1.757
10. History of self-harm	330	−1.173	0.228	−1.988
8. Parasuicide history	272	−0.700	0.232	−0.789
30. Refuses treatment	225	−0.301	0.240	*4.068*
77. Feels undervalued	195	−0.034	0.248	1.535
62. Hopelessness	189	0.021	0.249	−0.919
46. Suicidal ideation	142	0.504	0.270	−1.056
73. Insomnia	106	0.935	0.296	−0.742
82. Evidence of self-harm	101	1.016	0.302	−0.555
35. Clinically depressed	89	1.187	0.316	−1.109

Note
Overall model fit including item 30 = 28.87 $p < 0.01$, reliability = 0.85.
Overall model fit excluding item 30 = 12.38 ns, reliability = 0.91.

The reliability for the reduced scale is 0.91. Of course, removing the item, *Refuses Treatment,* from the self-harm scale does not imply that it is to be removed from the overall checklist. The refusal of treatment is clearly a vital piece of information in risk appraisal and carries great weight when considering the management of the client/patient. However, it is, apparently, not a feature specific to self-harming and does not provide useful information in generating a self-harm risk score.

At this point then, we have established that the nine-item self-harm scale conforms to a cumulative scale, and we can generate a summative score with some confidence that it properly discriminates between the cases. Nevertheless, in an idiographic context, we still need to ascertain that any particular case is properly represented by the score.

For illustration, we consider the profiles for three clients, A, B, and C (all drawn from the probation sample). These are presented in Table 7.4.

Client A manifests four features relevant to the self-harm scales and so s/he obtains a simple raw score of 4. The Rasch analysis provides a statistically derived score which turns out to have the value 1.67. This may be interpreted as a z-score with a mean of zero and a standard deviation of 1. Thus person A has a relatively high score in normative terms. Sato's Caution Index can be estimated from the information available in Tables 7.3 and 7.4 using formula 7.9 (see Appendix A for a worked example). This results in a value of 0.11 which is well below the value of 0.5 that Sato suggests as a cut-off, so it is apparent that the misfit index for this person A is not problematic. On the other hand, person B has a lower score but manifests a concerning caution index of 0.92. Person C, on the other hand, has a very high score implying a high-risk case and we can be confident that this profile conforms closely to the model.

The implication here is that person C should be considered closely as there is strong evidence that they represent a clear risk. Person B reveals a pretty low

Table 7.4 Self-harm profile from three cases

Risk feature	A	B	C
Risk to self	1	0	1
History of self-harm	1	0	1
Parasuicide history	0	0	1
Feels undervalued	1	0	1
Hopelessness	1	0	1
Suicidal ideation	0	1	1
Insomnia	0	0	1
Evidence of self-harm	0	0	1
Clinically depressed	0	1	0
Raw score	4	2	8
Derived score	1.67	−0.11	**4.82**
Misfit	0.11	0.92	0.00

Note
1 represents the presence of the indicator.
0 represents the absence of the indicator.

score and would probably be considered a low-risk case. However, the misfit is extremely high and this should alert the clinician to look carefully at the profile as the predictability of this case is unclear. Indeed, this person may manifest a high self-harm risk because of the particular combination of the only two symptoms he manifests, *Suicidal Ideation* and *Clinical Depression.*

Thus the use of the cumulative measurement model goes beyond the simple identification of a score and provides in addition an index of caution that, in a risk assessment context might better be labelled an *Index of Concern.* This index serves as a warning to the clinician to look more closely at the profile presented. More often than not the misfitting individual, upon more detailed examination, will be assigned a low risk label (high misfit does not imply high risk) but the index is important in order to check the potential over-reliance upon a simple scale score

Overall Conclusion

Risk assessment requires collation of information from many sources and, in order to ascertain the transparency of the collation process, clear and precise models for integrating data need to be applied. In psychological practice these are invariably measurement models of some sort. Unfortunately, complacency has become a feature in psychological measurement (Michell, 1999) and this has militated against a considered understanding of this most fundamental aspect of our practice.

Understandably, many practitioners find the technical underpinnings of their craft to be outside their comfort zone. Nevertheless, they are content to utilise, either directly or vicariously, these techniques without question. Ill-considered and suboptimal methods of collating risk assessment data, not only result in failures in public safety and/or individual injustices but also ultimately impact upon the credibility and reputation of the psychological profession.

This chapter does not purport to answer all of these problems but rather attempts to identify limitations in one aspect of common practice in risk assessment and to alert readers to the need for a detailed evaluation some of the technical underpinnings of the enterprise. It is not safe practice to rely upon the simple summation of risk factors – often with a blithe mention of alpha coefficients – without a detailed appraisal of the cumulative nature of those risk factors is undertaken. It is not safe practice to assume that a risk score is equally meaningful for each person being assessed without a clear understanding of the potential biases that accrue for that individual. Retrospectively defensible practice requires appraisal of the technical detail as much as the practical methodology applied in any profession.

Some Final Notes

The Rasch and Mokken models described here are often subsumed under the label Item Response Theory (IRT). However, not all IRT models are cumulative. The most commonly used IRT model is known as a two-parameter model and this relaxes the assumption of non-intersecting ICCs. As such it is analogous to a parametric version of Mokken's MH model and cannot be considered a cumulative model. Within the IRT framework the Rasch model is often termed a one-parameter model and Mokken's models are termed a Non-Parametric IRT models (NPIRT).

Another point worth mentioning is that, throughout this discussion of cumulative models, we have assumed that the item response is dichotomous (True-False, Present-Absent, etc.). This was for didactic purposes and we have not forgotten that many instruments use ordinal response formats such as Likert scaling. The cumulative modelling procedures of Rasch and Mokken may be readily applied to such data although the models may take on further complexity. For example, the basic Rasch approach can be extended to include partial credit and rating scale models. These are beyond the brief of the current chapter but the interested reader is referred to Bond et al. (2020) for an accessible introduction.

Available Free Software

The techniques described here are widely available in many data analysis packages although many of these may come at a cost. However, there are a number of free programmes available. The most notable of these are the packages made available through R (https://www.r-project.org/). This is a hugely comprehensive system covering all aspects of data analysis and a very accessible guide to the psychometric packages is Mair (2018).

References

Appelbaum, P. S. (2005). Dangerous severe personality disorders: England's experiment in using psychiatry for public protection. *Psychiatric Services, 56*(4), 397–399.

Beckett, C. (2008). Risk uncertainty and thresholds. In Calder, M. (Ed.). *Contemporary risk assessment in safeguarding children* (p. 46). Lyme Regis: Russell House.

Bedford, A., Watson, R., Lyne, J., Tibbles, J., Davies, F., & Deary, I. J. (2009). Mokken scaling and principal components analyses of the CORE-OM in a large clinical sample. *Clinical Psychology and Psychotherapy, 17*(1), 51–62. 10.1002/cpp.649

Bond, T., Yan, T., & Heene, M. (2020). *Applying the Rasch model: Fundamental measurement in the human sciences.* London: Routledge.

Carnovale, M., Sellbom, M., & Bagby, R. M. (2020). The Personality Inventory for ICD-11: Investigating reliability, structural and concurrent validity, and method variance. *Psychological Assessment, 32*(1), 8–17. https://doi.org/10.1037/pas0000776

Carson, D., & Bain, A. (2008). *Professional risk and working with people.* London: Jessica Kingsley.

Coid, J. W., Yang, M., Ullrich, S., Zhang, T., Sizmur, S., Farrington, D. P., Freestone, M., & Rogers, R. D. (2015). Improving accuracy of risk prediction for violence: Does changing the outcome matter? *International Journal of Forensic Mental Health, 14*(1), 23–32. 10.1080/14999013.2014.974085

Coombs, C. H., Coombs, L. C., & Lingoes, J. C. (1978). Stochastic cumulative scales. In S. Shye (Ed.). *Theory construction and data analysis in the behavioral sciences.* San Francisco: Jossey-Bass.

Dawes, R. M., Faust, D. F., & Meehl, P. E. (1989). Clinical versus actuarial judgment. *Science, 243*, 1668–1674.

Debelak, R. (2019). An evaluation of overall goodness-of-fit tests for the Rasch model. *Frontiers in Psychology, 9*, 2710. 10.3389/fpsyg.2018.02710

DeMatteo, D., Batastini, A., Foster, E., & Hunt, E. (2010). Individualizing risk assessment: Balancing idiographic and nomothetic data. *Journal of Forensic Psychology Practice, 10*(4), 360–371. 10.1080/15228932.2010.481244

Douglas, T., Pugh, J., Singh, I. et al. (2017). Risk assessment tools in criminal justice and forensic psychiatry: the need for better data. *European Psychiatry, 42*, 134–137.

Dunn-Rankin, P. (2004). *Scaling methods.* 2nd ed. Mahwah, N.J.: Lawrence Erlbaum.

Embretson, S. E., & Hershberger, S. L. Eds. (1999). *The new rules of measurement: What every psychologist and educator should know.* Mahwah, NJ: Lawrence Erlbaum Associates Publishers.

Fischer, G. H. (1985). Some consequences of specific objectivity for the measurement of change. In E. E. Roskam (Ed.). *Measurement and personality assessment* (pp. 39–55). Amsterdam: North-Holland.

Fischer, G. H., & Molenaar, I. W. editors (1995). *Rasch models: foundations, recent developments, and applications.* (pp. 69–95). New York: Springer-Verlag.

Glas, C. A. W., & Verhelst, N. D. (1995). Testing the Rasch model. In Fischer, G. H., & Molenaar, I. W. (Eds.), *Rasch models: Foundations, recent developments, and applications.* (pp. 69–95). New York: Springer-Verlag.

Goodenough, W. H. (1944). A Technique for Scale Analysis. *Educational and Psychological Measurement, 4*, 179–190.

Goodman, L. A. (1975). A new model for scaling response patterns: An application of the quasi-independence concept. *Journal of the American Statistical Association, 70*, 755–768.

Green, B. F. (1956). A method of scalogram analysis using summary statistics. *Psychometrika, 21*, 79–88.

Grove, W. M., & Meehl, P. E. (1996). Comparative efficiency of informal (subjective impressionistic) and formal (mechanical, algorithmic) prediction procedures: The clinical-statistical controversy. *Psychology, Public Policy and Law, 2*(3), 293–323.

Guttman, L. (1944). A basis for scaling qualitative data. *American Sociological Review, 9*, 139–150.

Hagquist, C., & Andrich, D. (2017). Recent advances in analysis of differential item functioning in health research using the Rasch model. *Health Quality of Life Outcomes, 15*, 181. 10.1186/s12955-017-0755-0

Hammond, S. M. (1995). An IRT investigation of the validity of non-patient analogue research using the Beck Depression Inventory. *European Journal of Psychological Assessment, 11*(1), 14–20. 10.1027/1015-5759.11.1.14

Karabatsos, G. (2003). Comparing the aberrant response detection performance of thirty-six person-fit statistics. *Applied Measurement in Education, 16*(4), 277–298.

Keating, D. M., & Boster, F. J. (2019). Nonlinear unidimensionality in communication science: Tests, examples, and implications. *Communication Research Reports, 36*(1), 67–77. 10.1080/08824096.2018.1555524

Mair, P. (2018). *Modern psychometrics with R.* Cham: Springer.

McDonald, R. P. (1999). *Test theory: A unified treatment.* Mahwah, NJ: Lawrence Erlbaum Associates Publishers.

Meehl, P. E. (1954). *Clinical versus statistical prediction.* Minneapolis: University of Minnesota Press.

Michell, J. (1999). *Measurement in psychology: A critical history of a methodological concept.* Cambridge: Cambridge University Press.

Mokken, R. J. (1971). *A theory and procedure of scale analysis.* Berlin: De Gruyter.

O'Rourke, M., Hammond, S., Smith, S., & Davies, J. (1996). *Risk Assessment, Management and Audit System (RAMAS). Professional Manual.* Surrey: Heathlands Mental Health Trust.

Proctor, C. H. (1970). A probabilistic formulation and statistical analysis of Guttman scaling. *Psychometrika, 35,* 73–78.

Quinsey, V. L., Harris, G. T., Rice, M. E., & Cormier, L. A. (1998). *Violent offenders: Appraising and managing risk.* Washington, DC: American Psychological Association Press.

Rasch, G. (1960). *Probabilistic models for some intelligence and attainment tests.* Copenhagen: Nielsen & Lydiche.

Rasch, G. (1977). On specific objectivity: An attempt of formalizing the generality and validity of scientific statements. *Danish Yearbook of Philosophy, 14,* 58–94.

Reed, J. (1997). Risk assessment and clinical risk management: The lessons from recent inquiries. *British Journal of psychiatry, 170,* 4–7.

Richie, J. H., Dick, D., & Lingham, R. (1994). *The report of the inquiry in the care and treatment of Christopher Clunis.* London: HMSO.

Sato, T. (1980). The S-P chart and the caution index, Tokyo, Japan: *NEC Educational Information Bulletin,* 80–1, C & C Systems Research Laboratories, Nippon Electric Co., Ltd.

Shepherd, S. M, & Lewis-Fernandez, R. (2016). Forensic risk assessment and culturaldiversity - contemporary challenges and future directions. *Psychol Public Policy Law, 22,* 427–438.

Sijtsma, K., & Meijer, R. R. (1992). A Method for Investigating the Intersection of Item Response Functions in Mokken's Nonparametric IRT Model. *Applied Psychological Measurement, 16*(2), 149–157. 10.1177/014662169201600204

Sijtsma, K., & Molenaar, I. W. (2002). *Introduction to nonparametric item response theory.* Thousand Oaks, CA: SAGE Publications.

Singh, J. P., Desmarais, S. L., Hurducas, C., Arbach-Lucioni, K., Condemarin, C., Dean, K., Doyle, M., Folino, J. O., Godoy-Cervera, V., Grann, M., & Ho, R. M. (2014). International perspectives on the practical application of violence risk assessment: A global survey of 44 countries. *International Journal of Forensic Mental Health, 13,* 193–206.

Siontis, G. C. M., Tzoulaki, I., Castaldi, P. J., & Ioannidis, J. P. A. (2015). External validation of new risk prediction models is infrequent and reveals worse prognostic discrimination. *Journal of Clinical Epidemiology, 68,* 25–34.

Tatsuoka, K. K. (1984). Caution indices based on item response theory. *Psychometrika, 49,* 95–110. 10.1007/BF02294208

Tatsuoka, K. K., & Linn, R. L. (1983). Indices for detecting unusual patterns: Links between two general approaches and potential applications. *Applied Psychological Measurement, 7*(1), 81–96.

van der Ark, L. A. (Andries) (2012). New developments in Mokken scale analysis in R. *Journal of Statistical Software, 48*(5). 10.18637/jss.v048.i05

van Schuur, W. (2003). Mokken scale analysis: Between the Guttman scale and parametric item response theory. *Political Analysis, 11*(2), 139–163. 10.1093/pan/mpg002

Walker, D. A. (1931). Answer-pattern and score-scatter in tests and examinations. *British Journal of Psychology, 22,* 73–86.

World Health Organisation (WHO). (1993). *The ICD-10 classification of mental and behavioural disorders.* Geneva: WHO.

Appendix A: Worked Example of Sato's Caution Index

We will work through the example using person A in Table 7.4. We will also use the item counts from Table 7.3. Firstly, we order the items according to their frequency with the most frequently endorsed item at position 1 and the item with the lowest frequency at position m (where *m* is the number of items).

For our example the item frequencies c_j are as follows:

366, 330, 272, 195, 189, 142, 106, 101, 89

For person A the response profile x_i is:

1	1	0	1	1	0	0	0	0

Person A has a score of 4 this is the value for *s*.

The formula for Sato's Caution Index shown above can be broken down into four terms.

$$T1 = \sum_{j=1}^{s} (1 - x_j)c_j$$

Term 1 takes the first *s* items and takes the sum of the products of 1 minus the item response and the item count.

$(1 - 1) \times 366 + (1 - 1) \times 330 + (1 - 0) \times 272 + (1 - 1) \times 195$ which equals 272.

$$T2 = \sum_{j=s+1}^{m} x_j c_j$$

For term 2 we take the last $(m - 4)$ items and calculate the sum of the products of the item response and the item count

$(1 \times 189) + (0 \times 142) + (0 \times 106) + (0 \times 101) + (0 \times 89)$ which equals 189.

$$T3 = \sum_{j=1}^{s} c_j$$

Term 3 is simply the sum of the item counts for the first *s* items:

366 + 330 + 272 + 195 which equals 1163.

$$T4 = \sum_{j=m+1-s}^{m} c_j$$

For term 4 we must solve $(m + 1 - s)$ which, in this case is $9 + 1 - 4 = 6$. We then calculate the sum of the sixth to the ninth item count:

$142 + 106 + 101 + 89$ which equals 438.

The caution index can now be calculated as:

$$SCI = \frac{T1 - T2}{T3 - T4} = \frac{272 - 189}{1163 - 438} = \frac{83}{725} = 0.114$$

This may seem a bit arduous by hand but it is a pretty trivial task to generate some code to do this.

8 What Works in the Digital Age? VR and Smartphone Applications for Forensic Psychology

Aniek M. Siezenga, Jean-Louis van Gelder, and Job van der Schalk

What Works in the Digital Age? VR and Smartphone Applications for Forensic Psychology

Forensic psychology lies at the intersection of criminal justice and mental health care (Vollm et al., 2018). Its main goal is to reduce the chance of re-cidivism and address treatment targets in relation to offence-related factors and psychiatric disorders (Kip et al., 2018; Vollm et al., 2018). The forensic po-pulation is characterised by various risk factors for recidivism, such as high psychiatric comorbidity (Fazel & Danesh, 2002; Van der Veeken et al., 2018), relatively low treatment motivation (Drieschner & Boomsma, 2008; Kip et al., 2019b) and low cognitive abilities (Kip et al., 2019b). The combination of these risk factors makes the forensic population both hard to reach and difficult to treat, which is reflected in high reoffending rates (Bengtson et al., 2019). As risk factors are diverse, the use of individualised therapy is essential for treatment efficacy (Bonta & Andrews, 2007). Implementing technology in treatment can support individualised therapy (Kip et al., 2019b). Furthermore, when applied in the right way, technology could reduce bias and increase inclusivity. Therefore, technologies could enhance the forensic field in the main elements of care: risk assessment, offender rehabilitation, and reintegration (Bonta & Andrews, 2007; Vollm et al., 2018). Two forms of eHealth with the potential for application with a forensic population include Virtual Reality (VR) and applications for mobile devices ("smartphone apps"). Both are discussed in this chapter.

VR has several features that can make it a valuable addition to the forensic psychology toolkit. In this chapter, we focus on immersive VR (also referred to as IVR) which is generally experienced through a head-mounted display (HMD) (Fox et al., 2009). For research and assessment purposes VR provides advantages over current methods. Among others, VR enables objective data gathering and standardised treatment, resulting in less biased and more individualised assessment. Consider roleplay exercises, which generally take place with real actors. Confederates or trained actors' verbal and non-verbal behaviour may cause unintentional variation in the treatment and they may vary in terms of

DOI: 10.4324/9781003230977-9

appearance and physique, dress, non-verbal cues, et cetera. All these aspects can be standardised using VR. Additionally, in VR, an avatar's or participant's characteristics (e.g., gender, age, skin colour, weight) can be experimentally changed and tailored to the needs of the specific target population.

Furthermore, clinical VR where simulated interactive learning environments are created that are difficult to realise in real life has been shown to be a powerful therapeutic tool (Hamilton et al., 2021). In these virtual settings, behaviour change can be supported without endangering others (Cornet & Van Gelder, 2020; Farley, 2018). Since VR environments are adaptive and do not require well-developed imaginative, verbal and cognitive skills, they can be tailored to the needs of diverse populations. Hence, they are an inclusive and engaging form of treatment compared to more conventional approaches and have the potential to be accepted by offenders (Kip et al., 2019b).

Smartphones have their own set of unique features. In the previous two decades smartphones have become an accessible and user-friendly form of technology with potential for research and intervention. Smartphone devices contain cameras, have GPS, internet connectivity, and various sensors (Miller, 2012). In addition, many different kinds of software applications can be run on these devices. Such features allow for efficient and individualised data collection, for example by registering participants' real-time location anywhere in the world, and administering interactive tests at any time of day (Kuntsche & Labhart, 2013; Miller, 2012). Furthermore, the potential of smartphones for forensic psychology extends to new possibilities for interventions, for example through serious gaming and via "portable" therapy (Bakker et al., 2016; Linardon et al., 2019). In addition, smartphones offer novel possibilities to engage with individuals living in remote areas or residential settings and provide opportunities to bring help and assistance within easier reach for a broader, and therefore more diverse, audience.

To summarise, both VR and apps can enhance treatment engagement and motivation (Kip et al., 2019b; Klein Tuente et al., 2020; Ticknor, 2019) and be tailored to individual user needs. Furthermore, both allow for objective data collection, which can reduce implicit bias in assessment. In addition, for an incarcerated population, VR and apps can support digital resocialisation. Yet, despite their potential, forensic psychology has not yet fully embraced the possibilities that these technologies offer (Cornet & Van Gelder, 2020; Kip et al., 2018; Ross, 2018; Ticknor, 2018). Our goal is twofold. First, we aim to provide a state-of-the-art review of smartphone and VR applications in forensic science. This updates the review for VR by Cornet and colleagues (2019). Second, we show the potential of these technologies beyond the current state of the art. Below, we start out with presenting the findings of our review.

Results

This review yielded 18 VR applications and 18 smartphone apps (see Tables 8.1 and 8.2 for details on the literature search). Based on these results, we conclude

Table 8.1 Search methods and eligibility criteria

The literature search included the databases of Web of Science, PsycINFO, PubMed, and Scopus in June 2021.

For VR, we replicated the search used in a previous review with the same keywords and databases (Cornet et al., 2019). We then conducted a similar search for apps. We used the following search terms: ("virtual reality" OR "augmented reality") / ("mobile app*") AND (judicial*, forensic*, crim*, delinquen*, aggress*, antisocial*, externali?ing, impuls*, violen*, prison*, "conduct disorder", psychopath*, offend*, detention, jail, parole, probation, victim*, police, "offender assessment", "offender correction", "offender rehabilitation").

To include VR and smartphone applications that were not reported on in scientific publications, we also conducted a web search with the Google Search Engine with keywords related to technology ("virtual reality" / "mobile app") in combination with a simpler search string of keywords related to a forensic population (e.g., "prison"/ "offender"/ "delinquent"). Finally, additional applications were located through browsing the reference sections of relevant articles.

Studies were selected if they were published in English or Dutch, and researched or described either VR or smartphone applications developed for or validated by a forensic population.

Table 8.2 Study selection

For VR, 3426 references were initially identified in the scientific databases. After duplicates were removed, this number was reduced to 2593. All references were screened by title and abstracts, which excluded a further 2542 articles. After selection, the remaining full-length articles were retrieved for further analysis resulting in the exclusion of another 41 studies. In total ten studies met the criteria to be included in this review. The web search yielded an additional eight VR applications, leading to final selection of 18 VR applications. For a schematic overview of the VR search, see Figure 8.1.

For smartphone apps, 1492 references were initially retrieved through the databases, which was reduced to 1204 after removing duplicates. After titles and abstracts were screened for eligibility, 39 articles were selected for further consideration. A total of six studies met the inclusion criteria and were included in this review. The web search yielded an additional 12 smartphone applications, leading to a total of 18 smartphone apps. For a schematic overview of the search see Figure 8.2.

---

that (1) the development and implementation of VR and smartphone applications for forensic populations are still in their infancy, but interest is increasing; (2) most VR applications have been developed for rehabilitation, whereas most smartphone apps have been developed for reintegration; and (3) scientific research investigating the effectiveness, feasibility and usability of VR and smartphone applications is scarce. Below we present an overview of the opportunities these technologies offer for supporting risk assessment, offender rehabilitation, and reintegration.

Method

Risk Assessment

VR for Risk Assessment

Forensic risk assessment refers to the process of predicting and evaluating the likelihood of future offending (Brown & Singh, 2014; Singh & Fazel, 2010). This involves the routine examination of individual, social, or contextual factors (Bogaerts et al., 2017; Brown & Singh, 2014).

VR offers several opportunities for forensic risk assessment. Firstly, exposing an individual to a virtual risk scenario does not pose actual risk to others or the user. Secondly, VR can provide insight into criminal decision-making processes which are usually covert due to the illegal nature of crime (Cornet & Van Gelder, 2020; Fromberger et al., 2018; Kip et al., 2019b). Thirdly, the lack of restrictions as to the kinds of different environments that can be developed allows for a wide

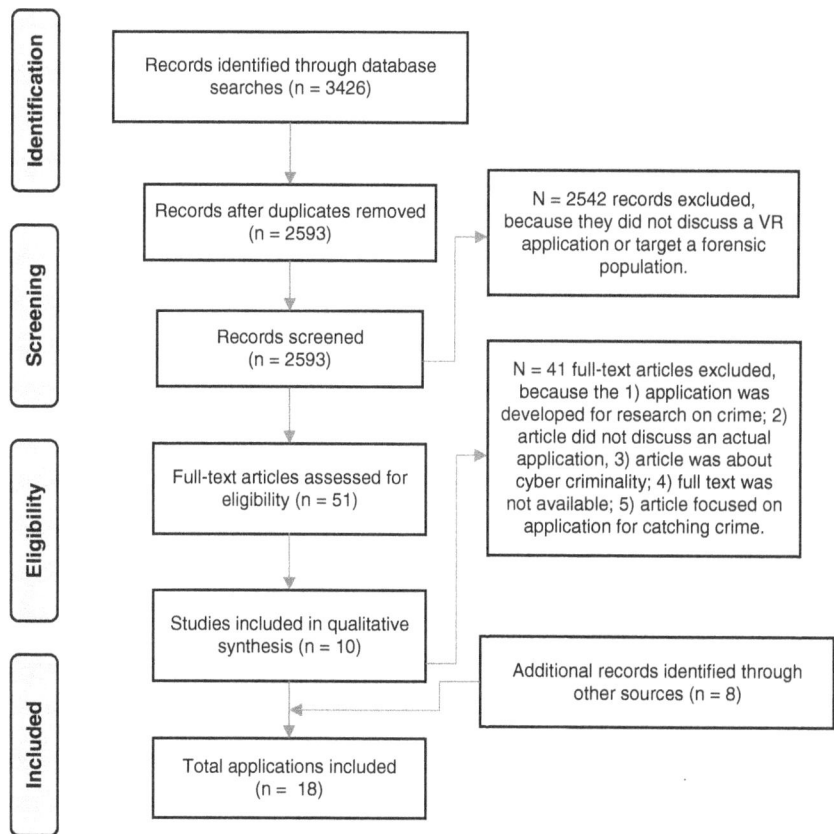

Figure 8.1 Schematic overview of the VR search.

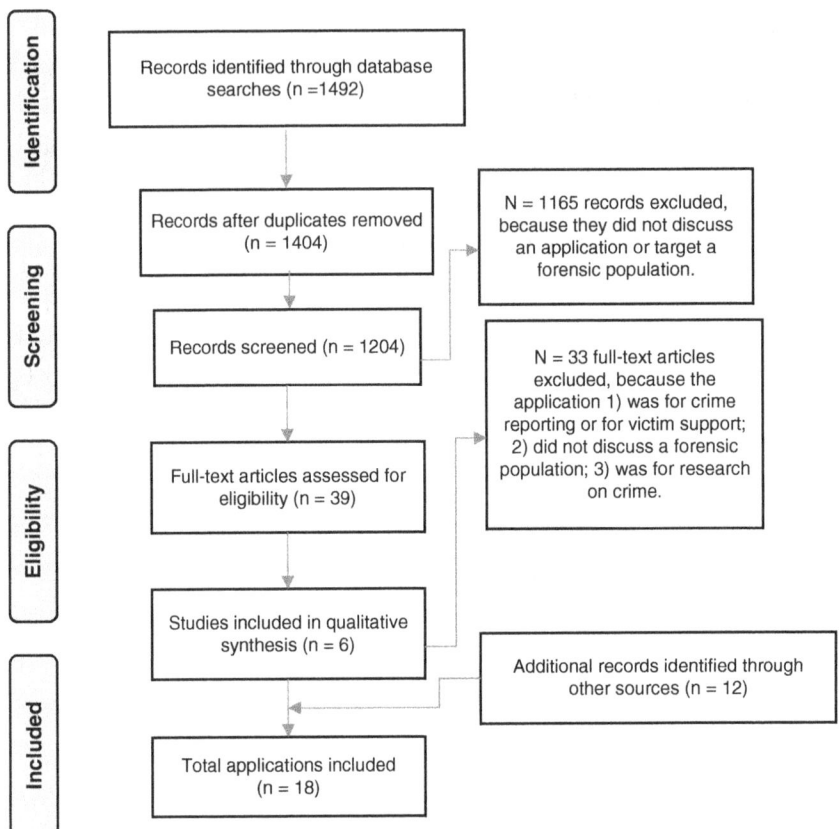

Figure 8.2 Schematic overview of the app search.

range of criminogenic situations to be assessed. Fourthly, VR offers high levels of researcher control. Besides the ability to test individualised scenarios, this enables exposing participants to the same virtual environment (VE) thus enabling highly standardised observation. Fifthly, VR allows for the measurement of physiological responses, which facilitates detailed measurement of behaviour (e.g., movement, eye gaze; see Nee et al. (2019) and Park & Lee (2021). Therefore, VR can provide a more thorough evaluation of behaviour, physiological processes and criminal decision-making processes (Parsey & Schmitter-Edgecombe, 2013). This may improve ecological validity of risk assessment and reduce implicit bias (Fromberger et al., 2014; Parsey & Schmitter-Edgecombe, 2013; Rizzo et al., 2000), because physiological measurements do not require data linked to individual factors as race or socioeconomic status (Haarsma et al., 2020).

Despite these advantages, the use of VR for risk assessment is still in its infancy. The located VR risk assessment tools and applications (see Table 8.3) make use of the advantages of VR in different ways. They share the aim to gain

Table 8.3 VR applications for risk assessment

Application/ authors	Target population	Goal	Description
(Renaud et al., 2014)	Sex offenders	Study the capacity of VR for the assessment of sexual profiles.	The erectile response of 22 sex offenders and 42 controls was measured with supplementary physiological measurements (penile plethysmography [PPG]) while they listened to audio stimuli and while immersed in a VE watching computer-generated avatars of males, females, boys and girls.
(Fromberger et al., 2018)	Sexual offenders against children (SOCs)	Study to investigate whether monitoring SOCs in virtual risk situations will yield additional information for risk assessment.	SOCs and non-offender controls walked through three VEs and were confronted with a virtual child character. They could choose to engage in approach or avoidance behaviour.
What's up? (Creemers, 2020)	Juveniles that enter residential youth institutions	Improve screening of juveniles in forensic care, optimise receiving the right treatment and test if VR can support forensic risk assessment among juveniles.	Neurobiological measurements are assessed in a VE to evaluate among others cognitive flexibility, pro-social behaviour, dealing with authority and pro-active aggression.
Virtual Reality Aggression Assessment (VRAA) (Sappelli et al., n.d.)	People with reactive aggression	Develop a VR assessment tool for reactive aggression.	Provoking scenarios are presented to people in order to reliably assess reactive aggression.

insight into decision-making processes but differ in the type of criminogenic environment they use for that purpose. These range from neutral environments like a supermarket (Fromberger et al., 2018), to provoking scenarios intended to trigger delinquent behaviour (Klein Tuente et al., 2020; Sappelli et al., n.d.; Smeijers & Koole, 2019). Furthermore, most of the located VR assessments only use virtual environments (VEs) to observe behaviour rather than supplementing VR with physiological measurements for objectively measuring behaviour. For example, to date only one research group used additional measurement equipment in their VR assessment of those convicted of sexual offences (Renaud et al., 2014).

VR offers a wide range of untapped opportunities for supporting forensic risk assessment. For example, supplementing VR assessment with additional equipment (e.g., to measure brain activity, heart rate, and/or skin conductance) may provide a more comprehensive image of behaviour and decision-making processes. Additionally, gamification can be used to make the assessment more interactive, attractive, and engaging. However, methods to quantify observed behaviour must be developed in order to be able to use VR for assessment purposes. In addition, even though research has shown that behaviour displayed in VR seems to correlate with how participants would behave in real-life (Fromberger et al., 2018; Nee et al., 2019; Renaud et al., 2013; Renaud et al., 2014), it is important to remain cautious about the generalisability of virtual forensic risk assessment to the real world. This generalisability depends on a series of factors, including the type of risk factor involved, the quality and character of the VR instrument, and the type of behaviour and offender under study. Until the external validity and diagnostic value of a specific risk assessment instrument has been unambiguously assessed, no claims towards generalisability can be made.

Smartphone Apps for Risk Assessment

In general, existing forensic risk assessment methods will occur in a clinical setting and are often dependent on retrospective self-reports. As retrospective self-reports cannot reliably capture fluctuations in behaviour, current methods appear restricted in how well they measure real-world behaviour (Parsey & Schmitter-Edgecombe, 2013). Compared to traditional forensic risk assessments, and also VR-based assessment, smartphones carry a number of advantages. Firstly, smartphones are an accessible and user-friendly technology that most people carry with them throughout the day. Secondly, smartphones have an extensive research potential, because they are equipped with a set of sensors (e.g., GPS, microphone, accelerometer, gyroscope) and features that can collect information about their user and their environment (Miller, 2012). The combination of these two characteristics enables efficient and frequent (even continuous) data collection in real time (e.g., ecological momentary assessments (EMA); Shiffman et al., 2008). These data can be collected in the user's natural living environment without temporal or spatial restrictions (Van Gelder, 2020), which reduces bias and increases ecological validity (Russell & Gajos, 2020; Shiffman et al., 2008).

However, developing apps for risk assessment and testing their effectiveness is challenging considering data can be affected by smartphones changing hands, and privacy and ethical issues (Keusch et al., 2019; Nicholas et al., 2019). In addition, even though computerised measurements make people feel more anonymous and therefore seem to reduce social desirability bias (Richman et al., 1999), a certain risk of social desirability when collecting data unsupervised cannot be excluded. The challenges in developing apps for forensic risk assessment are reflected in the limited number of apps for this specific purpose. There also seems to be a lack of apps targeted at the forensic population that use EMA methods to passively collect data through smartphone sensors.

Two of the forensic risk assessment apps that our review identified, QoL-ME and The *Zelfscore App* (see Table 8.4), have been developed to facilitate self-management for service users who wish to gain more insight into themselves and their progress. Therefore, these apps are self-report-based and require active user input.

Additionally, to actively collect self-report data, apps offer wider opportunities for forensic risk assessment (Areàn et al., 2016; Bush et al., 2019). Firstly, apps can include tasks or games which assess behaviour (e.g., neurological tasks or serious games) (Sobolev et al., 2021). Preliminary results even suggest that app-based serious games can predict reoffending or psychiatric relapse with predictive accuracy similar to commonly used risk assessments. Haarsma et al. (2020) developed a gamified set of neurocognitive tests administered on a tablet. To predict the chance of reoffending, test results were analysed with machine learning methods. Due to only neurocognitive input being required to predict recidivism levels, implicit bias and confounds of static factors (e.g., criminal history) are limited (Haarsma et al., 2020; Ormachea et al., 2016). Secondly, apps can collect data in an unobtrusive and highly individualised way (Parsey & Schmitter-Edgecombe, 2013). For example, smartphones can collect data on physical activity (accelerometers and pedometers), social network (Bluetooth, messaging services, or number of phone calls), sleep patterns (screen interaction), stress levels (additional wearables such as breast or wrist bands), and psychological well-being (facial emotion recognition through the front camera). Passively collecting such data enables evaluating the connection between measured factors (Russell & Gajos, 2020).

Offender Rehabilitation

VR for Rehabilitation

Treatment of patients in forensic settings focuses both on reducing criminogenic factors and treating psychiatric problems related to antisocial behaviour (Bonta & Andrews, 2007). For the efficacy of offender rehabilitation, it is essential to engage service users in their treatment and to support the transfer of cognitive skills to behaviour (Andrews & Bonta, 2010; Bonta & Andrews, 2007).

VEs have several characteristics that render them well-suited for training self-regulation skills and learning prosocial behaviour. Firstly, in VEs a situation can

Table 8.4 Smartphone applications for risk assessment

Application/ authors	Target population	Goal	Description
(McLoughlin et al., 2021)	Nursing staff on an all-male inpatient acute forensic psychiatry unit	Assess the internal and predictive validity of a mobile app risk assessment tool.	Developed for staff to assess risk of aggression. The app is based on the dynamic appraisal of situational aggression (DASA) risk assessment tool.
QoL-ME (Buitenweg et al., 2019)	People with severe mental health problems	Develop an app for quality of life (QoL) assessment.	An innovative, personalised, and visual app for QoL assessment. People treated in forensic psychiatry were involved in the development of the app.
Zelfscore App [self-score app] (Ter Horst et al., 2016)	Adult forensic inpatients	Make clients more aware of treatment goals and progress, and support shared decision making between inpatients and therapists.	Inpatients answer a combination of questions about different risk factors for reoffending. The results are visualised to map on in which domain progress has been made and which domain continues to carry risks.

be experienced that would otherwise involve risk, contain prohibitive ethical implications, or be impossible to create in real-life (Cornet & Van Gelder, 2020). Secondly, VEs can realistically reflect the real world, thus they do not pose high demands on imaginative skills, which may support transfer of skills learned in treatment to real life. In addition, it is important to consider that for VEs to realistically reflect the world of a diverse population as the forensic population, they must allow for a high level of customisation (e.g., VEs reflecting different kind of neighbourhoods, body types, gender identities, and skin colours). Thirdly, VR seems to provide higher self-reflectiveness compared to memory or imagination (Riva et al., 2016; Ventura et al., 2021). For example, individuals can embody another avatar in VR to increase perspective taking abilities (Ventura et al., 2021) and empathy levels (Schutte & Stilinović, 2017; Seinfeld et al., 2018; Ventura et al., 2021). Fourthly, the immersive character of VR and the possibilities of interaction and gamification are likely to be experienced as engaging (Klein Tuente et al., 2020; Ticknor, 2019), which supports therapy adherence and may reduce treatment drop-out (Andersson et al., 2018; Evans et al., 2009).

Multiple VR applications for offender rehabilitation have been developed (see Table 8.5). All of these focus on individual learning exercises, with aims ranging from learning practical skills (e.g., Virtual Mechanic) to aggression regulation skills (e.g., VR Aggression Prevention Training or VRAPT). Furthermore, there are differences in the methods used to achieve behaviour change. For example, VR-GAIME includes gamification, where Seinfeld et al. (2018) and FutureU include perspective changing exercises. Despite the variety in VR interventions for offender rehabilitation, only a limited number of efficacy studies have been undertaken. Two recent RCTs have been unable to prove the effectiveness of the VR interventions under study (Klein Tuente et al., 2020; Smeijers & Koole, 2019). More research is needed in different forensic settings (e.g., outpatient settings), with multiple research outcomes (e.g., behaviour and skills in social situations, treatment motivation, or emotion recognition) (Klein Tuente et al., 2020), different VEs, and with other behavioural change theories underlying the intervention. Furthermore, since technology as VR is suited for establishing virtual social connection, the potential of group learning could be explored. Especially for incarcerated populations the added value could be assessed of offering virtual group sessions, or virtually involving family members and peers to engage the offender's network in treatment.

Smartphone Apps for Rehabilitation

Whereas VR offers a safe environment for practicing skills and behaviour, this environment is generally physically bound to the treatment setting. To be able to continue the learning process beyond the treatment setting, smartphones could be used. Since these devices have become part of the daily routines of many, they offer unique advantages for delivering interventions (Stieger et al., 2018). They are accessible from almost anywhere and at any time. Therefore, they can reduce barriers to treatment adoption, increase acceptance of interventions, and

Table 8.5 VR applications for offender rehabilitation

Application/ authors	Target population	Goal	Description
Virtual reality aggression prevention training (VRAPT) (Klein Tuente et al., 2020)	Forensic psychiatric inpatients with low aggression regulation skills	Reduce reactive aggression.	In multiple guided interactive VE's forensic psychiatric inpatients are confronted with provocative social scenarios to practice aggression regulation skills.
"Vergeet mij niet" [Don't forget about me] (Enliven, n.d.)	Offenders of domestic violence	Enhance empathy, awareness, and behaviour change.	In 360° VR, domestic violence offenders take the perspective of a seven-year-old boy witnessing his parents arguing and physically fighting.
(Seinfeld et al., 2018)	Offenders of domestic violence	Test if changing perspective through immersive VR can change emotion recognition.	Participants take the perspective of a female and experience being a victim of domestic abuse.
Virtual Environment for the Treatment of Offenders (VETO) (Ticknor, 2017)	Juvenile offenders	Evaluate how VR can be deployed in juvenile correctional rehabilitation.	Juvenile offenders learn social coping skills in a cognitive behaviour-based VR group therapy, by controlling avatars in different VEs.
VR-Game for Aggression Impulse Management (VR-GAIME) (Smeijers & Koole, 2019)	Forensic psychiatric outpatients with aggression regulation problems	Reduce aggression.	This serious game targets implicit processes that are related to aggression. People have to avoid angry looking avatars and approach friendly looking avatars.
VR at De Waag (De Waag, 2020)	Forensic outpatients	Enhance social skills and regulation skills, get used to VR, practice meeting other people, and enhance perspective taking.	Three VR exercises are used in treatment: "Role plays" for enhancing social and regulation skills, "Walking around" to get used to VR, and "Changing perspectives" to enhance empathy and empathising skills (Hutten et al., 2021).

Virtual Mechanic (Collins et al., 2020; McLauchlan & Farley, 2019)	Prisoners with low literacy and numeracy skills	Improving learner engagement and progress with a VE.	A literacy and numeracy programme is contextualised within a virtual mechanic's workshop. Learners must identify various car parts, tools and features, manipulate components and follow instructions.
(Innovative Prison Systems, 2017)	Prisoners	Offender rehabilitation.	Various VR services, including formal education, vocational job training, and psychological rehabilitation.
FutureU (Van Gelder et al., 2022)	Young adult offenders	Enhance vividness of the future self and long-term thinking abilities, and reduce self-defeating behaviour.	Participants set goals and virtually travel through time to give advice from the perspective of their future self who had already achieved the goal.
Volver a Casa [Going Back Home] (Alarcón, 2020)	Inmates from different prisons	Give access to technology and to use VR as a bridge between the exterior and interior of prisons.	One of the work areas of Volver a Casa is connecting inmates with their family by having them virtually visit their homes in 360° VR.

enhance access to care (Zhang et al., 2015), either by providing stand-alone interventions, or by extending the reach of existing treatment methods (e.g., the My Companion App, see Table 8.6). Furthermore, app-based interventions can be highly individualised (Stieger et al., 2018) and offered at the right moment and place (ecological momentary interventions or EMIs; Heron & Smyth, 2010). Additionally, apps may improve transfer of skills acquired during treatment because interventions can be accessed and delivered in real time and in the natural living environment of the user (Heron & Smyth, 2010).

The apps that the current review yielded offer both EMIs that need to be actively accessed by users (e.g., chatting in the FutureU app), and EMIs that passively emerge (e.g., the GRiP app noticing heightened stress levels). However, even though smartphones contain sensors and features that can be used for EMA and EMI (e.g., accelerometers, GPS, and Bluetooth), the currently available apps only use a few of them. GPS is used in A-CHESS and BFO to locate the user and provide EMIs when the user enters a risk area. GRiP uses the microphone of the user's smartphone to capture their voice volume and external sensors (a heart or wrist band) to measure their heart rate variability. Furthermore, only a few apps offer educational and health care modules (e.g., A-CHESS and BFO), and they focus mostly on substance abuse.

To make better use of smartphones' potential for providing interventions for offender rehabilitation, intervention modules which focus on other aspects of behaviour change aside from addiction need to be developed. Another recommendation would be to further explore the possibilities of EMIs that use sensors and features to passively collect data. Offering support at the right moment and at the right place can assist a forensic population during stressful or risky situations. For example, through pre-programmed prompts or by offering the option of calling a therapist or peer. In such a manner, EMIs could afterwards support evaluating these risk situations to promote learning and support prevention. Therefore, it is worth looking into the possibilities of apps for offender rehabilitation and into the acceptance, feasibility, and usability of such interventions.

Reintegration

VR for Reintegration

Reintegration involves the process of re-entering society after having served a prison sentence or when released from a residential psychiatric institution. Empirical research into what elements and combinations of reintegration services prove most successful in reducing recidivism is scarce (Wormith et al., 2007). Since reintegration support and continuity of mental health treatment is often essential for preventing relapse and recidivism (Graffam et al., 2004; Ventura et al., 1998), support must necessarily enhance continuity of care and bridge the gap between life in prison and life on release. VR can reduce this gap in two ways. Firstly, VR can provide a realistic glimpse of the outside world while still in

Table 8.6 Smartphone applications for offender rehabilitation

Application / authors	Target population	Goal	Description
Goede Reactie is Preventie [Good reaction is prevention] (Hoogsteder et al., 2018)	Adult forensic psychiatric patients with aggression regulation problems, a high amount of arousal or stress, and low control skills	Learn to recognise stress and anger, and learn to monitor and control these feelings.	Biomarkers (wrist bands, breast bands or smartwatches) can be connected to the app to measure heart rate variability. The microphone measures voice volume. When stress levels or voice volume above certain values that are measured, the app offers an intervention.
A-CHESS (Gustafson et al., 2014; Johnson et al., 2016)	People suffering with alcohol addiction	Achieve and maintain recovery and prevent relapse in people suffering with alcohol addiction.	People have access to different kind of educational modules, GPS locates risk areas and will provide a micro intervention when the user is near a risk area. Weekly surveys gain information regarding well-being.
Breaking Free Online (BFO) – My Companion App (Elison et al., 2016)	For substance addicts. The programme was adapted to an internet-based intervention for substance-involved offenders	Strengthen resilience and build tools for recovery.	Different kinds of modules in the app support the BFO programme and help the user desist from substance misuse by providing relaxation exercises and EMIs if users enter risk areas.
Self-Control Training (SCT) app (Kip et al., 2021)	Populations with aggression regulation problems	Study if self-control could be improved and aggression be decreased via an app.	Users are asked to perform daily activities with their non-dominant hand.
FutureU (Mertens et al., 2022)	Young adult offenders	Reduce self-defeating behaviour by enhancing future orientation.	Consists of various modules: a gamified chat conversation with an aged avatar of the user, a time travel portal to take the perspective of your future self, and an implementation intention exercise.

custody. By virtually being exposed to the outside world, prisoners might be better prepared for what life looks like on the outside. Secondly, VR can support preparation for re-entry into the community by providing opportunities for practicing common "all-round" skills (e.g., opening a bank account; Dolven & Fidel, 2017) and learning how to avoid potential risk situations (e.g., how to reject an offer of drugs; Teng & Gordon, 2021).

The use of VR to support reintegration is already being explored, as is reflected in the various types of VR applications that this review yielded. Various prisons have implemented VR programmes to prepare for life after release (see Table 8.7). They offer virtual practice environments, ranging from navigating public transportation to shopping at a self-scan supermarket (Dolven & Fidel, 2017). By practicing these skills in a realistic and individualised environment, digital resocialisation is supported and offenders are better prepared for life after release, therefore reducing the gap between prison and society.

However, research investigating the effectiveness of using VR during reintegration is lacking. Since immersion in realistic looking scenarios (e.g., when practicing how to deal with risk situations after release) could potentially trigger traumas (Teng & Gordon, 2021), research is needed to avoid counterproductive effects.

Smartphone Apps for Reintegration

Since apps can be accessed at any place and any time they can function as a useful tool for assisting reintegration by supporting service users on probation. The majority of apps that the current review has yielded have been developed for the purpose of reintegration (see Table 8.8). Two types of reintegration apps can be broadly distinguished. Firstly, apps exist that function as an extended form of probation supervision. These apps can replace electronic ankle bracelets and reduce the number of physical check-ins, for example, by offering mobile check-ins with the probation officer and by providing probationers with Bluetooth breathalysers to measure alcohol levels at a distance (e.g., Outreach Smartphone Monitoring or OSM). Secondly, apps have been developed with the specific aim to facilitate the reintegration process without active supervision. To achieve the latter goal, apps can offer various possibilities, for example, gamification (e.g., MyNeon), or by offering educational modules (e.g., StaySafe and Mobile-Enhanced Prevention Support or MEPS), mental health support and crisis support (e.g., Utsikt and Changing Lives).

The reintegration apps we identified mostly provide educational modules or mental health support, which need to be actively accessed in the app. Ideally, reintegration apps should also contain EMA and provide EMI based on these data to facilitate continuity of care during reintegration. In addition, research on the uptake, feasibility, usability, and effectiveness of reintegration apps is lacking. Therefore, it would be valuable to study if probation officers and service users perceive the apps as useful, and if the apps support reducing recidivism.

Table 8.7 VR applications for reintegration

Application/ authors	Target population	Goal	Description
Colorado Prison Programme	Inmates convicted as juveniles and served at least 20 years of their sentence	Support inmates preparing for community entry.	To qualify for early release, inmates enrol in a three-year programme in which they use virtual reality to practice skills they never learned as teens, like doing laundry, grocery shopping, and navigating in public transport (Clarke, 2019).
Education Justice Project	Men incarcerated at the Danville Correctional Center	Introduce people who will soon be released meet challenges they can encounter after release.	The University of Illinois created various immersive reality scenarios: how to navigate public transportation, pay at the pump at a gas station or order from a digital kiosk at a fast-food restaurant (Heckel, 2018).
(Teng & Gordon, 2021)	Incarcerated women prior to their release	Practice acting in high-stress re-entry situations.	Female offenders practice various risk scenarios that might occur after release (e.g., during a job interview the manager asks about your criminal record).
VR Job Interview Training (VR-JIT) (Smith et al., 2020)	Returning citizens	Enhance interview skills and confidence, and increase the chance of receiving job offers.	Incarcerated individuals can practice job interviews with a virtual hiring manager. People receive immediate feedback if certain answers are correct or incorrect and the scenarios become more challenging over time.

Table 8.8 Smartphone applications for reintegration

Application/ authors	Target population	Goal	Description
Mobile-Enhanced Prevention Support (MEPS) (Edwards et al., 2020)	Gay or bisexual men and transgender women leaving jail	Support engagement in preventive health care during reintegration and reduce recidivism.	Provides tools for tracking and meeting goals, locating services, tracking and distribution of rewards, and receiving assistance of peer mentors.
StaySafe (Lehman et al., 2021)	People under community supervision or in residential settings	Help people make better decisions regarding health risk behaviours, especially those linked to HIV, viral hepatitis and other STDs.	Includes 12 weekly sessions in which users are guided through a series of steps, questions, and exercises aimed at promoting critical thinking about health risks associated with substance use and unprotected sex.
Changing Lives, Probation service Ireland (McGreevy, 2019)	For probationers suffering with addiction or mental health problems	Increase desistance by enabling probationers to identify problems; find support, information, advice and services.	Includes multiple modules, among others a journal to keep track of progress; a probation module where expectations and requirements of probation supervision are found; a mental health and addiction module that provides information, resources and support to probationers struggling with mental health problems or substance related problems.
Socrates 360 (Socrates Software, 2018)	Offenders in prison or during reintegration	Facilitate continuous independent learning opportunities.	Provides engaging and interactive educational modules, and access to health and well-being resources. Staff can upload documents such as medical records, which improves continuity of care.
Outreach Smartphone Monitoring (OSM) (Outreach Smartphone Monitoring, n.d.)	People on probation or parole	Decrease recidivism.	Contains various features to monitor and support people on probation: GPS to monitor inclusion/exclusion zones and curfews, and a Bluetooth breathalyser for self-measurement of alcohol levels. Furthermore, the app includes rehabilitative resources, court and event reminders, and incentives for compliance.

Scram (SCRAM TouchPoint, n.d.)	Probationers	Make community corrections programmes more efficient and to increase compliance by helping service users successfully complete their supervision.	Involves text-like messaging between probationer and officer, mobile check-ins, appointment reminders, and the ability to share documents.
MyNeon, (Mossler & Blank, 2014)	Probationers in the United States	Provide support, assistance and supervision upon release.	Community leaders enter community events or goals into the app (e.g., job training classes, specific courses, or volunteer opportunities. App users can earn points by engaging in these activities.
Utsikt ["View"] (Kriminalvården, n.d.)	Probationers in Sweden	Increase appointment attendance, and supplement and strengthen the probation treatment programme.	Utsikt contains appointment reminders, tools for managing thoughts, emotions, and actions in risk situations; a diary for writing down daily emotions and notes; and a goal section where users keep track of their goals.
VerlofHulp 2.0 [Leave Support 2.0], (Transfore, University of Twente, & Minddistrict, 2019)	Patients who have been institutionalised in clinical settings	To support professionals and inpatients during leave of absence.	At set times the patients get certain questions and propositions regarding the leave. Depending on the answers, the app will provide advice for supporting a good leave of absence.
Mijn Leven, Mijn Risico's, Mijn contacten [My life, My risks, My contacts]	Juvenile probationers in the Netherlands	Extend the reach of current probation methods.	The Dutch probation office developed three apps in which juveniles map their risk factors, their lifeline and their network of peers (Stichting Verslavingsreclassering GGZ, n.d.)

Discussion

The current review has identified VR and smartphone applications for forensic populations, with the specific aim of illustrating the possibilities that these technologies offer for research and intervention. The results indicate that few VR and app interventions have thus far been developed for this domain and that research on their feasibility, usability, and effectiveness is scarce. After an extensive review of the literature and a general web search, 18 VR and an equal number of smartphone applications were identified. We argue that both VR and smartphone apps nevertheless have much potential for this specific target group by offering novel ways for targeting treatment needs and supplementing standard therapies (Linardon et al., 2019). VR enables observation and training of behaviour in various criminogenic environments that are safe, cost-efficient, and easy to control (Van Gelder et al., 2014). Smartphone apps can provide cost-effective, easily accessible interventions that enable access to individualised treatment anytime, anywhere (Linardon et al., 2019; Zhang et al., 2015). In addition, both VR and smartphone apps entail the possibility of objectively collecting data, which can reduce implicit bias (Haarsma et al., 2020; Renaud et al., 2014) and therefore add to a more inclusive practice.

Among the identified VR and smartphone applications, their complementary use was hardly considered. This is a missed opportunity because the specific characteristics of VR and smartphone applications make them uniquely suitable for complementing each other. Whereas VR provides realistic and safe practice environments (Botella et al., 2015; Fox et al., 2009), it is only available at places where the required hardware is available. Smartphones, on the other hand, offer less of an immersive experience, but the portable nature of these devices facilitates the access to intervention material at any time and place. Furthermore, smartphones can track their users' real-world behaviour and can collect ecologically valid behavioural data (Bush et al., 2019; Miller, 2012). VR enables the objective observation of behaviour in simulated environments (Fox et al., 2009), although the extent to which this environment evokes real-world behaviour is yet to be determined. The combination of VR and smartphone apps in forensic psychology has the potential to increase learning effects in rehabilitation and reintegration, and the combined data of VR and smartphone apps can enrich assessments and research and ultimately tell us more about how we can better manage risk – with multiple benefits to society.

One example of complementary use of VR and apps is the FutureU intervention that is currently under development. This intervention aims to reduce self-defeating behaviour by enhancing future orientation and identification with the future self. In FutureU VR, participants are introduced to an avatar of their future selves with whom they interact. Taking the perspective of this future-self enhances future self-continuity (Ganschow et al., 2021) and has proven to reduce self-defeating behaviours among a student population (Van Gelder et al., 2013), and in a sample of convicted offenders (Van Gelder et al., 2021). FutureU also includes a smartphone application in which participants can interact with their future-self on a daily basis. An RCT to study the effectiveness of the FutureU smartphone application is currently underway (Mertens et al., 2022). Another RCT that will involve both VR and the smartphone application is planned for 2022.

Points of Attention Related to VR and Apps

The lack of development of VR and smartphone applications and their limited implementation in practice could be because of limitations related to the technology. The wearable nature of smartphones has the disadvantage that these devices can be lost, stolen, sold, or exchanged, leading to data loss or invalid data. Limitations related to software are high development costs and the expertise required for their development. In addition, once an application has been developed the involvement of software developers – and thus costs – does not necessarily stop, for example, because updates are required (Larsen et al., 2016). Therefore, VR and smartphone app development currently only seems available for research groups, forensic institutions, or individuals that have a certain amount of budget. That said, not too complex applications should be well within reach of the average research budget. Furthermore, this review also identified that for smartphone apps, research is scarce regarding what psychological mechanisms, behavioural change techniques, and features contribute to the application's efficacy (Bakker et al., 2016; Chib & Lin, 2018; Linardon et al., 2019). There is also a paucity of research on which features are essential to keep users engaged, preventing low uptake, and increasing retention rates (Bakker et al., 2016; Hennemann et al., 2017; Torous et al., 2018).

The implementation of VR and smartphone applications is a work in progress. Studies confirm that acceptance of eHealth among health care professionals is still limited (Hennemann et al., 2017; Kip et al., 2019a). It is therefore important to consider how the use of technology in forensic health practices is influenced by organisational culture, professional ideologies, values and working conditions (Graham & McIvor, 2017), and how increasing the use of technology will affect work within forensic health practices and the relationship between therapists and service users. Even though implementation is often only included in the final stages of intervention development, it is critical that the implementation process is carefully considered from the outset to ensure that VR and smartphone app interventions will be integrated in existing care (Kip et al., 2019a; Kip et al., 2021; Schueller & Torous, 2020).

Technologies like VR and smartphone applications have the potential to make the forensic field more inclusive. For example, VR and apps facilitate highly individualised data collection in real time that includes physiological measures. Such measurements are more objective compared to observations and questionnaire data. In addition, they can aid in explaining data from observations or questionnaires. Physiological measurements therefore have the potential to reduce the impact of blind spots and implicit bias in human judgement, which will support a more inclusive practice. To achieve inclusive design, it is important for researchers and software developers to design VR and smartphone applications with diversity in mind. For example, virtual avatars and VEs must reflect different cultural and social realities. To accomplish this, it is important that service users are involved during the development phase of the design. Furthermore, it is necessary that future research investigates how technology can facilitate the forensic context to become more inclusive, but also in what way technology can create additional barriers.

A final reason for the lack of development and usage of VR and smartphone applications for forensic populations is the various ethical concerns and privacy related questions that their usage raises (Schueller & Torous, 2020; Zhang et al., 2015). Firstly, forensic residential settings may resist access to smartphones and the internet, because of the adverse impact technology can have (e.g., access to the dark web, or opportunities for engaging in illegal activities). Secondly, ethical standards and professional guidance around the use of these technologies within health care practices is lagging behind their implementation. This creates both a gap and a grey area that impacts both the willingness and the ability of organisations and individual practitioners to implement. Furthermore, current laws regarding data privacy and security in mobile application research are lacking (Ross, 2018; Tovino, 2020). Both VR hardware and smartphones are provided by major technological companies who collect user data. Media coverage about some of these companies in recent years in relation to data sensitivity and security is likely to create barriers around engagement with technology in this field of work. For smartphone apps that collect background data, it is questionable how ethical it is to track people continuously, and possibly threaten the privacy of third-party bystanders (Miller, 2012; Tovino, 2020). For forensic populations in particular, the most important ethical concern is how the collected data will inform decision making. Hypothetically, fluctuations in mental state that previously would not have been noticed could now trigger rehospitalisation or reincarceration (Resnick & Appelbaum, 2019). Therefore, guidelines and protocols on how VR and apps will be applied to forensic psychology must be developed. Until then, it is important to be aware of data privacy and security and for what reasons data is being collected.

References

Alarcón, C. (2020). *Going back home*. Volver a Casa. Retrieved July 23, 2021, from https://volveracasavr.org/

Andersson, H. W., Steinsbekk, A., Walderhaug, E., Otterholt, E., & Nordfjærn, T. (2018). Predictors of dropout from inpatient substance use treatment: A prospective cohort study. *Substance Abuse: Research and Treatment, 12*, 1–10. 10.1177/1178221818760551

Andrews, D. A., & Bonta, J. (2010). Chapter 11 – prevention and rehabilitation. In D. A. Andrews & J. Bonta (Eds.). *The psychology of criminal conduct* (5th ed., pp. 345–392). Boston: Anderson Publishing, Ltd.

Areàn, P. A., Hoa Ly, K., & Andersson, G. (2016). Mobile technology for mental health assessment. *Dialogues in Clinical Neuroscience, 18*(2), 163–169. 10.31887/DCNS.2016.18.2/parean

Bakker, D., Kazantzis, N., Rickwood, D., & Rickard, N. (2016). Mental health smartphone apps: Review and evidence-based recommendations for future developments. *JMIR Mental Health, 3*(1), 1–31. 10.2196/mental.4984

Bengtson, S., Lund, J., Ibsen, M., & Långström, N. (2019). Long-term violent reoffending following forensic psychiatric treatment: Comparing forensic psychiatric examinees and general offender controls. *Frontiers in Psychiatry, 10*, 715. 10.3389/fpsyt.2019.00715

Bogaerts, S., Spreen, M., ter Horst, P., & Gerlsma, C. (2017). Predictive validity of the HKT-r risk assessment tool: Two and 5-year violent recidivism in a nationwide sample of Dutch forensic psychiatric patients. *International Journal of Offender Therapy and Comparative Criminology, 62*(8), 2259–2270. 10.1177/0306624X17717128

Bonta, J., & Andrews, D. A. (2007). Risk-need-responsivity model for offender assessment and rehabilitation. *Rehabilitation, 6*, 1–22. https://www.publicsafety.gc.ca/cnt/rsrcs/pblctns/rsk-nd-rspnsvty/rsk-nd-rspnsvty-eng.pdf

Botella, C., Serrano, B., Baños, R. M., & Garcia-Palacios, A. (2015). Virtual reality exposure-based therapy for the treatment of post-traumatic stress disorder: A review of its efficacy, the adequacy of the treatment protocol, and its acceptability. *Neuropsychiatric Disease and Treatment, 11*, 2533–2545. 10.2147/ndt.S89542

Brown, J., & Singh, J. P. (2014). Forensic risk assessment: A beginner's guide. *Archives of Forensic Psychology, 1*(1), 49–59. https://www.academia.edu/25597163/Forensic_Risk_Assessment_A_Beginners_Guide

Buitenweg, D. C., Bongers, I. L., van de Mheen, D., van Oers, H. A., & van Nieuwenhuizen, C. (2019). Cocreative development of the QoL-ME: A visual and personalized quality of life assessment app for people with severe mental health problems. *JMIR Mental Health, 6*(3), 12378. 10.2196/12378

Bush, N. E., Armstrong, C. M., & Hoyt, T. V. (2019). Smartphone apps for psychological health: A brief state of the science review. *Psychological Services, 16*(2), 188–195. 10.1037/ser0000286

Chib, A., & Lin, S. H. (2018). Theoretical advancements in mHealth: A systematic review of mobile apps. *Journal of Health Communication, 23*(10-11), 909–955. 10.1080/10810730.2018.1544676

Clarke, M. (2019, July 2). *Some prisons are using virtual reality for reentry and other programs.* Prison Legal News. Retrieved July 23, 2021, from https://www.prisonlegalnews.org/news/2019/jul/2/some-prisons-are-using-virtual-reality-reentry-and-other-programs/

Collins, J., Langlotz, T., & Regenbrecht, H. (2020). Virtual reality in education: A case study on exploring immersive learning for prisoners. *2020 IEEE international symposium on mixed and augmented reality adjunct (ISMAR-Adjunct)*, pp. 110–115. 10.1109/ISMAR-Adjunct51615.2020.00042

Cornet, L. J. M., Den Besten, A. L., & Van Gelder, J.-L. (2019). *Virtual reality en augmented reality in justitiële context.* Enschede: University of Twente.

Cornet, L. J. M., & Van Gelder, J.-L. (2020). Virtual reality: A use case for criminal justice practice. *Psychology, Crime & Law, 26*(7), 631–647. 10.1080/1068316x.2019.1708357

Creemers, H. E.(2020). *What's up? Virtual reality screening to inform treatment for juvenile offenders.* University of Amsterdam. Retrieved July 23, 2021, from https://cde.uva.nl/research/child-development/forensic-child--youth-care/forensic-child--youth-care.html?cb#Whats-Up-Virtual-Reality-screening-to-inform-treatment-for-juvenile-offenders

De Waag (2020). *Behandelaren getraind in VR.* Retrieved October 20, 2021 from https://dewaagnederland.nl/nieuws/de-waag/behandelaren-getraind-in-vr/

Dolven, T., & Fidel, E. (2017). This prison is using VR to teach inmates how to live on the outside. Retrieved July 23, 2021 from https://news.vice.com/en_us/article/bjym3w/this-prison-is-using-vr-to-teachinmates-how-to-live-on-the-outside

Drieschner, K., & Boomsma, A. (2008). The treatment engagement rating scale (TER) for forensic outpatient treatment: Description, psychometric properties, and norms. *Psychology Crime and Law*, *14*, 299–315. 10.1080/10683160701858206

Edwards, G. G., Reback, C. J., Cunningham, W. E., Hilliard, C. L., McWells, C., Mukherjee, S., Weiss, R. E., & Harawa, N. T. (2020). Mobile-enhanced prevention support study for men who have sex with men and transgender women leaving jail: Protocol for a randomized controlled trial. *JMIR Research Protocols*, *9*(9), 18106. 10.2196/18106

Elison, S., Weston, S., Davies, G., Dugdale, S., & Ward, J. (2016). Findings from mixed-methods feasibility and effectiveness evaluations of the "Breaking Free Online" treatment and recovery programme for substance misuse in prisons. *Drugs: Education, Prevention and Policy*, *23*(2), 176–185. 10.3109/09687637.2015.1090397

Enliven. (n.d.). *Huiselijk geweld.* Enliven. Retrieved July 23, 2021, from https://enliven.one/huiselijk-geweld/

Evans, E., Li, L., & Hser, Y.-I. (2009). Client and program factors associated with dropout from court mandated drug treatment. *Evaluation and Program Planning*, *32*(3), 204–212. 10.1016/j.evalprogplan.2008.12.003

Farley, H. (2018). Using 3D worlds in prison: Driving, learning and escape. *Journal For Virtual Worlds Research*, *11*(1). 10.4101/jvwr.v11i1.7304

Fazel, S., & Danesh, J. (2002). Serious mental disorder in 23000 prisoners: A systematic review of 62 surveys. *The Lancet*, *359*, 545–550. 10.1016/S0140-6736(02)07740-1

Fox, J., Arena, D., & Bailenson, J. (2009). Virtual reality: A survival guide for the social scientist. *Journal of Media Psychology: Theories, Methods, and Applications*, *21*, 95–113. 10.1027/1864-1105.21.3.95

Fromberger, P., Jordan, K., & Müller, J. L. (2014). Use of virtual reality in forensic psychiatry. A new paradigm? *Nervenarzt*, *85*(3), 298–303. 10.1007/s00115-013-3904-7

Fromberger, P., Meyer, S., Jordan, K., & Müller, J. L. (2018). Behavioral monitoring of sexual offenders against children in virtual risk situations: A feasibility study. *Frontiers in Psychology*, *9*, 224. 10.3389/fpsyg.2018.00224

Ganschow, B., Cornet, L., Zebel, S., & van Gelder, J.-L. (2021). Looking back from the future: Perspective taking in virtual reality increases future self-continuity. *Frontiers in Psychology*, *12*, 2204. 10.3389/fpsyg.2021.664687

Graffam, J., Shinkfield, A., Lavelle, B., & McPherson, W. (2004). Variables affecting successful reintegration as perceived by offenders and professionals. *Journal of Offender Rehabilitation*, *40*(1-2), 147–171. 10.1300/J076v40n01_08

Graham, H., & McIvor, G. (2017). Advancing electronic monitoring in Scotland: Understanding the influences of localism and professional ideologies. *European Journal of Probation*, *9*(1), 62–79. 10.1177/2066220317697659

Gustafson, D. H., McTavish, F. M., Chih, M.-Y., Atwood, A. K., Johnson, R. A., Boyle, M. G., Levy, M. S., Driscoll, H. D., Chisholm S. M., Dillenburg, L., Isham, A., & Shah, D. (2014). A smartphone application to support recovery from alcoholism: A randomized clinical trial. *JAMA Psychiatry*, *71*(5), 566–572. 10.1001/jamapsychiatry.2013.4642

Haarsma, G., Davenport, S., White, D. C., Ormachea, P. A., Sheena, E., & Eagleman, D. M. (2020). Assessing risk among correctional community probation populations: Predicting reoffense with mobile neurocognitive assessment software. *Frontiers in Psychology*, *10*, 2926. https://www.frontiersin.org/article/10.3389/fpsyg.2019.02926

Hamilton, D., McKechnie, J., Edgerton, E., & Wilson, C. (2021). Immersive virtual reality as a pedagogical tool in education: A systematic literature review of quantitative learning outcomes and experimental design. *Journal of Computers in Education*, *8*(1), 1–32. 10.1007/s40692-020-00169-2

Heckel, J. (2018, May 22). *Illinois design students create virtual reality scenarios for those soon to be released from prison*. Illinois News Bureau. https://news.illinois.edu/view/6367/653215

Hennemann, S., Beutel, M. E., & Zwerenz, R. (2017). Ready for eHealth? Health professionals' acceptance and adoption of ehealth interventions in inpatient routine care. *Journal of Health Communication*, *22*(3), 274–284. 10.1080/10810730.2017.1284286

Heron, K. E., & Smyth, J. M. (2010). Ecological momentary interventions: Incorporating mobile technology into psychosocial and health behaviour treatments. *British Journal of Health Psychology*, *15*(1), 1–39. 10.1348/135910709X466063

Hoogsteder, L., Van Horn, J., & Schipper, E. (2018). Goede Reactie Is Preventie – GRIP. Theoretische en technische achtergrond, Utrecht, Nederland: KFZ.

Hutten, J., Van Horn, J., Kuipers, F., de Man, G., & Wilpert, J. (2021). *Innovatieve behandelmethodes bij de Waag*. https://www.researchgate.net/publication/354464433_Innovatieve_behandelmethodes_bij_de_Waag

Innovative Prison Systems. (2017). *IPS_Innovative Prison Systems and Virtual Rehab establish partnership to support inmates' rehabilitation through the use of virtual reality*. Prison Systems. Retrieved July 22, 2021, from http://prisonsystems.eu/partnership-with-virtual-rehab/

Johnson, K., Richards, S., Chih, M.-Y., Moon, T. J., Curtis, H., & Gustafson, D. H. (2016). A pilot test of a mobile app for drug court participants. *Substance Abuse: Research and Treatment*, *10*, 1–7. 10.4137/SART.S33390

Keusch, F., Struminskaya, B., Antoun, C., Couper, M. P., & Kreuter, F. (2019). Willingness to participate in passive mobile data collection. *Public Opinion Quarterly*, *83*(S1), 210–235. 10.1093/poq/nfz007

Kip, H., Bouman, Y. H. A., Kelders, S. M., & van Gemert-Pijnen, L. (2018). eHealth in treatment of offenders in forensic mental health: A review of the current state. *Frontiers in Psychiatry*, *9*, 42. 10.3389/fpsyt.2018.00042

Kip, H., Kelders, S. M., Bouman, Y. H. A., & Van Gemert-Pijnen, L. J. E. W. C. (2019a). The importance of systematically reporting and reflecting on ehealth development: Participatory development process of a virtual reality application for forensic mental health care. *Journal of Medical Internet Research*, *21*(8), 12972. 10.2196/12972

Kip, H., Kelders, S. M., Weerink, K., Kuiper, A., Brüninghoff, I., Bouman, Y. H. A., Dijkslag, D., & Van Gemert-Pijnen, L. J. E. W. C. (2019b). Identifying the added value of virtual reality for treatment in forensic mental health: A scenario-based, qualitative approach. *Frontiers in Psychology*, *10*, 406. https://www.frontiersin.org/article/10.3389/fpsyg.2019.00406

Kip, H., Silva, M., Bouman, Y., Gemert-Pijnen, L., & Kelders, S. (2021). A self-control training app to increase self-control and reduce aggression – a full factorial design. *Internet Interventions*, *25*, 100392. 10.1016/j.invent.2021.100392

Klein Tuente, S., Bogaerts, S., Bulten, E., Keulen-de Vos, M., Vos, M., Bokern, H., Van IJzendoorn, S., Geraets, C. N. W., & Veling, W. (2020). Virtual Reality Aggression Prevention Therapy (VRAPT) versus waiting list control for forensic psychiatric inpatients: A multicenter randomized controlled trial. *Journal of Clinical Medicine*, *9*(7), 2258. https://doi.org/10.3390/jcm9072258

Kriminalvården. (n.d.). *The Swedish prison and probation service*. Kriminalvården. Retrieved July 15, 2021, from https://www.kriminalvarden.se/swedish-prison-and-probation-service/

Kuntsche, E., & Labhart, F. (2013). Using personal cell phones for ecological momentary assessment – an overview of current developments. *European Psychologist, 18*, 3–11. 10.1027/1016-9040/a000127

Larsen, M. E., Nicholas, J., & Christensen, H. (2016). Quantifying app store dynamics: Longitudinal tracking of mental health apps. *JMIR mHealth uHealth, 4*(3), 96. 10.2196/mhealth.6020

Lehman, W. E. K., Pankow, J., Muiruri, R., Joe, G. W., & Knight, K. (2021). An evaluation of StaySafe, a tablet app to improve health risk decision-making among people under community supervision. *Journal of Substance Abuse Treatment, 130*, 108480. 10.1016/j.jsat.2021.108480

Linardon, J., Cuijpers, P., Carlbring, P., Messer, M., & Fuller-Tyszkiewicz, M. (2019). The efficacy of app-supported smartphone interventions for mental health problems: A meta-analysis of randomized controlled trials. *World Psychiatry, 18*(3), 325–336. 10.1002/wps.20673

McGreevy, G. (2019). *Using technology to promote desistance in Northern Ireland: "Changing Lives" mobile app.* Justice Trends. Retrieved July 15, 2021, from https://justice-trends.press/using-technology-to-promote-desistance-in-northern-ireland-changing-lives-mobile-app/

McLauchlan, J., & Farley, H. (2019). Fast cars and fast learning: Using virtual reality to learn literacy and numeracy in prison. *Journal For Virtual Worlds Research, 12*(3). 10.4101/jvwr.v12i3.7391

McLoughlin, L., Carey, C., Dooley, S., Kennedy, H., & McLoughlin, I. (2021). An observational study of a cross platform risk assessment mobile application in a forensic inpatient setting. *Journal of Psychiatric Research, 138*, 388–392. 10.1016/j.jpsychires.2021.04.034

Mertens, E. C. A., Van der Schalk, J., Siezenga, A. M., & Van Gelder, J. L. (2022). Stimulating a future-oriented mindset and goal attainment through a smartphone-based intervention: Study protocol for a randomized controlled trial. *Internet Interventions, 27*, 100509. https://doi.org/10.1016/j.invent.2022.100509

Miller, G. (2012). The smartphone psychology manifesto. *Perspectives on Psychological Science, 7*(3), 221–237. 10.1177/1745691612441215

Mossler, L., & Blank, D. (2014, February 12). *Transforming probation with technology.* Data-Smart City Solutions. Retrieved July 15, 2021, from https://datasmart.ash.harvard.edu/news/article/changing-probation-in-new-york-city-with-an-app-383

Nee, C., Van Gelder, J.-L., Otte, M., Vernham, Z., & Meenaghan, A. (2019). Learning on the job: Studying expertise in residential burglars using virtual environments. *Criminology, 57*(3), 481–511. 10.1111/1745-9125.12210

Nicholas, J., Shilton, K., Schueller, S. M., Gray, E. L., Kwasny, M. J., & Mohr, D. C. (2019). The role of data type and recipient in individuals' perspectives on sharing passively collected smartphone data for mental health: Cross-sectional questionnaire study. *JMIR mHealth uHealth, 7*(4), 12578. 10.2196/12578

Ormachea, P. A., Davenport, S., Haarsma, G., Jarman, A., Henderson, H., & Eagleman, D. M. (2016). Enabling individualized criminal sentencing while reducing subjectivity: A tablet-based assessment of recidivism risk. *AMA Journal of Ethics, 18*(3), 243–251. 10.1001/journalofethics.2016.18.3.stas1-1603

Outreach Smartphone Monitoring. (n.d.). *What's this about?* OSM. Retrieved July 15, 2021, from https://www.osmnow.com/

Park, S. Y., & Lee, K. H. (2021). Burglars' choice of intrusion routes: A virtual reality experimental study. *Journal of Environmental Psychology, 74*, 101582. 10.1016/j.jenvp.2021.101582

Parsey, C. M., & Schmitter-Edgecombe, M. (2013). Applications of technology in neuropsychological assessment. *The Clinical Neuropsychologist, 27*(8), 1328–1361. 10.1080/13 854046.2013.834971

Renaud, P., Chartier, S., Rouleau, J.-L., Proulx, J., Goyette, M., Trottier, D., Fedoroff, P., Bradford, J.-P., Dassylva, B., & Bouchard, S. (2013). Using immersive virtual reality and ecological psychology to probe into child molesters' phenomenology. *Journal of Sexual Aggression, 19*(1), 102–120. 10.1080/13552600.2011.617014

Renaud, P., Trottier, D., Rouleau, J.-L., Goyette, M., Saumur, C., Boukhalfi, T., & Bouchard, S. (2014). Using immersive virtual reality and anatomically correct computer-generated characters in the forensic assessment of deviant sexual preferences. *Virtual Reality, 18*(1), 37–47. 10.1007/s10055-013-0235-8

Resnick, K. S., & Appelbaum, P. S. (2019). Passive monitoring of mental health status in the criminal forensic population. *The Journal of the American Academy of Psychiatry and the Law, 47*(4), 457–466. 10.29158/JAAPL.003865-19

Richman, W., Kiesler, S., Weisband, S., & Drasgow, F. (1999). A meta-analytic study of social desirability distortion in computer-administered questionnaires, traditional questionnaires, and interviews. *Journal of Applied Psychology, 84*, 754–775. 10.1037/0021-9010.84.5.754

Riva, G., Baños, R. M., Botella, C., Mantovani, F., & Gaggioli, A. (2016). Transforming experience: The potential of augmented reality and virtual reality for enhancing personal and clinical change. *Frontiers in psychiatry, 7*, 164. https://www.frontiersin.org/article/10.3389/fpsyt.2016.00164

Rizzo, A., Buckwalter, J., Bowerly, T., van der Zaag, C., Humphrey, L., Neumann, U., Chua, C., Kyriakakis C., Van Rooyen, A., & Sisemore, D. (2000). The virtual classroom: A virtual reality environment for the assessment and rehabilitation of attention deficits. *CyberPsychology & Behavior, 3*(3), 11–37. 10.1089/10949310050078940

Ross, S. (2018). Policy, practice and regulatory issues in mobile technology treatment for forensic clients. *European Journal of Probation, 10*(1), 44–58. 10.1177/2066220318761382

Russell, M. A., & Gajos, J. M. (2020). Annual research review: Ecological momentary assessment studies in child psychology and psychiatry. *Journal of Child Psychology and Psychiatry, 61*(3), 376–394. 10.1111/jcpp.13204

Sappelli, F., Verkes, R.-J., Bulten, E., & Smeijers, D. (n.d.) *Virtual reality agression assessment (VRAA)*. Pompestichting. Retrieved July 22, 2021, from https://www.pompestichting.nl/Onderzoek/Technologie-en-innovatie/Virtual-Reality%09/

Schueller, S. M., & Torous, J. (2020). Scaling evidence-based treatments through digital mental health. *American Psychologist, 75*(8), 1093–1104. 10.1037/amp0000654

Schutte, N. S., & Stilinović, E. J. (2017). Facilitating empathy through virtual reality. *Motivation and Emotion, 41*(6), 708–712. 10.1007/s11031-017-9641-7

SCRAM TouchPoint. (n.d.). *Mobile app for client monitoring and engagement*. Scram Systems. Retrieved July 15, 2021, from https://www.scramsystems.com/monitoring/scram-touchpoint/

Seinfeld, S., Arroyo-Palacios, J., Iruretagoyena, G., Hortensius, R., Zapata, L. E., Borland, D., De Gelder, B., Slater, M., & Sanchez-Vives, M. V. (2018). Offenders become the victim in virtual reality: Impact of changing perspective in domestic violence. *Scientific Reports, 8*, 2692. 10.1038/s41598-018-19987-7

Shiffman, S., Stone, A. A., & Hufford, M. R. (2008). Ecological momentary assessment. *Annual Review of Clinical Psychology, 4*, 1–32. 10.1146/annurev.clinpsy.3.022806.091415

Singh, J., & Fazel, S. (2010). Forensic risk assessment – a metareview. *Criminal Justice and Behavior, 37*, 965–988. 10.1177/0093854810374274

Smeijers, D., & Koole, S. L. (2019). Testing the effects of a virtual reality game for aggressive impulse management (VR-GAIME): Study protocol. *Frontiers in Psychiatry, 10,* 83–83. 10.3389/fpsyt.2019.00083

Smith, M. J., Mitchell, J. A., Blajeski, S., Parham, B., Harrington, M. M., Ross, B., Sinco, B., Brydon, D. M., Johnson, J.E., Cuddeback, G. S., Smith, J. D., Jordan, N., Bell, M. D., McGeorge, R., Kaminski, K., Suganuma, A., & Kubiak, S. P. (2020). Enhancing vocational training in corrections: A type 1 hybrid randomized controlled trial protocol for evaluating virtual reality job interview training among returning citizens preparing for community re-entry. *Contemporary Clinical Trials Communications, 19,* 100604. 10.1016/j.conctc.2020.100604

Sobolev, M., Vitale, R., Wen, H., Kizer, J., Leeman, R., Pollak, J. P., Baumel, A., Vadhan, N.P., Estrin, D., & Muench, F. (2021). The Digital Marshmallow Test (DMT) diagnostic and monitoring mobile health app for impulsive behavior: Development and validation study. *JMIR mHealth uHealth, 9*(1), 25018. 10.2196/25018

Socrates Software. (2018). *About us.* Socrates. Retrieved July 15, 2021, from https://www.socrates-software.com/app_privacy-html/

Stichting Verslavingsreclassering GGZ. (n.d.). *1,5 meter toezicht.* SVG. Retrieved July 24, 2021, from https://www.svg.nl/wat-doen-wij/blog/15-meter-toezicht

Stieger, M., Nißen, M., Rüegger, D., Kowatsch, T., Flückiger, C., & Allemand, M. (2018). PEACH, a smartphone- and conversational agent-based coaching intervention for intentional personality change: Study protocol of a randomized, wait-list controlled trial. *BMC Psychology, 6*(1). 10.1186/s40359-018-0257-9

Teng, M. Q., & Gordon, E. (2021). Therapeutic virtual reality in prison: Participatory design with incarcerated women. *New Media & Society, 23*(8), 2210–2229. 10.1177/1461444821993131

Ter Horst, P., De Vries, M. G., Kimpen, R., Peterse, J., & Kruijt, W. S. (2016). *Persoonsgebonden app voor het zelf scoren van protectieve en risicogebieden en het monitoren van voortgang hierop gedurende de behandeling.* https://docplayer.nl/60028658-De-hkt-r-en-hcr-20-v3-zelfscore-app.html

Ticknor, B. (2017). Creating a virtual environment for the treatment of offenders: Pilot 1.0. *Corrections Today, 58,* 46–50. https://www.thefreelibrary.com/Pilot+1.0%3A+Creating+a+virtual+environment+for+the+treatment+of...-a0491848170

Ticknor, B. (2018) Using virtual reality to treat offenders: an examination. *International Journal of Criminal Justice Sciences, 13*(2), 316–325. https://www.proquest.com/docview/2261031600

Ticknor, B. (2019). Virtual reality and correctional rehabilitation: A game changer. *Criminal Justice and Behavior, 46*(9), 1319–1336. 10.1177/0093854819842588

Torous, J., Nicholas, J., Larsen, M. E., Firth, J., & Christensen, H. (2018). Clinical review of user engagement with mental health smartphone apps: Evidence, theory and improvements. *Evidence-Based Mental Health, 21*(3), 116–119. 10.1136/eb-2018-102891

Tovino, S. A. (2020). Privacy and security issues with mobile health research applications. *The Journal of Law, Medicine & Ethics, 48*(1), 154–158. 10.1177/1073110520917041

Transfore, University of Twente, & Minddistrict. (2019). *Factsheet Verlofhulp 2.1.* Retrieved from https://www.transfore.nl/doe-mee-aan-het-project-verlofhulp-21

Van der Veeken, F. C. A., Lucieer, J., & Bogaerts, S. (2018). Forensic psychiatric treatment evaluation: The clinical evaluation of treatment progress with repeated forensic routine outcome monitoring measures. *International Journal of Law and Psychiatry, 57,* 9–16. 10.1016/j.ijlp.2017.12.002

Van Gelder, J.-L. (2020). Criminologie in de jaren twintig van de 21ᵉ eeuw. *Tijdschrift voor Criminologie*, *61*(4), 349–358. 10.5553/TvC/0165182X2019061004004

Van Gelder, J.-L., Cornet, L. J. M., Zwalua, N. P., Mertens, E. C. A., & Van der Schalk, J. (2022). Interaction with the future self in virtual reality reduces self-defeating behavior in a sample of convicted offenders. *Scientific Reports*, *12*, Article 2254, 10.1038/s415 98-022-06305-5.

Van Gelder, J.-L., Hershfield, H. E., & Nordgren, L. F. (2013). Vividness of the future self predicts delinquency. *Psychological Science*, *24*(6), 974–980. 10.1177/0956797612465197

Van Gelder, J.-L., Otte, M., & Luciano, E. C. (2014). Using virtual reality in criminological research. *Crime Science*, *3*(1), 10. 10.1186/s40163-014-0010-5

Ventura, L. A., Cassel, C. A., Jacoby, J. E., & Huang, B. (1998). Case management and recidivism of mentally ill persons released from jail. *Psychiatric Services*, *49*(10), 1330–1337. 10.1176/ps.49.10.1330

Ventura, S., Cardenas, G., Miragall, M., Riva, G., & Baños, R. (2021). How does it feel to be a woman victim of sexual harassment? The effect of 360°-video-based virtual reality on empathy and related variables. *Cyberpsychology, Behavior, and Social Networking*, *24*(4), 258–266. 10.1089/cyber.2020.0209

Vollm, B. A., Clarke, M., Herrando, V. T., Seppanen, A. O., Gosek, P., Heitzman, J., & Bulten, E. (2018). European Psychiatric Association (EPA) guidance on forensic psychiatry: Evidence based assessment and treatment of mentally disordered offenders. *European Psychiatry*, *51*, 58–73. 10.1016/j.eurpsy.2017.12.007

Wormith, J. S., Althouse, R., Simpson, M., Reitzel, L. R., Fagan, T. J., & Morgan, R. D. (2007). The rehabilitation and reintegration of offenders. *Criminal Justice and Behavior*, *34*(7), 879–892. 10.1177/0093854807301552

Zhang, M. W. B., Ho, C. S. H., Cheok, C. C. S., & Ho, R. C. M. (2015). Smartphone apps in mental healthcare: The state of the art and potential developments. *BJPsych Advances*, *21*(5), 354–358. 10.1192/apt.bp.114.013789

9 Assessment and Intervention Technologies in Juvenile Justice

Christopher M. King, Lauren Grove,
Rachel Bomysoad, Kenny Gonzalez, and
Loumarie Vasquez

Introduction

Justice-involved youth are a distinctive population in the justice system, with developmentally unique services needs and elevated rates of mental disorders (Beaudry et al., 2021; Shufelt & Cocozza, 2006). Such youth also confront and present with a range of barriers to access and engagement in behavioural health services, including concerns about expense, and low levels of motivation and utilisation (Abram et al., 2008; MacDonell & Prinz, 2017; Teplin et al., 2013; White et al., 2016). In addition, justice-involved youth are a diverse population, with evidence indicative of disproportionate rates of minority youth contact with the justice system (Development Services Group, Inc., 2014; Rovner, 2014; Zane & Pupo, 2021), and differential experiences and needs of justice-involved girls (Chesney-Lind et al., 2008; Walker et al., 2015; Zahn et al., 2009).

Many have recommended the Risk-Need-Responsivity (RNR) model (Bonta & Andrews, 2017) for guiding assessment and intervention efforts with justice-involved youth (Brogan et al., 2015; Guy et al., 2012; Hoge, 2016). Part of the RNR model's responsivity principle directs for the matching of youth to services that are tailored to their personal characteristics (McCormick et al., 2017; Singh et al., 2014; Vieira et al., 2009). For instance, services adapted for particular multicultural groups (Brogan et al., 2015; Gutierrez et al., 2018). Some have also noted that technology-facilitated services can be utilised in accordance with the RNR model and may entail certain advantages relative to other service modalities. In line with the specific responsivity principle, technology-facilitated services can correspond to youth's high rates of technology usage in general, and such solutions may have unique and flexible potential for helping to overcome barriers to access to care among justice-involved persons (Batastini, 2016; Kip & Bouman, 2021; McDougall et al., 2017).

Indeed, upon the onset of the COVID-19 pandemic, professionals involved in the case processing, management, and rehabilitation of justice-involved persons grew increasingly familiar with the flexible utility of videoconferencing-based services, such as telepsychiatry and telepsychology (Johnson et al., 2021; Kirschstein et al., 2021; Mulay et al., 2021). A broader suite of technological

DOI: 10.4324/9781003230977-10

options for behavioural health services has been termed *e-mental health* (Lal & Adair, 2014; Mucic & Hilty, 2016), with several such technologies being evident in the correctional and forensic assessment and treatment literatures (Kip et al., 2018; Kirschstein et al., 2021). However, to date, relatively little attention had been paid to e-mental health for juvenile justice. Moreover, despite the potential for e-mental health to variously expand access to care, threshold concerns have been noted about justice-involved youth, often members of historically marginalised groups and from socioeconomically disadvantaged communities, not having adequate access to technology that would be needed for e-mental health (Batastini, 2016) – a so-called *digital divide* (e.g., Her Majesty's Inspectorate of Probation, 2020).

e-Mental Health for Justice-Involved Adults as a Point of Comparison

A systematic review and meta-analysis of a handful of studies that investigated videoconferencing-facilitated psychological services with criminal justice or substance abuse samples found that this form of e-mental health evidenced generally comparable outcomes to that of traditional in-person services (Batastini et al., 2016). A subsequent meta-analysis of videoconferencing-facilitated psychological and psychiatric services included 17 studies that were conducted in correctional facilities (Batastini et al., 2021). The outcomes for these correctional studies in the aggregate were not statistically significantly different from in-person services. Another systematic review of 50 studies investigated or reviewed any form of e-mental health for the treatment of justice-involved persons (Kip et al., 2018). Besides tele-mental health, they reviewed studies of phone and text messaging facilitated interventions, the latter of which has been termed part of *mHealth* (Bath et al., 2018); digitised and online intervention programmes; exercise and therapeutic video games; online forums and social media; and simulation and virtual reality technologies (i.e., of criminogenic scenarios or stimuli, such as interpersonal irritants or children). The authors concluded that while the available evidence base as to effectiveness was variable and modest, such technologies were nonetheless promising.

None of the aforementioned reviews had focused specifically on juvenile justice. For instance, the systematic review by Kip et al. (2018) only reviewed three references that focused on justice-involved youth. And narrative reviews that have focused on juvenile justice were limited to a single type of e-mental health (Batastini, 2016; Bath et al., 2018). Accordingly, we conducted a systematic review focused specifically on e-mental health in juvenile justice contexts (Grove et al., 2021). We identified 36 primary study or review articles, dissertations, and theses, and observed four general categories of e-mental health that had been narratively discussed or investigated with justice-involved youth, or sometimes, their caregivers or juvenile justice professionals. In discussing each of these references below, we further subclassify the types of e-mental health involved. Of note, a few instances of technology reflected some degree of overlap across subcategories within one of the four general categories of e-mental health, or across two of the general categories (e.g., digitised intervention programmes involved some gaming or assessment elements). Studies were generally conducted in the United States, and the few exceptions are noted.

Telemental Health and mHealth

Telepsychology

Only one unpublished study had investigated a telepsychology service with justice-involved youth (Anderson, 2018). It entailed an evaluation of three solution-focused therapy sessions delivered via videoconferencing, with phone and text messaging contacts between sessions. The study used a multi-wave design with a sample of four youth who had been adjudicated delinquent. No significant changes were observed in either externalising behaviours or hopefulness post intervention.

Telepsychiatry

Five articles variously examined telepsychiatry services, with three using overlapping samples. Regarding the latter three studies, the first described the service as a telemedicine and referral programme (that included care of physical and behavioural health) between an academic medical centre and four custodial juvenile justice facilities located in rural areas (Fox et al., 2006). The study entailed an analysis of cost data for each facility before and one year after implementing the service. Some medical and total costs increased post-implementation, whereas other medical and transportation costs were not significantly higher after one year. Differences among sites were interpreted as suggesting that several cost variables were negatively related to level of utilisation of the service. The next study used a similar design to examine the time between referral and care, and the number of outpatient, inpatient, and emergency room appointments, one and two years after programme implementation at the four facilities (Fox et al., 2007). The authors found that some of the facilities exhibited significantly lower lags between referral and care, and significantly fewer outpatient and inpatient visits. In addition, there was a significant positive relationship between the frequency of outpatient and emergency room appointments and the per cent of those visits conducted via telemedicine. Finally, a third study, using a total sample of 190 youth from three of the four facilities, examined the number of youth's psychosocial goals and their completion of those goals at baseline and one and two years after programme implementation (Fox et al., 2008). The second year of the programme was significantly predictive of number and attainment of total goals. Youth sampled from year two had a higher number of total goals and most subcategories of goals. A higher proportion of those same youth also had completed several subcategories of goals.

Another telepsychiatry study used a design consisting of a review of chart records and administration of a satisfaction survey, with youth at a minimum-security juvenile justice facility (Myers et al., 2006). The telepsychiatry service consisted of videoconferencing sessions with a psychiatrist at an academic medical centre, and eventually, the addition of a nurse at the juvenile justice facility to provide on-site assistance. Over a study period of more than two years, 115 youth were served with 275 sessions. Certain mental disorder diagnoses were common and 80% of the youth received psychiatric medications. A majority of youth provided very good or outstanding ratings for all but one satisfaction item, and the overall satisfaction score was approximately 4 out of 5.

One article reported case studies for several different telepsychiatry programmes from four different states and different facilities within states (Kaliebe et al., 2011). The authors described the different telepsychiatry models that had been implemented and evident benefits and challenges. Another article provided a narrative review of two of the above described telepsychiatry studies; discussed the potential of telemental health for justice-involved youth within the context of the risk, need, and responsivity principles of the RNR model; and discussed some potential implementation challenges (Batastini, 2016).

Phone- and Text Messaging-Based Services

Three studies investigated a six-session cognitive-behavioural intervention called the *Real Victory Programme* that included an aftercare phone coaching component, with youth being provided with the phones as part of the programme. The phone coaching component consisted of two automated phone calls per day at times preferred by the participants for one year. The automated calls asked participants about their attainment of a primary goal and the effort they exerted towards accomplishing three daily tasks since the last call. Participants responded via their phone keypad, which would prompt pre-recorded messages of reinforcement from family, friends, or mentors for success inputs, and messages of encouragement for other inputs.

All three studies of the *Real Victory Programme* used a design consisting of a longitudinal follow-up with a services-as-usual comparison group. The first study used a sample of 70 youth on probation (Burraston et al., 2012). Participants in the experimental programme exhibited significantly lower rearrest rates than the comparison group at follow-up, regardless of whether the phone coaching component was included. The phone coaching component did, however, predict a longer time to rearrest relative to the comparison group. The next study involved additional analyses of the same sample and found that while the experimental programme predicted significantly fewer rearrests irrespective of the phone coaching component, answering more than half of the phone calls also predicted moderately reduced odds of any rearrest (Burraston et al., 2014). The final study involved a new sample of 256 youth who were on probation or living in group homes or secure facilities (Bahr et al., 2016). Although the experimental programme participants did not, as a group, exhibit lower rates of rearrests after one year, answering a higher number of phone calls was predictive of some reduction in felony rearrests at follow-up.

An unpublished study investigated a somewhat similar phone-based aftercare service called *Victory Seeker*, with youth being provided with phones as needed (Fowles, 2009). The service delivered automated daily prompts to participants for six months about effort towards and completion of a prosocial goal, along with personalised motivational or reinforcing messages from family and friends for successes, or else prompts to leave an explanatory voicemail about why one's personal goal was not accomplished. The study used a multi-wave design with a comparison group that received services as usual and one transitional aftercare session. The overall sample consisted of 68 youth drawn from a juvenile diversion programme. Results were mixed as to whether the experimental group exhibited fewer felony rearrests, and the experimental group exhibited significantly higher rates of drug use. Furthermore, better effects were not observed for participants who received the experimental service, nor for youth who presented with more deficits in executive functioning.

Another study examined a text messaging service that focused on facilitating attendance at behavioural healthcare appointments. The service consisted of the delivery of several reminders about upcoming appointments, a follow-up inquiry about whether the appointment was attended and why if not, and twice weekly motivational messages (Tolou-Shams et al., 2019). The study design consisted of interviews with seven caregivers and 15 juvenile justice professionals prior to development of the service, and then surveys with 15 justice-involved youth receiving mental health or substance use treatment, and two caregivers, about the service. Pre-implementation interviews yielded several themes: text messaging among justice-involved youth, their caregivers, and juvenile justice professionals was common but variable; privacy and stigma were concerns for the planned service; a preference for the service to be brief and simple, personally tailored, and positive. All the youth reported that the service was helpful in facilitating their attendance at appointments, and neither of the two interviewed caregivers reported that the service should be revised post implementation.

One other study investigated an intervention programme meant to improve sexual health among justice-involved girls (DiClemente et al., 2014). The programme consisted of three in-person sessions, four follow-up telephone sessions, and the provision, as needed, of medication for sexually transmitted illnesses to provide to a sexual partner. The study used a multi-wave design with a usual-care comparison group, sampling 188 African American girls at a juvenile detention facility. However, the design did not include efforts to isolate the effects of the phone sessions. Results of the programme were mixed: while participants in the experimental group reported significantly greater knowledge of sexual health and self-efficacy beliefs, as well as skills for condom use, there were no group differences as to number of sexual partners, condom use, or sexually transmitted diseases.

Another article provided a narrative description of a family systems aftercare intervention addressing family functioning and stress (Cervenka et al., 1996). The programme included monthly phone calls to high-risk youth at a juvenile justice assessment centre and their families for up to four years. An additional article provided a narrative review of mHealth for justice-involved youth (Bath et al., 2018). The authors reviewed studies of mHealth conducted with youth who were not justice involved, including a study involving youth with substance abuse problems. In addition, they suggested several potential applications of mHealth for justice-involved youth and caregivers, including reminders about court and treatment information, therapeutic information sharing, facilitating communication with and among providers, and facilitating large scale data analytics. Furthermore, the authors provided recommendations that included the development of standardised mHealth technologies with the input of justice-involved youth and their families and with consideration of ethical issues, investigating currently mHealth technologies and newly developed ones, and training professionals in the use of mHealth.

Online Forums and Social Media

A single study examined the feasibility of recruiting caregivers of justice-involved youth via Facebook, and then examined recruited caregivers' reported use of technology and social media, and opinions about e-mental health (Folk et al., 2020). Over the course of three weeks, about 12% of the 3,394 persons who clicked the study solicitation completed an online screening questionnaire. Ultimately about 5% completed a quantitative study survey. The results of that survey indicated that most caregivers reported having cellphones and computers, many reported using social media, and a majority indicated that they would probably or definitely enrol in a digital health intervention. Similar results were observed via qualitative interviews conducted with some participants. Moreover, most of the qualitative interviewees indicated that they would be willing to participate in family therapy via videoconferencing, a private Facebook support group for caregivers, and a text messaging intervention, after being presented with vignettes about these three types of e-mental health.

Primarily or Partially Digitised Intervention Programmes

Computerised Cognitive Behavioural Therapy (CBT)

Several studies examined different computerised CBT programmes or concepts. Two studies focused on programmes that would or did seek to treat depression among youth. One of the studies was descriptive in nature and involved focus groups and interviews with 40 human services providers in New Zealand, including some that worked with youth delinquency and gang involvement, about their attitudes towards such a service in general (Fleming & Merry, 2013). The participants – especially those working from a mental health orientation and who were shown a prototype of such technology – generally expressed interest in this type of e-mental health and opined about potential uses and needed training and resources.

The other study focusing on a computerised CBT programme for depression investigated a technology called *Guided Self-Help CPT Programme with Therapist Support* (Wannachaiyakul et al., 2017). The programme involved six weekly self-guided sessions of 45–60 minutes in duration using a computer, and brief in-person feedback and reinforcement about homework completion from a therapist. The study used a multi-wave design with a services-as-usual comparison group, and an overall sample of 84 youth at a juvenile vocational training centre in Thailand. The authors found that participants in the computerised CBT programme had significantly lower within-subjects depression scores at post and two follow-up timepoints (the comparison group's scores were significantly lower only at the two follow-ups), and significantly lower between-subjects depression scores at post relative to the comparison group.

A study conducted in New Zealand examined a self-directed computerised CBT programme called *Smart, Positive, Active, Realistic, X-Factor Thoughts* (*SPARX-R*), meant to improve cognitive behavioural skills for emotional regulation (Fleming et al., 2019). Youth used laptop computers for the programme, which consisted of a virtual therapist guide and exploratory play in a gamified digital environment to teach and rehearse cognitive behavioural skills. The sample consisted of 40 justice-involved boys who had been referred to a community-based day treatment programme. While the study design consisted of a multi-wave with a services-as-usual comparison group, planned between-subjects analyses were jettisoned in light of high rates of attrition. The authors also reported that the programme received several negative reports from youth and staff.

Another study was conducted in Canada and descriptively examined a computerised CBT programme called *Stop Now and Plan Youth Justice* (SNAP YJ), which aimed to enhanced cognitive behavioural skills towards reducing risk of delinquency and gang involvement (Sewell et al., 2019). The programme consisted of 12 hour-long sessions, administered with trained in-person facilitators and tablet and touchscreen devices. Participants were guided through digital modules comprised of instructional slides and educational videos, animated interactive roleplays, relaxation training, discussion questions and practice exercises, and live learning. The sample consisted of 15 boys residing in custodial juvenile justice facilities. Based on interviews conducted with the youth, the authors reported that all the participants acquired, to varying degrees, programme-related knowledge and skills, and particularly themes of self-awareness, emotional awareness, thinking about consequences, and prosocial skills and actions.

A final unpublished study investigated a computerised CBT programme called *The Students Managing Anger and Resolution Together* (SMART), which sought to improve anger management and conflict resolution skills to reduce aggression (Posick, 2009). The technology involved graphical simulations, games, and interactive interviews for instruction. The study used a repeated-measures design with a sample of 20 youth who were on probation. Participants completed four of the programme's eight modules. No significant results were found for anger, conflict resolution, or violence.

Other Digital Therapeutic Interventions

One descriptive study examined a computerised assessment-based motivational enhancement intervention programme for substance misuse and delinquency, of about 45 minutes to one hour in duration, based on the transtheoretical model of change (Levesque et al., 2012). The *Rise Above Your Situation* (*RAYS*) software administered a standardised assessment and delivered standardised feedback and a printed report to respondents, in addition to issuing a standardised report for counsellors with recommended intervention strategies. Based on a sample of 60 youth, some of whom were on probation, and eight counsellors, the authors reported that almost all the youth completed the programme, a large percentage of youth expressed agreement or strong agreement with acceptability items, and a large percentage of counsellors expressed similar agreement with helpfulness items.

A second study investigated eight one-hour sessions of listening to MP3 recordings of guided mindfulness meditations, which was compared to progressive muscle relaxation recordings, towards improving self-regulation abilities (Evans-Chase, 2015). The study used a between-within design with a sample of 60 youth residing at a juvenile detention facility. Those in the progressive muscle relaxation group scored significantly higher on multiple mindfulness measures at post, and a slightly higher percentage of those youth also reported greater reductions in stress. Youth in the mindfulness condition, however, reported greater use and more examples of mindfulness skills in their everyday lives.

A third study examined an online intervention programme for improving knowledge and skills around sexually transmitted illnesses (STIs), called *Sistas Informing, Healing, Living, and Empowering* (SiHLEWeb; Danielson et al., 2013). The programme presented five hypothetical characters whose lives were followed throughout the programme and utilised interactive videos to simulate in-person group sessions and deliver immediate feedback based on participants' responses to activities. The study involved a repeated measures design with 41 African American girls, ten of whom were recruited from a juvenile justice department. The authors found that about two-thirds of the girls completed the programme, with completers evidencing significantly improved condom use self-efficacy beliefs and knowledge about risk reduction practices, though relative improvements were not observed for partner communication skills, self-esteem, or ethnic pride.

A fourth study investigated an online adaption of the *Playing and Learning Strategies* (PALS) parenting programme (Feil et al., 2008). The Internet-adapted course consisted of interactive multimedia, uploaded recorded interactions between parent and infant, electronic communication with a professional, and a web-based monitoring system. The sample consisted of three justice-involved girls living in group foster care, who were furnished with laptops with webcams. Using a repeated measures design, the authors found that the participants demonstrated a 30–40% increase in knowledge about infant signs of needs and concomitant responsive parenting behaviours. They also reported that ratings of parent-child interaction videos recorded with both a camcorder and webcam resulted in high reliability, that the girls were able to utilise the programme with little assistance, and that the girls rated the technology to be highly usable and satisfactory.

An unpublished study examined a computerised empathy training programme, called *Mind Reading*, which consisted of emotions definitions, stories, quizzes, lessons, and games, administered via two-hour sessions for ten weeks (Brown, 2018). Using a between-within design with a services-as-usual comparison group and an overall sample of 14 youth drawn from a juvenile detention facility, the author did not observe any significant effects for the technology.

Computerised Educational Interventions

Two studies examined computerised literacy programmes. The first was an unpublished study that investigated self-paced instructional software involving tutorial lessons with videos, generated worksheets for practice, and supportive reading materials (Vigilante, 1994). Using a repeated-measures design with a sample of 43 youth at a juvenile detention facility, the author found an average increase of 9% in reading skills. In addition, 71% of the sample showed a positive gain in reading attitude. Moreover, all instructors yielded knowledge scores about the software of 80% or higher.

A more recent published study investigated a literacy programme, called *Read 180*, for students in grades 4 through 12 with reading deficits (Houchins et al., 2018). The programme included several technology elements, including computerised instructional materials and aids for teacher and student placement and monitoring. The study used a multi-wave design with a services-as-usual comparison group, with an overall sample of 464 boys residing in a long-term custodial juvenile justice facility. The boys who participated in the partially digitised programme achieved significantly higher scores on measures of reading comprehension and language, with effect sizes ranging from small to large, though not for measures of several other reading and spelling skills.

Computerised Cognitive Training

A single study investigated cognitive training exercises administered via tablet devices (*BrainHQ*) over the course of 10–30 hours of sessions (Rowlands et al., 2020). The study used a repeated measures design with a sample of 14 boys who had been diagnosed with conduct disorder alone or comorbid with other conditions, and who were at a maximum-security custodial juvenile justice facility for violent offending. The authors reported that most of the youth completed the programme and that it was regarded as tolerable and acceptable. Moreover, they found small to large significant pre-post improvements for multiple neurocognitive measures, including by virtue of total time using the technology.

Simulation Games

Only two articles and one dissertation reported on simulation video games for justice-involved youth. All the games involved youth making decisions about therapeutically relevant situations they might encounter in real life.

The first article narratively described a computerised therapeutic simulation board game called *BUSTED*, in which youth living in a group home or residential juvenile justice facility had to choose how to react to different life scenarios (Resnick, 1986). The purpose of the game was to reduce violence by improving self-awareness, interpersonal skills, and appreciation of consequences. Another article described a computerised simulation game meant to improve moral reasoning skills (Sherer, 1990). The game prompted Israeli "street corner" youth with histories of justice involvement to discuss and make choices about realistic moral dilemma scenarios. According to the authors, preliminary results were suggestive of the game's feasibility, in part due to positive feedback from the youth. Finally, an unpublished study surveyed a panel of four mental health professionals and researchers in the about a computerised intervention, called *Ethos*, that presented youth with moral dilemma scenarios for which they could make different choices and receive feedback about their choices (Caudle, 2011). The panelists regarded the game as evidencing content validity for moral reasoning and suggested that it may prove an effective intervention technology for enhancing involved skills.

Computerised Assessments

Only four studies had examined computerised assessment technologies with justice-involved youth. None of the studies investigated computerised assessment technology in the context of forensic mental health assessments for courts.

The first study examined self-reported information elicited via interactive multimedia software for biopsychosocial health risks screening and education (Paperny, 1997). Based on screening results, the software presented youth with feedback, video presentations, and printouts of their individual health results. Using a sample of 288 youth recruited from custodial juvenile justice facilities as well as runaway shelters, the authors found that both justice-involved and runaway youth yielded higher rates of several health risks relative to youth who were not justice involved.

A second study investigated the predictive validity for official delinquency records of technology-facilitated interviews conducted with 237 African American boys, with some of the sampled youth referred by juvenile court counsellors (Paschall et al., 2001). The interviews consisted of administration of questions via audio cassette recordings and the youth entering their responses via computer. The study used a single-group longitudinal design and found a significant and strong relationship between self-report and official court information concerning delinquency history.

A third study descriptively examined administrations of the *Voice Diagnostic Interview Schedule for Children* (Voice DISC-IV), which entailed administration via a computer and headphones (Wasserman et al., 2002). The sample consisted of 292 boys who were drawn from juvenile detention facilities. The authors reported that the rates of mental disorders yielded by the technology were similar to those observed in studies involving traditional clinical interviews with similarly situated youth.

The final study used a descriptive design to examine computer-assisted interviews about aggression and delinquency, whereby interviewers introduced the survey that youth completed via a provided computer (De Leeuw et al., 2003). The sample consisted of Dutch youth between the ages of 12–19, some of whom were receiving court-ordered treatment, though the sample size was not specified. The authors reported the preliminary results were suggestive of the method reducing stress around sensitive questions.

Systematic or Anecdotal Indicators of Advantages and Disadvantages of e-Mental Health

Advantages and disadvantages of e-mental health for justice involved youth were rarely systematically or rigorously studied in the reviewed references. Nevertheless, reports often included anecdotal mentions of both. The most frequently indicated advantages across the different types of e-mental health were positive opinions, enhanced access to care or specific responsivity, efficiency, and effectiveness or reliability and validity. Other occasionally indicated advantages were concerned with uniqueness, privacy, and fidelity. In contrast, the most commonly indicated disadvantages were the reverse of the most common advantages: negative opinions, barriers to access to care or service tailoring, lack of effectiveness or reliability and validity evidence, and inefficiency. Additionally indicated disadvantages concerned novelty, privacy and ethics, and fidelity, as well as a lack of in-person contact, negative consequences, and glitches.

Multicultural Diversity and the Available e-Mental Health Research for Juvenile Justice

Multicultural diversity and specific responsivity (e.g., a socioeconomic digital divide, linguistic diversity) have rarely been the primary focus of attention in a study of e-mental health for juvenile justice, or rigorously investigated. For instance, only five studies have been conducted outside North America. Most studies reported sex or gender data, with a sizable number of studies having exclusively sampled boys, and a handful only sampling girls. Seventeen of the studies reported information about the race or ethnicity of the sample, with a few studies having exclusively sampled African American youth, and one having sampled only white youth. The other studies had a relatively fair portion of white and non-white participants.

Few studies conducted significant difference testing based on sex or gender or race or ethnicity. Of these few studies, three did not find any sex or gender differences (Bahr et al., 2016; Burraston et al., 2014; Wannachaiyakul et al., 2017), whereas one study of a phone-based telehealth service found that girls were more likely to be arrested than boys (Burraston et al., 2012). As for race or ethnicity, three studies did not find any group differences (Brown, 2018; Fowles, 2009; Wasserman et al., 2002). In contrast, a study of phone-based telehealth found that white race was predictive of a higher number of felony arrests in one model (Bahr et al., 2016), and a study of a computerised educational programme found that African American and Latino youth evidenced significantly different effects primarily on baseline measures but also on some outcome measures, relative to white and mixed-race youth (Houchins et al., 2018).

Conclusion and Future Directions

Despite research on e-mental health for juvenile justice first emerging in the 1980s, an overall small number of studies have been conducted up to the present time, especially when considering increasingly specific types of e-mental health. Various design limitations of the available studies, mixed results, and the diversity of examined technologies caution against concluding that any type of e-mental health has yet been validated for assessment or treatment of justice-involved youth. Of note, validation is an especially complicated concept in this area, and one in need of much more research, including replication research, to inform the range of complex questions it entails. For example, e-mental health as an adjunctive or exclusive service? Expectations of equivalency with or incremental utility to similar in-person services? Replication evidence for the same technology?

There is also a pressing need for increased attention to and rigorous study of issues concerning multicultural diversity and potential digital divides for e-mental health and juvenile justice. As a starting point, more research of e-mental health for juvenile justice needs to separately examine effects for different demographic groups. Research examining the extent of digital divides along multicultural and socioeconomic lines is also sorely needed.

It can be anticipated, based on necessary shifts in practice during the COVID-19 pandemic towards wide uptake of secure videoconferencing platforms (e.g., American Psychological Association, 2020), that more research will soon be forthcoming, especially for telehealth. Relatedly, many psychological tests are available in computerised formats, including for secure remote administration. Though beyond the recent increase in the use of telehealth for assessment and treatment (presumably also in work with justice-involved youth), other types of e-mental health, and particularly those specifically developed for justice-involved youth, remain in the category of "emerging" technologies (see Kirschstein et al., 2021) that have yet to be widely disseminated to practitioners.

Looking forward, provisional practice guidelines and multidisciplinary trainings would be of assistance to practitioners. In addition, collaborations among practitioners, researchers, and technology specialists will likely be needed to support larger-scale telehealth implementations, to ensure that e-mental health generally is developed and implemented consistent with security measures (see, e.g., King et al., 2017) and for further development and evaluation of digitised intervention programmes and simulation games. Furthermore, funding and organisational policies supportive of additional development, evaluation, implementation, and sustainment of e-mental health for juvenile justice will be needed to facilitate the accrual of more evidence and expand this service modality more rapidly in the field. As a starting point, academic institutions often have good infrastructures for information technology, and promote research attentive to disadvantaged populations, such that initiatives involving researcher-practitioner partnerships may be the most feasible. Research could also be conducted to clarify and help overcome legal, administrative, and practical barriers to greater uptake of e-mental health in juvenile justice contexts. Subsequently, more evidence from researchers of the incremental benefits of e-mental health relative to traditional service modalities, and greater dissemination efforts by e-mental health product developers, would help to persuade administrators of the value and feasibility of investment in e-mental health.

References

Abram, K. M., Paskar, L. D., Washburn, J. J., & Teplin, L. A. (2008). Perceived barriers to mental health services among youths in detention. *Journal of the American Academy of Child and Adolescent Psychiatry*, *47*(3), 301–308. 10.1097/CHI.0b013e318160b3bb

American Psychological Association. (2020, June 5). *Psychologists embrace telehealth to prevent the spread of COVID-19*. American Psychological Association. https://www.apaservices.org/practice/legal/technology/psychologists-embrace-telehealth

Anderson, E. (2018). *Externalizing behavioral symptoms in adjudicated youth and solution-focused brief therapy delivered through video conferencing* (Publication No. 13420722) [Doctoral dissertation, University of Central Arkansas]. ProQuest Dissertations Publishing.

Bahr, S. J., Cherrington, D. J., & Erickson, L. D. (2016). An evaluation of the impact of goal setting and cell phone calls on juvenile rearrests. *International Journal of Offender Therapy and Comparative Criminology*, *60*(16), 1816–1835. 10.1177/0306624X15588549

Batastini, A. B. (2016). Improving rehabilitative efforts for juvenile offenders through the use of telemental healthcare. *Journal of Child and Adolescent Psychopharmacology*, *26*(3), 273–277. 10.1089/cap.2015.0011

Batastini, A. B., King, C. M., Morgan, R. D., & McDaniel, B. (2016). Telepsychological services with criminal justice and substance abuse clients: A systematic review and meta-analysis. *Psychological Services*, *13*(1), 20–30. 10.1037/ser0000042

Batastini, A. B., Paprzycki, P., Jones, A. C. T., & MacLean, N. (2021). Are videoconferenced mental and behavioral health services just as good as in-person? A meta-analysis of a fast-growing practice. *Clinical Psychology Review*, *83*, Article 101944. 10.1016/j.cpr.2020.101944

Bath, E., Tolou-Shams, M., & Farabee, D. (2018). Mobile health (mHealth): Building the case for adapting emerging technologies for justice-involved youth. *Journal of the American Academy of Child and Adolescent Psychiatry*, *57*(12), 903–905. 10.1016/j.jaac.2018.08.012

Beaudry, G., Yu, R., Långström, N., & Fazel, S. (2021). An updated systematic review and meta-regression analysis: Mental disorders among adolescents in juvenile detention and correctional facilities. *Journal of the American Academy of Child and Adolescent Psychiatry*, *60*(1), 46–60. 10.1016/j.jaac.2020.01.015

Bonta, J., & Andrews, D. A. (2017). *The psychology of criminal conduct* (6th ed.). New York, NY: Routledge. 10.4324/9781315677187

Brogan, L., Haney-Caron, E., NeMoyer, A., & DeMatteo, D. (2015). Applying the Risk-Needs-Responsivity (RNR) model to juvenile justice. *Criminal Justice Review*, *40*(3), 277–302. 10.1177/0734016814567312

Brown, E. L. (2018). *Developing a subcomponent of empathy in juvenile offenders* (Publication No. 10817599) [Doctoral dissertation, University of the Rockies]. ProQuest Dissertations Publishing.

Burraston, B. O., Bahr, S. J., & Cherrington, D. J. (2014). Reducing juvenile delinquency with automated cell phone calls. *International Journal of Offender Therapy and Comparative Criminology*, *58*(5), 522–536. 10.1177/0306624X13480947

Burraston, B. O., Cherrington, D. J., & Bahr, S. J. (2012). Reducing juvenile recidivism with cognitive training and a cell phone follow-up: An evaluation of the RealVictory Program. *International Journal of Offender Therapy and Comparative Criminology*, *56*(1), 61–80. 10.1177/0306624x10388635

Caudle, S. D. (2011). *Ethos: An original moral dilemma computer game and the testing of its content validity* (Publication No. 3463696) [Doctoral dissertation, North Carolina State University]. ProQuest Dissertations Publishing.

Cervenka, K. A., Dembo, R., & Brown, C. H. (1996). Family empowerment intervention for families of juvenile offenders. *Aggression and Violent Behavior*, *1*(3), 205–216. 10.1016/1359-1789(95)00007-0

Chesney-Lind, M., Morash, M., & Stevens, T. (2008). Girls' troubles, girls' delinquency, and gender responsive programming: A review. *Australian and New Zealand Journal of Criminology*, *41*(1, Spec Iss), 162–189. 10.1375/acri.41.1.162

Danielson, C. K., McCauley, J. L., Jones, A. M., Borkman, A. L., Miller, S., & Ruggiero, K. J. (2013). Feasibility of delivering evidence-based HIV/STI prevention programming to a community sample of African American teen girls via the internet. *Aids Education and Prevention*, *25*(5), 394–404. 10.1521/aeap.2013.25.5.394

De Leeuw, E., Hox, J., & Kef, S. (2003). Computer-assisted self-interviewing tailored for special populations and topics. *Field Methods*, *15*(3), 223–251. 10.1177/1525822X03254714

Development Services Group, Inc. (2014). *Disproportionate minority contact (DMC)*. Office of Juvenile Justice and Delinquency Prevention. https://ojjdp.ojp.gov/mpg/literature-review/disproportionate-minority-contact.pdf

DiClemente, R. J., Davis, T. L., Swartzendruber, A., Fasula, A. M., Boyce, L., Gelaude, D., Gray, S. C., Hardin, J., Rose, E., Carry, M., Sales, J. M., Brown, J. L., & Staples-Horne, M. (2014). Efficacy of an HIV/STI sexual risk-reduction intervention for African American adolescent girls in juvenile detention centers: A randomized controlled trial. *Women & Health*, *54*(8), 726–749. 10.1080/03630242.2014.932893

Evans-Chase, M. (2015). If they like it they can take it with them: A mixed methods examination of internet-based mindfulness meditation with incarcerated youth. *Advances in Social Work*, *16*(1), 90–106. 10.18060/17973

Feil, E. G., Baggett, K. M., Davis, B., Landry, S., Carter, J. J., Buzhardt, J., & Sheeber, L. (2008). Expanding the reach of preventive interventions: Development of an internet-based training for parents of infants. *Child Maltreatment*, *13*(4), 334–346. 10.1177/1077559508322446

Fleming, T., & Merry, S. (2013). Youth work service providers' attitudes towards computerized CBT for adolescents. *Behavioural and Cognitive Psychotherapy*, *41*(3), 265–279. 10.1017/S1352465812000306

Fleming, T. M., Gillham, B., Bavin, L. M., Stasiak, K., Lewycka, S., Moore, J., Shepherd, M., & Merry, S. N. (2019). SPARX-R computerized therapy among adolescents in youth offenders' program: Step-wise cohort study. *Internet Interventions, 18,* Article 100287. 10.1016/j.invent.2019.100287

Folk, J. B., Harrison, A., Rodriguez, C., Wallace, A., & Tolou-Shams, M. (2020). Feasibility of social media-based recruitment and perceived acceptability of digital health Interventions for caregivers of justice-involved youth: Mixed methods study. *Journal of Medical Internet Research, 22*(4), Article e16370. 10.2196/16370

Fowles, T. R. (2009). *Preventing recidivism with cell-phones: Telehealth aftercare for juvenile offenders* (Publication No. 3388388). [Doctoral dissertation, University of Utah]. ProQuest Dissertations Publishing.

Fox, K. C., Connor, P., McCullers, E., & Waters, T. (2008). Effect of a behavioural health and specialty care telemedicine programme on goal attainment for youths in juvenile detention. *Journal of Telemedicine and Telecare, 14*(5), 227–230. 10.1258/jtt.2008.071102

Fox, K. C., Somes, G., & Waters, T. M. (2006). The use of telemedicine technology and restructured referral patterns to reduce health care costs in a juvenile justice system. *Journal of Correctional Health Care, 12*(3), 214–221. 10.1177/1078345806292667

Fox, K. C., Somes, G. W., & Waters, T. M. (2007). Timeliness and access to healthcare services via telemedicine for adolescents in state correctional facilities. *Journal of Adolescent Health, 41*(2), 161–167. 10.1016/j.jadohealth.2007.05.001

Grove, L., King, C. M., Bomysoad, R., Vasquez, L., & Kois, L. E. (2021). Technology for assessment and treatment of justice-involved youth: A systematic literature review. *Law and Human Behavior, 45*(5), 413–426. https://doi.org/10.1037/lhb0000467

Gutierrez, L., Chadwick, N., & Wanamaker, K. A. (2018). Culturally relevant programming versus the status quo: A meta-analytic review of the effectiveness of treatment of indigenous offenders. *Canadian Journal of Criminology and Criminal Justice, 60*(3), 321–353. 10.3138/cjccj.2017-0020.r2

Guy, L. S., Packer, I. K., & Warnken, W. (2012). Assessing Risk of Violence Using Structured Professional Judgment Guidelines. *Journal of Forensic Psychology Practice, 12*(3), 270–283. https://doi.org/10.1080/15228932.2012.674471

Her Majesty's Inspectorate of Probation. (2020). *A thematic review of the work of youth offending services during the COVID-19 pandemic.* Her Majesty's Inspectorate of Probation. https:// www.justiceinspectorates.gov.uk/hmiprobation/wp-content/uploads/sites/5/2020/ 11/201110-A-thematic-review-of-the-work-of-youth-offending-services-during-the-COVID-19-pandemic.pdf

Hoge, R. D. (2016). Risk, need, and responsivity in juveniles. In K. Heilbrun, D. DeMatteo, & N. E. S. Goldstein (Eds.). *APA handbook of psychology and juvenile justice* (pp. 179–196). Washington DC: American Psychological Association. 10.1037/ 14643-009

Houchins, D. E., Gagnon, J. C., Lane, H. B., Lambert, R. G., & McCray, E. D. (2018). The efficacy of a literacy intervention for incarcerated adolescents. *Residential Treatment for Children & Youth, 35*(1), 60–91. 10.1080/0886571x.2018.1448739

Johnson, L., Gutridge, K., Parkes, J., Roy, A., & Plugge, E. (2021). Scoping review of mental health in prisons through the COVID-19 pandemic. *BMJ Open, 11,* e046547. 110.1136/bmjopen-2020-046547

Kaliebe, K. E., Heneghan, J., & Kim, T. J. (2011). Telepsychiatry in juvenile justice settings. *Child and Adolescent Psychiatric Clinics of North America, 20*(1), 113–123. 10.1016/ j.chc.2010.09.001

King, C. M., Heilbrun K., Kim, N. Y., McWilliams, K., Phillips, S., Barbera, J., & Fretz, R. (2017). Tablet computers and forensic and correctional psychological assessment: A randomized controlled study. *Law and Human Behavior, 41*(5), 468–477. 10.1037/lhb0000245

Kip, H., & Bouman, Y. H. A. (2021). A perspective on the integration of eHealth in treatment of offenders: Combining technology and the Risk-Need-Responsivity model. *Frontiers in Psychiatry, 12*, Article 703043. 10.3389/fpsyt.2021.703043.

Kip, H., Bouman, Y., Kelders, S. M., & van Gemert-Pijnen, L. (2018). eHealth in treatment of offenders in forensic mental health: A review of the current state. *Frontiers in Psychiatry, 9*, 42. 10.3389/fpsyt.2018.00042

Kirschstein, M. A., Singh, J. P., Rossegger, A., Endrass, J., & Graf, M. (2021). International survey on the use of emerging technologies among forensic and correctional mental health professionals. *Criminal Justice and Behavior.* Advance online publication. 10.1177/00938548211042057

Kois, L. E., Cox, J., & Peck, A. T. (2021). Forensic e-mental health: Review, research priorities, and policy directions. *Psychology, Public Policy, and Law, 27*(1), 1–16. 10.1037/law0000293

Lal, S., & Adair, C. E. (2014). E-mental health: A rapid review of the literature. *Psychiatric Services, 65*(1), 24 32. 10.1176/appi.ps.201300009

Levesque, D., Johnson, J., Welch, C., Prochaska, J., & Fernandez, A. (2012). Computer-tailored intervention for juvenile offenders. *Journal of Social Work Practice in the Addictions, 12*(4), 391–411. 10.1080/1533256X.2012.728107

MacDonell, K. W., & Prinz, R. J. (2017). A review of technology-based youth and family-focused interventions. *Clinical Child and Family Psychology Review, 20*(2), 185–200. 10.1007/s10567-016-0218-x

McCormick, S., Peterson-Badali, M., & Skilling, T. A. (2017). The role of mental health and specific responsivity in juvenile justice rehabilitation. *Law and Human Behavior, 41*(1), 55–67. https://doi.org/10.1037/lhb0000228

McDougall, C., Pearson, D. A. S., Torgerson, D. J., & Garcia-Reyes, M. (2017). The effect of digital technology on prisoner behavior and reoffending: A natural stepped-wedge design. *Journal of Experimental Criminology, 13*(4), 455–482. 10.1007/s11292-017-9303-5

Mucic, D., & Hilty, D. M. (Eds.) (2016). *e-mental health.* Switzerland: Springer. 10.1007/978-3-319-20852-7

Mulay, A. L., Gottfried, E. D., Mullis, D. M., & Vitacco, M. J. (2021). The use of videoconferencing in forensic evaluations: Moving forward in times of COVID-19. *Journal of Forensic Psychology Research and Practice, 21*(4), 338–354. 10.1080/24732850.2021.1877508

Myers, K., Valentine, J., Morganthaler, R., & Melzer, S. (2006). Telepsychiatry with incarcerated youth. *Journal of Adolescent Health, 38*(6), 643–648. 10.1016/j.jadohealth.2005.07.015

Paperny, D. M. (1997). Computerized health assessment and education for adolescent HIV and STD prevention in health care settings and schools. *Health Education & Behavior, 24*(1), 54–70. 10.1177/109019819702400107

Paschall, M. J., Ornstein, M. L., & Flewelling, R. L. (2001). African American male adolescents' involvement in the criminal justice system: The criterion validity of self-report measures in a prospective study. *Journal of Research in Crime and Delinquency, 38*(2), 174–187. 10.1177/0022427801038002004

Posick, C. M. (2009). *The use of computer-based interventions in cognitive behavioral therapy: Policy implications for violence and delinquency prevention in community corrections* (Publication No. 1463943) [Master's thesis, Rochester Institute of Technology]. ProQuest Dissertations Publishing.

Resnick, H. (1986). Electronic technology and rehabilitation: A computerized simulation game for youthful offenders. *Simulation & Games, 17*(4), 460–466. 10.1177/003755 0086174004

Rovner, J. (2014). *Disproportionate minority contact in the juvenile justice system.* The Sentencing Project. https://sentencingproject.org/wp-content/uploads/2015/11/Disproportionate-Minority-Contact-in-the-Juvenile-Justice-System.pdf

Rowlands, A., Fisher, M., Mishra, J., Nahum, M., Brandrett, B., Reinke, M., Caldwell, M., Kiehl, K. A., & Vinogradov, S. (2020). Cognitive training for very high risk incarcerated adolescent males. *Frontiers in Psychiatry, 11*, Article 225. 10.3389/fpsyt.2020.00225

Sewell, K. M., Woods, S., Bélisle, E., Walsh, M., & Augimeri, L. K. (2019). SNAP Youth Justice: Youth perceptions of their learning during a pilot of an evidence-informed intervention. *Journal of Evidence-Based Social Work, 16*(5), 478–496. 10.1080/26408066. 2019.1629139

Sherer, M. (1990). Computerized therapeutic games within the social work arena. *The International Journal of Sociology and Social Policy, 10*(4/5/6), 181–201. 10.1108/eb013111

Shufelt, J. L., & Cocozza, J. J. (2006). *Youth with mental health disorders in the juvenile justice system: Results from a multi-state prevalence study.* UNICEF. https://sites.unicef.org/tdad/usmentalhealthprevalence06.pdf

Singh, J. P., Desmarais, S. L., Sellers, B. G., Hylton, T., Tirotti, M., & Van Dorn, R. A. (2014). From risk assessment to risk management: Matching interventions to adolescent offenders' strengths and vulnerabilities. *Children and Youth Services Review, 47* (Part 1), 1–9. 10.1016/j.childyouth.2013.09.015

Teplin, L. A., Abram, K. M., Washburn, J. J., Welty, L. J., Hershfield, J. A., & Dulcan, M. K. (2013). *The Northwestern juvenile project: Overview.* Office of Juvenile Justice and Delinquency Prevention. https://ojjdp.ojp.gov/sites/g/files/xyckuh176/files/pubs/234522.pdf

Tolou-Shams, M., Yonek, J., Galbraith, K., & Bath, E. (2019). Text messaging to enhance behavioral health treatment engagement among justice-involved youth: Qualitative and user testing study. *JMIR mHealth and uHealth, 7*(4), Article e10904. 10.2196/10904

United Nations. (n.d.). *Fact sheet on juvenile justice.* https://www.un.org/esa/socdev/unyin/documents/wyr11/FactSheetonYouthandJuvenileJustice.pdf

United Nations Guidelines for the Prevention of Juvenile Delinquency (The Riyadh Guidelines), G.A. Res. 45/112, U.N. Doc. A/RES/45/112 (December 14, 1990), https://www.ohchr.org/en/ProfessionalInterest/Pages/PreventionOfJuvenileDelinquency.aspx

Vieira, T. A., Skilling, T. A., & Peterson-Badali, M. (2009). Matching court-ordered services with treatment needs: Predicting treatment success with young offenders. *Criminal Justice and Behavior, 36*(4), 385–401. 10.1177/0093854808331249

Vigilante, A. (1994). *Integrating computer-aided instruction for improving reading skills with juvenile delinquents* (ERIC Number ED367960) [Master's thesis, Nova University]. Institute of Education Sciences (ERIC).

Vincent, G. M., Guy, L. S., & Grisso, T. (2012). Risk assessment in juvenile justice: A guidebook for implementation. *Models for Change.* http://modelsforchange.net/publications/346/Risk_Assessment_in_Juvenile_Justice_A_Guidebook_for_Implementation.pdf

Walker, S. C., Muno, A., & Sullivan-Colglazier, C. (2015). Principles in practice: A multistate study of gender-responsive reforms in the juvenile justice system. *Crime & Delinquency, 61*(5), 742–766. 10.1177/0011128712449712

Wannachaiyakul, S., Thapinta, D., Sethabouppha, H., Thungjaroenkul, P., & Likhitsathian, S. (2017). Randomized controlled trial of computerized cognitive behavioral therapy program for adolescent offenders with depression. *Pacific Rim International Journal of Nursing Research*, *21*(1), 32–43.

Wasserman, G. A., McReynolds, L. S., Lucas, C. P., Fisher, P., & Santos, L. (2002). The Voice DISC-IV with incarcerated male youths: Prevalence of disorder. *Journal of the American Academy of Child & Adolescent Psychiatry*, *41*(3), 314–321. 10.1097/00004583-200203000-00011

White, L. M., Lau, K. S., & Aalsma, M. C. (2016). Detained adolescents: Mental health needs, treatment use, and recidivism. *The Journal of the American Academy of Psychiatry and the Law*, *44*(2), 200–212.

Zahn, M. A., Day, J. C., Mihalic, S. F., & Tichavsky, L. (2009). Determining what works for girls in the juvenile justice system. A summary of evaluation evidence. *Crime & Delinquency*, *55*(2), 266–293. 10.1177/0011128708330649

Zane, S. N., & Pupo, J. A. (2021). Disproportionate Minority Contact in the Juvenile Justice System: A Systematic Review and Meta-Analysis. *Justice Quarterly*, *38*(7), 1293–1318. https://doi.org/10.1080/07418825.2021.1915364

10 Implications and Considerations for Conducting Remote Forensic Evaluations in Underserved and Marginalised Communities

Ashley Batastini, Natalie Anumba, Michelle Guyon, and Meera Patel

Introduction

In 2013, the American Psychological Association published their *Guidelines for the Practice of Telepsychology*. In this chapter, telepsychology is defined as "the provision of psychological services using telecommunication technologies" which includes (among other modalities) "telephone, mobile devices, interactive videoconferencing, email, chat, text, and internet (e.g., self-help websites, blogs, and social media)". Similar definitions are used around the world. Today, telepsychological[1] approaches have become a necessity following the COVID-19 health crisis for sustaining clinical practices and safely engaging with clients. What many clinicians who are newer to the use of telepsychology may not realise is that attention on remote service delivery had been steadily increasing since around the 1990s. In the United States, this expansion was, in part, due a broader national interest on improving rural health care (e.g., via the Health Resources & Services Administration's Office of Rural Health Policy) that leaned on telehealth to connect geographically remote and historically impoverished communities to accessible, affordable, and good-quality services. In the United States, the boom in rural correctional facilities as a misguided attempt to boost economic growth (Glasmeier & Farrigan, 2007; Hooks et al., 2004), coupled with the general difficulty of recruiting providers to work in these settings, also led to an emphasis on telepractice to meet healthcare needs for incarcerated persons (see Ax et al., 2007; Manfredi et al. 2005).

However, as telecommunications became more normative in our daily lives with the proliferation of social media and videocall platforms like Skype, the use of telepsychology was promoted as an alternative for anyone with limited time, access, or financial means to seek mental health services. In a 2013 survey of practitioners regarding anticipated trends in psychotherapy by the year 2022, respondents endorsed telepsychology as having the highest likelihood of expansion (Norcross et al., 2013). While these practitioners could not have predicted the onset of a global pandemic, many scholars and advocates

DOI: 10.4324/9781003230977-11

underscored telecommunication services as a solution to the dueling problem of increased demand for services and provider shortages. In an invited commentary to the Australian Psychological Society, for example, Frueh (2015) asserted, "Technology is the key to solving mental healthcare access problems in the twenty-first century" (p. 304). The popularity of telepsychology led to other initiatives such as the establishment of the Psychology Interjurisdictional Compact (PSYPACT) in the United States that provided a mechanism for practicing across state lines, formal guidance from professional organisations and government agencies (e.g., American Psychological Association, 2013a, 2013b; American Psychiatric Association, 2018; Australia's National Digital Health Strategy, 2018; Digital Health & Care Scotland, 2018; United Kingdom National Health Service, 2019), and designated funding opportunities for research and training.

Among other pre-pandemic scholarships, a 2021 meta-analysis summarised two decades of empirical research comparing in-person and videoconference-based services across intervention and assessment outcomes, with articles published between 1997 and 2019 (Batastini et al., 2021). While these authors acknowledged several limitations in the available literature, findings consistently showed non-significant results suggesting that, in most cases, being in the same physical space with a client/examinee does not yield meaningfully different treatment progress or assessment decisions compared to synchronous video sessions. Notably, this analysis included research with adult clients who were seen in a variety of settings (e.g., in-home, university, medical facilities, veteran affairs centres/hospitals, prisons) for various types of services (e.g., counselling, psychiatric management, psychodiagnosis). These results added more rigorous support to the metaphorical green light that already existed for general telepsychological practice.

Yet, as mental health sectors were largely embracing telecommunication technologies, there appeared to be greater skepticism from forensic practitioners who expressed concern about whether data germane to certain psycholegal questions would be lost and whether courts would accept virtual evaluations (Batastini et al., 2019). There was also relatively little research specifically within forensic contexts to ease this hesitancy, though what data were available supported its use (see Batastini et al., 2016; Luxton et al., 2019; Manguno-Mire et al., 2007). Before the COVID-19 pandemic, an estimated one-third of forensic examiners had used videoconferencing to conduct an evaluation (Batastini et al., 2019; Daffern et al., 2021); however, an estimated 60% reportedly used videoconferencing after the onset of COVID-19 (Daffern et al., 2021). Another survey study found that 94% of forensic practitioners in more than 20 countries increased their use of videoconferencing in the wake of the pandemic (Kirschstein et al., 2021).

As much of the forensic practice community was jolted into a new normal, it is relevant to once again recognise that remote evaluations had already been on the rise in rural communities, where jails are overwhelmed with pretrial defendants who are more likely to be people of colour and/or have fewer resources to expend on their legal defence (Rabuy & Kopf, 2016; Sawyer, 2019), and local forensic examiners are harder to come by. Although the demand for forensic mental health assessments (FMHA) in many areas is disproportionate to the number of providers able to conduct them (Antonacci et al., 2008; Deslich et al., 2013), the need for such assessments in economically disadvantaged areas is particularly large (Ryba et al., 2003; Thomas et al., 2009). Lack of access to appropriately qualified forensic evaluators can lead to a host of problems, including long wait-times for evaluators from centralised state psychiatric hospitals, incentives to drop charges or offer quicker plea deals that may infringe on a defendant's rights (e.g., allowing a potentially incompetent defendant to accept a plea bargain), or retaining so-called "occasional experts" (i.e., mental health practitioners without specialised forensic training who are retained by courts that do not know better; Grisso, 1987). These outcomes may, in turn, lead to discrimination in the administration of justice.

While remote FMHA are one mechanism for alleviating many of the existing barriers that weigh on rural jurisdictions and defendants with fewer resources, there are several considerations and cautions regarding its use. This chapter first summarise the racial and economic imbalances in forensic mental health services and discuss the ways in which remote evaluations could improve equity in access to qualified evaluators and subsequent legal decisions. Despite respective guidelines for the practice of telepsychology and forensic work (e.g., *Specialty Guidelines for Forensic Psychology*, 2013), there is a need for guidance at the place where these areas overlap. As such, we offer recommendations for improving the efficiency and quality of remote FMHA, particularly when working with poorer, underserved, and/or marginalised agencies and examinees. Finally, we discuss relevant legal, policy, and advocacy considerations. Of note, the following sections focus on the use of technologies in criminal legal issues that use live audio-visual components (i.e., videoconferencing).

Forensic Mental Health Services in Rural and Economically Disadvantaged Regions

Causes and Consequences of Service Disparities: A Brief Lay of the Land

In general, multiple factors contribute to limited access of mental health services relative to need, including uneven dispersion of mental health professionals, smaller numbers of treatment facilities and psychiatric hospitals, having to travel significant distances for services, and poorer insurance coverage and limited public funding for mental health programmes (Backhaus, et al., 2012; Gale et al., 2019; Ellis, et al., 2009). Compounding broader issues of mental health treatment access is that communities of colour, immigrants and persons with limited English proficiency, older individuals, low-income individuals, and rural populations are less likely to receive mental health treatment than others (Thornicroft, 2008).

For many of these reasons, issues of mental illness, treatment access, and disparities are often concentrated in correctional settings, particularly local jails. In fact, despite not being a significant risk factor for crime (Peterson et al., 2014), the prevalence of mental health problems outpaces those of the general population, with up to 65% of jailed individuals reporting mood and anxiety related symptoms (Bronson & Berzofsky, 2021). In rural areas, people with mental illness may be more likely to receive care through contact with the criminal justice system than community mental resources (Gale et al., 2019) and rural Americans in general are more likely to end up in jail than their urban counterparts (Kang-Brown et al., 2019). Poverty, which includes a higher proportion of rural residents than urban (Dobis et al., 2021), is also associated with risk of involvement with the criminal justice system, with incarceration further fuelling socio-economic marginalisation (see Martin, 2011; Rabuy & Kopf, 2015). Further, black and Hispanic/Latinx Americans are overrepresented among those incarcerated (Bronson & Berzofsky, 2021) and those in poverty compared to white Americans (Shrider et al., 2021). Indigenous persons, many of whom reside in rural and low-income areas (Dewees & Marks, 2017), are also overrepresented in the United States, Canadian, Australian, and New Zealand justice systems (Papalia et al., 2019).

Correction facilities in remote locations face a unique set of struggles related to recruiting and retaining qualified professionals, facing daunting security considerations that complicate the transportation of correctional clients for treatment, and managing individuals with challenging presentations and high needs (Batastini et al., 2016). Shortages in mental health care and providers have particular consequences for pretrial detainees, including decreased availability of state hospital beds for transfer and prolonged incarceration related to slow-to-process charges in facilities that are ill-equipped to treat them, which may constitute a violation of one's rights (Callahan & Pinals, 2020; Gowensmith, 2019). There are also implications for due process; compared to pretrial defendants who are not detained, those who are incarcerated may have more restricted access to private meeting spaces and communications with attorneys. Additionally, these defendants may be served by attorneys who are overloaded with cases and face the burden of travelling to remote sites (Kalb, 2018). Throughout the European Union, an estimated one in five incarcerated persons is awaiting court action. In the United States, this number is approximately six out of ten jailed individuals (Zheng & Milton, 2021). Given the financial resources needed to be released from jail while awaiting trial and research suggesting people of colour are less likely to be granted released than white people (see Digard & Swavola, 2019), forensic examiners have a greater chance of encountering examinees from marginalised communities in jail rather than on bail or bond.

High rates of mental illness in pretrial correctional settings can give rise to legal questions regarding pretrial detainees' competence to stand trial. Competence to stand trial evaluation referrals are not only the most often ordered by courts, but they have also increased in recent years to crisis levels (Gowensmith, 2019), resulting in a high demand for forensic mental health assessments, added strain on state-provided mental health services, continued detention for individuals requiring hospital level of care, and delay in the resolution of criminal cases (Murrie et al., 2020). For example, if concerns emerge about a pretrial detainee's competence to stand trial or if a detainee is adjudicated incompetent to stand trial, the detainee is likely to experience long waits for admission to state hospital for an in-person evaluation or restoration treatment (Thornicroft, 2008). The specialised nature and cost of forensic mental health evaluations exacerbates disparities in rural and economically disadvantaged regions, where access to qualified evaluators and budgets are especially strained (Luxton & Lexcen, 2018).

A high demand for pretrial FMHA, including not only adjudicative competency but also issues such as mental state at the time of the offense, could lead to retention of unqualified evaluators and/or poor-quality evaluations, particularly given the lack of clear and legally enforceable standards of care to regulate forensic mental health evaluations in many jurisdictions (Heilbrun et al, 2008; McCallum & Gowensmith, 2019). The backlog of competency and other pretrial referrals has caught the attention of the media, legislatures, and the courts, resulting in lawsuits and significant contempt of court fines (e.g., *Trueblood et al. v. Washington State DHSH*, 2014). If incompetent defendants remain confined for extensive periods of time, or if they are deemed unrestorable, charges may ultimately be dropped. When psychiatric bed space or outpatient services are unavailable, individuals may be released from jail to the community without adequate care. These decisions can cost jurisdictions the opportunity to pursue justice for alleged wrongdoing to society as well as the opportunity to prevent decompensation and future criminal justice contacts.

The Role of Technology in Closing the Gap

In recent decades, technology has emerged as a way to address concerns about access to mental health services and may be especially applicable in regions where internet use is growing, such as parts of Latin America, the Middle East, and Africa (Hilty et al., 2017). Technology-based health services have a lengthy history in correctional settings (see Batastini et al., 2013 for a review). Aimed at addressing these disparities in rural counties, Miller et al. (2005) published one of the earliest known descriptions of a telepsychiatry clinic for forensic evaluation and consultation services. Despite ongoing questions regarding the acceptability of such technology to the courts and the lack of case law discussing the admissibility of remote forensic evaluations (Goldenson & Josefowitz, 2021), video-conferencing has been used in criminal and civil court proceedings for at least two decades (Drogin, 2020; Luxton & Lexcen, 2018; e.g., see *Thornton v. Snyder*, 2005; *United States v. Baker*, 1995). To date, there are no known constitutional challenges to the use of remote FMHA. Although research and guidance specific to the practice of forensic psychology remain limited at the time of this writing, what is available suggests that remote FMHA are a viable and valid option (Luxton & Lexcen, 2018; Luxton et al., 2019; Manguno-Mire et al., 2007).

Benefits of Remote FMHA

The integration of technology in FMHA comes with multiple notable benefits. These include decreases in costs associated with examiner travel to facilities and transportation of incarcerated individuals. Without having to account for travel time, forensic examiners may be able to increase the number of evaluations they can reasonably conduct and/or dedicate more time to report-writing, thereby improving quality and turnaround times. In addition to time and cost-related factors, eliminating the need to transport in-custody defendants reduces security and safety concerns, as conducting evaluations remotely maintains the physical safety of the evaluator while possibly reducing the need for physical restraints (particularly if technological equipment is protected), which can be uncomfortable or distracting. Elderly defendants or those with physical disabilities may also be more difficult to transport. Additionally, remote evaluations can create greater flexibility in scheduling evaluations and facilitating the presence of the examinee's attorney to observe interviews or the use of court-approved interpreters. The ability to conduct high-quality evaluations in a timelier and confidential manner may help preserve the defendant's right to a speedy trial or, if the defendant is incompetent or otherwise experiencing acute mental illness, facilitate an efficient referral for psychiatric services. In rural areas that are often mental healthcare deserts, such services may likewise be conducted via telehealth (e.g., connecting virtually to larger medical centres to oversee medication management).

Within the context of interjurisdictional policies (see discussion below), the use of videoconferencing to conduct FMHA remotely may also encourage national and international networking, thereby increasing courts' and examinees' access to mental health professionals who have specialised expertise or who match the examinee in terms of race, ethnicity, or language. Certain technologies may also be more accommodating for certain types of examinees. For example, the ability to use closed captioning or simply turn up the volume may improve engagement or cooperation for those with hearing impairment. Finally, remote FMHA may improve trainee participation by allowing trainees to join virtual interview session and/or expanding access to expertly trained supervisors in the field via tele-supervision. Broadening opportunities for trainees may enhance education of forensic mental health professionals, particularly as virtual evaluations have become more normative post-pandemic and serve as a means of recruitment to more geographically remote and/or underserved areas (Drogin, 2020; Luxton & Lexcen, 2018; Luxton et al., 2019).

Remote FMHA Is Not a Universal Remedy

It is relevant to acknowledge that remote FMHA is not a perfect solution. Several drawbacks and concerns have been identified (Batastini et al., 2019; Chen, et al., 2021; Drogin, 2020; Luxton et al., 2019; Ralston et al., 2020) including the following:

- High initial expenses for technology in jails or courts that do not already have necessary equipment.
- Variable facility infrastructure to support videoconferencing (e.g., availability of private consultation/interviewing space, stability of internet connection).
- Concerns about providing incarcerated examinees unsupervised access to expensive equipment or to the internet.
- The potential for technological problems (such as audio delay or video failure), necessity of staff training and willingness to use technology.
- The possibility that a person not visible to the examiner may be present and influence or coach the examinee.
- The inability to assess aspects of an examinee's presentation (e.g., eye contact; olfactory information, responses to internal stimuli) or administer certain types of test instruments.
- Examinee reactions to the use of technology that may impact response style.
- Limits in the ability to manage immediate safety issues (e.g., medical emergencies, suicidality, damage to property) from a remote location.
- Jurisdictional/licensure considerations.

Batastini et al. (2019) found that examiners who had prior experience conducting remote FMHA endorsed significantly fewer concerns about its use compared to those who had never conducted remote evaluations, suggesting that at least some of these concerns may not translate to real-world issues that impact the administration of FMHA. However, more empirical research is needed (see Bernhard et al., 2021). Further, there is limited guidance regarding how to ensure telepsychology, including FMHA, is practiced in a culturally appropriate and equitable manner (Ralston et al., 2020; Yellowlees et al., 2008). Some examinees, particularly those belonging to vulnerable populations, vary in their access to appropriate internet-connected devices or reliable internet connection, attitudes towards technology, and exposure to and comfort using technology. Finally, as discussed in further detail below, remote FMHA will not fix the shortage of qualified forensic examiners. Telepsychology expands *who* people have access to, not necessarily how many providers are available.

Managing an Effective Remote FMHA Practice

Recommended Training and Credentials

Currently, there are no specific certifications or other credentials for using technology to conduct remote FMHA. However, practitioners conducting such evaluations should always consider ethical guidelines and recommendations regarding competency in their country, region, or jurisdiction and apply these to their use of technology in forensic evaluations (e.g., *Guidelines for Practice of Telepsychology* [APA, 2013]; *Providing Psychological Services via Electronic Media* [CPA, 2020]; *The Practice of Telepsychology* [NZPB, 2013]). Other professionals (e.g., see Algahtani et al., 2021, for telepsychology guidelines with Arabic communities) and groups representing practitioners (e.g., Divisions 12 and 41 of the American Psychological Association) have also been disseminating resources related to use of technology in response to the COVID-19 pandemic and beyond. Practitioners are strongly encouraged to not only seek out these materials and relevant practice updates, but to also attend regular continuing education trainings on tele-psychology, including those focused on remote testing and assessment, as well as familiarise themselves with telepsychology laws and policies in their jurisdiction. Further, forensic practitioners should remain current on recommendations and empirical literature regarding various populations, develop an understanding of the structures that marginalise individuals and communities, and engage in culturally responsive practices (e.g., see *APA Guidelines on Race and Ethnicity in Psychology* [APA, 2019]; Council of National Psychological Associations for the Advancement of Ethnic Minority Interests, 2016).

Initiating a Remote System, Environment, and Workflow

Basic Videosystem Set-Up

Practitioners should consider the extent to which they anticipate using tele-psychology methods in their work. A practitioner who interacts only with one agency may need to invest less in their set-up than a practitioner who interacts with multiple agencies and settings, all of whom are likely to have different technology demands. Therefore, if telepsychology is or will be a major propor-tion of the practitioner's workload, they should consider adopting several modalities (e.g., access to several common videoconferencing programmes) to facilitate practice. Having access to multiple platforms is also useful in the event an examinee experiences difficulties with one platform and needs to switch to another.

One of the major considerations in determining which platform(s) to use for virtual connection is the location of the examinee. Some agencies, such as jails, prisons, or court settings may already have appropriate technology in place and use certain programmes or software. While it may be simplest to adopt these same programmes, some operate as closed systems within an institution making it more difficult for outside users to gain access. Thus, it is recommended that practitioners first consult with the outside agency's information technology staff to determine if access is possible. Practitioners may also conduct FMHA with people not living in a secure care setting. Provided access to a stable internet connection, a device that allows audio and video streaming, and a private and quiet location, people in remote areas can participate in an evaluation. When practitioners need to select their own software platforms, either for connections with facilities or community-released examinees, they should review associated privacy protections, ease of access, and cost. Many platforms are or can be compliant with national data protection standards such as the Health Insurance Portability and Accessibility Act (HIPAA) in the United States and General Data Protection Regulation (GDPR) in the European Union.

In addition to examinee location, the practitioner's space should be quiet, private, and have lighting that allows the examinee to see them clearly. As the examiner's immediate environment will be visible to the examinee, care should also be taken to consider which personal items (e.g., photos, diplomas, memorabilia) are in camera view. A web camera separate from the built-in computer cameras can offer an increased number of options for angling, lighting, and placement to create a more ideal frame of the examiner. Headphones with a microphone are encouraged to promote clearer audio communication.

Remote Evaluations Involving Jail Staff or Court Personnel

Secure care agencies will differ in the extent to which they are familiar and already using telecommunication technology (Mulay et al., 2021). It will likely be easier for agencies already using telecommunications for other court purposes (e.g., video arraignments), to adopt telepsychology practices than those who are not. The practitioner should determine who at the facility is involved with technology, noting this may not be the staff member who schedules visits. When facilities are reluctant to shift to virtual evaluations, the practitioner may use this hesitancy as an opportunity to engage in ongoing communications with jail staff about the benefits of virtual evaluations and help troubleshooting to the extent appropriate. When feasible, the evaluator or their agency may consider providing hardware for the jail such as a tablet in a hardcase protector or wireless headphones (wireless to reduce ligature risk) that can be stored and used exclusively for virtual evaluations. Additionally, the evaluator should obtain contact information for staff who are able to facilitate and troubleshoot during the evaluation.

As with in-person evaluations, the privacy afforded by the secure environment is another consideration. Rooms that are readily accessible, private, and free from external distractions are a rarity in most in-custody and at-home settings. With telepsychology, however, it can be harder to discern the extent to which privacy (or lack thereof) exists or how the space itself (e.g., windows in the room, thin walls, volume of the computer or monitor) facilitates distraction or reluctance to engage in the evaluation. Practitioners may want to work with agency staff to understand the layout of the room and mitigate any possible intrusions on privacy before the first evaluation.

Additionally, staff in secure settings may be reluctant to leave examinees in the room alone with technology hardware. Even for examinees with reasonable behavioural stability, facilities may insist on prohibitions that preclude privacy such as requiring security staff members be present during the evaluation or that a door be left open where staff can monitor the examinee. The practitioner should consider the context of their evaluation and their capacity to negotiate with the agency to circumvent these concerns. For example, an insanity evaluation should not be conducted with outside individuals in the room given concern for privacy around disclosures of criminal activity. Some settings have

implemented solutions such as protecting the computer technology behind ac-
rylic glass, similar to that used in non-contact visiting booths, or place correctional staff in line of sight of the examinee through a window but ensuring they
are unable to hear the evaluation.

Remote Evaluations with Examinees in the Community

In setting up evaluations with examinees in the community, practitioners should
develop and disseminate a standard set of instructions outlining basic necessities
and requirements for participating in the evaluation before the evaluation takes
place. People unfamiliar with forensic evaluations may not understand they
cannot have family members present or listening, or that the evaluation may take
multiple hours unlike a therapy or primary care session. Additionally, practitioners should gather several pieces of information from the examinee at the start
of the evaluation, such as confirming their identity and obtaining their physical
address and phone number in case of emergency or the provider needs to initiate
a welfare check. It is also recommended that the examiner and examinee develop
a code word the examinee can say if their privacy is compromised so the
practitioner will know to pause questioning related to the evaluation. Examinees
should be instructed to silence or turn off other devices and close out any other
windows on their computer screen.

Modifying the Evaluation Procedure for Virtual Administration

While technological aspects with respect to software, hardware, and environment
are important to consider, practitioners must also think through how to modify
their typical procedures to fit a telepsychology model. First, informed consent
procedures need to be adapted (TrustPARMA offers samples for general telepsychology and teleneuropsychology practice). In addition to the typical notifi-
cations, examinees should be informed about the use of the virtual platform and
the steps taken to secure their communications and data. During in-person
evaluations, examinees usually sign the notification/consent form but remote
evaluations make this process more challenging. Practitioners may consider
online document signing software (e.g., Docusign) if the examinee is allowed
access to a keyboard. Other options may include sending the informed consent
by mail with return envelope. In court-ordered evaluations, informed consent is
not a requirement (see *APA's Specialty Guidelines for Forensic Psychology*, 2013);
however, we nonetheless suggest at least documenting that notification was
provided and verbal consent or assent was obtained or declined.

Testing needs may dictate whether a remote evaluation is possible. Some
testing instruments can be adapted to telepsychology either because they are
verbally administered or testing companies have developed online methods for
their use. However, some secure care agencies may prohibit examinees from
interacting with the computer or its accessories other than through the video

stream, so these online methods may be of limited use in criminal forensic contexts. Testing that requires use of manipulatives or visual stimuli may be particularly difficult if not impossible to implement via a virtual platform without computerised or digital adaptations. Procedures that deviate significantly and/or do not have empirical backing to demonstrate their utility in a virtual space, place the psychologist at risk for having their work not accepted by courts. Practitioners should continue to review relevant literature, attend trainings, and consult with colleagues in determining whether procedural modifications are appropriate. Additional recommendations for remote psychological testing are published elsewhere (Corey & Ben-Porath, 2020; Luxton et al., 2014).

Psychologists should also consider augmentation of their behavioural observation procedures given the limited ability to view the examinee's behaviour in some respects. For example, examiners may ask the examinee to explicitly demonstrate some movements (e.g., walking, holding their hands up to assess for tremor) or ask about behaviours in a self-report format (e.g., "do you tend to move more slowly than other people?" or "how often do you shower?"). Examiners should be especially cautious about attributing limited-quality observations to mental health, medical, or cultural causes. For example, eye contact or vocal tone/inflections may be influenced by the remote setting and may not be indicative of a characteristic abnormality or deviation from expected behaviour. Finally, psychologists should adapt their case tracking procedures to document which evaluations are conducted remotely vs. in-person, where examinees were located, as well as case outcomes and process notes. In fact, we advocate for jurisdictions and/or forensic service departments to track these outcomes more broadly (e.g., at the state or region level) to inform policy surrounding remote forensic evaluations.

Improving Court Communications

As in all evaluations, evaluators must strive for transparency in their reports (Otto et al., 2014). Most forensic evaluations include a description of the evaluation procedures, such as the length of the interview and data sources used. For remote evaluations, the practitioner should additionally explain that the evaluation was conducted virtually, with appropriate details about the remote environment, and discuss whether the virtual format impacted the quality of the communication. The following is an example of such documentation:

> This evaluation was conducted remotely using a HIPAA-compliant version of Zoom, an online videoconferencing platform. The examinee was at her home and I was at my office. The virtual platform featured a passcode, waiting room, and meeting lock oncethe meeting began to ensure privacy. The examinee indicated she was alone at home and no distractions within the home were noted. She did notappear distracted by other elements on the computer screen. She and I were able to hear and see each other well and the format did not noticeably impact the nature or quality of data collection.

Additionally, any augmentation of testing procedures should be well documented in descriptions of the test administration. The psychologist should state what changes were made, how these differ from typical practice, and any potential impact on the testing results and interpretation.

The ability to explain these modifications is also relevant for any subsequent testimony, as attorneys may be more likely to try to scrutinise remote evaluation procedures. It can be challenging enough to discuss test procedures and results to a lay audience; discussing the ins and outs of test validity at the interface of technology with only a burgeoning research base heightens the difficulty. Cross examination may involve technical questions about how it is possible to know virtual assessments are acceptable if there is inadequate guidance to support procedural adjustments such as subtest substitution or how certain tests perform in a virtual format. Keeping up with research literature, ethical principles, and evolving practice guidelines about remote evaluations will aid examiners in making defensible methodological choices and later justifying them to the court.

To Conduct a Remote Evaluation or Not: Making an Informed Decision

Just because remote evaluations can be conducted in many cases does not always mean they should be. Several factors should be considered when determining whether to proceed with a virtual evaluation. Table 10.1 outlines several questions forensic examiners may want to ask themselves before proceeding with a remote evaluation.

Policy and Advocacy Considerations

Despite the benefits of remote FMHA, two key issues remain: (1) the limited number of providers formally trained in FMHA and (2) the availability of both community and inpatient mental health services. Additional pressures in the system, particularly for pretrial individuals, may be alleviated by reallocating taxpayer dollars (e.g., from "tough-on-crime" initiatives to more community-based crisis interventions and diversion), use of jail-based restoration services (including via virtual formats) for defendants with less severe impairment, expansions in interjurisdictional policies, and better incentives to recruit and retain newly trained psychologists to work in remote or underserved areas. In this last section, we focus on issues of interjurisdictional practice and briefly discuss training and recruitment needs within the context of remote FMHA.

Enhancing Interjurisdictional Practice

Interjurisdictional practice, which refers to the provision of psychological services across jurisdictions, may be one solution to help connect rural areas to qualified forensic experts and deter the retainment of "occasional experts" in these areas. The United States Association of State and Provincial Psychology Boards

Table 10.1 Pre-evaluation questions to assess appropriateness of forensic telepractice

Question	Example/rationale
Does the environment allow the evaluation to proceed withintegrity and without significant insult to thevalidity of the procedures?	If an individual is unable to attend and focus on the evaluation because they are disrupted by a lack of privacy, outside stimuli that demand their attention, or significant limitations imposed by the agency, the quality of the data may be too disrupted to yield reasonably confident opinions.
Is adequate technology available for all parties involved?	All parties would require adequate access to sufficient technology, as poor connectivity (e.g., low bandwidth internet, devices with unreliable audio-visual components) can disrupt a smooth, quality communication and interfere with information-gathering. While internet access is increasing in many areas, people in more rural or frontier areas may have less consistent internet service. Individuals living in the community may also be using their own data plans for which the cost of a multi-hour streaming event may be significant. Examiners may suggest that examinees use a private room at their attorney's office, the local courthouse, or at a public library or other community centre where WiFi access is free.
Does the examinee present with unique characteristics that are notwell suited for a virtual evaluation?	For example, telepractice may not be feasible for examinees who are physically incapable of using or learning the equipment, community-released examinees who are houseless and have little access to private personal space, or those with visual, hearing, or language barriers if the inclusion of interpreters or closed-captioning features are not possible. Individuals with significant cognitive impairments may also have challenges following instructions remotely if there is no caregiver present to help with set up and troubleshooting. While clinical lore has suggested concern about teleassessment with individuals who have paranoid beliefs regarding technology, this has not borne out in the research literature (Santesteban-Echarri et al., 2020). That is not to say that all individuals who hold these beliefs could participate effectively, but this is not a factor that would automatically nix a remote evaluation. However, some people with severe psychotic symptoms may be unable to attend effectively to the video screen. In some cases, these challenges do not become apparent until sometime after the remote evaluation begins.

(Continued)

Table 10.1 (Continued)

Question	Example/rationale
	In one example, an in-custody examinee was so distracted by what he reportedly saw and heard through a window that he was unable to continue answering questions. While what he reportedly saw and heard (e.g., correctional officers making faces, saying bad things about him) was unlikely to be true and in line with some of his delusional beliefs, the psychologist elected to rule out that uncertainty by completing the evaluation in person. In essence, examinees need to have basic cognitive skills to understand the circumstances, interact with the psychologist and the technology, and develop sufficient rapport.
Are there suspected legal issues that would be difficult to mitigate or overcome?	Psychologists need to consider the admissibility of testing procedures that have been adapted from standard procedures for remote administration and whether this would be subjected to legal scrutiny. Certain psycholegal questions may dictate the need for significant psychological testing that requires an in-person meeting to administer. Additionally, some high stake cases may increase the likelihood the expert's methods will be vulnerable to aggressive cross-examination. In these cases, an in-person evaluation may be conducted to ensure the utmost confidence in providing opinions that involve significant liberty and safety issues. The acceptability of remote evaluations may also be weighed against an individual's rights. This consideration is especially relevant for examinees from rural and underserved populations who are more likely to await the outcome of their cases in jail or other secure placements than in the community.

(ASPPB, n.d.) created the Psychology Interjurisdictional Compact (PSYPACT) to "facilitate telehealth and temporary in-person, face-to-face practice of psychology across jurisdictional boundaries" without needing additional licensure (2015). PSYPACT has increased the accessibility of psychological services (including FMHA), but it cannot be fully implemented until it is legislated within a state (i.e., a psychologist licensed in a PSYPACT state can only provide services to other PSYPACT states). To date, 26 US states participate in PSYPACT, 11 of which joined in 2021 alone, likely due to the increased demand for psychological services and decreased willingness to receive services in-person during the pandemic. Beyond health safety concerns, PSYPACT is beneficial for allowing rural

communities to be connected to more qualified forensic experts, thereby reducing docket backlogs and maintaining a person's right to a speedy trial (Dale &
Smith, 2021; Neal, 2020). However, some rural states with lowest number of
licensed psychologists per capita (e.g., Mississippi, Louisiana; Lin et al., 2020)
have not enacted or initiated PSYPACT legislation.

In Europe, the European Federation of Psychologists' Association (n. d.)
created EuroPsy to facilitate cross-border mobility by setting a standard for
professional training and education for psychologists that culminates in a
European Certificate in Psychology (2021). Although not one of the available
specialised certifications, forensic practice is included in the curriculum. There
are 39 European countries participating in EuroPsy. However, because countries
have varying licensure requirements and laws pertaining to psychological and
forensic practice, EuroPsy (unlike PSYPACT) is not a mechanism by which
psychologists are allowed to practice across countries without licensure. EuroPsy
accelerates the process of licensure in other countries by signifying a psychologist
has completed a nationally accredited curriculum in psychology along with
at least one year of full-time work as a psychologist trainee. Across the globe,
increasing awareness and advocacy related to interjurisdictional and cross-border
practice is crucial to ensure more accessible FMHA from those qualified to
provide them.

Recruiting and Retaining New Talent and Early Career Professionals

Opening borders to access forensic examiners in other jurisdictions will likely do
little to reduce the demand for evaluations if there is not an accompanying increase
in the pool of available providers. To promote professional investment and competence in remote FMHA and improve their quality, graduate programmes are
encouraged to offer didactic and practicum activities related to remote psycho-
diagnostic evaluations and those that address psycholegal questions, with an emphasis on navigating ethical and procedural differences. To meet social justice
objectives, ensuring trainees have experience working directly with rural or
otherwise underserved clients is strongly encouraged. Cultivating interest in rural
and economically disadvantaged areas early on may help recruit and retain newly
licensed psychologists to offer services in these areas in the long term.

The new "norm" of conducting remote evaluations in particular may make
rural areas more attractive for psychologists looking to start or expand their
business who would otherwise be dissuaded by the need to relocate to a more
remote region. Though some challenges may be mitigated by the use of remote
technologies, forensic practitioners who are new to working with rural or economically disadvantaged examinees or court systems should be prepared to
address unique challenges such as:

- The likelihood of dual relationships or associations (e.g., the first author
  [A.B.B.] conducted a competency evaluation with an examinee who was

later a therapy client of a practicum student A.B.B. was supervising at the state prison).

- The possibility of needing to educate unfamiliar attorneys or judges about forensic psychology principles or procedures.
- Connecting with professionals or organisations outside their region of practice for consultation or continuing education.
- The need to remain attentive to a wide range of cultural and economic differences that may impact rapport, data gathering, and/or bias the forensic opinion.

Practitioners should also have an awareness about the types of forensic and general mental health services that are available in the region to better understand systemic constraints and help inform recommendations when applicable. Beyond providers themselves, areas with a high scarcity of trained forensic psychologists must also engage in recruitment and retention efforts by actively seeking and welcoming qualified practitioners, advocating for more competitive financial incentives, helping to create a professional network of rural providers (Briggs, 2015), and being open to the use of remote FMHA.

Note

1 This chapter will predominately use the term "telepsychology" to refer to remote, telecommunication services. However, other terms such as telemental health or tele-practice may be used interchangeably.

References

Algahtani, F. D., Hassan, S., Alsaif, B., & Zrieq, R. (2021). Assessment of the quality of life during COVID-19 pandemic: A cross-sectional survey from the Kingdom of Saudi Arabia. *International Journal of Environmental Research and Public Health, 18*(3), 847. 10.33 90/ijerph18030847

American Psychiatric Association. (2018). Annual Meeting | AJMC. (n.d.) Retrieved January 18, 2022, from https://www.ajmc.com/conferences/apa-2018

American Psychological Association. (2013a). Guidelines for the practice of tele-psychology. *American Psychologist, 68*(9), 791–800. 10.1037/a0035001

American Psychological Association. (2013b). Specialty guidelines for forensic psychology. *American Psychologist, 68*(1), 7–19. 10.1037/a0029889

American Psychological Association. (2019). APA guidelines on race and ethnicity in psychology: Promoting responsiveness and equity. https://www.apa.org/about/policy/guidelines-race-ethnicity.pdf

Antonacci, D. J., Bloch, R. M., Saeed, S. A., Yildirim, Y., & Talley, J. (2008). Empirical evidence on the use and effectiveness of telepsychiatry via videoconferencing: Implications for forensic and correctional psychiatry. *Behavioral Sciences & the Law, 26*(3), 253–269. 10.1002/bsl.812

Association of State and Provincial Psychology Boards. (n.d.). *Psychology interjurisdictional compact.* https://www.asppb.net/page/PSYPACT

Australia's National Digital Health Strategy. (2018). Safe, seamless, and secure: Australia's national digital health strategy. https://conversation.digitalhealth.gov.au/sites/default/files/adha-strategy-doc-2ndaug_0_1.pdf.

Ax, R. K., Fagan, T. J., Magaletta, P. R., Morgan, R. D., Nussbaum, D., & White, T. W. (2007). Innovations in correctional assessment and treatment. *Criminal Justice and Behavior, 34*(7), 893–905. 10.1177/0093854807301555

Backhaus, A., Agha, Z., Maglione, M. L., Repp, A., Ross, B., Zuest, D., & Rice-Thorp, N. M. (2012). Videoconferencing psychotherapy: A systematic review. *Psychological Services, 9*(2), 111–131. 10.1037/a0027924

Batastini, A. B., King, C. M., Morgan, R. D., & McDaniel, B. (2016). Telepsychological services with criminal justice and substance abuse clients: A systematic review and meta-analysis. *Psychological Services, 13*(1), 20–30. 10.1037/ser0000042

Batastini, A. B., McDonald, B. R., & Morgan, R. D. (2013). Videoteleconferencing in forensic and correctional practice. In K. Myers & C Turvey (Eds.). *Telemental health: Clinical, technical, and administrative foundations for evidence-based practice.* Eslevier Inc. (pp. 251–271).

Batastini, A. B., Paprzycki, P., Jones, A. C., & MacLean, N. (2021). Are videoconferenced mental and behavioral health services just as good as in-person? A meta-analysis of a fast-growing practice. *Clinical Psychology Review, 83*, 101944. 10.1016/j.cpr.2020.101944

Batastini, A. B., Pike, M., Thoen, M. A., Jones, A. C., Davis, R. M., & Escalera, E. (2019). Perceptions and use of videoconferencing in forensic mental health assessments: A survey of evaluators and legal personnel. *Psychology, Crime & Law, 26*(6), 593–613. 10.1080/1068316x.2019.1708355

Bernhard, P. A., McDowell, L., & Vincent, G. M. (2021). Forensic practitioners' use and perceptions of telepsychology before and during COVID-19. *Law and Human Behavior, 45*(5), 468–480. 10.1037/lhb0000464

Briggs, B. (2015). *Solutions for recruitment and retention of rural psychologists by rural psychologists* (Doctoral dissertation, Antioch University).

Bronson, J., & Berzofsky, M. (2021). *Indicators of mental health problems reported by prisoners and Jail Inmates, 2011-12.* (Washington, D.C.: U.S. Department of Justice, Office of Justice Programs, Bureau of Justice Statistics, 2017), at 1–4.

Callahan, L., & Pinals, D. A. (2020). Challenges to reforming the competence to stand trial and competence restoration system. *Psychiatric Services, 71*(7), 691–697. 10.1176/appi.ps.201900483

Canadian Psychological Association. (2020). Providing psychological services via electronic media. https://cpa.ca/aboutcpa/committees/ethics/psychserviceselectronically/

Chen, C. K., Palfrey, A., Shreck, E., Silvestri, B., Wash, L., Nehrig, N., Baer, A. L., Schneider, J. A., Ashkenazi, S., Sherman, S. E., & Chodosh, J. (2021). Implementation of telemental health (TMH) psychological services for rural veterans at the VA New York harbor healthcare system. *Psychological Services, 18*(1), 1–10. 10.1037/ser0000323

Corey, D. M., & Ben-Porath, Y. S. (2020). Practical guidance on the use of the MMPI instruments in remote psychological testing. *Professional Psychology: Research and Practice, 51*(3), 199–204. 10.1037/pro0000329

Council of National Psychological Associations for the Advancement of Ethnic Minority Interests. (2016). Testing and assessment with persons and communities of color. https://www.apa.org/pi/oema

Daffern, M., Shea, D. E., & Ogloff, J. R. (2021). Remote forensic evaluations and treatment in the time of COVID-19: An international survey of psychologists and psychiatrists. *Psychology, Public Policy, and Law, 27*(3), 354–369. 10.1037/law0000308

Dale, M. D., & Smith, D. (2021). Making the case for videoconferencing and remote child custody evaluations (RCCEs): The empirical, ethical, and evidentiary arguments for accepting new technology. *Psychology, Public Policy, and Law, 27*(1), 30–44. 10.1037/ law0000280

Deslich, S., Stec, B., Tomblin, S., & Coustasse, A. (2013). Telepsychiatry in the 21st century: Transforming healthcare with technology. *Perspectives in Health Information Management, 10*. 1f.

Dewees, S., & Marks, B. (2017). *Twice invisible: Understanding rural Native America*. First Nations Development Institute. https://www.usetinc.org/wp-content/uploads/bvenuti/WWS/ 2017/May%202017/May%208/Twice%20Invisible%20 -%20Research%20Note.pdf

Digard, L., & Swavola, E. (2019, April). *Justice denied: The harmful and lasting effects of pretrial detention*. Vera Institute of Justice. https://www.vera.org/downloads/publications/ Justice-Denied-Evidence-Brief.pdf

Digital Health & Care Scotland. (2018). Scotland's digital health and care strategy: Enabling, connecting and empowering. April 25. https://www.gov.scot/publications/ scotlands-digital-health-care-strategy-enabling-connecting-empowering/

Dobis, E. A., Krumel, Jr. T. P., Cromartie, J., Conley, K. L., Sanders, A., & Ortiz, R. (2021). Rural America at a glance: 2021 edition. U.S. Department of Agriculture.

Drogin, E. Y. (2020). Forensic mental telehealth assessment (FMTA) in the context of COVID-19. *International Journal of Law and Psychiatry, 71*, 101595. 10.1016/j.ijlp.2020. 101595

Ellis, A. R., Konrad, T. R., Thomas, K. C., & Morrissey, J. P. (2009). County-level estimates of mental health professional supply in the United States. *Psychiatric Services, 60*(10), 1315–1322. 10.1176/ps.2009.60.10.1315

European Federation of Psychologists' Association. (n.d.). *EuroPsy. EuroPsy*. https://www. europsy.eu/

Frueh, B. C. (2015). Solving mental healthcare access problems in the twenty-first century. *Australian Psychologist, 50*(4), 304–306. 10.1111/ap.12140

Gale, J., Janis, J., Coburn, A., & Rochford, H. (2019). *Behavioral health in rural America: Challenges and opportunities*. Iowa City, Iowa: Rural Policy Research Institute. https:// rupri.org/contact-us/

Glasmeier, A. K., & Farrigan, T. (2007). The economic impacts of the prison development boom on persistently poor rural places. *International Regional Science Review, 30*(3), 274–299. 10.1177/0160017607301608

Goldenson, J., & Josefowitz, N. (2021). Remote forensic psychological assessment in civil cases: Considerations for experts assessing harms from early life abuse. *Psychological Injury and Law, 14*(2), 89–103. 10.1007/s12207-021-09404-2

Gowensmith, W. N. (2019). Resolution or resignation: The role of forensic mental health professionals amidst the competency services crisis. *Psychology, Public Policy, and Law, 25*(1), 1–14. 10.1037/law0000190

Grisso, T. (1987). The economic and scientific future of forensic psychological assessment. *American Psychologist, 42*(9), 831–839. 10.1037/0003-066x.42.9.831

Heilbrun, K., DeMatteo, D., Marczyk, G., & Goldstein, A. M. (2008). Standards of practice and care in forensic mental health assessment. *Psychology, Public Policy, and Law, 14*, 1–26.

Hilty, D. M., Chan, S., Hwang, T., Wong, A., & Bauer, A. M. (2017). Advances in mobile mental health: Opportunities and implications for the spectrum of E-mEntal health services. *mHealth, 3*, 34. 10.21037/mhealth.2017.06.02

Hooks, G., Mosher, C., Rotolo, T., & Lobao, L. (2004). The prison industry: Carceral expansion and employment in U.S. counties, 1969–1994. *Social Science Quarterly, 85*(1), 37–57. 10.1111/j.0038-4941.2004.08501004.x

Kalb, J. (2018). Gideon incarcerated: Access to counsel in pretrial detention. *UC Irvine Law Review, 9*(1), 101–140.

Kang-Brown, J., Hinds, O., Schattner-Elmaleh, E., & Wallace-Lee, J. (2019, December). People in Jail in 2019. *Vera Institute of Justice.* https://www.vera.org/downloads/publications/people-in-jail-in-2019.pdf

Kirschstein, M. A., Singh, J. P., Rossegger, A., Endrass, J., & Graf, M. (2021). International survey on the use of emerging technologies among forensic and correctional mental health professionals. *Criminal Justice and Behavior*, 009385482110420. 10.1177/00938548211042057

Lin, L., Conroy, J., & Christidis, P. (2020, January 1). Datapoint: Which states have the most licensed psychologists? *Monitor on Psychology, 51*(1), 19.

Luxton, D. D., & Lexcen, F. J. (2018). Forensic competency evaluations via videoconferencing: A feasibility review and best practice recommendations. *Professional Psychology: Research and Practice, 49*(2), 124–131. 10.1037/pro0000179

Luxton, D. D., Lexcen, F. J., & McIntyre, K. A. (2019). Forensic competency assessment with digital technologies. *Current Psychiatry Reports, 21*(7). 10.1007/s11920-019-1037-9

Luxton, D. D., Pruitt, L. D., & Osenbach, J. E. (2014). Best practices for remote psychological assessment via Telehealth technologies. *Professional Psychology: Research and Practice, 45*(1), 27–35. 10.1037/a0034547

Manfredi, L., Shupe, J., & Batki, S. L. (2005). Rural jail telepsychiatry: A pilot feasibility study. *Telemedicine and e-Health, 11*(5), 574–577. 10.1089/tmj.2005.11.574

Manguno-Mire, G. M., Thompson, J. W., Shore, J. H., Croy, C. D., Artecona, J. F., & Pickering, J. W. (2007). The use of telemedicine to evaluate competency to stand trial: A preliminary randomized controlled study. *Journal of the American Academy of Psychiatry and the Law Online, 35*(4), 481–489.

Martin, L. L. (2011). Debt to society: Asset poverty and prisoner reentry. *The Review of Black Political Economy, 38*(2), 131–143. 10.1007/s12114-011-9087-1

McCallum, K. E., & Gowensmith, W. N. (2019). Tipping the scales of justice: The role of forensic evaluations in the criminalization of mental illness. *CNS Spectrums, 25*(2), 154–160. 10.1017/s1092852919001275

Miller, T. W., Burton, D. C., Hill, K., Luftman, G., Veltkemp, L. J., & Swope, M. (2005). Telepsychiatry: Critical dimensions for forensic services. *The Journal of the American Academy of Psychiatry and Law, 33*, 539–546.

Mulay, A. L., Gottfried, E. D., Mullis, D. M., & Vitacco, M. J. (2021). The use of videoconferencing in forensic evaluations: Moving forward in times of COVID-19. *Journal of Forensic Psychology Research and Practice, 21*(4), 338–354. 10.1080/24732850.2021.1877508.

Murrie, D. C., Gardner, B. O., & Torres, A. N. (2020). The impact of misdemeanor arrests on forensic mental health services: A state-wide review of Virginia competence to stand trial evaluations. *Psychology, Public Policy, and Law.* 10.1037/law0000296

Neal, T. (2020, December 27). *Courts see case backlogs due to COVID-19 delays.* Arkansas Democrat Gazette. https://www.arkansasonline.com/news/2020/dec/27/covid-19-impacting-courts/

New Zealand Psychologist Board. (2013). The practice of telepsychology. https://psychologistsboard.org.nz/wpontent/uploads/2021/06/BPG_The_Practice_of_Telepsychology_FINAL_131212.pdf

Norcross, J. C., Pfund, R. A., & Prochaska, J. O. (2013). Psychotherapy in 2022: A Delphi poll on its future. *Professional Psychology: Research and Practice, 44*(5), 363–370. 10.1037/a0034633

Otto, R. K., DeMier, R., & Boccaccini, M. T. (2014). *Forensic reports and testimony: A guide to effective communication for psychologists and psychiatrists.* Hoboken, New Jersey: John Wiley & Sons.

Papalia, N., Shepherd, S. M., Spivak, B., Luebbers, S., Shea, D. E., & Fullam, R. (2019). Disparities in criminal justice system responses to first-time juvenile offenders according to Indigenous status. *Criminal Justice and Behavior, 46*(8), 1067–1087. 10.1177/0093854 819851830

Peterson, J. K., Skeem, J., Kennealy, P., Bray, B., & Zvonkovic, A. (2014). How often and how consistently do symptoms directly precede criminal behavior among offenders with mental illness? *Law and Human Behavior, 38*(5), 439–449. 10.1037/lhb0000075

Rabuy, B., & Kopf, D. (2015, July 9). *Prisons of poverty: Uncovering the pre-incarceration incomes of the imprisoned.* Prison Policy Initiative. https://www.prisonpolicy.org/reports/income.html

Rabuy, B., & Kopf, D. (2016, May 10). *Detaining the poor: How money bail perpetuates an endless cycle of poverty and jail time.* Prison Policy Initiative. https://www.prisonpolicy.org/reports/incomejails.html

Ralston, A. L., Holt, N. R., & Hope, D. A. (2020). Tele-mental health with marginalized communities in rural locales: Trainee and supervisor perspectives. *Journal of Rural Mental Health, 44*(4), 268–273. 10.1037/rmh0000142

Ryba, N. L., Cooper, V. G., & Zapf, P. A. (2003). Juvenile competence to stand trial evaluations: A survey of current practices and test usage among psychologists. *Professional Psychology: Research and Practice, 34*(5), 499–507. 10.1037/0735-7028.34.5.499

Santesteban-Echarri, O., Piskulic, D. Nyman, R.K., & Addington, J. (2020). *Telehealth Interventions* for schizophrenia-spectrum disorders and clinical high-risk for psychosis individuals: A scoping review. *Journal of Telemedicine & Telecare, 26*(1-2), 14–20.

Sawyer, W. (2019, October 9). How race impacts who is detained pretrial. *Prison Policy Initiative.* https://www.prisonpolicy.org/blog/2019/10/09/pretrial_race/

Shrider, E. A., Kollar, M., Chen, F., & Semega, J. (2021). *Income and poverty in the United States: 2020 (P60-273).* United States Census Bureau.

Thomas, K. C., Ellis, A. R., Konrad, T. R., Holzer, C. E., & Morrissey, J. P. (2009). County-level estimates of mental health professional shortage in the United States. *Psychiatric Services, 60*(10), 1323–1328. 10.1176/ps.2009.60.10.1323

Thornicroft, G. (2008). Stigma and discrimination limit access to mental health care. *Epidemiologia e Psichiatria Sociale, 17*(1), 14–19. 10.1017/s1121189x00002621

Thornton v. Snyder, 428 F.3d 690 (7th Cir. 2005). https://scholar.google.com/scholar_case?case=17988380564578469841&q=Thornton+v.+Snyder,+2005&hl=en&as_sdt=6,43&as_vis=1

Trueblood et al. v. Washington State DSHS. (2014). Washington State Department of Social and Health Services. https://www.dshs.wa.gov/bha/trueblood-et-al-v-washington-state-dshs

United Kingdom National Health Service. The NHD long term plan. (2019, August 21). https://www.longtermplan.nhs.uk

United States v. Baker, 45 F.3d 837 (4th Cir. 1995). https://casetext.com/case/us-v-baker-69

Yellowlees, P., Marks, S., Hilty, D., & Shore, J. H. (2008). Using e-Health to enable culturally appropriate mental healthcare in rural areas. *Telemedicine and e-Health, 14*(5), 486–492. 10.1089/tmj.2007.0070

Zheng, Z., & Milton, T. D. (2021). *Jail Inmates in 2019 (NCJ 255608).* Bureau of Justice Statistics. https://bjs.ojp.gov/content/pub/pdf/ji19.pdf

Part II

Forensic Practice and Working with Biases

11 Supervising Assessment Practice

Jason Davies

Introduction

Forensic psychologists are expected to be objective and impartial in their work and to mitigate the impacts of sources of difference and bias in their practice. For example, the registration body in the United Kingdom includes within its standards of proficiency, that forensic psychologists must "be aware of the impact of culture, equality and diversity on practice" and "be able to practice in a non-discriminatory manner" (standards 5 & 6; https://www.hcpc-uk.org/standards/standards-of-proficiency/practitioner-psychologists/; accessed 06/09/21[1]). In addition, explicit assumptions about impartiality are widely accepted specifically in relation to assessment practice; "Given the significant weight placed by the court on the opinions of forensic evaluators, objectivity and accuracy are crucial" (Zappala et al., 2018, p. 46). Whilst these broad standards and assumptions are readily accepted, achieving these is much more complicated than their simple (and laudable) wording might suggest. Central reasons for this include that the factors which might impact our ability to accomplish these might be outside of our awareness, and that specific psychological processes may hamper our efforts to scrutinise our own views and beliefs. Consequently, such "deaf, dumb, blind and numb spots – things that are not (or once were but are no longer) heard, spoken about, noticed or felt" (Davies, 2015, p. 138) are often outside of conscious awareness, or where recognised may be viewed as "shameful" to admit to and discuss. This can result in such factors having a hidden, covert, or secret influence on our practice and decision making.

Within the supervision literature, the notions of hidden or overlooked influences have been considered in relation to boundary crossing and violations in forensic settings (Davies, 2015). However, these features appear to be also pertinent to impartiality lapses and breaches resulting from (intended or unintended) bias when undertaking assessment and testing tasks. For example, the term "ethical blindness" (Barnao et al., 2012) has been used to describe those situations in which ethical issues are ignored, overlooked, or missed. Giving rise to such ethical blindness may be the biases arising in individual practice. Research in the area of susceptibility to bias has shown that the "bias blind spot" – the tendency for individuals to consider themselves to be less biased or influenced by

DOI: 10.4324/9781003230977-13

bias than others–may be part of the "human condition" (Pronin et al., 2002). Importantly for us here is that this bias blind spot has been demonstrated with a range of groups, including forensic psychologists (Zappala et al., 2018). It is important to stress that areas of bias which have lower availability (i.e., for which we have less information and evidence readily accessible to us) and higher negative desirability (i.e., are biases or shortcomings that are less palatable to accept) are likely to be those we are most guarded against recognising (Pronin et al., 2002). This seems to be exacerbated if we see ourselves as less susceptible to bias (the "better than average effect").

The bias blind spot appears to be rooted in the introspection illusion, i.e., the tendency to over value one's own thoughts, feelings, and interpretations over behavioural evidence when assessing bias in ourselves and doing the opposite when considering other people's biases, and failing to recognise the limitations of one's introspective activity (Pronin & Kugler, 2007). Consequently, simple introspection – thinking and reviewing one's own thinking – has been identified as an ineffective mechanism for identifying and addressing bias (Zappala et al., 2018). However, this same "distortion" may place an outsider in a good position to provide scrutiny and feedback in relation to bias. These ideas of bias and the underlying processes need to be held in mind as we consider the role (and limits) of supervision in this area.

The role of motivation is important when considering bias, especially as there is an implied assumption that people are unaware of, and would be moved to address their biases should they become aware of them (Noon, 2018). Whilst there may be some practitioners for whom bias is something they are aware of but have no intention of addressing, research would suggest that in most cases, practitioners indicate a willingness to overcome bias in their practice; "the more clinicians identify with their role as a forensic psychologist, the more motivated they are to find ways to mitigate their biases" (Neal & Brodsky, 2016, p. 71). Despite this intent, it should be recognised that experts concede it is likely to be impossible to remove all bias (Zapf & Dror, 2017); however, it seems right and proper that we should strive to get as close to bias free practice as is possible. To this end, this chapter explores how self and other supervision (e.g., Davies, 2015) might be applied to the assessment and testing aspects of forensic psychology practice with the specific intent to assist with recognising and responding to bias. However, in keeping with supervision as an action oriented activity, the key issue is minimising the impact of bias on the actions and behaviour of the practitioner (Noon, 2018) rather than changing attitudes or belief per se. To assist with this, both the practitioner and supervisor should routinely attend to power and privilege whilst working within the scope of their expertise and recognising the limits of their competence (Ivers et al., 2017).

An Overview of Practice Supervision

Practice supervision aims to provide a formalised relationship in which psychologists can maintain, develop and evaluate practice skills and professional competence and attend to complex ethical challenges and dilemmas (Davies, in press). Whilst supervision can take many forms, this chapter focuses on 1-1 supervision in which a practitioner (supervisee[2]) meets with a supervisor on a regular basis. For UK-based psychologists[3] supervision offers a mechanism by which the professional registration requirement of "being able to reflect on and review practice" (standard 11; https://www.hcpc-uk.org/standards/standards-of-proficiency/practitioner-psychologists/; accessed 06/09/21), can be enacted, and through which forensic psychologists are able to receive support and development. Whilst there are a multitude of models and approaches to supervision (for an introduction see Davies, 2015), three functions – learning or formative; managerial or normative, and supportive or restorative (Kadushin, 1992; Proctor, 1988) are generally agreed upon. These take place within a "supervisory working alliance" (Bordin, 1983). Developing a safe, containing and functional supervisory alliance is a necessary condition to enable open exploration of an individual's practice. The alliance is particularly important when the content of supervision might focus on delicate, difficult or challenging aspects of the supervisees work or their individual approach to their work. An effective supervisory relationship can help to mitigate defensiveness or avoidance, which may arise because of vulnerability experienced during such explorations. However, it is important to note here that supervision is not therapy or counselling, and therefore the focus is on the ways in which specific factors might impact the work being undertaken by the supervisee. Fostering an effective supervisory working alliance (for more details on how this might be achieved see Davies, 2015; Davies, in press) is therefore the foundation onto which examination of sources of bias in assessment and testing practice in supervision can take place.

An Overview of Assessment Practice

Psychological assessment covers a range of activities which typically take place through direct contact with the assessee (e.g., interviewing and psychometric testing); via formal and informal behavioural observation and by drawing on information gathered from third party sources such as relatives, victims, carers, and family. Each of these avenues presents unique opportunities and challenge for bias to influence and be mitigated in forensic assessment practice.

When psychological assessment and testing is concerned with collecting information directly from the assessee, the model for evidence-based clinical forensic interviewing proposed by Davies (2019) may be useful. This provides a framework in which the multitude of factors which need to be considered are described. Particularly relevant to our considerations here are the potential for examiner/interviewer bias and how these might affect the *content and tasks* of the interview, might be exacerbated by or impact the interviewers *personal style*, and how *supervision* might be used to provide audit, skills monitoring, and quality control.

Undertaking psychological assessment within forensic contexts requires a range of skills, knowledge, and competencies. These include interpersonal skills (e.g., engaging the person(s) being assessed or third party's providing information); task skills (i.e., knowledge and skills to perform the specific assessment) and decision-making skills (i.e., ability to process information and decide on the next course of action), all of which will be influenced and informed by the assessors' individual style. Typically assessment and testing information is collected in order to inform other processes such as forensic case formulation (e.g., Hart et al., 2011; Sturmey & McMurran, 2011) or to lay the foundation for further work such as therapy (Davies & Nagi, 2017). At each point of the process there is opportunity for bias to impact in ways which could lead to harms such as suboptimal decision making and inappropriate conclusions being drawn.

Although the potential for bias may be present in any piece of assessment or testing practice, there may be some factors which are particularly relevant to priming bias. It is therefore important that the practitioner explicitly identify and consider *client characteristics* (e.g., gender, racial and cultural background, educational and social experience); *demands or expectations* of the setting, service or "commissioner of the work"; the *prior information* they have about the client, and the *purpose* of their assessment, before, during or after the assessment task. Doing so can assist both the practitioner and their supervisor when seeking to use supervision to support the practitioner to understand and address possible bias in their assessment and testing practice.

Supervising Assessment and Testing Practice

Supervision can provide an avenue for ongoing "socialisation" into objectivity within practice (Neal & Brodsky, 2014). As already noted, the supervisory working alliance creates the context for supervision of assessment and testing practice to take place. When considering the alliance as a foundation from which to examine bias within assessment practice, the following conditions may be particularly important: (a) an acceptance on the part of the supervisor and the practitioner that bias is ubiquitous and part of the human condition and thus to be expected (despite how strongly you believe yourself to be different or immune!); (b) given (a), bias is not something to be embarrassed about, but is to be considered and understood; (c) recognition that bias is unlikely to be static as it is influenced by a multitude of personal, organisational and systemic factors and thus it may be helpful to assume that "objectivity is compromised unless proven otherwise" (Goldyne, 2007, p. 65); (d) the willingness of supervisor to be, and for the practitioner to accept the supervisor as a "critical friend" offering challenge and scrutiny in a supportive and empowering way; (e) for the supervisor and supervisee to examine practice in the spirit of curiosity and openness. Thus, effective supervision of assessment and testing practice requires a willingness to examine our own hidden views and beliefs (Teal et al., 2012) and an awareness that we might (unintentionally) attempt to "neutralise" the information we receive where it contradicts our inner view (Pronin et al., 2002).

Attempting to identify and counter potential sources of bias is not a new endeavour in forensic practice. Although almost 30 years old, a very helpful (and easy to read) way to begin exploring sources of bias and possible ways to counter these is provided by Borum et al. (1993). In this paper the authors describe a number of issues which can impact clinical judgement and decision making (e.g., overreliance on memory; confirmatory bias; misestimation of covariation) and describe ways in which these might be identified and addressed. In addition, other papers which provide descriptions of possible sources of bias and how these might be managed may serve as a helpful starting point for supervisors and practitioners. For example, Neal and Grisso (2014) identify and describe some of the common types of bias which may be found in forensic psychology evaluations (e.g., representativeness, availability, and anchoring; see also Tversky & Kahneman, 1974, for the seminal work detailing cognitive biases arising from judgemental heuristics). These authors also discuss several ways in which supervisors can assist the supervisee by using strategies such as *attention to base rates*; presenting or considering the *opposite or alternative* opinion, view or conclusion; using appropriate *structured* methods to guide the process of assessment and testing (recognising the challenge in identifying appropriate); and identifying the most *pertinent/essential pieces of information* to collect (usually four to six pieces). A very comprehensive list and discussion of possible strategies for managing bias (tested and yet to be examined) which were identified through research with forensic psychologists is presented by Neal and Brodsky (2016), whilst Goldyne (2007) considers emotionally driven motivations that may lead to bias and details a range of strategies for proactively detecting and minimising bias. Finally, Croskerry et al. (2013; tables 1 and 2) describe educational and workplace strategies (e.g., structured data collection, slowing down decision making, creating a supporting environment) and the notion of forcing functions – rules which direct or dictate an action based on an algorithm, flowchart, or decision matrix – in relation to medical education. Together these papers and the information contained within this chapter provide a resource of ideas and actions that can be applied in self and other supervision.

It is important to recognise that the ways in which we might be influenced can be subtle and very difficult to identify and quantify. For example, the use of the term "bias" may itself lead individuals to become unintentionally guarded or defensive and, it may be that the use of more neutral terms (e.g., "effect", "tendency"; Pronin et al., 2002) can make it easier for practitioners to consider those forces (including their beliefs and judgements) which may impact their work. Further, processes such as the anchoring bias, i.e., the first information received influencing how we interpret and understand later information (Zapf & Dror, 2017) may be shaped by formal information (e.g., the request for the assessment) or other immediately available information (e.g., the gender, age, or racial background of the client). This can be exacerbated by the tendency for an independent opinion to move towards the position held by the "commissioner" of the work (adversarial allegiance) which has been demonstrated in a range of practice areas (Zapf & Dror, 2017). In addition, there may be overt or subtle collective pressures, institutional practices or social values, and assumptions which might lead to bias (Noon, 2018). Recognising this fundamental challenge is important as the behavioural consequences of bias can be subtle and difficult to link directly to sources of bias (Noon, 2018). For example, we may be unaware of how particular information has led to assumptions which have impacted our selection of tests, the application of test norms or the wording used within a report.

A general way in which supervision may be used to pre-empt, identify, and address bias is through making the assessment process explicit, transparent, and pre-planned. In some ways, adapting the approach to Open Science which is being adopted in many areas of research (e.g., https://www.apa.org/science/about/psa/2019/02/open-science; https://osf.io/; accessed 29/09/21) may provide a template for increasing transparency and mitigating the impacts of bias. The general open science approach includes pre-registration (developing and making public the research protocol before engaging in research); making data public (to allow others to analyse the information and compare their conclusions with yours) and open access (making reports and papers widely accessible). Within assessment and testing practice this could include using supervision to be explicit about *why* the assessment is being undertaken and *who* requested it; specifying *what* information/test data will be collected, in what order and for what reason; and describing *how* information/test data will be analysed. With respect to data (e.g., test results) it would also be possible to ask someone else to independently score and interpret the findings so that these can be compared with your own. However, whilst arriving at the same conclusion may be used to indicate some level of reliability, it is important to recognise that the source material being used may contain the bias which leads to a particular conclusion. In addition, it can be helpful to keep a decision log (as is done in qualitative research), and to ask others (e.g., a supervisor) to review and critique the decisions you have made along the way – especially where these represent a deviation from your plan. Through supervision we might also consider how our personal and professional *values* and *beliefs* impact on the assessment being undertaken, and the role that the selected *theories and models* being utilised inform or influence our decision making (and may themselves be affected by bias). Finally, subjecting your reports to scrutiny and challenge from your supervisor (or others) can help to detect bias within the writing style, sequencing, and structure of the document.

Addressing the Limitations of Practitioner Self-Report

The way supervision is practiced by many people means that much of the material accessible within supervision relies on supervisee recall and self-report. This is a potentially limiting factor especially when we wish to consider and address potential bias. However, there are a number of strategies that a supervisor can draw upon to help the practitioner recognise and subsequently examine and address potential bias.

Use of evidence-based assumptions: Familiarity with the literature on bias and experience from other sources (e.g., own practice, training) provides the supervisor with a wealth of information from which to openly make assumptions. This may take the form of applying general principles to the work of the supervisee, e.g., how does the research on the bias blind spot and the introspection illusion apply to you and this piece of work; drawing on personal experience, e.g., "traps I've fallen into – what traps are you aware of for you in this case and how can they be managed"; making observations about differences between the supervisee and the client, e.g., how might the differences in your education level/gender/cultural experiences be impacting the assessment process and how are these being addressed; making assumptions about the likely influence of extraneous material or the sequence in which information was gained, e.g., how did reading the previous report by Prof. XX shape your thinking and decision making; and using base rate information to assume alternative (more optimistic or pessimistic) outcomes (such as the scenario planning component of the HCR-20; Douglas et al., 2013). When the supervisor uses assumptions as a way to prompt the supervisee to consider where bias may lurk, it is important that these are linked to evidence/data, are specific and are pertinent to the work being undertaken.

Use of challenge: Constructive challenge is a key part of supervision and is often coupled with using evidence-based assumptions. Some ways in which challenge can be used effectively are for the supervisor to present an alternative or opposite hypothesis based on the available evidence; for the supervisor to highlight existing evidence which might not fit or might undermine aspects of the assessment conclusions and encouraging the practitioner to do this as well (i.e., looking for information that may support *or* refute the current view); for the supervisor and supervisee to consider what piece(s) of evidence that have not been collected might undermine the current hypotheses or formulation. It is also possible to challenge *why information is being collected* in order to minimise the opportunity for cognitive contamination, i.e., collecting wider information which may influence/bias decisions even though the information gathered is not directly relevant (Zapf & Dror, 2017). Questions such as "why is gathering this information relevant", "how will this piece of information assist in the assessment task", can be helpful for this. It is important for the supervisor to also be mindful that cognitive contamination can also be introduced through the questions/discussions had in supervision and thus these questions should also be applied by the supervisor to their supervisory practice. The purpose of challenge within supervision as described here is to help the supervisee "step back" from their current position and to re-evaluate the information, the way it has been collated, integrated, or formulated and to review the conclusions drawn.

Use of test material: Selecting relevant and appropriate test materials requires skilled and often subtle decision making to maximise the likelihood that the information gleaned will be "fit for purpose". Here the supervisor should help the supervisee scrutinise decisions about test selection and use, and the approach to testing being adopted (e.g., where, how, when, and why a test is being used). The supervisor and supervisee might also take time to set out what conclusions might be drawn from different possible outcomes from the test (e.g., if the scale shows X or Y; if the test provides limited information or if indices indicate the test result may be invalid). Wherever possible, conversations about testing should begin before the assessment takes place and continues through to the point where conclusions are finalised. It is essential for the practitioner to examine the person-test fit – how well does this test fit the question to be addressed, with this client, at this time and in this circumstance/ setting. Within the supervision context this can be supported through the supervisors asking specific questions such as "given information within the manual/publications about the way this test was developed what safeguards are in place to maintain its validity; which test or version of the test might be most relevant in this instance; what normative data is likely to be most valid in this instance and why; what factors need to be considered (e.g., literacy, cultural assumption) for this application of the test to be valid and useful". It is important to remember that factors which compromise test validity will ultimately undermine the conclusions we can draw and thus the value, relevance and robustness of our findings.

Use of direct observation: Addressing unconscious bias within practice has been described using stages of change type models (e.g., Croskerry et al., 2013) with some describing ways in which movement from denial through acceptance to adaptation and integration may be achieved (Teal et al., 2012). Developmental models of supervision (e.g., Stoltenberg & McNeill, 2011) recognise that those at an early stage of skill/competence development may have limited awareness and capacity to observe and report their actions, thoughts and emotions both during and after a piece of work. For this reason, "live supervision", direct observation of the supervisees practice, or opportunities to record the work of the practitioner can be essential for the supervisor to be effective in their role. Recording of practice can also enable the use of other supervisory methods and techniques to guide reflection such as Interpersonal Process Recall (Ivers et al., 2017). It is important to note that developmental models recognise that individuals will differ in the extent of their development across different competencies, knowledge, and skill. Thus, experienced practitioners may be in an "early stage" of development in relation to cultural competence and recognising and addressing bias and thus benefit from live supervision. Indeed, despite its association with early stages of development, direct observation can be helpful for all supervisees from time to time. In common with developmental models, some authors have described phases.

Use of third parties: Where it is not possible or appropriate to directly observe or to record the work of the practitioner (or as a supplement to other forms of information), there may be ways to obtain helpful feedback from others either routinely or when specifically requested. This may be in the form of feedback from colleagues or clients, to the practitioner or directly to the supervisor. At its most basic level it may be possible to *ask the client* about their experience of the assessment and any ways in which they consider you or the assessment approach might be biased towards/against them or the assessment purpose, and/or to *ask colleagues* about any evidence or examples they might have for possible bias in your assessment and testing practice. More formally it may be possible to adapt a *360° feedback* approach (widely used as part of staff appraisals) to examine specific aspects of practice such as the possible experience of/management of bias in assessment practice.

Supervisor Skills and Competence in Identifying and Addressing Bias

The ability of the supervisor to assist the practitioner in identifying and addressing or mitigating sources of bias is reliant on the skills and expertise of the supervisor in this area. It must be acknowledged that supervisors will have their own (known and unconscious) biases and will be subject to the processes that have been described. Supervisors will be at a point of development in relation to their bias awareness and competence; however, it is important for supervisors to strive towards competence in the areas of unconscious bias and cultural sensitivity (Teal et al., 2012) if they are to be able to assist the practitioner in this area. Just as the practitioner can be impacted by effects such as anchoring and allegiance, these can influence and affect the supervisor and the process of supervision. In addition to relevant training, the supervisor themselves need to have a forum (e.g., their own supervision) in which they can examine their competence with regard to identifying and addressing bias in others, have an opportunity to examine and address their own biases and understand how these might impact on the supervision they provide. Disclosure to the practitioner about the supervisor's own biases may also be appropriate especially where this might provide a helpful context for the practitioner to consider themselves and their work or where there may be learning that can be drawn from this. Supervisors should also encourage the supervisee to notice and challenge them when supervisor bias is identified. This can provide an excellent opportunity for the supervisor to model openness and learning through reflective practice ("reflect *in* action"), by accepting and acknowledging the challenge, openly recognising and describing the discomfort that can result from bias being detected, and addressing how learning from this might take place (including how practice may need to be changed).

Monitoring through Self-Supervision

As we have noted earlier, research has shown that simple introspection provides no specific remedy for bias reduction and consequently one might be drawn to the conclusion that any form of self-supervision would be of limited value. However, there may be ways to enable us to make use of self-supervision alongside engaging in supervision with others. First, knowing about the fallibility of our own appraisals and ability to recognise bias may help us to reappraise our introspective ability and seek (and accept) other forms of evidence about our own biases; "When participants were taught that valuing introspections is likely to lead one astray in making judgements about influences on the self, they ceased claiming that they were less susceptible to bias than their peers" (Pronin & Kugler, 2007, p. 575). It is important to note here, however, that simply reading an article on the limits of introspection may not be sufficient to counter the "bias blind spot" (Zappala et al., 2018). Second, it may be that adding structure to the way in which an individual critically reviews their own work could provide opportunities for an individual to do at least some monitoring and responding themselves. Having a simple list or workbook of questions may provide an approach to self-supervision that can move us away from simple introspection. Such an approach might help us to "step into the shoes of another" in order to see our practice from other viewpoints. For example, the list of questions and task provided by Goldyne (2007; table 2) and the supervisor strategies contained within this chapter might provide a useful starting point for self-supervision questions. We can also consider a number of behavioural indicators which might be revealed through considering your approach "in this instance" with your "usual or typical approach". For example, am I doing what I usually do; sequencing the interview/tasks as I typically do; approaching the assessment as I normally do; what, if any, adaptations am I making (or failing to make) and why; what, if any, hypotheses do I have (or not have) and why. As with all supervision, candour during the task and a focus on developing concrete next steps or actions upon which to act are necessary to ensure supervision might help address bias where this is present.

Unconscious Bias and Cultural Competence

Whilst we have considered bias generally, and examined how supervision might be used to assist with identifying and mitigating various forms of unconscious bias, bias associated with cultural and racial factors merit specific consideration. It is increasingly being recognised that *becoming* culturally competent (Campinha-Bacote & Munoz, 2001) and working towards individual and institutional *cultural proficiency* (Wells, 2000) are essential although, as has been shown in supervisee research, most of us will be susceptible to overestimating the extent of our multicultural competence (Ladany et al., 1997).

Although targeting health care and those seeking treatment, the model of the proposed mechanisms through which health and human service providers can influence race/ethnicity disparities in treatment, and the eight hypotheses of the ways in which factors such as race can impact decisions and actions these can be readily adapted for use in supervision (Van Ryn & Fu, 2003).

At the most basic level, supervision can provide a forum in which the practitioner can be encouraged to consider the role and impact of a person's culture in relation to the assessment task (Burkard et al., 2006) and collecting culturally relevant data pertinent to the reason for the assessment (Campinha-Bacote & Munoz, 2001). Practitioners can also be supported to maintain "a broad, objective, and open attitude toward individuals and their culture" (Wells, 2000, p. 194). This could include explicitly monitoring cultural responsiveness within supervision and promoting discussions about race and culture. For example, research suggests that supervisor direction to consider multicultural issues may be useful; "supervisees from all racial groups became more adept at conceptualizing treatment strategies when instructed to focus on multicultural issues … [although this] did not lead to more sophisticated etiology-based multicultural conceptualizations" (Ladany et al., 1997, p. 291). Further, supervisors can help the practitioner to focus on the uniqueness of each client and to provide guided reflection and review when the practitioner is exposed to difference and potential triggers which may make bias explicit (Teal et al., 2012). It is also likely that strategies designed for attending to and addressing personal bias in general (e.g., Marcelin et al., 2019, figure 3) can be readily adapted and utilised within self and other supervision.

Actively engaging with people from different backgrounds and with different beliefs and education provide opportunities for the development of cultural competence. Whilst research on cross-cultural supervision is limited (e.g., Burkard et al., 2006; Burkard et al., 2014), securing supervision from a supervisor from a distinctly different background to oneself may be helpful to practitioners. However, it is recognised that in any country, there is (a numerical) challenge for a practitioner from a majority ethnic group to access supervision with someone from a minority group. It may be that remote/online working presents a unique opportunity for this limitation to be addressed by enabling practitioners and supervisors from different background and even countries to be brought together.

Is the Potential for Bias Always a Problem?

Having considered the possible problems that can arise from bias we need to consider if we can, or perhaps should, strive to remove all sources and forms of bias whenever they do (or, pre-emptively thinking, could) arise. "Chasing" bias and possible sources of bias in our practice might have a range of unintended consequences such as paralysing us from acting or limiting the scope of our thinking and ideas to those which are "safe" or of which we can assure ourselves are free from any form of bias. Further, despite the association of bias with harmful omnipotence, bias might have little, if any, meaningful impact on many of the decisions we make or conclusions we reach. This is likely to be the case where other evidence provides us with direction or outweighs any impact that bias might be able to exert.

In most assessment situations we are likely to have to prioritise the collection of some information over other information and make decisions about how much assessment information to collect – when can we say we have enough information to draw a conclusion or how can we make the "best" judgement/decision in the time, resources, and information available? Often, such questions are likely to result in practitioners using heuristics (mental short cuts) to guide practice and decision making. However, the use of heuristics has generally been considered as potentially problematic, associated with bias and sub-optimal performance and decision making. However, heuristics are generally adopted because they are expedient and efficient in spite of the possibility these might have for introducing error. Indeed, heuristics, whilst often requiring much less information than other decision-making strategies may be more accurate in some circumstances (for a more detailed discussion see Gigerenzer & Gaissmaier, 2011).

Supervision may be particularly valuable to us in our attempts to formalise our heuristics in order to make them explicit and testable. Supervision should also provide us with a space in which we can be mindful of bias and responsive to addressing it, whilst accepting that much of our activity (and processes) as forensic psychologists are not linear, pre-planned and carefully selected, but are real world (and real time) interactions in which much of the information is unknown and where we are shaped by both prior knowledge and experience as well as the current situation. Indeed, whilst we may strive towards a rational (and statistical) approach to assessment and formulation, we frequently need to rely on heuristics to allow us to engage with and complete assessment tasks; with heuristics often resulting in high levels of "accuracy". This position should not be seen as an acceptance of intentionally biased, discriminatory, or harmful practice but instead a recognition that bias presents one of the many competing challenges (and perhaps opportunities) we face when seeking to deliver ethical and equitable assessment practice.

Conclusion

Bias is a largely hidden yet powerful force which can impact assessment practice in a multitude of ways. By accepting our susceptibility to being influenced by factors outside our conscious control and our bias blind spots we can set the scene for being able to use supervision to help us mitigate the impact of bias on our practice. Supervision can also assist us in maintaining our curiosity (about ourselves, our practice, and others) attending to "hard to hear" information and seeking out opportunities for exploring bias and embracing diversity. Whilst there is a need for research to be specifically focussed on supervision as a mechanism for managing bias, we have seen in this chapter how supervision might be employed to provide scrutiny and support to those undertaking assessment tasks. However, it is incumbent on supervisors to develop and maintain their own competences (e.g., research on bias and decision making) and to strive towards cultural (and diversity) proficiency if they are to assist supervisees in this area.

Notes

1 Similar registration or licence requirements exist in other territories where forensic psychology is practiced.
2 The terms "practitioner" and "supervisee" are used interchangeably with selection based on maximising the clarity and flow of the text.
3 Similar registration or licence requirements exist in other territories where forensic psychology is practiced.

References

Barnao, M., Robertson, P., & Ward, T. (2012). Ethical decision making and forensic practice. *The British Journal of Forensic Practice, 14*, 81–91.
Bordin, E. S. (1983). A working alliance based model of supervision. *The Counseling psychologist, 11*(1), 35–42.
Borum, R., Otto, R. K., & Golding, S. (1993). Improving clinical judgment and decision making in forensic evaluation. *Journal of psychiatry & law, 21*(1), 35.

Burkard, A. W., Johnson, A. J., Madson, M. B., Pruitt, N. T., Contreras-Tadych, D. A., Kozlowski, J. M., Hess, S. A., & Knox, S. (2006). Supervisor cultural responsiveness and unresponsiveness in cross-cultural supervision. *Journal of Counseling Psychology, 53*(3), 288–301. 10.1037/0022-0167.53.3.288

Burkard, A. W., Knox, S., Clarke, R. D., Phelps, D. L., & Inman, A. G. (2014). Supervisors' experiences of providing difficult feedback in cross-ethnic/racial supervision. *The Counseling psychologist, 42*(3), 314–344. 10.1177/0011000012461157

Campinha-Bacote, J., & Munoz, C. (2001). A guiding framework for delivering culturally competent services in case management. *The Case manager, 12*(2), 48–52. 10.1067/mcm.2001.114902

Croskerry, P., Singhal, G., & Mamede, S. (2013). Cognitive debiasing 2: Impediments to and strategies for change. *BMJ Quality & Safety, 22*(Suppl 2), ii65–ii72.

Davies, J. (2015). *Supervision for forensic practitioners*. London: Routledge.

Davies, J. (2019). Developing a model for evidence-based clinical forensic interviewing. *International Journal of Forensic Mental Health, 18*(1), 3–11.

Davies, J., & Nagi, C. (2017). *Individual psychological therapies in forensic settings: Research and practice*. Abingdon: Taylor & Francis.

Davies, J. (in press). Staff supervision in forensic contexts. In J. M. Brown (Ed.). *Cambridge handbook of forensic psychology*. Cambridge: Cambridge University Press.

Gigerenzer, G., & Gaissmaier, W. (2011). Heuristic decision making. *Annual Review of Psychology, 62*(1), 451–482. 10.1146/annurev-psych-120709-145346

Goldyne, A. J. (2007). Minimizing the influence of unconscious bias in evaluations: A practical guide. *Journal American Academy Of Psychiatry And The Law, 35*(1), 60.

Hart, S., Sturmey, P., Logan, C., & McMurran, M. (2011). Forensic case formulation. *International Journal of Forensic Mental Health, 10*(2), 118–126.

Ivers, N. N., Rogers, J. L., Borders, L. D., & Turner, A. (2017). Using interpersonal process recall in clinical supervision to enhance supervisees' multicultural awareness. *The Clinical Supervisor, 36*(2), 282–303.

Kadushin, A. (1992). *Supervision in social work* (3rd ed.). New York: Columbia University Press.

Ladany, N., Inman, A. G., Constantine, M. G., & Hofheinz, E. W. (1997). Supervisee multicultural case conceptualization ability and self-reported multicultural competence as functions of supervisee racial identity and supervisor focus. *Journal of counseling psychology, 44*(3), 284.

Marcelin, J. R., Siraj, D. S., Victor, R., Kotadia, S., & Maldonado, Y. A. (2019). The impact of unconscious bias in healthcare: How to recognize and mitigate It. *The Journal of Infectious Diseases, 220*(Suppl. 2), S62–S73. 10.1093/infdis/jiz214

Neal, T. M. S., & Brodsky, S. L. (2014). Occupational socialization's role in forensic psychologists' objectivity. *Journal of Forensic Psychology Practice, 14*(1), 24–44. 10.1080/15228932.2013.863054

Neal, T. M. S., & Brodsky, S. L. (2016). Forensic psychologists' perceptions of bias and potential correction strategies in forensic mental health evaluations. *Psychology, Public Policy, and Law, 22*(1), 58–76. 10.1037/law0000077

Neal, T. M. S., & Grisso, T. (2014). The cognitive underpinnings of bias in forensic mental health evaluations. *Psychology, Public Policy, and Law, 20*(2), 200–211. 10.1037/a0035824

Noon, M. (2018). Pointless diversity training: Unconscious bias, new racism and agency. *Work, Employment and Society, 32*(1), 198–209.

Proctor, B. (1988). A co-operative exercise in accountability. In M. Marken & M. Payne (Eds.). *Enabling and ensuring: Supervision in practice* (2nd ed.), pp. 21–34. Leicester: Leicester National Youth Bureau and Council for Education and Training in Youth and Community Work.

Pronin, E., & Kugler, M. B. (2007). Valuing thoughts, ignoring behavior: The introspection illusion as a source of the bias blind spot. *Journal of Experimental Social Psychology, 43*(4), 565–578. 10.1016/j.jesp.2006.05.011

Pronin, E., Lin, D. Y., & Ross, L. (2002). The bias blind spot: Perceptions of bias in self versus others. *Personality & Social Psychology Bulletin, 28*(3), 369–381. 10.1177/01461672 02286008

Stoltenberg, C. D., & McNeill, B. W. (2011). *IDM supervision: An integrative developmental model for supervising counselors and therapists.* Abingdon: Routledge.

Sturmey, P., & McMurran, M. (2011). *Forensic case formulation* (Vol. 49). Chichester: John Wiley & Sons.

Teal, C. R., Gill, A. C., Green, A. R., & Crandall, S. (2012). Helping medical learners recognise and manage unconscious bias toward certain patient groups. *Medical Education, 46*(1), 80–88. 10.1111/j.1365-2923.2011.04101.x

Tversky, A., & Kahneman, D. (1974). Judgment under Uncertainty: Heuristics and Biases, *Science, 185*, 1124–1131.

Van Ryn, M., & Fu, S. S. (2003). Paved with good intentions: Do public health and human service providers contribute to racial/ethnic disparities in health? *American Journal of Public Health, 93*(2), 248–255.

Wells, M. I. (2000). Beyond cultural competence: A model for individual and institutional cultural development. *Journal of Community Health Nursing, 17*(4), 189–199. 10.1207/S15327655JCHN1704_1

Zapf, P. A., & Dror, I. E. (2017). Understanding and mitigating bias in forensic evaluation: Lessons from forensic science. *International Journal of Forensic Mental Health, 16*(3), 227–238. 10.1080/14999013.2017.1317302

Zappala, M., Reed, A. L., Beltrani, A., Zapf, P. A., & Otto, R. K. (2018). Anything you can do, I can do better: Bias awareness in forensic evaluators. *Journal of Forensic Psychology Research and Practice, 18*(1), 45–56. 10.1080/24732850.2017.1413532

12 The Power Threat Meaning Framework: Implications for Practice within the Criminal Justice System

Jo Ramsden and Kerry Beckley

Introduction

The Power Threat Meaning Framework (PTMF; BPS, 2018) is a document which aims to provide people with a resource for making sense of internal distress, unusual experiences, and any other phenomena which might otherwise be understood as symptomatic of a mental health problem. The framework strives to provide an alternative to a diagnostic classification system by offering explanatory narrative structures which work to contextualise difficult, upsetting internal experiences and to situate them as intelligible (threat based) responses to life events. Importantly, the PTMF discusses how power can operate problematically within relationships and within our wider society in a way that harms individuals and groups. The framework specifically considers how groups within society are devalued, oppressed or marginalised, and denied the opportunity to make sense of their own experiences due to unequal power relations and lack of shared social resources. Thus it seeks to make explicit links between personal distress and troubled or troubling behaviour at an individual level, and within wider institutional, social, economic, and political contexts.

The framework radically challenges us to consider the wider systemic and practice implications of accepting that people are shaped by their circumstances to respond to the world in destructive and dangerous ways. It draws our attention to the adverse conditions that individuals survive, and asks us to intervene in a manner that is less focused on individual "pathology" in order to facilitate access to social justice. For those of us concerned with public protection, the framework invites us as individuals, and wider society, whether that be families, communities, or systems within criminal justice and health services, to understand the interaction between power and threat, to inform our assessment, "treatment" and management of risk and offending. In doing so, the PTMF encourages us to move away from biased assessments that ignore context and fail to account for trauma stemming from adverse childhood events (ACEs), and wider factors such as poverty, deprivation, racism, and ideological forces.

To have currency and utility within criminal justice systems (CJS) in the United Kingdom, the PTMF has to not only explain risk (as it relates to public protection) but also guide us to work more effectively with it. It is the ultimate

DOI: 10.4324/9781003230977-14

aim of this chapter to articulate how the PTMF can inform practice. We suggest that application of the PTMF within the CJS requires examination of how we work and how the system itself has the potential to induce threat responses – to exacerbate risk. We will discuss how the PTMF should be used to challenge our professionally biased attention which tends to be turned towards the classification of risk and the assessment of individuals, and away from our own threat responses. This chapter is interested in how the PTMF facilitates an understanding of the CJS as a traumatised system, and how the "core questions" can be used to structure a narrative which highlights these issues. Whilst we have used our experience of the CJS in England and Wales, perhaps most specifically within the consideration of Imprisonment for Public Protection (IPP) sentences, the PTMF can equally apply to other countries, and so we invite the reader to consider these ideas in the context of their own experience.

We use the terminology of "prisoner" and "worker" throughout the chapter to reflect the reality of individual's status within the CJS. These terms are not considered to be a reflection of personhood. We acknowledge that they may be problematic and that people otherwise described by these terms may prefer alternative definitions.

Case Example

Adedayo is a 25-year-old man who received an Imprisonment for Public Protection (IPP) sentence with a three-year tariff for a violent robbery which occurred in the context of a history of acquisitive offending.

The IPP sentence was introduced in 2003 under the Criminal Justice Act, created to increase the power the courts had in sentencing those deemed to be "dangerous", and so effectively subject to an indeterminate sentence akin to a life sentence. The IPP sentence came into force in April 2005, and by September 2012, nearly 8500 individuals had received this sentence.

The brief circumstances of the index offence were that Adedayo attacked and robbed a female stranger whilst intoxicated with drugs and alcohol. Within prison he is experienced by staff as hostile and "non- compliant" often using his role as a "diversity rep" within the prison to air grievances and to accuse others of racism. He is repeatedly rejected by the Parole Board for release, despite being a number of years over tariff because his attitude within the prison is seen as evidence of him continuing to present a risk to the public.

- Below is a case example which is explored using the core questions that the PTMF invites us to use. These are:
  - What has happened to you? (How has power operated in your life?)
  - How did it affect you? (What kinds of threats does this pose?)
  - What sense did you make of it?(What is the meaning of these situations and experiences to you?)
  - What did you have to do to survive? (What kinds of threat responses are you using?)

In applying a PTMF perspective to Adedayo, we start with the question "what has happened to you?" Adedayo was raised in both the United Kingdom and Nigeria, taken into care in the United Kingdom initially due to emotional and physical neglect as his parents were drug users, and consequently his aunt took him back to Nigeria. Whilst in Nigeria, his emotional and behavioural difficulties were considered evidence of witchcraft. He returned to the United Kingdom aged 17, as his aunt was no longer willing to offer him a home. He had no real connection with family members living in the United Kingdom, and consequently ended up homeless. Adedayo was briefly admitted to hospital following an episode of "drug induced psychosis". Whilst there, he attracted the labels of antisocial and narcissistic personality disorder on the basis of relatively brief professional involvement.

When asked "How did this affect you?" (What kind of threats does this pose?), Adedayo recognised that he had difficulty trusting other people, and experienced an absence of close relationships. He tended to keep others at a distance, and was dismissive of the need for help and support. Adedayo described struggling to identify with both British and Nigerian cultures, feeling ostracised by both to some extent. In terms of "meaning", (what sense do you make of this?) his narrative was one of being different to others, that there was something wrong with him. He spoke of being treated differently and unfairly. Adedayo was profoundly aware of the injustice of the IPP sentence which he saw as discriminating against him. He talked about men entering prison with determinate sentences (meaning they may be released before him) but having committed far more serious crimes.

When considering what Adedayo did in order to survive his early life experiences (what kinds of threat response are you using?), he recognised that his sense of autonomy was necessary, as he could not rely on others, and also recognised that he was wary of disclosing any personal distress or need given that this had been conceptualised as "evil" when in Nigeria. Upon reflection, he recognised that he was scared, angry and felt of little importance to anyone. He was essentially alone. Offending was, for Adedayo a means of funding the drugs he was using to manage profound feelings of hopelessness, disconnection, and powerlessness. In terms of his custodial experiences, Adedayo perceived that he was treated as a "large black man", who was somewhat different to the majority of white males whom he was located with, and that his physical appearance and demeanour was seen as evidence of his continuing risk to others. Adedayo described experiencing both overt racism, in terms of white prisoners being afforded more opportunity for employment and privilege over BAME individuals, and on a personal level in terms of how he was spoken to by both peers and staff. In explicitly raising his concerns, he was experienced as accusatory, and punished or dismissed accordingly, his communication being experienced as a threat by the system. Having given up hope of being able to progress, Adedayo effectively disengaged with staff, whilst remaining behaviourally compliant.

Assessments of Risk Which Fail to Account for Trauma

The case example shows how the PTMF can deepen our understanding of how and why people offend and the nature of the distress which underpins destructive acts. We can also begin to see how readily risk assessments fail to take account of the person's lived experience. Adedayo might be described as problematically "non-compliant", for example, without any understanding of the very under-standable reasons which underpin his hostility and "disengagement". The PTMF also encourages us to be aware of Adedayo's strengths, which too often get obscured by the identity of "offender". He is intelligent, reflective, and feels passionately about the rights of those who are discriminated against.

Understanding how threat responses manifest provides us with an opportunity to develop a more sophisticated formulation of risk in individual cases. But ap-plying a PTMF perspective to this endeavour allows us to better understand some of the biased assumptions we may make in our routine practice. As workers, we need to be aware of the fact that many of the tools and resources at our disposal are not neutral and are, instead, shaped by vested interests (e.g., economic, organisational, political) and poorly attuned to the impact of living in a world which is impoverished, unequal, racist, misogynistic (Larcombe, 2012; Mayson, 2019; Woldgabreal et al., 2020). As workers, therefore, we are often ill equipped to understand those who approach the social world from a *survival perspective*. We are guided, by our tools and our organisational cultures, to base our risk assessments on inaccurate assumptions which are grounded in the logical position of those with power and privilege. When we don't notice this, we risk inadvertently maintaining an unjust status quo.

Rapid assumptive errors (Murphy & McVey, 2010) are common when working with people who, through early adversity, struggle to trust that relational encounters are important and relevant for them. Below we illustrate how *logical* assumptions that are embedded within common CJS practice tend to ignore meaning and position us poorly as workers to both understand and manage risk effectively (Ramsden & Lowton, 2014).

We Confuse Non-Compliance with Risk

The PTMF may help us to understand that many of the things that traumatised people with offending histories do which is classed as "non-compliant" is, in fact, driven by an emotional, threat-based short circuit of reason and reflection. In some cases we might argue that it constitutes the only access to power that an individual has when all other sources of influence or efficacy have been removed. Our assumptions about what we refer to as "non-compliance" bring with it the possibility of unreasonable expectations about how people can evidence a re-duction in risk. Phrases such as "he chose not to use his skills" are commonly made, and seen as evidence that the person requires a "further period of con-solidation" before progression can occur. In Adedayo's case, we can see the potential for the "system" to consider his hostility and dismissiveness as indicative of the fact that his risk has not been addressed, as opposed to considering the impact of his continued incarceration in an environment which poses considerable threats to him. This can result in unrealistic, non-trauma informed expectations upon individuals to evidence risk reduction (to comply). Remaining in custody may be compounding of Adedayo's stress and shame, and potentially of his risk. The social injustice of his sentence is also left unaddressed (see later in this chapter) meaning that the system fails to work effectively with the trust issues which underpin his risk to the public.

We Assume What Others Want or Need

Implicit assumptions (about people finding safety in, for example, work, family, individualism) which underpin much of our risk assessment and service delivery can mean that we make incorrect assessments about what is motivating for people. For example, there is an implicit assumption that release to the community is more desirable than remaining in custody. When one considers the paucity of resources available to many individuals in the community, however, this is certainly not a universal position. We may also assume, for example, that an individual who struggles without structure and purpose will find employment highly protective, and a "power resource". In assuming this, we fail to understand the position of a traumatised individual who struggles to form effective interpersonal relationships with bosses or colleagues. There may be stresses too when "survival" in the community means having a lifestyle which is valued and admired by peers (and less likely to induce ridicule or shame). Under these circumstances, failing to earn enough money (*in a way that is approved by peers*) to fund the desired lifestyle, or being under pressure to succeed, or to be seen as successful may be deeply problematic.

We Confuse Ruptures to the Relationship with Risk

For many of us, working within the CJS is to have experienced hostility, aggression, and even violence. The logical assumption made by many workers (given the frameworks we have for understanding other humans) is that that people act in prosocial ways to preserve and protect relationships that they want to maintain and nurture. This is, however, to overlook the impact of trauma or oppression and to forget the fact that another human being (even one as well-meaning and benign as we see ourselves to be) has the capacity to represent a powerful threat. Human beings have the capacity to act defensively and aggressively when they perceive a relationship to bring with it the dangers that have been experienced before, such as abandonment, abuse, humiliation, and invalidation. It is often the case that these dangers are more present in a relationship which has been (or has the potential to be) important.

Application of the PTMF to difficult and sometimes dangerous encounters is not to suggest that workers can insulate themselves from feeling threat or that they should experience nothing but compassion for someone who is frightening.

To do so would be to deny the impact of the misuse of power that people within the system can inflict on workers. Instead, we can try to apply the PTMF to recognise when our own threat responses, as workers, have been triggered and when those responses lead us make assumptive errors; to misunderstand or to act without reason or compassion. The application of the framework may help us to notice when we might misuse our societally sanctioned power to silence or disavow. This is a process which may only be possible later and with reflection, but the importance of this understanding and of the repair that it makes possible cannot be overstated.

Misunderstanding the threat-based origins of relational ruptures also brings with it the possibility that we will overlook what are important aspects of risk management located within the threat response. For example, an individual who acts dismissively towards workers for fear of abandonment may well be evidencing offence paralleling behaviour which is relevant to the management of his risk of intimate partner violence. This individual may have repeat changes of workers because it is assumed that none of these relationships are helping him to reduce his risk when, in fact, the ruptures are an inevitable part of his relationship pattern. Risk for this individual may be better managed through creating opportunities for understanding the significance of the rupture, for example, that attaching to others is triggering past relational experiences. Application of a trauma informed framework such as the PTMF is essential to help workers and organisations to feel brave and confident enough to move towards the rupture, to explore and understand it collaboratively and with compassion.

We Make Incorrect Assumptions about the Meaning of What People Say or Don't Say

It is often the case that workers within the CJS make problematic assumptions about narratives. We assume that prisoners are consciously "minimising" their offence or that their accounts demonstrate a "lack of victim empathy". We may assume that denial of an offence is deeply problematic from a risk management perspective or that a sparse, benign account of childhood is a direct representation of a lack of trauma. It is important to understand narratives from a threat response perspective and to draw assumptions about the impact of trauma on language, memory, and speech. We know, for example, that childhood accounts which lack balance and detail are indicative of an insecure attachment strategy (Harkins, 1995). We may also assume that victim blaming, minimisation, and denial are functional strategies to manage deeply feared threats of recrimination and shame (Blagden et al., 2014; Harkins et al., 2015; Walton, 2019). One limitation of trauma informed approaches are that they lack a critical race lens, and consideration of how someone's culture may influence their personal narrative. Our understanding of the threat based function of these behaviours and how they serve to protect the individual (and what they protect him/her from) is arguably more informative than the behaviour itself. Without that understanding we may straightforwardly demand changes to the behaviour to evidence a decrease in risk without putting forward a more meaningful risk management strategy which looks to reduce the threats on which they are based.

Offence accounts can become "dead" stories (Spence, 1982), with the person feeling traumatised by the continual recounting of significant adverse events in their life. It can be helpful for workers to reflect upon their most shameful or embarrassing experience, and what it would be like to tell this repeatedly to strangers. Individuals who have committed acts of serious harm often find their behaviour deeply shaming and result in them feeling worthless and expecting rejection from others. Additionally, when individuals focus on their own personal trauma as a means of making sense of their trajectory into violence, they can be dismissed as minimising, or failing to take responsibility, as opposed to constructing a narrative which makes sense and is meaningful. Evolving evidence has resulted in a move away from these ideas being central to risk reduction, with strength based approaches coming to the fore, from which the individual has opportunity to tell their story from a position of relative personal power and resource. There is also an increased focus on trauma focused interventions, although an apparent rejection of the possibility that such work can reduce the person's risk to others. This is nonsensical, given that when one looks at the risk factors associated with violence and sexual violence, they originate from early trauma, poor attachments, and social inequality. Whilst the evidence for any effective intervention with this population remains in its infancy, there is evolving evidence that trauma focused approaches, for example, schema therapy (Bernstein et al., 2021), can be considered to be "risk-reducing".

The importance is, therefore, underscored of applying the PTMF to the *process* of storytelling, and not just to the content. We can see how traumatised individuals may employ a range of protective strategies in response to questions such as "what happened to you"? Arguably, it may be more important to apply a trauma informed understanding to the way in which histories and events are remembered and re-told rather than to assume that the content is a reliable and important account of the trauma. It is, perhaps, the mark of a truly trauma informed service when we can *assume* trauma based on a person's presentation rather than requiring us to tell them about it.

Biased Attention within the CJS

Returning to the example of Adedayo, this is a young man who would have set out in the world with relatively few social, emotional, and interpersonal resources. Adedayo would have utilised the only forms of power available to him. As with many people with a similar history, those forms of power were socially unacceptable and harmful. It is, therefore, understandable that the criminal justice system took action to protect the public and to prevent Adedayo from creating more victims. However, it is questionable that the way in which the CJS acted ultimately led Adedayo to becoming less risky. The misuse of power in this case has not been made visible by the system or responded to restoratively to enable Adedayo to access social justice. As this case illustrates, risk assessment of the individual tends to obscure systemic failings which may compound risk.

Application of the PTMF means we are invited to explore how other forms of power have impacted upon Adedayo and our meaning-based narrative of his life should include the impact of the IPP sentence. *The IPP sentence was abolished in 2012 by the Legal Aid, Sentencing and Punishment of Offenders Act, as the European Court of Human Rights ruled that the sentence breached prisoner's human rights. (Although uniquely British, the IPP sentence is used here to illustrate how the system has the capacity to perpetuate trauma. There will be different examples in other countries.)*

Effectively, therefore, it has been already recognised that keeping Adedayo in custody on indeterminate sentence is an abuse of power, and yet he still has to prove to an independent body (i.e., Parole Board), that his risk to the public has reduced. This illogical position will no doubt pose a significant threat to Adedayo: in effect he is expected to deny the social injustice he has encountered (to publicly accept that his risk is his responsibility alone) and acquiesce to the very body that poses a threat to him. Adedayo's success in this stressful endeavour relies on his capacity to access the very resources (emotion regulation, interpersonal effectiveness, assertiveness, confidence) that we understand to be unavailable to him through early adverse childhood experiences.

One group of individuals who hold power in Adedayo's situation are prison psychologists, who are required to assess how risks and needs could be reduced through the completion of some form of offending behaviour programme or therapeutic intervention. Whilst this chapter does not aim to provide a full analysis of these options, it is fair to say that there is very little robust evidence to suggest that any of the interventions offered in a custodial environment will, with any certainty, impact upon the reasons why an individual may offend in the first place. As we have discussed, this is, in part because they focus on individual "deficits" as opposed to social and political factors. The concept of "outstanding core risk reduction work" is a source of power held by the CJS to prevent progression. In effect, these interventions once again locate the responsibility for risk within Adedayo as an individual (with little emphasis on the need for restorative action by the CJS in relation to the IPP sentence). The propensity for power to be misused by professional assessment remains, potentially compounding Adedayo's trauma by failing to acknowledge the social injustice he has suffered.

A Traumatised CJS?

As we have illustrated throughout this chapter, the CJS can readily fail to account for trauma and context when considering individuals who have offending histories. Positively, the new suite of offending behaviour programmes (MOJ & HMPPS, 2018) offer a strengths-based approach which aims to provide individuals with greater resources as opposed to an elimination of attitudes and behaviours that may contribute a risk to the public. In other words, these programmes shift the rehabilitation focus onto social capital and away from problematically requiring individuals to not be experiencing the symptoms of trauma. They also place more focus on personal meaning in terms of the individual's narrative around how their life came to be. However, these continue to be delivered in an environment which (arguably) routinely obscures misuses of power within the CJS and utilises biased tools and assessments. As a consequence, these positive developments are not immediately leading to cultural changes, meaning that assumptive errors continue to be made about threat responses which are then experienced within the system as challenges to progression and as evidence of continuing risk. Whilst these errors and biases continue, the system itself is able to perpetuate trauma and abuse. The following is taken from the report of the scrutiny visit to HMP Long Lartin by HM Chief Inspector of Prisons 2nd and 9th February 2021 (HM Inspectorate of Prisons, 2021):

> The segregation unit subjected prisoners to a very austere regime for long periods without any reintegration planning. Planned used of force was very high, largely because of the excessive use of handcuffs...

> the regime on the unit was poor with prisoners only receiving a telephone call and shower on alternate days.

Application of the PTMF to the system itself can potentially help us to re-frame these injustices as organisational threat responses. The psychodynamic literature on organisational stress contains much to help us reflect upon how this happens. For example, Isabel Menzies, in her seminal paper (Menzies, 1960) discusses how a large teaching hospital in London developed a range of practices as a way of managing systemic anxiety associated with the task of caring for other human beings. Other authors indicate how groups and organisations may direct behaviour and resources towards the unconscious needs of group members (e.g., Stokes, 1994) and inflict "unconscious abuses" (Hinshelwood, 2014) towards prisoners as a consequence. If we accept that organisations have an unconscious life which exists alongside its observable functions and structures (e.g., Barrett, 2020; Obholzer & Roberts, 2019) then it is, perhaps, not that difficult to speculate about the threats the CJS unconsciously has to manage. To begin with there are public expectations about elimination of risk and victimhood – expectations that place the CJS in the anxious position of both being unable to perfectly eliminate risk whilst also acting to reassure society about danger. Workers are, of course, subjected routinely to dangerous and frightening individuals and to histories of both victimisation and offending that are often unimaginably awful. It would be, perhaps, unsurprising if, in its attempts to unconsciously manage the stress that the system is under, threat based practices emerged which worked to serve the anxiety within the system at the expense of those incarcerated within it. This may be particularly the case given that prisoners lack both public sympathy and a powerful "survivor" discourse meaning there is both a failure to support the system to engage with the victimisation of its inhabitants and a lack of pressure to change.

The PTMF suggests some provisional ways of grouping together common narratives based on the assumption that people facing typical constellations of threats and power abuses (within a particular set of historical and cultural contexts), are likely to share meanings and survival responses. These general patterns are informed by, and can be used to inform, personal narratives. One of these general patterns is titled "Surviving social exclusion, shame, and coercive power" (*Provisional General Pattern 6*). It is described as "characteristic of a large number of (individuals) … in the criminal justice system" (p. 67) and indicates how many people with histories of offending have survived similar backgrounds of trauma and oppression. The people described by this pattern are understood, therefore, to be vigilant to threats consistent with these early experiences and to have often antisocial responses to these threats.

Arguably, the CJS might be seen to employ practices which are characteristic of this pattern suggesting these practices might be understood as organisational threat responses. These organisational threat responses (with their capacity to dominate, humiliate, ignore, disempower, etc.) potentially exacerbate threat responses in the people forced to use the CJS and – ultimately, potentially, fail to serve the public by decreasing risk. As we have already discussed, the application of the PTMF is not to eliminate threat but to notice it and its impact (*and to drive social action to address what is threatening*). The CJS culture that exists, however, tends not to notice and comment and, therefore, meaningful risk reduction strategies associated with culture change within the system are left unexplored. The PTMF helps us to identify these links and to debunk the (publicly supported) narrative that brutal, punitive regimes are required for effective risk management.

How Workers Can Take Up Roles within a Traumatised CJS – Fictional Examples

John is a new prison officer, who has decided to take up a career in the prison service. John grew up with parents who were separated. His mother remarried a man who showed little interest in John and his brother and, over the years became a violent and unpredictable alcoholic. John's earliest years were spent in a chaotic and emotionally deprived environment which was ill equipped to meet his own emotional development needs. John has little experience of working effectively with individuals with complex emotional needs who have used violence of varying forms, including sexual violence. John's own experiences mean that he has heightened threat based vigilance to being perceived as the "weak link", and has been told that he will be manipulated or coerced by prisoners if he lets his guard down. John may well have fewer resources for being effective interpersonally because he is male and because power operates ideologically within society to instil notions of masculinity which privilege the importance of dominance and/or control within interpersonal encounters. Around all of this are other forms of ideological power which insist that prisoners should be harshly treated and punished. John is, therefore, having to manage a threatening situation with few resources. He is unlikely to feel in any way supported to assert his authority confidently and effectively in a way that is characterised by understanding and kindness. In doing so he is, perhaps, predisposed to respond with hostility and indifference to traumatised men or women who have also experienced varying degrees of trauma and who have well established, problematic, ways of responding to these threats, and in many ways is in a parallel position to most of the individuals he is charged to manage. As a consequence, we might expect John to practice in a way which is ill attuned to the needs of those he serves but which are nonetheless organisationally sanctioned by a traumatised system and protective for John. In his own attempts to survive, John may inadvertently rely on institutionally sanctioned responses which replicate the abuse that the prisoners have already experienced in their own lives, as he has.

Take the example of Sally, a young female forensic psychologist in training, who occupies a different power position in the environment than John. She may feel the need to overcompensate for her youth and femininity in the context of a male prison by being overly assertive, and potentially punitive towards those who challenge her in order to protect herself. It would not be uncommon for someone in Sally's position to find herself undertaking an assessment of risk or personality disorder with a male prisoner who manages his anxiety of being judged negatively or misunderstood through verbal challenge, disengagement or even hostility, resulting in Sally's narrative being one of an imposed authority, with descriptions of interpersonal functioning being "narcissistic" or "psychopathic" traits. Beckley (2010) outlines how this "schema chemistry" (Young, 2009) can be crucial in order to make sense of interpersonal dynamics which may, or may not, having a bearing on future risk.

The roles as articulated above are shaped and encouraged and able to exist within a CJS which has no narrative framework for understanding the importance of its own unconscious life and the impact on it of repeated, sustained and horrific trauma. This system has biased attention towards the individuals who use its services and, currently, few structures for thinking about and noticing itself. One of the important aspects of the PTMF is its availability as a resource for everyone. It is a principle which is upheld by the framework that we should all be able to access a way of understanding ourselves which accounts not only for trauma but also for how power has operated in our lives. It is, therefore, both acceptable and meaningful to apply the framework to the system itself and for workers within it to use it to help them understand how and why they may practice as they do.

Implications for Practice

Reframe Offending as a Threat Response

The PTMF promotes practice which leads to restorative social action. This is, perhaps, the most challenging requirement for workers who might be lacking resources and organisational support to properly practice in a way that addresses the injustices their prisoners have experienced. It would be a brave offender manager, for example, who presents a case to the parole board that Adedayo's risk is compounded by the IPP sentence.

Nonetheless, it is perhaps incumbent on us as workers to continually reframe offending as a threat response, *where this is relevant*. With individuals, workers may be able to use an explicit PTMF approach to help develop a narrative understanding of the person and to co-construct a formulation of behaviour and offending. Within this process it is, perhaps, empowering to help individuals to consider the dynamic with the system – how others might respond poorly towards them on the basis of their own threat responses.

Working with individuals to reframe offending as a threat response is to allow us the opportunity to prepare for parole hearings, for court appearances or for offending behaviour programmes and to anticipate threats within these forums and to plan for how to respond.

For the wider system it is, perhaps, a radical act to continually reframe offending as a threat response. For many workers who are used to and familiar with the myriad of organisationally sanctioned methods for positioning prisoners as individually pathological and responsible, the use of the PTMF is, potentially, to be re-programmed! Consider the widespread use of the word "disengaged". For Adedayo and for so many like him, disengagement is a useful strategy for protecting himself from services which are, at best, meaningless and, at worst, disempowering and abusive. It requires vigilance on the part of the worker to notice and adjust the mechanisms through which we continually disavow trauma and adversity.

Nonetheless, it is possible for us as workers to engage in this process of re-framing in all activities such as documenting incidents, report writing, and giving evidence to parole boards and courts. In doing so, we potentially engage in the very practices which the PTMF would support – practice which potentially leads to social action. If we comment, for example, on the limitations of an offending behaviour programme (rather than talk about individual disengagement), we potentially stimulate scrutiny of that programme and of ways in which it might be adjusted to make it more meaningful to people with particular needs.

Workers can bring this re-framing of threat responses not just into written tasks but into supervision, reflective spaces and formulation sessions with colleagues. Being explicit about the task – of understanding behaviour through a trauma informed lens – will enable others to question, challenge and notice each other's language and interpretation. It is perhaps more in keeping with the need for radical culture change (and the telling truth to power that this necessitates) that we look to create trauma informed discussion spaces rather than assuming that individuals may expertly model a new way of thinking.

Talk Explicitly about Power

The PTMF invites us to be explicit about power and threat issues (or coping and surviving) which might be considered a new and unexplored discourse within criminal justice settings. The importance of creating space for exploring the implications of this cannot be overstated.

Workers can use the PTMF with prisoners to begin to talk about where power lies and where it might be used or misused. Undoubtedly, this will be new and difficult terrain for workers for whom a conversation about power is to acknowledge the very aspect of their relationship with prisoners that is often the source of mistrust – the power to inform the system about this person's risk and, ultimately, to deny them their liberty. We would suggest that the very acknowledgement of this power, how that feels and how and why it might be problematic will work restoratively where social injustices have been perpetrated.

Talking about power will also, potentially, be difficult for workers who are themselves afraid or traumatised. Talking about power begins a process of sharing power and this might feel – for the frightened or overwhelmed worker – as if the one thing they have to keep them safe is being eroded. Supervision is key here to help workers to move towards these types of conversations with prisoners.

Naming and talking about power with prisoners allows us as workers to negotiate and share power in a way that is potentially highly relevant and useful for risk management. The application of the PTMF, for example, may allow us to talk about what powers we – individual workers and the wider system – have over this person and when those powers would be used. We may be able to talk about systemic threat responses (when coercive or restrictive risk management strategies will feel necessary) and what could happen to trigger those. We may be able to invite the individual prisoner to consider how we might communicate better when threat responses are heightened and how we might seek to understand risk under those conditions. These are exciting and fruitful areas for those of us concerned with public protection to explore.

Finally, in this section, explicit discussions about power potentially better enable involvement and co-production activities given the potential for franker discussions about organisational anxiety associated with the sharing of power with people who have offended in the past. It has been argued by many prisoner activists and lived experience practitioners (e.g., Ball, 2020) that it is apprehensive services and workers which obstruct meaningful involvement. An explicit and collaborative approach to managing the risks associated with the co-production task is likely to be containing for workers (and prisoners). This type of approach invites those with both lived and professional experience to talk openly about what might go wrong and what enacted power would look like should these feared events occur. Workers are invited to consider how they may jointly (and with compassion and respect) work together to manage these risks.

Use It to Help a Traumatised System

We have argued in this chapter that one of the main obstacles to the type of culture change that the PTMF requires is the unacknowledged anxiety which exists within the criminal justice system and all the services and organisations and workers that it comprises. Arguably, therefore, one of the most important applications of the PTMF has to be to the system itself. Applying the PTMF in this way requires workers to understand themselves as a product of the system and not independently, expertly immune to the anxiety. Considering how the system enacts unconscious disquiet requires us to create the conditions for noticing and exploring how this happens. It requires us to use the PTMF to facilitate discussion and exploration; to challenge each other and to observe ourselves bravely. The task would be to notice social defences (threat responses) and how these operate to help us manage unease within the system at the expense of the prisoner. Taking this further, the task is then to think about what we need to practice differently and, ultimately, to build compassion, understanding and healing within the CJS. Beyond this, the aim is to drive social action and to change revenge driven ideologies within society which understand only punishment as a means of delivering justice and safety.

Acknowledgements

With thanks to Anjula Gupta and Lucy Johnstone.

References

Ball, M. A. (2020). Service user involvement and co-production in personality disorder services: An invitation to transcend re-traumatising power politics. In J. Ramsden, S. Prince, & J. Blazdell (Eds.). *Working effectively with personality disorder: Contemporary and critical approaches to clinical and organisational practice.* West Sussex: Pavilion Publishing.

Barrett, J. (2020). The organisation and it's discontents: In search of the fallible and 'good enough' care enterprise. In J. Ramsden, S. Prince, & J. Blazdell (Eds.). *Working effectively with personality disorder: Contemporary and critical approaches to clinical and organisational practice.* West Sussex: Pavilion Publishing.

Beckley, K. A. (2010). Team dynamics: A schema focused approach. In P. Willmot & N. Gordon (Eds.). *Working positively with personality disorder.* Chichester: Wiley Blackwell and Sons.

Bernstein, D., Keulen-de Vos, M., Clercx, M., De Vogel, V., Kersten, G., Lancel, M.,…, Arntz, A. (2021). Schema therapy for violent PD offenders: A randomized clinical trial. *Psychological Medicine*, 1–15. 10.1017/S0033291721001161

Blagden, N., Winder, B., Thorne, K., & Gregson, M. (2014). Making sense of denial in sexual offenders: A qualitative phenomenological and repertory grid analysis. *Journal of Interpersonal Violence, 29*(9), 1698–1731.

Harkins, L., Howard, P., Barnett, G., Wakeling, H., & Miles, C. (2015). Relationships between denial, risk, and recidivism in sexual offenders. *Archives of sexual behavior, 44*(1), 157–166.

Harkins, M. M. (1995). Recent studies in attachment: Overview, with selected implications for clinical work. In S. Goldberg, R. Muir, & J. Kerr (Eds.). *Attachment theory: Social, developmental, and clinical perspectives* (pp. 407–474). Hillsdale, New Jersey: Analytic Press, Inc.

Hinshelwood, R. D. (2014). Abusive help – helping abuse: The psychodynamic impact of severe personality disorder on caring institutions. *Criminal Behaviour and Mental Health, 12*(2), S20–S30.

HM Inspectorate of Prisons. (2021). https://www.justiceinspectorates.gov.uk/hmiprisons/inspections/hmp-long-lartin-4

Johnstone, L., Boyle, M., Cromby, J., Dillon, J., Harper, D., Kinderman, P., Longden, E., Pilgrim, D., & Read, J. (2018). *The power threat meaning framework: Towards the identification of patterns in emotional distress, unusual experiences and troubled or troubling behaviour, as an alternative to functional psychiatric diagnosis.* Leicester: British Psychological Society.

Larcombe, W. (2012). Sex offender risk assessment: The need to place recidivism research in the context of attrition in the CJS. *Violence against Women, 18*(4), 482–501. 10.1177/1077801212452249

Mayson, S. (2019). Bias in, bias out. Available at http://digitalcommons.law.uga.edu/fac_artehop/1293

Menzies, I. E. P (1960). A case-study in the functioning of social systems as a defence against anxiety: A report on a study of the nursing service of a general hospital. *Human Relations, 13*(2), 95–121.

MOJ & HMPPS. (2018). https://www.gov.uk/guidance/offending-behaviour-programmes-and-interventions

Murphy, N., & McVey, D. (2010). *Treating personality disorder: Creating robust services for people with complex mental health needs.* Hove, New York: Routledge.

Obholzer, A., & Roberts, V. Z. (2019). *The unconscious at work: A Tavistock approach to making sense of organizational life.* Abingdon: Routledge.

Ramsden, J., & Lowton, M. (2014). Probation practice with offenders: The importance of avoiding errors of logic. *Probation Journal, 61*(2), 148–160.

Spence, D. P. (1982). *Narrative truth and historical truth.* New York: W.W. Norton.

Stokes, J. (1994). Problems in multidisciplinary teams: The unconscious at work. *Journal of Social Work Practice, 8*(2), 161–167.

Walton, J. (2019). The evolutionary basis of belonging: Its relevance to denial of offending and labelling those who offend. *Journal of Forensic Practice, 22*, 202–211.

Woldgabreal, Y., Day, A., & Tamatea, A. (2020). Do risk assessments play a role in the enduring 'color line'? *Advancing Corrections Journal, 10*(2020), 18–28.

Young, J. (2009). Personal communication. August 11.

13 Individual Bias in Forensic Practice

Todd E. Hogue and Mats Dernevik

Overview

This chapter examines how individual biases impact on forensic psychology practice. The intention is to encourage practitioners to better understand the factors that impact on their decision making, and to reflect on those factors unique to the individual which may introduce bias into their forensic practice. Registering as a practitioner psychologist, forensic, clinical, or otherwise requires undertaking a training process focused on developing the competencies to act as a practitioner psychologist. This training pathway is focused on obtaining the experience, knowledge, and skills development necessary to undertake the explicit tasks of working as a forensic or clinical psychologist. There is, however, less focus given to considering those more implicit factors which may impact idiographically on forensic clinical judgements.

Many of these factors are directly relevant to other areas of clinical decision making but some have specific implications for working in forensic practice. Some of the research examining biases in forensic practice is presented, as well as an overview of Dror's (2020) model for understanding fallacies and bias in forensic science practice. We argue that this model should equally be applied to forensic psychology practice, and how forensic psychology practice could be improved. We then focus in more detail on how the attitudes and the experiences and beliefs of individual forensic practitioners may specifically impact on their practice and then suggest some steps that could be taken to reduce the individual level of bias in forensic practice.

Introduction: A central aspect of forensic work focuses on risk, and the extent that the risk of current and future offending can be predicted. Over the last five decades there has been an increasing body of work focused on refining the practice of effectively predicting risk of future violence. Paul Meelh's (Meehl, 1954) seminal work contrasting clinical versus statistical approaches to the prediction of future behaviour (see Grove, 2005, for a summary), started the focus on how to improve the accuracy of the prediction of future behaviour. In forensic practice this has led to the development of a range of risk assessment approaches (Monahan & Skeem, 2014), and the development of structured professional judgement as an alternative methodology (Douglas et al., 1999). The main focus

DOI: 10.4324/9781003230977-15

has been on increasing the accuracy of prediction through refining the processes undertaken to make predictions and evaluating the efficacy of those methods.

For all the focus on increasing the accuracy of prediction, there has been an increasing awareness of a range of factors which continue to impact on the accuracy of forensic decision making (Neal, 2016, 2018; Neal & Grisso, 2014; Shepherd & Sullivan, 2017; Zapf et al., 2018). Shepherd and Sullivan (2017) highlight implicit and explicit factors that impact on the interpretation of future violence risk. Risk prediction instruments are able to effectively predict future risk, but have yet to be effective in the management and reduction of risk. They argue there is a tendency to overvalue the effectiveness of risk instruments, a potential for authorship bias, the possibility that the typical use ROC analysis underestimates risk, and that they are full of methodological errors.

They make the argument for greater clarity and understanding about the assumptions and research evidence upon which risk prediction tools are based. This includes contrasting the nomothetic nature of the evidence which measure are validated on, with the idiographic nature of the use of most risk prediction processes (Fazel et al., 2012). They also highlight a number of limitations in the prediction of violence literature and point out that,

> Risk instruments add a level of structure and transparency to estimations of violence. A range of clinician biases may be minimised as a result. However, the process is not immune to harmful subjectivity and prejudices, not just in the course of assessment but also in the interpretation of results. (Shepherd & Sullivan, 2017, p. 297)

This concern over the impact of individual variation even when using standardised risk tools is echoed by Beech and colleagues (2016) who indicate that, "Principally, professionals need to be aware of their own biases, and any tendency they have towards over, or underestimating, risk level" (p. 74). This impact of the effect of the individual assessor is also seen in the introduction of subjective adjustments to risk scores, where adjusted scores are less predictive than unadjusted scores (Hanson & Morton-Bourgon, 2009) which leads them to conclude that "this is an argument to say that introducing subjective opinion into the assessment, made the assessment less valid" (Beech et al., 2016, p. 73). Critically important in terms of considering the role of the assessor in the assessment, they conclude that "Ratings of change may be affected by the relationship the assessor has with the individual in question, the importance the assessor places on various aspects of change, and their personal opinion of the individual" (Beech et al., 2016, p. 73). To ensure consistent and accurate decisions in forensic cases it is critical that individual variation due to assessor behaviour should be minimised.

Bias in Decision Making

When undertaking assessment and presenting expert opinion in forensic cases, the assumption is that the forensic psychologist or psychiatrist is providing their expert opinion in a clear and unbiased manner. However, there is increasing evidence that the decisions made are often biased, and what underpins these biases should be examined more closely.

Models for decision making from other fields of psychology are likely to apply also to forensic assessments and violence risk decision making. From economics and the behavioural economics of decision making, "Prospect Theory" (Kahneman & Tversky, 1979) is of particular interest as it explains a loss aversion bias. The theory is useful for explaining apparent irrational behaviour, as it describes how individuals assess their loss and gain perspectives in an asymmetric manner. The prospective "pain" of losing money outweighs the "pleasure" of winning when making decisions in uncertain situations. Decisions about violence risk are generally different from economic theories as there is rarely a defined gain. The gain is, at best, implicit and sometimes not considered at all. However, the gains of forensic decisions are still relevant for the individual being assessed: less deprivation of liberties, better quality of life, etc. The gains for the decision maker are usually even more obscure: making secure beds available, lowering costs of care, etc. Violence risk decisions are vicarious by nature; it is not the assessor who personally risks being a victim of violence, but rather undefined members of the public, family and acquaintances of perpetrators who are at risk. However different the nature of decisions might be, one study, using vignettes of release decision making for forensic patients, generally supported the usefulness of Prospect Theory to understand decisions accepting or rejecting violence risk (Dernevik et al., 2015).

This study used two different groups of forensic decision-makers (clinicians and judiciary) and a control group (teachers). Perceived gains had a small impact ($\eta2 = .17$) on decisions, while perceived losses had a large impact ($\eta2 = .58$), accounting for more than half of the variance in risk acceptance. The effect of perceived loss was equal across the three groups, supporting the global functioning of prospect theory. Another study of clinician's perception of risk and protective factors suggested clinicians preferred clinical factors before non-clinical factors, put more weight on individual than on contextual factors and more weight on risk factors than on protective factors, also supporting Prospect Theory (Sturidsson et al., 2004).

A number of studies have highlighted the extent to which external factors impact the selection of cases undertaken, as well as the actions taken by the forensic professional including how the views of forensic experts may skew the type of forensic assessments that they undertake (Neal, 2016). This study examined how the views of forensic psychologists may filter the types of cases that they take on, which in turn may impact on the type of assessments undertaken and thus the evidence provided. A total of 206 forensic psychologists took on capital case assessments in jurisdictions where the death penalty applies. The psychologists were asked for their views of capital punishment and the cases they agreed to take on. Those with strong views against capital punishment were more willing to work for the defence and likely to reject other cases. Those more supportive of capital punishment were more likely to be involved in capital cases more generally. The findings suggest that there may be a self-filtering effect of cases such that those individuals with strong anti-capital punishment views end up working predominately for the defence and that this may contribute to an "allegiance effect" in adversarial cases. The important thing here is that attitudes about issues related to the case potentially impacted on the judgements being made.

Several studies have found that expert opinion may be influenced by the extent to which the expert is instructed by the prosecution or defence (Murrie et al., 2008, 2009). When examining 23 real world cases it was found that scores on the Psychopathy Checklist Revised (PCL-R; Hare, 2003) varied in relation to who instructed the expert (Murrie et al., 2009). When instructed by the prosecution, PCL-R scores on the same patient were higher than when instructed by the defence, and the difference was more than the standard error of measurement for the tool. A similar pattern was also obtained when examining assessments undertaken using actuarial risk tools. Once again, when instructed by the prosecution scores were higher than when instructed by the defence. Both studies indicate that experts are biased by who is instructing them to undertake the assessment.

Other factors may also impact on the way that forensic assessments are undertaken. Neal and Grisso (2014) conducted an international survey of 434 experts on how forensic examinations were undertaken and the different tools used in these assessments. This survey identified a wide range of tools used in forensics assessments and raised questions about the extent to which appropriate tools were available to assess the identified areas of need for the range of different populations being assessed. On average, four different assessment tools were used on each case, which raised question about the impact of the assessor identifying appropriate tools for a particular case, the impact of different tools being used and what to do when different measures have divergent outcomes. As they point out, "…the lack of guidance for forensic evaluators leads to subjective decisions in every case about what these variables should be and how they should be indexed" (Neal & Grisso, 2014, p. 1418).

To evidence implicit bias in assessors, Neal (2016) undertook to measure indicators of bias in forensic mental health assessments related to insanity evaluations. It was hypothesised that differences in the style of writing, emotional tone, and length of report would act as proxy variables to indicate the underlying attitudes of the assessor as expressed in the way that the reports were written. Some of their hypotheses were supported, indicating that some observed proxies (e.g., emotional content of language, length of report etc.) may be indicative of bias. However, the applied nature of the research meant that it was not fully possible to test the true extent of the impact of such bias on practice. They concluded that future research exploring bias should attempt to maintain experimental controls so as to more clearly study and identify the link between behaviour and potential bias when undertaking mental health assessments.

Bias in the Cognitive Processes of Decision Making

Possible biases in the cognitive processes underlying decision making has long been identified as a possible source of concern when undertaking forensic assessments (Borum et al., 1993), and different types of possible cognitive biases have also been identified. The extent to which forensic evaluators acknowledge their potential biases was examined in a study of 80 forensic mental health professionals (Zappala et al., 2018). Individuals were asked about four different types of potential cognitive biases which might apply (illusory correlation, hindsight bias, fundamental attribution error, and confirmation error), and the extent to which this applied to others and to themselves. Individuals showed evidence of blind spot bias (Pronin et al., 2002) where individuals fail to recognise their own potential for bias in comparison to the bias of others. Interventions to impact on this observed bias did not have an effect and the authors concluded that it is essential that individuals find methods to reduce the impact of bias on their professional work and that "bias awareness is necessary for improving clinical decision-making in the field of forensic psychology …" (Zappala et al., 2018, p. 54).

To examine the extent to which mental health professionals recognised and considered the role of cognitive bias in their work (Zapf et al., 2018), Zapf undertook an international survey of 1099 individuals who undertook assessments for court. Participants were asked about the accuracy of forensic assessments, and the scope and nature of bias as it applied to their and to other individual's assessments. Respondents were generally aware of the issue of cognitive bias, and that this needed to be considered in forensic practice. They were more likely, however, to think that this was an issue for others more than for themselves, and that simply recognising it as an issue was thought to be sufficient for address the effects. Overall, there was support for blind spot bias with individuals thinking this was more of an issue for others than for themselves.

Summary of the Research

To better understand the types of bias impacting on forensic psychiatric assessments, Meyer and Valença (2021) undertook a systematic review to identify factors related to bias in forensic assessments. While this paper is focused on forensic psychiatric assessments it is still relevant in understanding the impact of bias within forensic assessments. Of the 30 articles which they included in the review they were able to classify them into three broad areas: (1) legal elements and wording, (2) psychometric tools, and (3) expert technique and inter-rater agreement.

On legal elements, there was seen to be a lack of clear terminology and correspondence between legal definitions and diagnoses, low inter-rater reliability of between experts, and the use of hyperbolic clinical language which exacerbated clinical-legal and inter-examiner disagreement (Meyer & Valença, 2021). While psychometric tools tend to be developed to increase the consistency of assessment, they found limited evidence that this was the case, and low inter-examiner agreement while using a relevant psychometric tool. Interestingly, they came to the conclusion that psychometric tools in a checklist format were particularly vulnerable to interviewer bias. They highlighted a lack of standardisation and the use of a common theoretical framework, which resulted in reduced consistency in the area, and high inter-examiner disagreement. They drew attention to a number of areas where the views and attitudes of the forensic assessors were likely to interfere with the accuracy of the assessment. This included, that which related to the type of offence committed or the psychiatric diagnosis given, interviewer biases in the completing of structured checklists, and the inclusion of extraneous clinical or criminological variables which in turn biased the assessment. The authors argued for the identification, control and avoidance of those issues which introduce bias to improve forensic practice. Critical to this is clinicians recognising this is an issue and the need for a better framework for understanding how biases should be examined and addressed.

A Model to Consider Biases in Forensic Practice

To better understand the impact of bias on practice it is necessary to develop a framework to assist with the consideration of this. Dror, in developing a Hierarchy of Expert Performance (Dror, 2016, 2018, 2020) argues the necessity for developing a theoretical framework to better understand, quantify, and evaluate, biases in forensic practice. Dror (2020) outlines a number of cognitive and human factors which potentially impact in the decision-making process. Although Dror is approaching this with reference of forensic science expertise (i.e., the assessment of fingerprints and other evidence this type), we would argue that the framework also relates to applying psychological/psychiatric expertise in forensic practice. As such, in describing Dror's model we will highlight how fallacies or sources of bias would equally apply to a forensic psychological/psychiatric assessment.

Dror (2020) argues that there are six common fallacies or ways of thinking about the data which lead to biases.

First Fallacy

Ethical Issues

This is the misbelief that expressing bias in decision making is an ethical issue resulting from unscrupulous or unethical behaviour on the part of the professional rather than understanding what cognitive bias is truly about. It isn't related to intentional or unscrupulous behaviour but rather broader unintentional biases. An example of this might be where the content, findings and recommendations of an assessment are dismissed because the forensic assessor is working independently, or instructed by the defendant, and therefore seen to be intentionally unethically biased in their work.

Second Fallacy

Bad Apples

This is the assumption that observation bias in expert opinion is due to the competency and ability of the expert involved rather than a recognition that cognitive biases are much more implicit and widespread, and more importantly, not due to a lack of competency on the part of the expert. An example would be assuming that errors in an assessment are due to the incompetence of the assessor rather than potentially due to more general cognitive biases.

Third Fallacy

Expert Immunity

This is the belief that "experts" are impartial and immune from biases in their decision-making process. However, this is not the case, and some of the processes used by the expert may in themselves be particularly susceptible to cognitive biases (e.g., relying on heuristics or schemas in decision making). An example would be where the individual perceives themselves as an expert in the area, and subsequently uses shortcuts, data-chunking, and other heuristics to inform their judgements – which in turn introduces bias into the judgement. This might, for example, apply to an individual who completes training on how to use a risk or personality assessment – but then uses shortcuts when implementing it because of their "expertise".

Fourth Fallacy

Technological Protection

The assumption that the inclusion of technology, tests, instrumentation, artificial intelligence, or automation of the process will ensure an unbiased process. An example in forensic practice is the overreliance on individual assessments or measures, which in turn leads to an error in prediction, such as only using certain tools to predict risk where other factors might be applicable but sit outside the scope of the agreed and more commonly used "risk tools".

Fifth Fallacy

Blind Spot

This is the bias that others may be biased, but I am not. The expert is happy to accept that others may be affected by implicit biases, but that this does not happen to them, and does not impact on their expert practice. An example of this is where the individual considers their assessment, or the assessment of those in their organisation or service to be accurate while alternative assessments from other individuals or contrasting organisations are biased, such as with opposing Parole Board reports or admission reports arguing different outcomes.

Sixth Fallacy

Illusion of Control

This is the belief that experts who acknowledge that they could be biased have an "illusion of control" such that they believe that they will be able to control bias simply through the exertion of their willpower and desire to control the bias in that situation. An example of this often applies where the individual has a long established professional/therapeutic relationship with the individual which may have a positive or negative biasing on resulting assessments. However, the individual practitioner considers that because they are professional, they are able to manage any bias in their forensic practice.

While these fallacies have a distinct impact on the way that the decision-making process is evaluated, perhaps a more important consideration is where the source of the bias is seen to emanate from. In Dror's model, the second domain to consider is where the source of the bias arises from. For Dror (2020), the sources of bias range from those which are very case specific such as the actual available data on the case itself – through to biases due to human nature, such as information processing errors, which are mainly related to the individuals undertaking the assessment.

In Dror's model one should consider the possible sources of bias across these levels.

1   *The data:* The starting point is the data that is known about the case. For example, in a forensic science analysis this might be something like a voice recording of the potential perpetrator, while in a forensic psychology assessment this might be an interview or recorded interview with the alleged perpetrator including their accent, etc. In both cases there is scope for the information about the interview to introduce bias into the interpretation of the data.

2   *Reference materials:* This relates to the extent to which reference material that the data is being compared to may bias the interpretation of the data. A forensic science example would be confirming that a particular individual matches an expected or desired outcome, such as a fingerprint or DNA match, where there is room for assessor interpretation and bias. In forensic psychology this might relate to looking for evidence of item factors on personality or psychopathy assessments where there is an expectation at the outset about the likely score or diagnoses – which might then in part become self-fulfilling. This might also apply to searching for offence paralleling behaviours rather than observing behaviours in a more impartial way.

3   *Contextual information:* This relates to experts being exposed to or knowing other information which is irrelevant for the decision being made but which may still influence judgements about the case. In a forensic science case this might be something like knowing that there is an identified suspect, or that someone has confessed influences judgements around something like fingerprint identification.

In a forensic psychology case, an example might be knowing an individual's current institutional behaviour and this impacting on the way that historical data is interpreted and coded in a risk or personality disorder assessment.

4   *Base rate bias:* This is the extent to which expected base rates from other similar cases influence expectations and judgement of the current case that they are unrelated to. In a forensic science case this would be where observed physical evidence is most often indicative of a particular offence (the high base rate) and this knowledge impacts on the investigation/assessment such that the less common finding is overlooked due to assuming the base rate cause is applied. In forensic psychology this might apply to assuming that because an individual had a particular offence history, or scores high on a measure such as the PCL-r, that the individual is responsible for future offending and this base rate assumption impacts on expert opinion and the extent to which alternative explanations are explored.

5   *Organisational factors:* This applies to the extent that the organisation, and the expectations and processes within that organisation, may impact on the professional judgements which are made. The example that Dror (2020) proposes for forensic science is where there is "a senior person who 'signs off' on reports or analyses, there can be the danger of 'writing what that person wants to read' and a lack of challenge of their scientific decisions" (p. 8002). This can similarly apply in a forensic psychology context where the assessor's view and expectations of the individual supervising reports impacts on the findings and tone of the report independent of the actual aspects of the case.

6   *Education and training:* This is where the forensic science expert must have the appropriate training and expertise to conduct the investigation, and is often an issue where there may be multiple areas of expertise necessary to appropriately assess the case. This same issue applies to forensic psychology. Training and education may narrow the focus of expectations about a case where only one focus or hypothesis is being considered, whereas a wider range of training and knowledge is necessary to understand the case fully. For example, a lack of neuro-psychological or other specialist knowledge could limit the assessment or formulation being undertaken.

7   *Personal factors:* Dror (2020) identifies these as including " … motivation, personal ideology and beliefs" (p. 8002), and goes on to describe a number of situations where idiographic differences between forensic scientists on a range of factors might bias and impact on their professional practice. This can equally be the case within the context of forensic practice where individual beliefs and expectations about particular individuals or groups of "offenders" might impact disproportionally on professional judgements being made. For example, a strong belief that there is no treatment for individuals with personality disorder, or a strong dislike for those who have committed sexual offences may significantly impact on professional work done with either of these groups of individuals. We will discuss this in more detail in the next section.

8   *Human and cognitive factors, and the human brain:* These are the wider factors which apply to the broader understanding of how the human brain works. They

include that information is encoded and decoded, and how there are a range of biases which apply to all humans in terms of information retrieval and understanding, and as such should also apply to forensic psychological expertise.

Considering Personal Factors Biases: Attitudes

The purpose of presenting Dror's (2020) model is not to argue the detail of how this applies to forensic practice, but to raise awareness about the need for a more comprehensive examination about the extent to which this may be the case. While, as outlined above, there has been some recent work looking at biases in forensic practice, there is by no means a coherent or comprehensive understanding of the area. While Dror raises the potential impact of personal factors in his model, there is a dearth of research examining how such individual beliefs, experiences or values may impact on forensic judgements.

One way that this might impact practice is where strongly held attitudes impact on judgements about related topics or individuals. This could happen either because they didn't like a particular individual, or because they hold strong negative attitudes towards a group of individuals. There is relatively little research examining the effect of individual differences on how forensic practitioners make judgements. In one study, however, (Dernevik et al., 2001) practitioners were asked to rate patients using a measure of how they feel about the patient on the Feeling Word Checklist (see Holmqvist & Armelius, 1994), and then to complete an HCR-20 (Webster et al., 1997) assessment of the same patient. What they found was that how the practitioner felt about the patient on the Feeling Word Checklist significantly predicted the level of risk as reported on the HCR-20 with a multiple regression of .659, an R square of .433 – with 43% of the risk rating being accounted for by how the practitioner feels about the patient. Dernevik's study is worrying as it questions the impartiality of risk assessments.

In a similar way, attitudes towards anyone who commits a sexual offence may impact on judgements. Sexual offending often results in a strong emotional reaction from the public and professionals alike (see Harper et al., 2017), and this emotional reaction may impact on one's professional practice. A consistent finding in the area is that the more experience or training you have had with or about those who have committed sexual offences, the more positive you're attitudes will be. However, one would not expect this to be related to how one makes professional judgements. To examine this, Tan (2014) and Hogue and Tan (2016) asked 35 forensic assessors, most of whom were chartered forensic psychologists, to complete the ATS-21 (Hogue & Harper, 2019), which measures attitudes towards those convicted of sexual offences (Harper et al., 2017), and to rate a vignette describing sexual offence behaviour. A significant $-.315$ correlation was found such that those individuals with more negative attitudes rated the offender as at a greater risk of reoffending.

More recently, a much larger study examined the relationship between attitudes towards sexual offending (ATS-21) and risk of reoffending (Harper & Hicks, 2021); however, they used samples of both students (N = 341) and forensic professionals (n = 186). As expected, they found that forensic professionals had significantly more positive attitudes towards those who have committed sexual offences than students. However, what wasn't expected was that 48% of the variance of the risk ratings was accounted for by the score on the ATS, the more positive rating on the ATS the lower rating of perceived risk. Importantly, there wasn't a significant difference in the risk ratings of the student or the forensic professionals indicating that in both groups 48% of the variance relating to the rating of risk was down to their pre-existing attitudes to those who have committed sexual offences. The potential implications for forensic practice are quite significant given that the risk rating of an individual should be independent of the views that the forensic practitioner holds about the client group.

Considering Personal Factors Biases: Attitudes

While attitudes clearly play a potential part in how forensic practitioners make judgements there may be other types of experience which equally have an impact on forensic practice. Miller and Brodsky (2011) raise the issue of needing to consider a number of factors which potentially impact on judgements and practice when making predictions of violence. They suggest that a range of psychological factors may impact on violence assessments including:

- Mental heuristics, e.g., confirmation bias, illusory correlation
- Pre-existing attitudes, e.g., punishment or rehabilitation
- Past personal or professional experience, professional training experience
- Witnessing consequences of inaccurate prediction
- Adversarial alliance
- Fear of making a risk judgement error
- "Clinical lore" typically "err on the side of safety"

This suggests that such outside factors can have a significant effect on forensic judgements. They argue that attitudes, values and experiences both personal and professional have the capacity to impact on judgements and that this impact may not be straightforward, with the potential for such attitudes to have a negative or positive impact on judgements and practice. To start to address this potential they offer a self-assessment guide for helping the individual consider those factors which might impact on an individual undertaking violence prediction. They suggest that considering such questions may promote discussion, act to promote regular reflection, and possibly help structure supervision.

Miller and Brodsky (2011) suggest that it might be appropriate to turn the topics for consideration on the assessment into a more formal checklist for use when considering the impact of different factors on violence judgements. Tan (2014) did this by developing the Evaluator Specific Factor Scale (ESF; Hogue & Tan, 2016[1]) and asked forensic practitioners to reflect on their practice. Although this was a very small sample (N = 35) there were a number of interesting findings. A number of the questions formed natural subscales. As an example, the scales reflected the practitioner's affective reaction (alpha = .786) with questions relating to:

- My colleagues have commented that my personal attitudes affect my work.
- My supervisor(s) has commented that my personal attitudes affect my professional judgement.
- I often find myself feeling emotionally involved in cases.
- I have strong reactions/feelings towards the assessee during risk assessments.

As well as the inclusion of Gut Level reactions (alpha =.692) which asks:

- I always ask myself "what is my gut instinct about a case".
- I follow my gut instinct in cases.
- I rarely question my gut instinct (−).

Interestingly in terms of affective reaction, 42% indicated some agreement that they feel emotionally involved in cases, and 23% indicated some agreement that they have strong reactions/feelings towards the assessee. In terms of Gut Level Response, 68% indicate some agreement that they always ask themselves about their gut instinct about the case and 32% provide some agreement that they always follow their gut instinct. While Tan (2014) doesn't provide a more detailed analysis of the checklist or its impact on practice it does provide a route to better analyse and study the way that the assessment of violence is undertaken and the type of factors which may impact on individual differences in forensic practice.

Addressing Individual Biases

Once there is a recognition that an individual may have biases which are individual to them it is important to consider how these might then be addressed. In doing so it is good to consider the following issues which might drive individual bias.

Reflecting Capacity

This relates to the ability for a person to self-reflect on what they're doing and the comparison here is like a metacognition around those with and without self-reflection. So, the question is, does the individual think about and reflect on their decision-making process sufficiently and about the right things?

Types of Possible Bias

This relates to whether any bias is either internally or externally driven for the individual. This is similar to how structured and unstructured professional biases work in risk assessments and relates to how some biases are likely to be driven by a range of errors in decision making, and others by the structure placed around the decision making. The important issue here is to acknowledge a bias is possible – and then engage in the process of identifying where this bias comes from and how to not be impacted by it.

Anxiety States

To what extent is the individual's decision making impacted by anxiety around the case and the decisions that are being made? You can see this being manifested in a number of ways relating to the experience, confidence, and knowledge base that an individual has.

An example of where the anxiety of the professional is likely to have a high impact is related to making judgements of offender risk. This is especially the case in those release judgements from secure environments where there is a risk of future offending. In these cases, there is an implicit bias towards being overly cautious in the risk judgement being made. This in turn is likely to ensure that the professional errs towards a conservative judgement – resulting in more false positives than false negatives resulting in individuals being kept in security longer than necessary.

Attitudes

An individual's attitudes towards a particular group, behaviour, or type of crime or a specific individual can impact their judgements. An obvious example would be attitudes to those convicted of sexual offences, where it is known that differing attitudes are consistently shown to impact on perceptions of risk, appropriate levels of punishment, or treatment interventions. The importance here is that professionals need to be self-aware of their attitudes towards particular groups or individuals, with a need to then reflect on how this might impact inappropriately on their decision making.

Diversity

It is critically important to acknowledge and recognise that factors related to diversity may impact and bias judgement. Recognition of the factors relating to diversity including social, cultural, and racial factors as they apply both to the forensic practitioner and the diversity of the population they are working with needs to be considered. This also applies to recognising that the literature and research upon which many decisions are based may not be sufficiently diverse to ensure that it does not introduce or support bias in forensic judgements.

Trauma

While there is an increasing recognition that trauma has a major impact on the clients seen in forensic settings, with the need for this to be considered in forensic practice, it is also critically important to consider how primary or secondary trauma experienced by the forensic practitioner may impact on or bias their judgements also.

Personality

While we recognise the importance of the personality of the forensic client it may also be important to recognise the personality of the forensic practitioner and the impact that this may have on biasing judgements and practice. For example, personality style my impact on the extent to which the practitioner is open to alternative explanations, or are overly conservative about the judgements that they make.

Professional and Organisational Biases

Professionals need to also recognise that their professions and the organisations that they work for may implicitly impact and bias the judgements that they make. This relates to the implicit bias related to the way in which expertise or information from other professions (e.g., nursing, psychiatry, etc.) may be considered, or the extent to which those working in health and prison services may be considered or weighted differently than those in private practice or working in a different organisation.

Ways of Considering Types of Bias

1 *Personal bias:* Relates to the type of biases that an individual may hold which is related to their training experience and personal beliefs. In this way it is an idiographic bias, although groups of individuals with a similar experience or background may have similar kinds of biases. These biases will also be influenced by the personality of the practitioner and their individual views. Personal biases may relate to the extent to which an individual may hold specific attitudes or have had an experience which impacts on how they make judgements about the type of individual or type of problem being considered.

2 *Professional bias:* This is related to how professions may see particular topics in a certain way. In this case you can think about it in terms of what is seen to be the professional thing to do in a situation, the guidance about the kinds of training, and a consideration of the different risk factor theories which are seen to be prevalent in the area etc. Their being from that particular professional background might result in dismissing information and judgements from other professionals because they come from a different professional background even though the information presented is accurate.

3 *Organisational bias:* This relates to the biases that an individual has related to working within a particular organisation. Examples of this would be the extent to which decisions are impacted on by organisational structures, expectations and standards. Examples of this would be working within a specific prison or health service and the extent to which this impacts on professional judgements. This potentially impacts at multiple levels. At a high level it effects standards of work behaviour and the types of assessments and activities allowed to occur. At a lower level it impacts on the expected behaviour that is part of the culture of an individual ward or unit.

Examples of where organisational biases are likely to impact on professional judgements are those situations where organisational practice and policy might clash with or influence the clinical judgement that would otherwise be made. This can be seen where organisations dictate what the acceptable assessment or risk measures to be used are – possibly influenced by cost, the availability or lack of workforce training – all which then clashes with what would be best practice from a professional perspective.

Taking It Forwards – Think before You Write!

The focus of this chapter has been to highlight to the reader the need to think about the possible influences that may impact on their decision making before they put pen to paper and commit to the assessment or other clinical work that is being undertaken. Traditionally, clinicians are concerned about the information that is available both about, and from, the client and the extent that external biases or absences in the information impact on their professional judgement. The current argument is different, in that it asks the forensic practitioner to consider the extent to which their internal, individual biases and experiences impact on the clinical/ forensic decisions they make. This understanding of reflective practice needs to be increasingly recognised and integrated into forensic practice.

Note

1 For more information contact thogue@lincoln.ac.uk

References

Beech, A. R., Wakeling, H. C., Szumski, F., & Freemantle, N. (2016). Problems in the measurement of dynamic risk factors in sexual offenders. *Psychology, Crime & Law*, *22*(1–2), 68–83. 10.1080/1068316X.2015.1109095

Borum, R., Otto, R., & Golding, S. (1993). Improving clinical judgment and decision making in forensic evalution. *The Journal of Psychiatry & Law*, *21*(1), 35–76. 10.1177/009318539302100104

Dernevik, M., Falkheim, M., Holmqvist, R., & Sandell, R. (2001). Implementing risk assessment procedures in a forensic psychiatric setting: Clinical judgement revisited. In Farrington, D. P., Hollin, C. R., & McMurran, M. (Eds.), *Sex and violence: The psychology of crime and risk assessment* (pp. 83–101). London: Routledge.

Dernevik, M., Singh-Dernekik, S., & Grann, M. (2015, March 4). Factors influencing decisions about risk of violence. Faculty of Forensic Psychiatry Annual Conference, Budapest.

Douglas, K. S., Cox, D. N., & Webster, C. D. (1999). Violence risk assessment: Science and practice. *Legal and Criminological Psychology*, *4*(2), 149–184. 10.1348/135532599167824

Dror, I. E. (2016). A hierarchy of expert performance. *Journal of Applied Research in Memory and Cognition*, *5*(2), 121–127. 10.1016/j.jarmac.2016.03.001

Dror, I. E. (2018). Biases in forensic experts. *Science*, *360*(6386), 243–243. 10.1126/science.aat8443

Dror, I. E. (2020). Cognitive and human factors in expert decision making: Six fallacies and the eight sources of bias. *Analytical Chemistry, 92*(12), 7998–8004. 10.1021/acs.analchem. 0c00704

Fazel, S., Singh, J. P., Doll, H., & Grann, M. (2012). Use of risk assessment instruments to predict violence and antisocial behaviour in 73 samples involving 24 827 people: Systematic review and meta-analysis. *BMJ, 345*(July 24), e4692–e4692. 10.1136/bmj.e4692

Grove, W. M. (2005). Clinical versus statistical prediction: The contribution of Paul E. Meehl. *Journal of Clinical Psychology, 61*(10), 1233–1243. 10.1002/jclp.20179

Hanson, R. K., & Morton-Bourgon, K. E. (2009). The accuracy of recidivism risk assessments for sexual offenders: A meta-analysis of 118 prediction studies. *Psychological Assessment, 21*(1), 1–21. 10.1037/a0014421

Hare, R. D. (2003). *The Hare psychopathy checklist—revised* (2nd ed.). Multi-Health Systems: Toronto, Canada.

Harper, C. A., & Hicks, R. (2021). *The effect of attitudes towards individuals with sexual convictions on professional and student risk judgments* [Preprint]. PsyArXiv. 10.31234/osf.io/rjt5h

Harper, C. A., Hogue, T. E., & Bartels, R. M. (2017). Attitudes towards sexual offenders: What do we know, and why are they important? *Aggression and Violent Behavior, 34*, 201–213. 10.1016/j.avb.2017.01.011

Hogue, T. E., & Harper, C. A. (2019). Development of a 21-item short form of the Attitudes to Sexual Offenders (ATS) Scale. *Law and Human Behavior, 43*, 117–130.

Hogue, T. E., & Tan, J. (2016, November 2). The impact of attitudes towards sexual offenders on clinical judgments of risk. Presented at the Association for the Treatment of Sexual Abusers Annual Conference, Orlando, Florida.

Holmqvist, R., & Armelius, B. (1994). Emotional reactions to psychiatric patients: Analysis of a feeling checklist. *Acta Psychiatrica Scandinavica, 90*(3), 204–209.

Kahneman, D., & Tversky, A. (1979). Prospect theory: An analysis of decision under risk. *Econometrica, 47*(2), 263–291. 10.2307/1914185

Meehl, P. E. (1954). *Clinical versus statistical prediction: A theoretical analysis and a review of the evidence.* University of Minnesota Press: Minneapolis MN. 10.1037/11281-000

Meyer, L. F., & Valença, A. M. (2021). Factors related to bias in forensic psychiatric assessments in criminal matters: A systematic review. *International Journal of Law and Psychiatry, 75*, 101681. 10.1016/j.ijlp.2021.101681

Miller, S. L., & Brodsky, S. L. (2011). Risky business: Addressing the consequences of predicting violence. *The Journal of the American Academy of Psychiatry and the Law, 39*(3), 6.

Monahan, J., & Skeem, J. L. (2014). The evolution of violence risk assessment. *CNS Spectrums, 19*(05), 419–424. 10.1017/S1092852914000145

Murrie, D. C., Boccaccini, M. T., Johnson, J. T., & Janke, C. (2008). Does interrater (dis) agreement on Psychopathy Checklist scores in sexually violent predator trials suggest partisan allegiance in forensic evaluations? *Law and Human Behavior, 32*(4), 352–362. 10.1007/s10979-007-9097-5

Murrie, D. C., Boccaccini, M. T., Turner, D. B., Meeks, M., Woods, C., & Tussey, C. (2009). Rater (dis)agreement on risk assessment measures in sexually violent predator proceedings: Evidence of adversarial allegiance in forensic evaluation? *Psychology, Public Policy, and Law, 15*(1), 19–53. 10.1037/a0014897

Neal, T. M. S. (2016). Are forensic experts already biased before adversarial legal parties hire them? *PLoS One, 11*(4), e0154434. 10.1371/journal.pone.0154434

Neal, T. M. S. (2018). Discerning bias in forensic psychological reports in insanity cases. *Behavioral Sciences & the Law, 36*(3), 325–338. 10.1002/bsl.2346

Neal, T. M. S., & Grisso, T. (2014). Assessment practices and expert judgment methods in forensic psychology and psychiatry: An international snapshot. *Criminal Justice and Behavior*, *41*(12), 1406–1421. 10.1177/0093854814548449

Pronin, E., Lin, D. Y., & Ross, L. (2002). The bias blind spot: Perceptions of bias in self versus others. *Personality and Social Psychology Bulletin*, *28*(3), 369–381. 10.1177/01461672 02286008

Shepherd, S. M., & Sullivan, D. (2017). Covert and implicit influences on the interpretation of violence risk instruments. *Psychiatry, Psychology and Law*, *24*(2), 292–301. 10. 1080/13218719.2016.1197817

Sturidsson, K., Haggård-Grann, U., Lotterberg, M., Dernevik, M., & Grann, M. (2004). Clinicians' perceptions of which factors increase or decrease the risk of violence among forensic out-patients. *International Journal of Forensic Mental Health*, *3*(1), 23–36. 10. 1080/14999013.2004.10471194

Tan, J. (2014). *The role of evaluators in forensic risk assessments: Investigating the influence of personal experiences and attitudes.* (Unpublished dissertation). University of Lincoln: Lincoln, UK.

Webster, C.; Simon Fraser University. Mental Health, Law and Policy Institute, & Forensic Psychiatric Services Commission of British Columbia. (1997). *HCR-20: Assessing risk for violence.* Mental Health, Law, and Policy Institute, Simon Fraser University, in cooperation with the British Columbia Forensic Psychiatric Services Commission. http://www.worldcat.org/isbn/0864911572

Zapf, P. A., Kukucka, J., Kassin, S. M., & Dror, I. E. (2018). Cognitive bias in forensic mental health assessment: Evaluator beliefs about its nature and scope. *Psychology, Public Policy, and Law*, *24*(1), 1–10. 10.1037/law0000153

Zappala, M., Reed, A. L., Beltrani, A., Zapf, P. A., & Otto, R. K. (2018). Anything you can do, I can do better: Bias awareness in forensic evaluators. *Journal of Forensic Psychology Research and Practice*, *18*(1), 45–56. 10.1080/24732850.2017.1413532

14 Cultural Bias in Forensic Assessment: Considerations and Suggestions

Andrew Day, Yilma Woldgabreal, and Luke Butcher

Introduction

Assessment is quite rightly considered to be the cornerstone of effective forensic practice. Forensic assessment is best understood as a systematic process of collecting and integrating all relevant information about an individual's presenting needs, in a way that can then inform judgements about appropriate intervention, development, and management strategies. Given that the results of almost every forensic assessment can have a profound impact on a person's life, there is a clear ethical responsibility for the assessing clinician to ensure that all enquiries are meaningful and appropriate and, importantly, that evidence can be produced to support any opinions or recommendations that are put forward. At the same time, the forensic assessment is inherently a subjective task that involves a high level of personal judgement. Different hypotheses about a presenting problem should be considered throughout the assessment process until a coherent understanding emerges. As such there is always potential for bias to occur, whether this be conscious or unconscious.

The aim of this chapter is to explore just some of the ways in which cultural and/or racial bias might impact on the forensic assessment. This is perhaps not something that practising forensic clinicians will always consider; possibly because they have been trained to approach assessment in ways that have come to be accepted as conventions in their respective professions, even when these have not adequately considered issues of bias. And yet, a legal claim brought by Mr Jeffrey Ewert against multiple representatives of Correctional Services Canada has drawn worldwide attention to the problem of cultural bias in forensic assessments. Mr Ewert is a Canadian Aboriginal man who was, at the time, serving two life sentences for second-degree murder and attempted murder. He repeatedly waived his right to apply for parole on the grounds that he believed that he was unlikely to be successful in light of forensic assessments which concluded he remained at "high risk" of reoffending. In *Ewert v Canada* [2015], Mr Ewert successfully argued that the assessment tools that were used to assess his level of risk lacked validity for use with persons of Aboriginal descent and were thus inappropriate. His case, and the discussion that followed (see Haag et al., 2016; Hart, 2016), highlighted just how important it is for assessors to consider the

DOI: 10.4324/9781003230977-16

influence of cultural factors and, specifically, ways in which the identity of the service user[1] and the cultural context in which the assessment occurs influence both the quality and admissibility of the findings. The tools in question (the Hare Psychopathy Checklist – Revised [PCL–R see Hart et al., 1992]; the Violence Risk Appraisal Guide [VRAG] and the Sex Offender Risk Appraisal Guide [SORAG, see Rice et al., 2013]; the Static 99 see Hanson & Thornton, 2000; and the Violence Risk Scale–Sex Offender version [VRS–SO, see Olver et al., 2007]) are all well known to forensic professionals and are widely used to assess the risk of both interpersonal and sexual violence.

Since the judgement was handed down in the *Ewert v Canada* case, the Black Lives Matter movement has drawn further attention to the much broader issue of the representation of people of colour in criminal justice systems across the Western world. Woldgabreal et al. (2020), for example, have reported statistics showing that in the United States, African Americans make up nearly 40% of the incarcerated population but only around 13% of the general population (United States Census Bureau, 2015), and that in England and Wales, black, Asian, and minority ethnic men and women make up just 14% of the population, but 25% of the adult prisoner population – and over 40% of young people in custody (Ministry of Justice, 2016). The statistics relating to the over-representation of Indigenous or First Nations peoples are even more confronting (see Australian Bureau of Statistics, 2018; Government of Canada, Office of the Correctional Investigator, 2017; New Zealand Department of Corrections, 2018), prompting ongoing discussion about the systemic nature of racism and discrimination across all levels of the criminal justice system (e.g., Koziol, 2018). Given that the over-representation of people of colour in Western countries appears to be increasing rather than decreasing (e.g., an independent review of the treatment of people of colour in the England and Wales criminal justice system by Lammy, 2017, found that the proportion of young adult people of colour in prison rose from 11% in 2006 to 19% in 2016, and during the same time period the proportion of juveniles of colour rose from 25% to 41%), there is growing pressure on *everyone* who works in the criminal justice system to critically reflect on the role that their work plays in maintaining this status quo and in perpetuating discrimination. Given our assertion that assessment is the cornerstone of effective forensic practice, it seems reasonable then to ask how cultural and racial bias might present in the forensic assessment.

Bias in Racial Difference

Before considering some specific sources of racial bias that can arise during the assessment process, it is important to first draw attention to some of the more general drivers of discriminatory practice. Social psychology reminds us that our racial identity and the mere existence of group categories create prejudice, and that this is reflected in a tendency to favour and prefer those who are like us (ingroup members) over those who are dissimilar (outgroup members) (Amodio & Cikara, 2021; Chekroud et al., 2014); a phenomenon that has been linked to implicit bias and discriminatory behaviour (Krosch & Amodio, 2019). In this regard, numerous studies that seek to answer questions about racial prejudice using the tools of cognitive neuroscience and psychophysiology have now been published (e.g., Brown et al., 2006; Cikara et al., 2011; Cikara et al., 2017; Han, 2018; Mattan et al., 2018; Vanman et al., 2013; Van Bavel et al., 2008). The results cumulatively show that race serves as a powerful interpretive lens, often implicitly or unconsciously, and that we are all more likely to favour ingroup members and less likely to empathise with those from outgroups. Racial bias arising from this type of social categorisation may, on the surface, seem benign, but can impede our ability to embrace and understand outgroup members objectively. In other words, this means that race essentially influences how we all interpret and experience the environment on an everyday basis, and that "our beliefs and attitudes can become so strongly associated with the category that they are automatically triggered, affecting our behavior and decision making" (Eberhardt, 2020, p. 32). So, when conducting a forensic assessment, a clinician from a dominant culture who is working with a person of colour might automatically base their opinion on a range of assumptions which may or may not be true but easily result in misinterpretations of significant risk (e.g., the presence of socio-economic disadvantages, such as unemployment, lower level of educational achievement and impoverished neighbourhoods). In the United Kingdom, for example, young African and Caribbean men are known to be more likely to have police involvement in their admission to psychiatric services, more likely to be admitted to secure or forensic services, and are more likely to be given higher or longer acting doses of psychotropic drugs. It is easy to see how implicit racial bias can contribute to these treatment pathways and outcomes, potentially demonstrating a western stereotype of black psychiatric patients as both volatile and dangerous (see Johnstone & Boyle, 2018). By contrast, when assessing someone who is similar to us, it is more likely that the person will be appraised positively at an unconscious level. Indeed, this tendency has been observed in a recent study by the current authors that compared post-intervention violence risk assessment scores between Aboriginal and Caucasian prisoners in an Australian jurisdiction (Woldgabreal et al., in press). The results showed that Aboriginal people in prison were scored as at higher risk and assessed as having fewer protective factors than Caucasians. It seems that two different types of biases are at play here – a bias that can arise from socio-economic inequalities and reduce protective factors, and a bias that can occur as a result of practitioners' inability to see such disadvantages.

It is also, of course, worth remembering that racial bias can be conscious. It may even arise as a form of resistance to difficult confrontations with racial inequality. A good example of this is the "All Lives Matter" movement that has emerged in response to the "Black Lives Matter" protests (Gallegos, 2018). This type of active resistance has been referred to as "white fragility"; a "state in which even a minimum amount of racial stress becomes intolerable, triggering a range of defensive moves" (DiAngelo, 2011, p. 54). The same narrative can exist in forensic assessments, with proponents of established approaches often advocating strongly to protect the status quo. In our view this may partly explain why contemporary forensic assessments have largely remained anglophonic in their orientation and development and have largely neglected the specific historical contexts, disadvantages, and concerns of people of colour. The inference here is that forensic mental health and correctional practitioners who conduct assessments based on such a hegemonistic perspective will be susceptible to operating from the assumption that these tools can be applied to all populations, preserving the myths of culture neutrality, colour blindness, and closed-mindedness.

Different Types of Assessment

We now turn to considering how bias might present in different approaches to the actual assessment. It is possible to describe at least four different approaches to forensic assessment, as follows: (1) unstructured professional judgement – an approach where clinicians use their professional judgement and experience to make a determination; (2) actuarial assessment – where specific, empirically derived factors are used to provide cut-off scores that inform predictions about future behaviour; (3) structured professional judgement where a clinician applies their knowledge of the literature to inform the assessment; and (4) anamnestic assessment which is a highly individual-specific approach that seeks to contextualise the presenting problem (e.g., Whittington et al., 2013). In practice, of course, any decision about which assessment approach is most appropriate should be largely determined by the goals of the assessment rather than the personal preferences of the clinician. Hunsley and Mash (2008) have identified a number of quite distinctive purposes for assessment in mental health settings, which Day (2019) has argued also translate into the forensic setting. The forensic clinician might be asked, for example, to assess whether a person is currently at risk of harm to self or others (diagnosis and screening), whether they present a significant future risk to others (prognosis), how any risk might best be mitigated (case conceptualisation and treatment planning), or whether attending treatment has proven effective (monitoring and evaluation). Whilst different approaches will clearly be required to answer these different questions (notwithstanding some attempts to streamline the process through, for example, the emergence of "risk-needs" assessment tools), in practice the forensic assessment will nearly always rely heavily on the use of a clinical interview (or series of interviews), often supplemented with some type of more structured assessment or psychometric testing and, wherever possible, the gathering of collateral information. There are opportunities for racial bias to enter the assessment process when using each of these approaches, either through the inappropriate application of assessment tools (as was the case in *Ewert v Canada*), or by ignoring relevant cultural factors in the interview (see Allnutt et al., 2010).

Bias in the Interview

As the clinical interview will often serve as the main source of information, it is important to be aware of all potential sources of bias, as well as those that relate specifically to culture or race. Day et al. (2019) have, for example, recently discussed how some forensic service users are seen as having little insight into the causes of their behaviour, whilst others are seen as having only a limited capacity to accurately self-report, perhaps due to attention and concentration issues or to memory problems. Others may, of course, actively seek to create a certain impression – and there is certainly a view that many forensic service users will have a tendency to minimise responsibility for any behaviour linked to offending (e.g., Tan & Grace, 2008). Nesca and Dalby (2013) state this very clearly when they recommend that "all forensic interviews must begin with the assumption that the interviewee is motivated to lie or distort information and, as a result, cannot be completely trusted" (p. 40). Professional discussions of these sources of bias in the forensic assessment are of particular interest because they almost exclusively describe the source of assessment bias as being in the person being assessed, rather than in the person conducting the assessment or in the methods that are employed. In other words, the clinician is exempt from acting in any way other than being objective and fair.

This is not to suggest, of course, that impression management should not be a consideration in every assessment interview, but rather that cultural factors may also have an impact on how a person presents in an interview. Perhaps the most obvious example here arises when an interview is conducted with someone for whom English is a second (or perhaps third) language, when an apparent inability to self-report may simply reflect difficulties in understanding what is being asked rather than any defensiveness or deliberate intent to mislead. Translating feelings and forms of expression from one language can also be challenging and, at times, impossible, particularly if there is no similar word in the assessor's language (see Lomas, 2020). For example, the experience of shame or anger is known to be quite different for those from collectivist cultural groups (see Bolger et al., 2013). Adherence to cultural norms may also influence the way people present themselves in an assessment, particularly in relation to being interviewed about offending behaviour. Family and domestic violence, for example, has different meanings and functions in some cultures than in Western cultures; it may, for example, be normalised or accepted in different ways which will influence the ways in which a person talks about (personal) responsibility (World Health Organization, 2009).

A much broader set of issues may also arise in relation to the level of trust that exists between those who are conducting an assessment on behalf of the state and those from a minority culture who may have had negative experiences of government agencies, either in their current country or in their country of origin. Take, for example, those who have been granted asylum following political persecution and the expectation that is often placed on them to participate openly and honestly in a forensic assessment that is conducted in their new country. Even though Greenberg and Shuman (2007) rightly argue that the forensic assessment should essentially be evaluative and that the stance taken by the assessor should be objective and dispassionate (rather than collaborative and helpful), in practice there is also a need to work in a manner that promotes the development of trust, even when this may take time to build. Simply asking about previous experiences of being interviewed and criminal justice/mental health system involvement is likely to be helpful in this regard, especially when the assessor is open to the possibility that responses to these questions will be relevant to their understanding of other information gathered over the course of the assessment. This also requires, at some level, the assessor to trust the person who is being assessed as a legitimate source of knowledge. Crewe (2020) has described this in terms of how easy it is to unfairly discriminate against those in the criminal justice system in their capacity as "knowers", based on pre-existing prejudices. This is sometimes referred to as epistemic injustice and can be profoundly disempowering for forensic service users. A cultural example of this from our own practice in Australia is when we consider the spirituality that underpins behaviour in some Aboriginal cultures – when the term "black magic" is used to explain why certain behaviours (such as child sexual offending) have occurred. An obvious risk here is that, rather than seeking to understand the cultural significance and relevance of this attribution for the offending behaviour, the dominant culture assessor will simply dismiss the idea of "black magic" as an attempt to deflect personal responsibility or as knowledge that in some way lacks credibility or legitimacy. In fact, dismissing or reattributing meaning in this instance becomes an attractive option for the assessor who will nearly always not have access to the cultural knowledge that is required to understand its spiritual meaning (some topics are taboo and cannot be discussed between certain family members or with those of different genders, let alone with those from outside cultures). Other examples described in the literature by Barber Rioja and Rosenfeld (2018) include culturally unique experiences, such as "sinking heart" described by Punjabi Sikh's (Krause, 1989), or the phenomenon of "wind" among Cambodian trauma survivors (Hinton & Otto, 2006).

Bias in Psychometric Assessment

Perhaps the most identified examples of bias occur when psychometric assessment tools (including risk assessment tools as in the *Ewert* case) are used that have been developed for use with a dominant cultural group but then applied to those from different cultures without sufficient validation. This is what Van de Vijver and Tanzer (2004) have referred to as construct bias; when assessments are informed by majority experiences and values that are likely to be inappropriate and unfamiliar to minority groups. In this regard, one only needs to be reminded of the controversies that have arisen in relation to the intelligence testing of those from minority groups and the different ways in which group-level comparisons have been used to support racist ideologies in psychological research and practice (see Ford, 2004). Bias of this type can, however, occur in more subtle ways. There is, for example, a view in disciplines such as psychology that practitioners should always opt for assessment instruments that are psychometrically strong; that, in addition to evidence of reliability and validity, measures should also have appropriate data for norm-referenced interpretation and/or supporting evidence regarding their accuracy (i.e., sensitivity, specificity, predictive power in risk assessment; Hunsley & Mash, 2008). This extends to individual characteristics, where it is accepted that psychometric tests should be sensitive to race, ethnicity, as well as to specific cultural factors, although this type of information is simply not available. Even the most established and best validated forensic assessment tools have limited norms for minority cultural groups, and even the idea of a norm can serve to homogenise and stereotype in a way that overlooks the diversity that exists within most cultural groups. The result is that the practitioner is often left trying to apply group data that has been collected from dominant culture populations.

Vincent and Viljoen (2018) have argued that an instrument is not necessarily racially biased if one group (e.g., people of colour) score higher, on average, than another group (e.g., Caucasian people), pointing to the ethical standards that now apply regarding the validation of our instruments which state that test bias is only present when scores *function differently* for different groups of people. In this way it is argued that the bias is not in the test, but in the way in which any results are interpreted or applied. Thus, their argument is that the real concern is when significant mean score or error rate differences on instruments by race result in harsher system-related responses (see Skeem & Lowenkamp, 2016). In other words, the problem is mainly one of interpretation, rather than of bias inherent in any assessment tool. This does, however, appear to minimise the realities of people of colour in the Western world as statistically generated true means (latent means) difference assumes equality or a "level playing field" across population groups when it is clear that this is far from the reality. For example, people of colour do typically experience significant socio-economic disadvantage (e.g., unemployment and lower levels of education) and differential treatment by criminal justice systems (e.g., higher rates of unlawful stops, searches, arrest, and charges by police; see Delsol & Shiner, 2015).

Discussion

Our aim in writing this chapter was to explore just some of the ways in which cultural or racial bias might impact on the forensic assessment. It is also important, however, to offer some suggestions for advancing practice in this area. One possibility here – and one that has proven helpful in our own practice – is to understand and engage with the idea of the cultural interface. This is a term that is used to refer to the space between people of colour and Western practitioners, where knowledge is shared and common ground and innovation are established (e.g., Maakrun & Maher, 2016; Nakata, 2007). Working at the cultural interface requires clinicians to deploy critical reflexivity to explore the culturally bound nature of their approaches and protocols, and how these contribute to bias. This inevitably requires explicit consideration of how inherent power relations are enacted between the clinician and service user (at structural, systemic, relational, and clinical levels), an appreciation and exploration of the historical, social, and political contexts of persons of colour, of intergenerational trauma or cultural dislocation, and developing an understanding of the inter-sectional nature of justice involvement for minority cultural groups and for people of colour. The deployment of critical reflexivity of this type can help the clinician to better understand why they are asking for certain information and the purpose it will be used (Morley, 2015). Accordingly, we suggest that reflex-ivity – at both the personal and disciplinary levels – is critical to minimising bias and that the first step is to recognise how often these important cultural con-siderations are ignored, disregarded, or simply not asked about in current as-sessment protocols. Of course, this brings with it a level of uncertainty to professional practice, requiring the clinician to question both personal claims of knowledge (i.e., expertise), and the processes through which their knowledge has been created.

On a more practical level, guidance is available about how to actually ask questions about culture. Aggarwal et al. (2020), for example, have described the development of the Cultural Formulation Interview (American Psychiatric Association Press, 2013), along with implementation instructions and standar-dised questions around common topics. This was developed as part of the DSM-IV revision for the DSM-5 by the Cross-Cultural Issues Subgroup for use in mental health settings. Shepherd (2021) has also recently identified a series of simple questions that are likely to be useful in building trust and eliciting cultural information. These include questions such as "how would your community view your problem?", "are people with your problems normally helped or punished in your community?", "do you think your friends and family would be upset if you spoke to forensic professionals about your problems?", and so on. Shepherd also offers helpful examples of how to ask about cultural background (e.g., "have you or your parents ever lived in a different country?") and acculturation experiences (e.g., "how close do you feel towards your community?"). Asking questions of this type can be particularly helpful in understanding more about the culture of the person being assessed and, in this way, reduce any tendency for stereotypes to be imposed on the person's experience. It may be important nonetheless to draw on the expertise of those with cultural knowledge to ensure that any interpretation of this information is correct (see next).

A bigger challenge perhaps lies at the disciplinary level. This relates to the suggestion that the outcomes of many forensic assessments simply reflect the historical, socio-economic, and political disadvantages experienced by people of colour in the Western societies, lending themselves to the differential treatment of people of colour across both the forensic mental health and criminal justice systems (e.g., Gillies, 2013; Klingele, 2020). The argument that many assessment instruments neglect the specific historical contexts, disadvantages, and concerns of people of colour in the Western nations is a powerful one, as are charges that our assessment tools are based on a hegemonistic perspective that operates from the assumption that they can be applied to all populations. Our suggestion here is to encourage clinicians to be both cautious and careful in their interpretation of evidence that is derived from more formal structured assessment tools and to take care when judging whether the assumption of true mean difference in assessment scores between the majority and minority is conceptually plausible or whether it simply continues to undermine and perpetuate the disadvantages experienced by people of colour. There is a real problem here with assessing people as if they are independent from their social and cultural context, and it is here that preparing carefully for the assessment and involving cultural knowledge holders, both service users and cultural consultants, is likely to be key.

Background Research on Culture

It is perhaps a truism to state that having more knowledge about a person's cultural background will increase the accuracy of any evaluation, but we hope that this chapter provides some rationale for why this is important. As Barber Rioja and Rosenfeld (2018) have argued, "culturally responsive assessment practices ... require familiarity with the culture of the evaluatee" (p. 2). However, given that there is relatively little published guidance about how best to gather information about someone's cultural history an obvious solution is to simply ask the person being assessed and other relevant stakeholders (e.g., family member, community leaders and representatives).

Service User Involvement and Cultural Consultants

The benefits of service user involvement in health, mental health, disability, and human services are now well established. For example, this has been shown to improve quality of life, empowerment, sense of control, community belonging, self-efficacy, and social integration (e.g., Miler et al., 2020; Rosenberg & Argentzell, 2018). At its core, service user involvement is a mechanism to break down traditional barriers, assumptions, and exclusionary practices, and thus, to bring about an emancipation from dominant service paradigms at a "personal and policy level" (Beresford & McLaughlin, 2021, p. 2). At a clinical level, bringing a service user orientation to the assessment allows each person to play a more active role in the decisions about them (Beresford & Branfield, 2006; Lammers & Happell, 2003). This is sometimes referred to as "co-production", whereby clinicians and service users make better use of each other's knowledge, assets, and resources by focusing more on outcomes than service delivery outputs (Weaver et al., 2019).

This approach requires clinicians to move away from a "cultural competence"–based approach to a "lack of competence"–based approach (Gray & Hetherington, 2007) that directly challenges the notion that someone can be competent in another's culture. In short, it requires the assessor to adopt a novice position in their efforts to understand an individual's cultural identity and context, and it is through this process that they can come to appreciate the personal, interpersonal, and larger social context in which any problematic behaviour occurs (Lewis-Fernandez & Kirmayer, 2020). In an important sense, this will simply mean spending more time listening to service-users and other holders of cultural knowledge and understanding the ways in which their culture is relevant to their experience.

Despite significant progress being made in other areas, service user involvement in justice services remains underdeveloped (Barr & Montgomery, 2016; Weaver et al., 2019) and there are tensions and contradictions that arise when providing opportunities for involvement by service users of the criminal justice system. There are, however, examples of service user involvement in the forensic assessment (e.g., self-risk prediction), with some studies showing that this enhances engagement and results in greater accuracy (Hall & Duperouzel, 2011; Kroner, 2012; Kroner et al., 2020). More broadly, there are also many examples of where clinicians, policy makers, and administrators have involved service users and community groups in co-producing policy and intervention programmes to provide stronger outcomes for service users, victims, and their communities (see Butcher et al., 2020).

Conclusion

It is clearly the responsibility of the forensic professional to establish how the different types of information that are collected over the course of an assessment should inform the opinion. And it is here that a degree of reflexivity is required to be deployed to identify and avoid cultural bias. A simple conclusion from this chapter is that we should be very careful about overattributing meanings to assessment data that lack cross-cultural validity. By carefully preparing for an assessment and engaging and listening to the advice of service users, the clinician will be better placed to complete assessments that have greater validity and, ultimately, are more useful.

The main conclusion from this chapter is that cultural and racial bias – conditioned through our experience, values, and beliefs – can negatively influence the processes and outcomes of every forensic assessment. It operates at an unconscious level and forensic clinicians are not exempt! As such there is a need to be very careful about overattributing meanings to assessment data that lack cross-cultural validity and, by carefully preparing for an assessment and engaging and listening to the advice of service users, the clinician will be better placed to complete assessments that have greater validity and, ultimately, are more useful. The good news is that the same research that has uncovered the neurological pathways of racial bias also offers solutions, with studies showing that completing tasks as simple as connecting with racially diverse groups and gaining awareness of racial issues and discrimination can make those in a privileged position in society more open-minded, reflective, and act more fairly (Eberhardt, 2020). Done well, training can increase practitioners' competence. We may not ever eliminate racial bias in forensic assessments, but we can educate ourselves and others to buffer some of the detrimental effects of racial bias on people of colour.

Note

1 The term "service user" has been chosen to describe people who are in contact with justice services.

References

Aggarwal, N. K., Lam, P., Diaz, S., Cruz, A. G., & Lewis-Fernandez, R. (2020). Clinician perceptions of implementing the cultural formulation interview on a mixed forensic unit. *Journal of the American Academy of Psychiatry and Law*, *48*(2), 216–225. 10.29158/JAAPL.003914-20

Allnutt, S., O'Driscoll, C., Ogloff, J., Daffern, M., & Adams, J. (2010). *Clinical risk assessment & management: A practical manual for mental health clinicians.* Sydney, NSW: Justice Health.

American Psychiatric Association. (2013). *Diagnostic and statistical manual of mental disorders* (5th ed.). Arlington, VA: American Psychiatric Publishing.

Amodio, D. M., & Cikara, M. (2021). The social neuroscience of prejudice. *Annual Review of Psychology*, *72*, 439–469. 10.1146/annurev-psych-010419-050928

Australian Bureau of Statistics. (2018). *Aboriginal & torres strait islander prisoner characteristics.* Retrieved from https://www.abs.gov.au/AUSSTATS/abs@.nsf/DetailsPage/4517.02018?OpenDocument

Barber Rioja, V., & Rosenfeld, B. (2018). Addressing linguistic and cultural differences in the forensic interview. *International Journal of Forensic Mental Health*, *17*, 377–386. 10.1080/14999013.2018.1495280

Barr, N., & Montgomery, G. (2016). Service user involvement in service planning in the criminal justice system: Rhetoric or reality? *Irish Probation Journal*, *13*, 143–155.

Beresford, P., & Branfield, F. (2006). Developing inclusive partnerships: User-defined outcomes, networking and knowledge – a case study. *Health and Social Care in the Community*, *14*(5). 436–444. 10.1111/j.1365-2524.2006.00654.x

Beresford. P., & McLaughlin, H. (2021). Introduction. In H. McLaughlin, P. Beresford, C. Cameron, H. Casey, & J. Duffy (Eds.). *The Routledge handbook of service user involvement in human services research and education* (pp. 1–5). Abingdon: Routledge.

Bolger, M., De Deyne, S., & Mesquita, B. (2013). Emotions in "the world": Cultural practices, products, and meanings of anger and shame in two individualist cultures. *Frontiers in Psychology*, *4*(867), 1–14. 10.3389/fpsyg.2013.00867

Brown, L. M., Bradley, M. M., & Lang, P. J. (2006). Affective reactions to pictures of ingroup and outgroup members. *Biological Psychology*, *71*, 303–311. 10.1016/j.biopsycho.2005.06.003

Butcher, L., Day, A., Miles, D., Kidd, G., & Stanton, S. (2020). Community engagement in Youth Justice program design. *Australian New Zealand Journal of Criminology*, *53*, 369–386. 10.1177/0004865820933332

Chekroud, A. M., Everett, J. A., Bridge, H., & Hewstone, M. (2014). A review of neuroimaging studies of race-related prejudice: Does amygdala response reflect threat? *Frontiers in Human Neuroscience*, *8*(179), 1–11. 10.3389/fnhum.2014.00179

Cikara, M., Botvinick, M. M., & Fiske, S. T. (2011). Us versus them: Social identity shapes neural responses to intergroup competition and harm. *Psychological Science*, *22*, 306–313. 10.1177/0956797610397667

Cikara, M., Van Bavel, J. J., Ingbretsen, Z. A., & Lau, T. (2017). Decoding "us" and "them": Neural representations of generalized group concepts. *Journal of Experimental Psychology General*, *146*(5), 621–631. 10.1037/xge0000287

Crewe, B. (2020). *Innovative models of offender management and intervention: Creating a rehabilitative culture.* ICPA Online Learning Academy, 2nd November.

Day, A. (2019). Psychological assessment in the correctional setting. In Polaschek, D. L. L., Day, A., & Hollin, C. R. (Eds.). *The international handbook of correctional psychology* (pp. 488–498). Chichester: Wiley.

Day, A., Daffern, M., Dunne, A., Papalia, N., & Thomson, K. (2019). Interviewing forensic mental health patients who have a history of aggression: Considerations and suggestions. *International Journal of Forensic Mental Health, 18*, 12–20. 10.1080/14999013. 2018.1504353

Delsol, R., & Shiner, M. (Eds.). (2015). *Stop and search: The anatomy of a police power.* London: Palgrave Macmillan.

DiAngelo, R. (2011). "White fragility". *International Journal of Critical Pedagogy, 3*(3), 54–70.

Eberhardt, J. (2020). *Biased: The new science of race and inequality.* London: William Heinemann.

Ewert v. Canada. (2015). FC 1093 (CanLII). Ottawa: The Canadian Legal Information Institute. Retrieved from http://can lii.ca/t/gl9d9

Ford, D. Y. (2004). *Intelligence testing and cultural diversity: Concerns, cautions, and considerations.* The National Research Center on the Gifted and Talented (NRC/GT). University of Connecticut.

Gallegos, L. (2018). Unconscious racial prejudice as psychological resistance: A limitation of the implicit bias model. *Critical Philosophy of Race, 6*(2), 262–279.

Gillies, C. (2013). Establishing the United Nations' declaration on the rights of Indigenous peoples as the minimum standard for all forensic practice with Australian Indigenous peoples. *Australian Psychologist, 48*(1), 14–27. 10.1111/ap.12003

Government of Canada, Office of the Correctional Investigator. (2017). *Annual report 2016–2017.* Retrieved from https://www.oci-bec.gc.ca/cnt/rpt/annrpt/annrpt20162017-eng.aspx

Gray, M., & Hetherington, T. (2007). Hearing indigenous voices in mainstream social work. *Families in Society: The Journal of Contemporary Social Services, 88*(1), 55–66. 10.1606/1 044-3894.3592

Greenberg, S. A., & Shuman, D. W. (2007). When worlds collide: Therapeutic and forensic roles. *Professional Psychology: Research and Practice, 38*(2), 129–132. 10.1037/0735-7028.38.2.129.

Haag, A., Boyes, A., Cheng, J., McNeil, A., & Wirove, R. (2016). An introduction to the issues of cross-cultural assessment inspired by Ewert v. Canada. *Journal of Threat Assessment and Management, 3*, 65–75. 10.1037/tam0000067

Hall, S., & Duperouzel, H. (2011). "We know about our risks, so we should be asked." A tool to support service user involvement in the risk assessment process in forensic services for people with intellectual disabilities. *Journal of Learning Disabilities and Offending Behaviour, 2*(3), 122–126. 10.1108/20420921111186598

Han, S. (2018). Neurocognitive basis of racial ingroup bias in empathy. *Trends in Cognitive Sciences, 22*(5), 400–421. 10.1016/j.tics.2018.02.013

Hanson, R. K., & Thornton, D. (2000). Improving risk assessments for sex offenders: A comparison of three actuarial scales. *Law and Human Behavior, 24*(1), 119–136. 10.1023/A:1005482921333

Hart, S. D. (2016). Culture and violence risk assessment: The case of Ewert v Canada. *Journal of Threat Assessment and Management, 3*(2), 76–96. 10.1037/tam0000068

Hart, S. D., Hare, R. D., & Harpur, T. J. (1992). The Psychopathy Checklist—Revised (PCL–R): An overview for researchers and clinicians. In J. C. Rosen & P. McReynolds (Eds.). *Advances in psychological assessment* (Vol. 8, pp. 103–130). New York: Plenum Press. 10.1007/978-1-4757-9101-3_4

Hinton, D., & Otto, M. W. (2006). Symptom presentation and symptom meaning among traumatized Cambodian refugees: Relevance to somatically focused cognitive-behavioral therapy. *Cognitive Behavioral Practice, 13*(4), 249–260. 10.1016/j.cbpra.2006.04.006

Hunsley, J., & Mash, E. J. (Eds.). (2008). *A guide to assessments that work.* Oxford: Oxford University Press.

Johnstone, L. & Boyle, M. (2018). *The power threat meaning framework: Towards the identification of patterns in emotional distress, unusual experiences and troubled or troubling behaviour, as an alternative to functional psychiatric diagnosis.* Leicester: British Psychological Society.

Klingele, C. (2020). Making sense of risk. *Behavioral Sciences & the Law, 38*(3), 218–225. 10.1 002/bsl.2458

Koziol, M. (2018). 'Systemic racism' fueling skyrocketing rates of Indigenous imprisonment, says peak law body. *Sydney Morning Herald.* Retrieved from https://www.smh. com.au/politics/federal/systemic-racism-fueling-skyrocketing-rates-of-indigenous-imprisonment-says-peak-law-body-20180314-p4z4aj.html

Krause, I. B. (1989). Sinking heart: A Punjabi communication of distress. *Social Science & Medicine, 29*(4), 563–575. 10.1016/0277-9536(89)90202-5.

Kroner, D. (2012). Service user involvement in risk assessment and management: The transition inventory. *Criminal Behaviour and Mental Health, 22,* 136–147. 10.1002/cbm. 1825;

Kroner, D., Morgan, R., Mills, J., & Maeda, K. (2020). Risk assessment tool floundering? Let's ask the client to self-predict. *International Journal of Law and Psychiatry, 16,* Epub. 10.1016/j.ijlp.2020

Krosch, A. R., & Amodio, D. M. (2019). Scarcity disrupts the neural encoding of Black faces: A socio-perceptual pathway to discrimination. *Journal of Personality and Social Psychology, 117*(5), 859–875. 10.1037/pspa0000168

Lammers, J., & Happell, B. (2003). Consumer participation in mental health services: Looking from a consumer perspective. *Journal of Psychiatric and Mental Health Nursing, 10*(4), 385–392. 10.1046/j.1365-2850.2003.00598.x

Lammy, D. (2017). *An independent review into the treatment of, and outcomes for black, Asian and minority ethnic individuals in the criminal justice system.* Retrieved from https://www.gov.uk/ government/publications/lammy-review-final-report

Lewis-Fernandez, R., & Kirmayer, L. (2020). The cultural formulation interview: Progress to date and future directions. *Transcultural Psychiatry, 57*(4), 487–496. 10.1177/13634 61520938273

Lomas, T. (2020). Towards a cross cultural map of lexical map of wellbeing. *The Journal of Positive Psychology.* 10.1080/17439760.2020.1791944

Maakrun, J., & Maher, M. (2016). Cultural interface theory in the Kenya context and beyond. *Issues in Educational Research and Beyond, 26*(2), 298–314.

Mattan, B. D., Wei, K. Y., Cloutier, J., & Kubota, J. T. (2018). The social neuroscience of race-based and status-based prejudice. *Current Opinion in Psychology, 24,* 27–34. 10.1016/ j.copsyc.2018.04.010

Miler, J., Carver, H., Foster, R., & Parkes, T. (2020). Provision of peer support at the intersection of homelessness and problem substance use services: A systematic 'state of the art' review. *BMC Public Health, 20*(641). 10.1186/s12889-020-8407-4

Ministry of Justice. (2016). *Black, Asian and minority ethnic disproportionality in the criminal justice system in England and Wales.* Retrieved from https://www.gov.uk/crime-justice-and-law

Morley, C. (2015). Critical reflexivity and social work practice. In J. D. Wright (Ed.). *International encyclopedia of the social and behavioral sciences* (2nd ed., pp. 281–286). London: Elsevier Health Services.

Nakata, M. (2007). The cultural interface. *The Australian Journal of Indigenous Education, 36S,* 7–14.

Nesca, M., & Dalby, J. T. (2013). *Forensic interviewing in criminal court matters.* Springfield, IL: C.C. Thomas Publishers.

New Zealand Department of Corrections. (2018). *Prison statistics.* Retrieved from https:// www.corrections.govt.nz/resources/research_and_statistics/quarterly_prison_statistic

Olver, M. E., Wong, S. C. P., Nicholaichuk, T., & Gordon, A. (2007). The validity and reliability of the violence risk scale-sexual offender version: Assessing sex offender risk and evaluating therapeutic change. *Psychological Assessment, 19*, 318–329. 10.1037/1040-3590.19.3.318

Rice, M. E., Harris, G. T., & Lang, C. (2013). Validation of and revision to the VRAG and SORAG: the Violence Risk Appraisal Guide-Revised (VRAG-R). *Psychological Assessment, 25*, 951–965. 10.1037/a0032878.

Rosenberg, D., & Argentzell, E. (2018). Service users experience in peer support in Swedish mental health care: A "tipping point" in the care giving culture? *Journal of Psychosocial Rehabilitation and Mental Health, 5*, 53–61. 10.1007/s40737-018-0109-1

Shepherd, S. (2021). *Working with justice-involved culturally and linguistically diverse populations.* APS College of Forensic Psychologists Professional Development Webinar.

Skeem, J. L., & Lowenkamp, C. T. (2016). Risk, race, and recidivism: Predictive bias and disparate impact. *Criminology, 54*(4), 680–712. 10.1111/1745-9125.12123

Tan, L., & Grace, R. (2008). Social desirability and sexual offenders: A review. *Sexual Abuse: A Journal of Research and Treatment, 20*(1), 61–87. 10.1177/1079063208314820

United States Census Bureau. (2015). *State & County QuickFacts.* Washington, DC. Retrieved from http://www.census.gov/quickfacts/map/PST045215/12

Van Bavel, J. J., Packer, D. J., & Cunningham, W. A. (2008). The neural substrates of in-group bias: A functional magnetic resonance imaging investigation. *Psychological Science, 19*, 1131–1139.

Van de Vijver, F., & Tanzer, N. K. (2004). Bias and equivalence in cross-cultural as-sessment: An overview. European Review of Applied Psychology/Revue *Européenne de Psychologie Appliquée, 54*(2), 119–135. 10.1016/j.erap.2003.12.004

Vanman, E. J., Ryan, J. P., Wiliam P., & Ito, T. A. (2013). Probing prejudice with startle eyeblink modification: A marker of attention, emotion, or both? *International Journal of Psychological Research, 6*(Special Issue), 30–41. 10.21500/20112084.717

Vincent, G. M., & Viljoen, J. L. (2018). Racist algorithms or systemic problems? Risk assessments and racial disparities. *Criminal Justice and Behavior, 47*, 1576–1584. o1gdr/.o/i/p:stht0.1177/0093854820954501

Weaver, B., Lightowler, C., & Moodie, K. (2019). *Inclusive justice: Coproducing change.* Children and Young People's Centre for Justice. Retrieved from https://www.cycj.org.uk/resource/inclusive-justice-co-producing-change/

Whittington, R., Hockenhull, J. C., McGuire, J., et al. (2013). A systematic review of risk assessment strategies for populations at high risk of engaging in violent behaviour: Update 2002–8. Retrieved from https://www.ncbi.nlm.nih.gov/books/NBK261197/

Woldgabreal, Y., Day, A., Daffern, M., Lloyd, C., & Graffam, J. (in press). An empirical test of the factor structure of the violence risk scale and its measurement invariance across time and cultural groups. *Criminal Justice and Behavior.* Published online April 2022 https://doi.org/10.1177/00938548221084984

Woldgabreal, Y., Day, A., & Tamatea, A. (2020). Do risk assessments play a role in the enduring 'color line'? *Journal of the International Corrections and Prisons Association, 10*, 18–28.

World Health Organization. (2009). *Violence prevention: The evidence.* Geneva: WHO.

15 Personal Construct Psychology and Repertory Grids: Acknowledging and Exploring Perspectives

Nicholas Blagden and Adrian Needs

Introduction

The central tenet of personal construct psychology (PCP) is that people's processes are psychologically channelised by the ways in which they anticipate events. Anticipations direct and mobilise the person, enabling more or less appropriate action and comprehension based on a structured and usually evolving network of pathways. They are, in effect, hypotheses about the world that are put to the test of experience and operate in systems. The epistemological position with which founder George Kelly (1955) introduced PCP is "constructive alternativism", which asserts that people make sense of (or "construe") reality in different ways. There will be commonality amongst people's construing as well as individuality. The emphasis in constructive alternativism, however, is that we can always construe things differently (Walker & Winter, 2007). As Kelly argued in the second volume of his magnum opus: "there is nothing in the world which is not subject to some form of reconstruction" (p. 937).

We cannot ever fully understand an individual's construing, but we can seek to improve our understanding of pivotal aspects of their understanding and help them to reveal to us their own ways of making sense (Shotter, 2007). Although PCP has different methods of achieving this, the most well-known and utilised is the repertory grid. Kelly developed this approach as a way to understand his clients' psychological difficulties, whilst enabling them to gain insight into their construing, including its implications and consequences (Burr et al, 2020). It can also be used as part of a joint focus on elaborating changes in construing and associated patterns of behaviour.

Despite demonstrable utility for forensic clinical practice (Houston, 1998; Needs & Jones, 2017), PCP has had limited traction within the area (Blagden et al., 2012). This chapter offers an exploration of PCP, its focus on the meaning-making of individuals, and its main assessment/research method of repertory grids. It is a collaborative venture, characterised by the experience of inter-subjectivity – of making sense "with". This can itself nurture a sense that both personal change and connectedness beyond the self are possible, something that can be particularly relevant to clients from a background of disadvantage and inequality. The chapter examines the applications and value of PCP and its

DOI: 10.4324/9781003230977-17

methods in forensic clinical practice, whilst suggesting its compatibility with holistic approaches within complexity science and other emerging perspectives which have the potential to transform the discipline.

These include the recent move within clinical psychology to focus more on context, meaning-making, and social influences (Boyle, 2020). Indeed, the Power, Threat, Meaning Framework, an alternative approach to clinical assessment replaces the traditional diagnostic question of "What is wrong with you?" with: "What has happened to you?"; "How did it affect you?"; "What sense did you make of it?" and "What did you have to do to survive?". PCP can be construed as a psychology of human concern (Shotter, 2007). It deals with issues that matter to the person concerned rather than those of the academic or professional fraternity.

Whose Meanings?

One of the most radical features of George Kelly's *The Psychology of Personal Constructs* (1955) is its emphasis on continuity of functioning between psychologists and other people. Kelly noticed that psychology textbooks typically presented two versions of humankind. One was the kind of person who was composed of chapter heading categories such as "perception", "learning" and "motivation", who reacted to stimuli and obeyed scientific principles tested in the laboratory, not always with human participants. The other, more implicit version was the author of the text. This privileged being was able to formulate and act in terms of theories and hypotheses, even testing them and modifying them according to outcomes. Kelly suggested that the mode of functioning of the second kind of person might be seen as a formalised version of what all people do. Perhaps, he continued, if we wish to understand a person, we should try to understand his or her sense-making rather than regarding our own sense-making as sacrosanct; people behave, think and feel in terms of what makes sense to them, within the contexts of their lives, rather than in terms of what makes sense to us as professionals. This realisation itself necessitates a concern with diversity, equality, and inclusion.

As such it encourages recognition of culturally embedded experience and understanding. An individual's construing will have developed to enable anticipation in a nexus of circumstances, routines, opportunities, threats, interpretations, tropes, and idioms – and the actions and perspectives of other people, including towards him or herself. These perspectives are available for adoption in personal sense-making and agency (Gillespie, 2012) but can also constrain or invalidate, including in ways relevant to identity that instil a sense of shame (Mascolo & Mancuso, 1990). Cultural conditions can also, for example, confront with historical legacies such as those of slavery (Mitchell, 2021), impart a rhetoric of moral unacceptability or incapacity which obscures structural disadvantage in society (Becker, 1964; Harré, 1984), or diminish through social exclusion the will to self-regulation (DeWall, 2013). Standardised psychological approaches might try to take a person out of context but cannot take the context out of a person (Wijsen, 2020).

Not that we have to agree with an individual's sense-making, or regard it as legitimising actions that harm others. Understanding where a person is "coming from" is not the same as making excuses, any more than construing those with whom we are engaged from the external, "third person" standpoint of conventional professional procedures and protocols necessarily precludes the exercise of empathy. However, an approach based on construing by its very nature takes empathy and, for that matter, consideration of contexts beyond a sporadic level. It provides a cogent perspective to, for example, enable a client troubled by traumatic memories to find (in the words of Stolorow, 2007) a "relational home" for emotional experiences which are difficult to construe.

PCT was ahead of its time in many respects. In 1955, widespread acceptance of the idea that organised "cognition" might be a determinant of behaviour lay in the future. The advent of cognitive then cognitive behavioural therapy three decades later satisfied many who had or would have felt little affinity with the side-lining as mere epiphenomena of cognitive processes and products by radical behaviourists. Undoubtedly, some of PCP's thunder was stolen. Yet there was always far more to PCP than advocacy of the importance of cognition. Kelly did not even teach PCP routinely to his students, preferring to help them develop their construing from their own starting points (Don Bannister, personal communication). In a rather similar manner, PCP does not attempt to train, impose or measure against "correct" (some would say white middle class) thinking. It does not regard cognition in terms of collections of more or less isolated beliefs, schemas, or self-statements that can be changed like spark plugs. Construing comes from engaging in situated action of systemically organised anticipations (Needs & Jones, 2017).

This can widen our views of what might be necessary to facilitate personal change. Failure to assess, for example, the "hidden" implications of what clients believe they might become can be a major source of lack of generalisation and maintenance of treatment gains (Kirchner et al., 1979; Tschudi, 1977; Winter, 1992). More widely, failure to take into account the personal meanings of recipients can lead to interventions being experienced by them as largely meaningless (Needs, 1988a; Yardley, 1979). Practitioners who proceed in this way might also be seen, ironically, as rather psychopathic (Winter, 1992).

"One size fits all" makes little sense from a PCP perspective. It engages with where the individual is coming from in every respect – the sense-making and anticipations behind current behaviour and the influences (such as social, cultural, and socio-economic) behind these. In this, it is not immediately compatible with "new public management"/ "managerialist" imperatives, associated with tensions with a more personal approach in a range of contexts (Bryans, 2000; Fortier & Malloy, 2019). A preoccupation with professional constructs at the expense of the construing of clients has additional origins. The common currency of psychological research and practice is the "variable". It is easy to forget that variables are shorthand labels standing in for often complex and contextually based processes (Polaschek, 2012), frequently conceptualised more as "isolated building blocks" than as parts of a "network of relations" (Capra, 1982). Much of the relevant knowledge base is derived from contrived situations, group averages (McNeill, 2012), is "immediacy fixated" (Dreier, 2009), and assumes linear relationships between variables although these are far from always found in the real world. (The size of a fire rarely depends on the number of matches used to start it.) In fact, many of the statistics we commonly use in psychology were developed for agriculture (Bodmer et al., 2021).

What Dreier (2009) termed "the standard arrangement" provides a metaphor as well as a knowledge base for a form of science based on procedures rather than processes, adherence to prescriptive rules, and the detachment of a third-person perspective. This is a less developed form of expertise than the flexible responsiveness to individual perspectives, specific situations, and culture required of autonomous professionals working to create optimal outcomes in complex situations (Sookermany, 2012). This is not to say that practitioners should play fast and loose with procedures. There are, for example, established arguments for preserving "programme integrity" or fidelity in the use of risk assessment protocols. However, there are times in assessment and formulation (not to say intervention) when practitioners need to engage with complexity in a way that is sensitive, creative, and innovative, engaging in information-gathering and problem-solving in a way that does more than pave the way to what the practitioner is familiar with or the organisation provides in bulk. These are times when engagement should be "contextualized" rather than "routinized" (Athay & Darley, 1981) or, in PCP terms, involve "circumspection" rather than "preemption" (Kelly, 1955; Reid, 1979).

An Integrative Approach

The holistic and embedded nature of Kelly's vision is suggested by PCP's Fundamental Postulate: "A person's processes are psychologically channelised by the ways in which he anticipates events" (Kelly, 1955, p. 46). He was clearly not talking about detached information-processing, representation, or symbolic manipulation: his "person" is engaged fundamentally with the environment. He suggested that we must move away from a focus on events or meanings inside the heads of individuals and move towards a focus on events occurring "out there" in relation to their interactive behaviour; as contended by Mead, meaning can be regarded as present in the social act before emergence in consciousness (Shotter, 2007). This is consistent with contemporary developments in science and philosophy, notably an "enactive" approach to mind:

> Natural cognitive systems are simply not in the business of accessing their world in order to build accurate pictures of it. They participate in the generation of meaning through their bodies and action often engaging in transformational and not merely informational interactions; *they enact a world*.
> (Di Paolo et al., 2014, p. 39)

What has been termed an embodied, embedded, and enactive ("3e") approach (Dent et al., 2020) has drawn together developments from cognitive and complexity science into an integrated account of human functioning that leaves behind a cognitive psychology based largely on static, unrealistic experimental displays and speculative flow charts of putative processes that at best provide a fragmented view of human action in real-life contexts (Neisser, 1976). Such contemporary developments might usefully be combined with practice and theoretical insights from PCT to explore more deeply what can be invested in personal action.

Compelling concerns from such developments include "the extent to which a situation affects the viability of a self-sustaining and precarious network of processes that generates an identity...... Encounters will be good or bad depending on their effects on autopoiesis" (Di Paolo et al., 2014 p. 48). An autopoietic system, such as a person or other living organism, is one that is self-generating and self-sustaining (Varela, 1979). Supported by sense-making and the capacity to adapt (De Jaegher & Froese, 2009), necessary characteristics of an autopoietic system are unity and continuity, sense-making and purpose, agency and self-efficacy, connectedness and reciprocity. Kelly (1955) famously viewed individuals as a "form of motion" and these can be seen as corresponding to the needs activated by transition summarised respectively by Ashforth (2001) as identity, meaning, control, and belonging (Needs, 2020). These aspects are implicated in many areas of actual or potential concern to forensic psychologists including transitional states relevant to trauma, major life events, and responses to interventions as well as offending and desistance (Needs, 2018, 2020; Needs & Adair-Stantiall, 2018).

Related concerns can often be glimpsed in the use of "laddering" in exploring accounts of offences such as homicides (Needs, 1988b; Needs & Jones, 2017). This involves comparing, in pairs, stages of an offence and preceding circumstances (identified through interview) written on small cards. When an aspect of similarity or difference (and contrast) is suggested by the individual, he or she is then asked why that aspect might be important. When an answer is given, the individual is asked why that, too, might be important – and so on, until a final abstraction (the top of the "ladder" is reached). Of course, rapport is essential, as like other PCT techniques it is very much a process of joint exploration. It can be helpful, for example, to introduce the method by saying that it involves the practitioner sounding like a rather annoying child who keeps asking "why?". It is also important to give the individual time to unwind before the end of the session (Rowe, 1983). In forensic applications, the process may have exposed core values and meanings entangled in a personal crisis and catastrophic event, of which the person may previously have been only dimly aware.

Offences such as homicide can be poorly understood and traumatic, using the term advisedly, to the perpetrator (Ferrito et al., 2017). In exploration by laddering, themes that one's identity had been or was about to be massively undermined and that the world has lost all coherence can figure prominently. At times there appear to have been desperate attempts to forestall uncertainty, perhaps by attempts to impose constructions, even switching to the opposite poles of bipolar constructs (Howells, 1981; Winter, 2003). Such work can help get beyond vocabularies of motive that are not far removed from journalistic cliches, descriptions rather than explanations, processes reified into things, the kinds of "proxy-level" variables suggested by Polaschek (2012). There is also a possibility that this form of exploration may encourage or even constitute a form of "processing" of trauma at a level of meaning perhaps missed in largely visualisation-based exposure therapies.

From an assessment perspective, piecing together the enactment of the offence episode can suggest how "intent" can be complex, fluctuating, and multifaceted (Briscoe, 1975). Although there are many offences that are planned and acted out accordingly, some do involve escalation or a step-by-step progression towards an outcome that may not have been envisaged. In this respect they are like many, if not most, forms of human behaviour. Radley (1977) used the analogy of an artist painting a picture, typically without a clear image of the end product in mind but responding to each brushstroke and the emerging array on the canvas. It will be apparent that, to use Di Paolo et al.'s (2014) term, this is very much a transformational process.

In some violent offences, personal concerns intertwined in offending can be part of a "criminal spin" (Ronel, 2011). Caught in an ever-decreasing circle of deteriorating circumstances and preoccupation, "components" of the individual (as an autopoietic system) might come to interact more with each other than in adaptive exchanges with the environment (Laroche et al., 2014). Such a perspective suggests interesting hypotheses concerning the antecedents of, for example, serial homicides (Needs, 2022) and reminds us that construing always takes place in a context (Bannister, 1979). With some exceptions (Needs & Adair-Stantiall, 2018; Zemel et al., 2018), the study of proximal life events and their impact prior to offending remains an under-developed area in forensic psychology, despite its clear relevance to risk assessment. Methods such as laddering can help open up this important contextual area along with the personal significance of offence dynamics. In terms of risk assessment and management, they can help to identify relevant "stimulus and response equivalences" (Mischel, 1973). They might also tell us something of how anticipations based on past environments might continue to exert an influence, something that can be particularly relevant in the context of trauma-informed care (Jones, 2018). The latter example highlights how ways in which views and intentions of authority figures and others in a custodial environment are construed can resonate strongly with negative experiences in the past, compounding distress in the present and potentially limiting constructive engagement.

Making Sense "with", Not Just "of"

When one person construes another person, this usually includes construing of that other person's construing. Put simply, we see people in part according to what we believe to be their outlooks and views. Although research into construing has identified developmental and individual differences in this capacity, this provides a basis for social interaction. Kelly's (1955) Sociality Corollary states: "To the extent that one person construes the construction processes of another, he may play a role in a social process involving the other person." In a social interaction this is usually two-way, something both (or more, in a group) the participants are doing. This could be seen as giving rise to a Laingian regress where person A construes person B and vice versa, but person A's construing of B includes B's construing of A and so forth (Laing et al., 1966). This is not a trivial point. The reciprocal influence of interviewer and interviewee can play out in the manner of a "Betari box" in, for example, a risk assessment interview (Shingler & Needs, 2018). Prisoners sometimes complain that in this setting psychologists can focus on rushing through protocols and appear to show little interest in them as individuals, whilst psychologists can talk of regret at lack of time and limited opportunities to get to know a prisoner (Shingler et al, 2020a & b). A consequence is that both prisoners and psychologists may experience an invalidation of identity, possibly accompanied by validation of stereotypical (or in PCT terms, "constellatory") construing of the other. Meanwhile, co-construction of what should be a shared and exploratory task is limited and we are left with an example of how construing influences rather than just predicts reality.

Such conditions inevitably pose difficulties for engaging in a genuine, facilitative social process incorporating a degree of mutual understanding (Stringer, 1979) and "interconnected action" or "praxis" (Radley, 1979). Radley explained the latter term: "people relate to one another through their coordinated activities, directed towards the situations in which they find themselves" (Radley, 1979 p. 85). The information gained elicited through a joint, collaborative approach can be more relevant, comprehensive, and accurate than that obtained through naïve objectivity (Daston, 1992) or an adversarial approach dominated by suspicion. Parallels can be drawn with qualitative research (e.g., Murakami, 2003).

Making sense "with" instead of just "of" a person (De Jaegher et al, 2010) can be a powerful process. Intersubjectivity, with the coming together and acknowledgement of subjectivities in coordinated action and shared meaning, is central to the emergence of new perspectives and patterns of behaviour in ordinary social development (Stevanovic & Koski, 2018) and contexts such as psychotherapy (Boston Change Process Study Group, 2002, 2013), including finding a "relational home" for trauma (Stolorow, 2007). It can also help development away from the profound and often long-standing sense of lack of connectedness to other people or mainstream society that characterises many of our service users (Molino, 2021; Needs, 2020). Conversely, failure to engage with the nature and referents of an individual's construction processes may compound this sense of lack of connectedness and marginality and does little to foster new development.

Repertory Grids

Repertory grids have been described as a form of structured interview (Bannister & Fransella, 2019); if so, it is one which is subtle, collaborative, and nuanced. The repertory grid is the most widely used technique of personal construct theory and even nearly 20 years ago had been used in approximately 3000 different studies (Neimeyer, 2004), including counselling and clinical (Randal et al., 2016), education and social work (Borell, et al, 2003) and forensic applications (Blagden et al., 2014; Houston, 1998; Needs & Jones, 2017). Grids allow a unique insight into the ways an individual construes an aspect of their world (Houston, 1998); in essence, they are a technique for studying personal and interpersonal systems of meaning (Neimeyer, 2004).

The basic grid consists of four component parts: topic, elements, constructs, and ratings. Each grid is conducted in relation to a particular "***topic***", whether it is for clinical or research purposes. "***Elements***" are examples from within a topic and can take many forms such as people, roles, situations (such as those that evoke anger or anxiety, or stages of an offence) or objects. When selecting elements, the clinician/researcher must give careful consideration to the relevance of elements; for example, "spouse" would not be an appropriate element for unmarried individuals (Bell et al., 2004). In clinical and forensic settings where most work has centred on identity and personal change, the elements are representative people and those that are salient to that individual. Kelly preferred a range of elements that took the form of many roles such as authority figure, parent/family, role model/admired person, and person they do not like. In Blagden et al.'s (2014) research on denial in men with sexual convictions the elements in the grids consisted of mother, father, prisoner admitting offence, prisoner maintaining their innocence, police officer, person convicted of a sexual offence, "victim", person you like, person you don't like, self now, self as you'd like to be and self before arrest. The elements were chosen as they reflected the topic under investigation and were seen to be the most suitable for the aims.

The third component of a repertory grid is the "***constructs***". Constructs can be conceptualised as ways which individuals make sense within a particular topic. For Kelly (1955) personal constructs are bipolar discriminations which anticipate or help make sense of an event. For example, in a construct of "hot-cold", hot can only make sense in relation (or in contrast) to cold, whilst the discrimination carries implications for what is likely to be encountered in an element construed in this way. The main method of construct elicitation is the triadic method.

This involves presenting three elements (usually written on cards) to the participant and asking them something along the lines of: "*For you personally, how are two alike but somehow different from the third?*" For example, a person may be presented with the element cards "self now", "self as offender" and "self ideally" and they may say "'self now' and 'self ideally' are the two that are alike because they 'can trust people'" (so "trust people" would become one, sometimes referred to as the "emergent" pole) whereas "'self as offender' was unable to trust" (the contrast or "implicit" pole would then be "unable to trust"). Elements can be selected at random (though they can be sequential: see Tan & Hunter, 2002) and once a construct is elicited the cards are then replaced ready for the next iteration. The elicitation process continues until the researcher is satisfied that all meaningful constructs have been elicited for that topic. Previous research suggests around 10–12 constructs is usually sufficient for gaining an understanding of an individual's construing of a particular topic (Ryle & Breen, 1972; Tan & Hunter, 2002).

This triadic process of elicitation requires skills and can be complex as it requires participants to provide psychological rather than "dictionary definition" opposites. In clinical settings this may mean that clients struggle to articulate their discriminations; the process is one of making explicit what is implicit and quite possibly never before verbalised. Patience is needed, perhaps with encouraging the client to talk a little about the elements in question. Valuable information can often be gained in this way and this kind of intersubjective focus can ease the crystallising of the client's meaning. One possibility with the triadic method is producing "bent" constructs, which combine different constructs within a single dimension such as "ambitious" and "athletic" (Neimeyer et al., 2005). In research involving individuals with intellectual disabilities in particular, some acknowledge that participants can struggle to consider the differences between people and are only able to think of the similarities (Mason, 2003; Kitson-Boyce et al, 2018). In cases such as this, a simpler dyadic elicitation method may be used whereby only two elements are presented to the participant. They are then asked to describe two ways in which they are similar, such as "how are your brother and father like each other?" Following this, they are asked to consider contrast or implicit poles of the elicited constructs; for example, the contrast of "ambitious" might be "lazy" (Walker & Winter, 2007). This approach can also be used with particularly abstract elements such as situations. Both elicitation methods facilitate communication and a laddering process can be used, whereby participants are asked which construct they prefer, which they associate themselves with and why. This enables higher-order constructs to be explored and elicited (Gaines-Hardison & Neimeyer, 2012).

Once constructs have been elicited, they are used to evaluate the elements. A seven-point rating scale provides meaningful data for statistical analysis (Grice, 2002) but is not the only possibility. For example, depending on the client group – for example with those with intellectual disabilities – and the degree of abstraction of the constructs – rank ordering of elements, from the most to the least in terms of the characteristic indicated by the construct, can also be a useful option. When the ratings are complete the resulting grid, in which each element is evaluated on every construct, will resemble Figure 15.1 and be ready for input into a statistical package for analysing repertory grids such as Idiogrid (Grice, 2007).

An initial "eyeball" analysis can be valuable (see Jankowicz, 2004). For example, in the above grid, "me now" indicates an individual who sees himself as pessimistic and aggressive, who struggles to consider other perspectives.

Tight and Loose Construing

Analysis of repertory grids allows an understanding of an individual's construct system that goes beyond what is immediately apparent. Pearson correlations and Euclidean distances, respectively, enable an understanding of the relationships between pairs of constructs and pairs of elements. A structural measure often

Construct (left pole)	Me Now	Police Officer	Father	Me Ideally	Alleged Victim	Prisoner Admitting Offence	Peson You Don't Like	Mother	Sexual Offender	Me Before Arrest	Prisoner Maintaining Innocence	Person You Like	Construct (right pole)
Positive outlook on life	6	1	6	2	2	4	1	7	3	3	3	2	Down/depressed
Successful (in life)	5	2	6	4	3	3	2	5	1	3	3	2	Layabout (waster)
Wants to get on (Progress)	2	4	2	6	4	6	6	6	4	4	4	3	Stubborn
Blinkered	3	5	6	3	6	5	4	1	4	4	4	6	Looks at different perspectives
Truthful	4	2	3	5	2	4	2	6	2	3	3	2	Bullshitter (liar)
Can admit wrongdoing	3	2	1	4	2	3	2	6	1	2	2	1	Arrogant
Respectful and curtious	4	2	2	3	2	2	2	7	2	2	2	2	Ignorant
thoughtful (listens)	2	2	2	3	3	3	2	7	2	3	3	2	Not attentive
Caring	5	1	2	5	3	4	2	6	2	3	3	2	Not bothered (selfish)
Trustworthy	3	2	2	4	2	3	2	7	2	3	3	2	Can't be trusted (bad person)
Agressive	2	6	6	3	6	4	6	5	4	5	5	6	Calm

Notes:

Constructs: 11   # Elements: 12.

Grid Type: Rating   Scale Range: 1.00 to   7.00.

Figure 15.1 Example of completed repertory grid.

used when analysing grid data is Principal component analysis (PCA). PCA provides a two-dimensional graphical display of the components of a participant's construal system, where the elements are represented as points and the constructs are represented as lines from the origin. Figure 15.2 is an example of a PCA output.

Of note within this grid is that the construing of "sexual self" and "future sexual self" is not well defined by the grid as revealed by their position close to the origin. This may indicate that "sexual self" and "future sexual self" are ambiguous or ambivalently construed and that the participant is struggling to make sense of both their current and future sexual self (see Winter, 2003). This is potentially useful information for those working with this individual.

PCA of repertory grids also gives an indication of a person's degree of cognitive simplicity or tight construing (Fransella et al, 2004). In PCP terms, cognitive complexity can be witnessed in an integrated and elaborated construct system, whereas cognitive simplicity is seen in overly tight construct systems and is characterised by dichotomous, "all or nothing" thinking (Houston, 1998; Winter, 1992). The loosening and tightening of construing forms part of the creativity cycle (Kelly, 1955), in which loose construing allows the generation of new ideas which are then tested by the person through tight construing (Winter, 1992). People who are functioning at normal levels of psychological wellbeing will move fluently through each phase of the cycle.

The most widely used measure of cognitive complexity/differentiation is the calculation of the percentage of variance accounted for by the first component (Smith, 2000), with a high percentage indicating cognitive simplicity. Ryle and Breen (1972) found, using relatively large grids, that in a sample of "normal" participants the mean variance accounted for by the first principal component was 39.4%. In a case study by Garcıa-Mieres et al., (2016), the corresponding measure was 56%, indicative of tight construing. Interestingly, the grid in Figure 15.1 was indicative of tight construing as it was found that 63.63% of the variance was accounted for in the first component (Blagden, 2011). There is debate as to how accurate such variance of the 1st component is as a measure of cognitive complexity (it will also be influenced by the number of constructs and elements), although Smith (2000) found rep grids to have good test-retest reliability.

Making Sense of Culture, Tackling Bias, and Negotiating Change

One of the advantages of PCP and repertory grids is that they privilege the individual's own culture, meanings, and experiences, attempting proactively to understand the individual's world. Repertory grids should be seen as an open-ended method, tailored to the context, concerns, and culture of the individual rather than a standardised test. PCP research has previously focused on culturally sensitive topics such as immigration (Burr et al., 2014), citizenship and national identity (Kalekin-Fishman, 2009), experiences of BAME in clinical

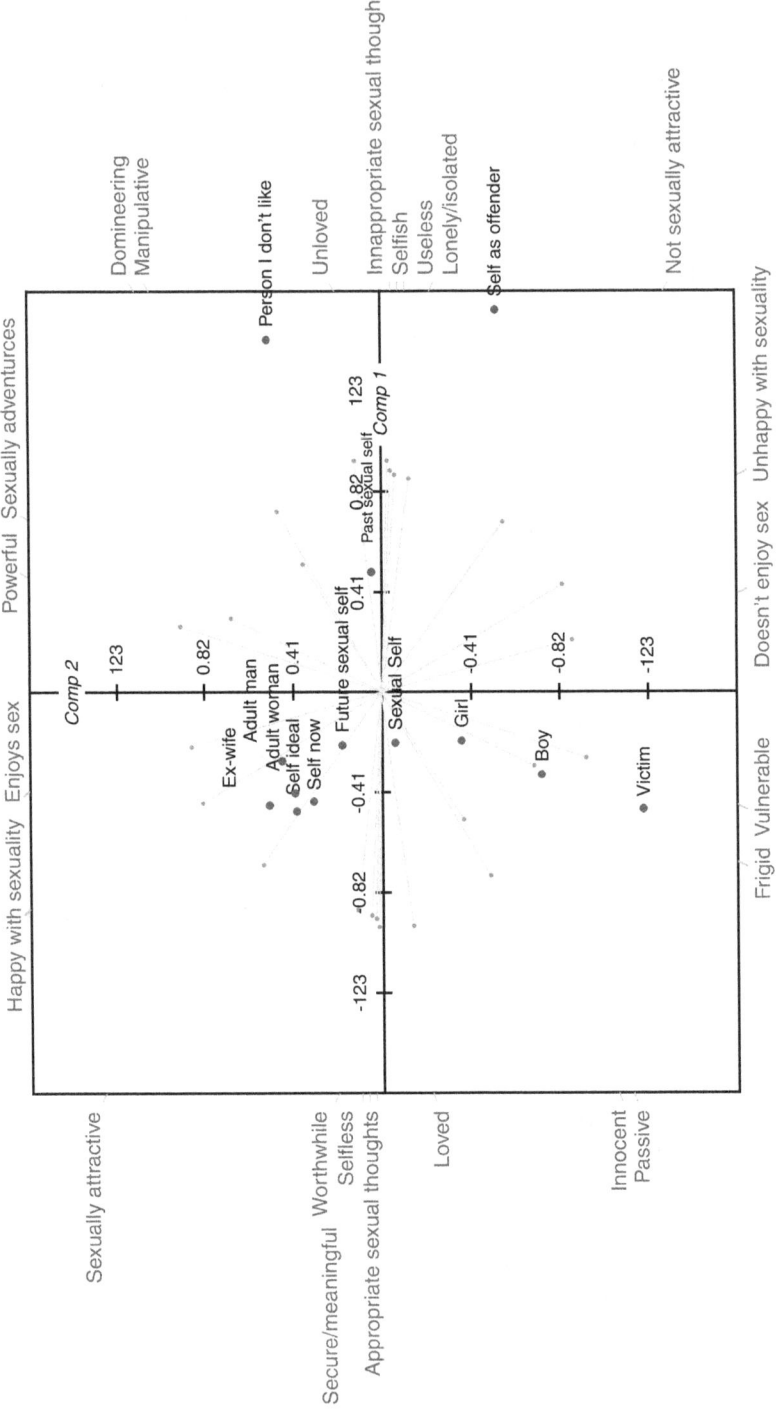

Figure 15.2 PCA output of person with sexual convictions making sense of their sexual selves.

psychology (Odusanya et al., 2018) resettlement of refugees (Naffi & Davidson, 2017), terrorism (Canter et al., 2014). As Canter et al. (2014) argue, the use of repertory grids for exploring sense-making, particularly in culturally sensitive research, should not be undervalued. Repertory grids allow individuals to give meaning to their experiences rather than the frames that society's dominant discourses may impose (Odusanya et al., 2018).

An additional advantage of grids is that the process is an indirect or opaque one; this can help minimise response bias or conscious dissimulation, as it is difficult to "see through" the aims of the grid (Blagden et al., 2012; Hicks, 1999; Mason, 2003). The indirectness of the method also allows for more fundamental positions to be uncovered and interviewing techniques like laddering (which illuminates values that underlie a person's construing) can help make sense of people's resistance to change (Hicks, 1999; Fransella et al, 2004). PCP reminds us that the process of change is hard and that hostility, resistance, relapse are part of the ebb and flow of change. Kelly (1958) suggested that hostility is usually a product of the experience of guilt, with guilt described as the dislodgement from a core role construct. In essence, a person gets a glimpse of a "new self" and becomes aware that they have gone too far in their psychological change (Fransella, 2005). Hostility stops the process of change and prevents the person from having to face that guilt (at not being the person they thought they were). This may result in the client regressing to a previous state. While some may regard this "relapse" as negative, Fransella (2005) argues that it can be beneficial to go a few steps back in their process of change to a position where they feel more familiar, before resuming the elaboration of new possibilities.

Repertory grids are useful for illuminating an individual's underlying thinking, but it is important that they are not mistaken for a sort of psychic x-ray, which offers privileged access to the exact workings of a person's mind (Butt & Burr, 2004). Many psychologists, if they become aware of them at all, encounter repertory grids detached from their theory of origin. It was largely because of this that PCP legend Don Bannister declared at a PCP conference in 1985 that it might take until he was on his deathbed before he finally decided that the benefits of grids to clinical practice and research, which he knew more than most, outweighed this potential diversion from true understanding of the theory (unfortunately, he passed away a year later and the answer to the obvious question is that we don't know). There was some discussion at a later PCP conference (in 1990) where an audience member described having been asked by a psychiatrist to "do" a patient's constructs, in a similar way to how a nurse might have been asked to "do" (test) a patient's blood. The ensuing statement that in this sense we don't "have" constructs – we construe – met with visible and emphatic consensus. Grids and associated techniques have enormous value as tools for exploration, for providing nuanced insights, and opening up communication with clients about non-obvious but often pivotal areas. However, they are best used in rather out of context and that context includes the innovative and radical vision of PCP itself.

Conclusion

PCP's focus on individuals attempts to make sense of the world they experience lends itself to a concern with diversity. Trying to understand people and their problems in their own terms is a collaborative, holistic enterprise but in these respects is compatible with advances in the fields of cognition, social interaction, and complex systems; this may be a source of mutual benefit in years to come and contribute to a more integrated psychology overall. Despite the value and utility PCP and repertory grids can have for forensic clinical practice, it has had limited application in those settings in recent years due largely to the dominance of standardised and didactic approaches to thinking and meaning based on nomothetic science (and, it should be said, a content which at early readings may seem unfamiliar and abstract). It has demonstrable potential in identifying and construing often hidden and elusive patterns and dynamics in areas such as offending, trauma, and the maintenance of psychological problems.

Repertory grid methods allow individualised data to be collected in relation to how an individual construes a certain part of their world (Bell, 2005). There are numerous advantages to this when considering understanding individual experiences. For example, the overall aim of procedure is difficult to see through so socially desirable response sets are likely to be reduced; they are also highly flexible. The technique can also be applied to neurodiverse populations and can be adapted to suit the needs of the client. Several studies have adapted repertory grids for clients with intellectual or learning disabilities (Kitson-Boyce et al, 2018; Mason, 2008; McNair et al., 2016; Ryle & Lunghi, 1970). Indeed, the strength of repertory grids is that they are administered "with" people with learning disabilities, rather than "to" them, and as such also provide a collaborative and person-centred tool to measure change (McNair et al., 2016).

Alan Radley pointed out that "the nature of persons is inexplicable by reference to individuals taken separately" (Radley, 1979 p. 81). We are not, as Radley goes on to say, "tucked away inside our 'private subjectivities'". A major implication of this is that we should always be mindful of the social circumstances, past and present, of the individual in front of us. This should include consideration of "intersubjective webs" (Nolan and Walsh, 2012) and the identities, perceived standpoints, and opportunities for autonomy which are available to a person (Radley, 1979). It follows that we should also reflect upon how we are similarly constituted and how this may influence our practice.

References

Ashforth, B. E. (2001). *Role transitions in organizational life: An identity-based perspective.* Mahwah NJ: Lawrence Erlbaum Associates.

Athay, M., & Darley, J. M. (1981). Toward an interaction-centered theory of personality. In J. T. Tedeschi (Ed.), *Impression management theory and social psychological research.* Academic Press.

Bannister, D. (1979). Personal construct theory and politics. In P. Stringer, & D. Bannister (Eds.) *Constructs of sociality and individuality.* Academic Press.

Bannister, D., & Fransella, F . (2019). *Inquiring man: The psychology of personal constructs.* Routledge.

Becker, E. (1964). *Revolution in psychiatry: The new understanding of man.* Free Press, Macmillan.

Bell, R.C. (2005) The repertory grid technique In F. Fransella, (Ed.), *International handbook of personal construct psychology.* John Wiley & Sons Ltd.

Bell, R., Bannister, D., & Fransella, F. (2004).*A manual for repertory grid technique.* John Wiley & Sons.

Blagden, N., Winder, B., Gregson, M., & Thorne, K. (2012). The practical utility of using repertory grids with sexual offenders maintaining their innocence: A case study. *The British Journal of Forensic Practice, 14*(4), 269–280.

Blagden, N., Winder, B., Gregson, M., & Thorne, K. (2014). Making sense of denial in sexual offenders: A qualitative phenomenological and repertory grid analysis. *Journal of Interpersonal Violence, 29*(9), 1698–1634. 10.1177/0886260513511530

Blagden, N. J., Mann, R., Webster, S., Lee, R., & Williams, F. (2018). "It's not something I chose you know": Making sense of pedophiles' sexual interest in children and the impact on their psychosexual identity. *Sexual Abuse, 30*(6), 728–754.

Blagden, N. J. (2011). *Understanding denial in sexual offenders: The implications for policy and practice.* Nottingham Trent University (United Kingdom).

Butt, T. W., & Burr, V. (2004). *Invitation to personal construct psychology* (2nd edn.). Whurr Publishers.

Bodmer, W., Bailey, R. A., Charlesworth, B., Eyre-Walker, A., Farewell, V., Mead, A., & Senn, S. (2021). The outstanding scientist, R.A. Fisher: His views on genetics and race. *Heredity, 126,* 565–576.

Boston Change Process Study Group (2002). Explicating the implicit: The local level and the microprocess of change in the analytic situation. *International Journal of Psychoanalysis, 83,* 1051–1062.

Boston Change Process Study Group (2013). Enactment and the emergence of new relational organization. *Journal of the American Psychoanalytic Association, 61*(4), 727–749.

Borell, Klas, Espwall, Majen, Pryce, Joanna, & Brenner, Sten-Olof (2003). The repertory grid technique in social work research, practice, and education. *Qualitative Social Work,* 2(4), 477–491. 10.1177/1473325003024006.

Briscoe, O. V. (1975). Assessment of intent—an approach to the preparation of court reports. *The British Journal of Psychiatry, 5,* 461–465.

Bryans, S. (2000). The managerialisation of prisons: Efficiency without a purpose? *Prison Service Journal, 134,* 8–10.

Burr, V., Giliberto, M., & Butt, T. (2014). Construing the cultural other and the self: A Personal Construct analysis of English and Italian perceptions of national character. *International Journal of Intercultural Relations, 39,* 53–65.

Canter, D., Sarangi, S., & Youngs, D. (2014). Terrorists' personal constructs and their roles: A comparison of the three I slamic terrorists. *Legal and Criminological Psychology, 19*(1), 160–178.

Capra, F. (1982). *The turning point.* Bantam Books.

Daston, L. (1992). Objectivity and the escape from perspective. *Social Studies of Science, 22*(4), 597–618.

Dent, H., Nielsen, K., & Ward, T. (2020). Correctional rehabilitation and human functioning: An embodied, embedded, and enactive approach. *Aggression and Violent Behavior, 51,* 101383.

De Jaegher H., Di Paolo, E., & Gallagher, S. (2010). Can social interaction constitute social cognition? *Trends in Cognitive Sciences, 14*(10), 441–447.

De Jaegher, H., & Froese, T. (2009). On the role of social interaction in individual agency. *Adaptive Behavior, 17* (5), 444–460.

De Wall, C. N., & Twenge, J. M. (2013). Rejection and aggression: Explaining the paradox. In C. N. De Wall (Ed.), *The Oxford handbook of social exclusion.* Oxford University Press.

DeWall, C.N. (Ed). (2013). *Oxford handbook of social exclusion.* New York: Oxford University Press.

Di Paolo, E.A., Rohde, M., & De Jaegher, H. (2014). Horizons for the enactive mind: Values, Social interaction and play. In J. Stewart, O. Gapenne, & E. A. Di Paolo (Eds), *Enaction: Towards a new paradigm for cognitive science.* A Bradford Book, The MIT Press.

Dreier, O. (2009). Persons in structures of social practice. *Theory & Psychology, 19,* 93–112.

Ferrito, M., Needs, A., & Adshead, G. (2017). Unveiling the shadows of meaning: Meaning making for perpetrators of homicide. *Aggression and Violent Behavior, 34,* 263–272.

Fortier, E., & Malloy, D. (2019). Moral agency, bureaucracy and nurses: A qualitative study. *Canadian Journal of Practical Philosophy, 3,* 1–14.

Fransella, F. E. (2005). *The essential practitioner's handbook of personal construct psychology.* John Wiley & Sons Ltd.

Gaines-Hardison, H., & Neimeyer, R. (2012). Assessment of personal constructs: Features and functions of constructivist techniques. In P. Caputi, L. Viney, B. Walker, & N. Crittenden (Eds.), *Personal construct methodology* (pp. 3–51). Wiley-Blackwell.

Garcıa-Mieres, H., Ochoa, S., Salla, M., Lopez-Carrilero, R., & Feixas, G. (2016). Understanding the paranoid psychosis of James: Use of the repertory grid technique for case conceptualization. *World Journal of Psychiatry, 6*(3), 381–390. 10.5498/wjp.v6.i3.381.

Gillespie, A. (2012). Position exchange: The social development of agency. *New Ideas in Psychology, 30,* 32–46.

Grice, J. W. (2002). Idiogrid: Software for the management and analysis of repertory grids. *Behavior Research Methods, Instruments, & Computers: A Journal of the Psychonomic Society, Inc, 34*(3), 338–341. 10.3758/bf03195461

Grice, J. W. (2007). Idiogrid (version 2.4)[computer software]. Stillwater, Oklahoma: Idiogrid Software.

Harré, R. (1984). Public-collective psychological processes and social skills. In P. Trower (Ed.), *Radical approaches to social skills training.* Croom Helm.

Hicks, C. (1999). *Research methods for clinical therapists: Applied project design and analysis.* Churchill Livingstone.

Horley, J. (2008). *Sexual offenders: Personal construct theory and deviant sexual behavior.* Routledge.

Houston, J. (1998). *Making sense with offenders: Personal constructs, therapy and change.* John Wiley & Sons Ltd.

Howells, K. (1981). Social construing and violent behaviour in mentally disordered offenders. In J. Hinton (Ed.), *Dangerousness: Problems of assessment and prediction.* Allen & Unwin.

Jankowicz, D. (2004). *The easy guide to repertory grids.* John Wiley & Sons Ltd.

Jones. L. (2018). Trauma-informed care and 'good lives' in confinement: Acknowledging and offsetting adverse impacts of chronic trauma and loss of liberty. In G. Akerman, A. Needs, & C. Bainbridge (Eds.). *Transforming environments and rehabilitation: A guide for practitioners in forensic settings and criminal justice.* Routledge.

Kalekin-Fishman, D. (2009). Blood-Territory-Rights-Duties: Constructing and construing citizenship as a form of life. In Personal constructivism: Theory and applications (pp. 89–113). Pace University Press New York.

Kelly, G.A. (1955). *The psychology of personal constructs* Vols 1 & 2. Norton.

Kelly, G.   (1958). *Personal construct theory and the psychotherapeutic interview. Clinical psychology and personality.* New York: Wiley.

Kirchner, E. P., Kennedy, R. E., & Draguns, J. G. (1979). Assertion and aggression in adult offenders. *Behavior Therapy, 10,* 452–471.

Kitson-Boyce, R., Blagden, N., Winder, B., & Dillon, G. (2018). This time it's different – preparing for release through CoSA (The prison model): A phenomenological and repertory grid analysis. *Sexual Abuse, 31*(8), 886–822. 10.1177/1079063218775969

Laing, R. D., Phillipson, H., & Lee, A. R. (1966). *Interpersonal perception: A theory and a method of research.* Tavistock.

Landfield, A.W. (1971) *Personal construct systems in psychotherapy.* Rand-McNally.

Laroche, J., Berardi, A. M., & Brangier, E. (2014). Embodiment of intersubjective time: Relational dynamics as attractors in the temporal coordination of interpersonal behaviors and experiences. *Frontiers in Psychology, 10,* 3389.

Mascolo, M. F., & Mancuso, J. C. (1990). Functioning of epigenetically evolved emotion systems. *International Journal of Personal Construct Psychology, 3,* 205–222.

Mason, J. (2003). The use of a repertory grid as an aid to assessment and formulation in a sex offender with a learning disability. *The British Journal of Forensic Practice, 5*(3), 13–20. 10.1108/14636646200300016.

Mason, J. (2008). Measuring psychological change in offenders with intellectual disabilities and alcohol misuse using repertory grids: Two case examples. *The British Journal of Forensic Practice, 10*(4), 37–44.

McNair, L., Woodrow, C., & Hare, D. (2016). Using repertory grid techniques to measure change following dialectical behaviour therapy with adults with learning disabilities: Two case studies. *British Journal of Learning Disabilities, 44*(3), 247–256.

McNeill, F. (2012). Four forms of 'offender' rehabilitation: Towards an interdisciplinary perspective. *Legal and Criminological Psychology, 17,* 1–19.

Mischel, W. (1973). Towards a cognitive social learning reconceptualization of personality. *Psychological Review, 80,* 252–283.

Mitchell, L. (2021). *Living with indirect exposure to street gang youth violence in a 6th form college community.* Unpub. D.Foren.Psy thesis, University of Portsmouth.

Molino, S. D. (2021). *An exploration of constructions of connectedness and the role of intersubjectivity in personality disorder.* Unpub. D.Foren.Psy thesis, University of Portsmouth.

Murakami, K. (2003). Orientation to the setting: Discursively accomplished intersubjectivity. *Culture & Psychology, 9*(3), 233–248.

Naffi, N., & Davidson, A. L. (2017). Engaging host society youth in exploring how they construe the influence of social media on the resettlement of Syrian refugees. *Personal Construct Theory and Practice, 14,* 116–128.

Needs, A. (1988a). *The subjective context of social difficulty.* Unpub. D.Phil thesis, University of York.

Needs, A. (1988b). Psychological investigation of offending behaviour. In F. Fransella, & L. Thomas (Eds.) *Experimenting with personal construct psychology.* Routledge.

Needs, A. (2018). Only connect: Implications of social processes and contexts for understanding trauma. In G. Akerman, A. Needs & C. Bainbridge (Eds.). #Needs, A. (2020). Veterans, horses and the rediscovery of "with". *The Psychologist,* September, 54–58.

Needs, A. (2020). Veterans, horses and the rediscovery of "with". *The Psychologist,* September, 54–58.

Needs, A. (2022). Serial and mass murders. In C. Byrne, & S. Gayathri (Eds.), *Encyclopedia of violence, peace & conflict* (3rd edn.). Elsevier.

Needs, A., & Adair-Stantiall, A. (2018). The social context of transition and rehabilitation. In G. Akerman, A. Needs & C. Bainbridge (Eds).

Needs, A., & Jones, L. (2017). Personal construct psychotherapy. In J. Davies, & C. Nagi (Eds.), *Individual psychotherapy with clients in forensic settings*. Wiley.

Neisser, U. (1976). *Cognition and reality: Principles and implications of cognitive psychology*. Freeman.

Neimeyer, G. J., Bowman, J. Z., & Saferstein, J. (2005). The effects of elicitation techniques on repertory grid outcomes: Difference, opposite, and contrast methods. *Journal of Constructivist Psychology*, 18(3), 237–252. 10.1080/10720530590948791.

Neimeyer, R. A. (2004). Repertory grid methods. [online] available at: http://www.pcp-net.org/encyclopaedia/repgrid-methods.htmlaccessed 28th May 2022.

Nolan, G., & Walsh, E. (2012). Caring in prison: The intersubjective web of professional relationships. *Journal of Forensic Nursing, 8*, 163–169.

Odusanya, S. O., Winter, D., Nolte, L., & Shah, S. (2018). The experience of being a qualified female BME clinical psychologist in a National Health Service: An interpretative phenomenological and repertory grid analysis. *Journal of Constructivist Psychology, 31*(3), 273–291.

Polaschek, D. L. (2012). An appraisal of the risk–need–responsivity (RNR) model of offender rehabilitation and its application in correctional treatment. *Legal and Criminological Psychology, 17*(1), 1–17.

Radley, A. R. (1977). Living on the horizon. In Bannister, D. (Ed.), *New perspectives in personal construct theory*. Academic Press.

Radley, A. R. (1979). Construing as praxis. In (Eds.), p. 86.P. StringerD. Bannister

Randal, C., Bucci, S., Morera, T., Barrett, M., & Pratt, D. (2016). Mindfulness-based cognitive therapy for psychosis: Measuring psychological change using repertory grids. *Clinical Psychology & Psychotherapy, 23*(6), 496–508.

Reid, F. (1979). Personal constructs and social competence. In P. Stringer, & D. Bannister (Eds.), *Constructs of sociality and individuality*. London: Academic Press.

Ronel, N. (2011). Criminal behavior, criminal mind: Being caught in a "criminal spin". *International Journal of Offender Therapy and Comparative Criminology, 55*(8), 1208–1233.

Rowe, D. (1983). *Depression: The way out of your prison*. Routledge and Kegan Paul.

Ryle, A., & Breen, D. (1972). Some differences in the personal constructs of neurotic and normal subjects. *The British Journal of Psychiatry, 120*(558), 483–489. 10.1192/bjp.120.558.483

Ryle, A., & Lunghi, M. (1970) The dyad grid: A modification of repertory grid technique *British Journal of Psychiatry, 117*, 323–327.

Shingler, J., Sonnenberg, S. J., & Needs, A. (2020a). Psychologists as 'the quiet ones with the power': Understanding indeterminate sentenced prisoners' experiences of psychological risk assessment in the United Kingdom. *Psychology, Crime & Law, 26*(6), 571–592.

Shingler, J., Sonnenberg, S. J., & Needs, A. (2020b). 'Their life in your hands': the experiences of prison-based psychologists conducting risk assessments with indeterminate sentenced prisoners in the United Kingdom. *Psychology, Crime & Law, 26*(4), 311–326.

Shingler, J., & Needs, A. (2018). Contextual influences in prison based psychological risk assessment: Problems and solutions. In G. Akerman, A. Needs, & C. Bainbridge (Eds.), *Transforming environments and rehabilitation* (pp. 323–347). Taylor & Francis.

Shotter, J. (2007) Re-visiting George Kelly: Social constructionism, social ecology and social justice – all unfinished projects. *Personal Construct Theory & Practice, 4*, 68–83.

Smith, H. J. (2000). The reliability and validity of structural measures derived from repertory grids. *Journal of Constructivist Psychology*, 13(3), 221–230.

Sookermany, A. M. (2012). What Is a skillful soldier? An epistemological foundation for understanding military skill acquisition in (post) modernized armed forces. *Armed Forces & Society*, *38*(4), 582–603.

Stevanovic, M., & Koski, S. E. (2018). Intersubjectivity and the domains of social interaction: Proposal of a cross-sectional approach. *Psychology of Language and Communication*, *22*(1), 39–70.

Stolorow, R. D. (2007). *Trauma and human existence: Autobiographical, psychoanalytic, and philosophical reflections*. The Analytic Press.

Stringer, P. (1979). Individuals, roles and persons. In P. Stringer & D. Bannister (Eds.), *Constructs of sociality and individuality* (pp. 91–112). New York: Academic Press.

Tan, F. B., & Hunter, M. G. (2002). The repertory grid technique: A method for the study of cognition in information systems. *MIS Quarterly*, *26*(1), 39–57. 10.2307/4132340

Tschudi, F. (1977). Loaded and honest questions: A construct theory view of symptoms and therapy. In Bannister, D. (Ed.) *New perspectives in personal construct theory*. London: Academic Press.

Varela, F. J. (1979). *Principles of biological autonomy*. Elsevier North Holland.

Walker, B. M., & Winter, D. A. (2007). The elaboration of personal construct psychology. *Annual Review of Psychology*, 58, 453–477. 10.1146/annurev.psych.58.110405.085535.

Wheatley, R., Winder, B., & Kuss, D. (2020a). Using a visually adapted repertory grid technique (VARGT) with men who stalk. *The Journal of Forensic Practice*, *22*(2), 109–121. 10.1108/JFP-10-2019-0048

Wijsen, F. (2020). Beyond global apartheid: Polarization and (de)radicalisation in Tanzania, *Journal of Constructivist Psychology*, *33*(3), 307–319. 10.1080/10720537.2019. 1676341

Winter, D. A. (1992). A personal construct theory view of social skills training. In P. Maitland, & D. Brennan (Eds.), *Personal construct theory, deviancy and social work* (2nd edn.). Inner London Probation Service/Centre for Personal Construct Psychology.

Winter, D. (1992). *Personal construct psychology in clinical practice*. Routledge.

Winter, D. A. (2003). A credulous approach to violence and homicide. In J. Horley (Ed.). *Personal construct perspectives on forensic psychology* (pp. 15–53). London: Routledge.

Yardley, K. M. (1979). Social skills training – A critique. *British Journal of Medical Psychology*, *52*, 55–62.

Zemel, O., Einat, T., & Ronel, N. (2018). Criminal spin, self-control, and desistance from crime among juvenile delinquents: Determinism versus free will in a qualitative perspective. *International Journal of Offender Therapy and Comparative Criminology*, *62*(15), 4739–4757.

16 Using Social Media Data in Forensic Evaluations: Addressing Bias

Ashley Batastini, Madison Lord, and Michael Vitacco

Using Social Media Data in Forensic Evaluations: Addressing Bias

How do you decide whether information is credible or trustworthy? Does the content of the message matter (e.g., whether it seems plausible, cites appropriate references, aligns with your worldview)? Does it matter who said it (e.g., a celebrity/influencer, politician, healthcare provider, national news source, relative)? What about where it came from or the method of exposure? Consider the following scenario: your neighbour tells you she heard the government approved a new drug that can prolong life expectancy by as much as 5 years. Whether you find this information believable may depend on myriad factors; for example, your appraisal of how likely it is such a drug exists given the current state of medical science, how often your neighbour seems to be correct about other topics, her known or suspected sociopolitical ideologies, level of education or occupation, the availability of corroborating evidence, etc. Now consider: would the extent to which you believed this information change if, instead, you saw your neighbour post about the new drug on her Facebook page?

In the year before Y2K, David Bowie[1] nearly proved his otherworldliness by predicting the current state of the internet in a BBC interview. A quick online search will queue the video clip for interested readers. At a time when the internet was little more than AOL email and AskJeeves.com (a rudimentary search engine), Bowie foresaw what was coming: a juxtaposition of progress and chaos. Even as the interviewer scoffs at the idea, Bowie remains adamant the internet will "change things". As of October 2021, just under 5 billion people worldwide were estimated to be active social media users (https://datareportal.com/social-media-users). These sites have become a daily depository of personal data, most of which are accessible to a public audience. Your strategy for determining the veracity of any data or data source most likely includes some combination of objective and subjective reasoning. Yet, determining truth on social media can be particularly challenging. Although some sites are working to diffuse interactions with so-called "fake news", we know social media platforms like Facebook, Instagram, Twitter, TikTok, and WhatsApp can perpetuate the spread of misinformation and misrepresentation (Allcott, Gentzkow, & Yu, 2019). The process

DOI: 10.4324/9781003230977-18

of parsing apart what information is real or has significance to a given purpose is more subjective.

Decisions to keep or retain information based on personal feelings, experiences, assumptions, or preferences are vulnerable to bias. However, the decision to ignore information from social media because of its inherent challenges also has the potential to widen the margin of error in drawing conclusions or predictions about a person's intent or behaviour.

Although a thorough review is beyond the scope of this chapter, it is necessary to acknowledge the robust research on cognitive biases in forensic mental health assessment (FMHA; e.g., Murrie & Warren, 2005; Neal & Brodsky, 2016; Neal & Grisso, 2014; Neal, 2017). In one seminal study, Murrie et al. (2013) showed compelling evidence for adversarial allegiance – a subconscious tendency to provide opinions that support the retaining party. While forensic professionals can acknowledge cognitive biases exist, they falsely believe that (a) sheer willpower or introspection can reduce biases and (b) others are more suspectable to biases than they are (Zapf et al., 2018). In separate but relevant academic areas, research on bias in evaluating credibility of information on social media is increasing. In Gearhart et al. (2019), for example, participants saw a Facebook news story (either about abortion or gun legislation) with comments posted by other (mock) users that were congruent or incongruent with their expressed views on these topics. As might be expected, participants exposed to news stories with like-minded commentary rated the story, its writer, and the publication outlet as less biased and more credible than participants who saw commentary with dissimilar sentiments. Some studies have also begun exploring biases related to the racial/ethnicity of the source or user. In Spence et al. (2013), for example, participants were asked to read a Facebook post about heart disease that was posted by either a White "avatar" or an African American "avatar". Contrary to what might be expected, the African American avatar was seen as more trustworthy and caring but not more competent than the White avatar regardless of participant race.

Hsieh-Yee (2021) argues that people's determination of social media trustworthiness can be broken down to their judgements about the source's integrity (is it honest?), ability (does the source have necessary skills/knowledge related to the content), and benevolence (does the source have good intentions?). The weight placed on these dimensions can also depend on level of risk (e.g., a report on vaccine efficacy vs. a cat video), with greater consideration of each dimension as risk increases. Drawing on trust literature, Hsieh-Yee (2021) recommends users take care not to "rely on social categorization, reputation, institutional affiliation, wishful thinking, fear or the urgency of a situation to rush their decision on whether to trust the information found on social media" (p. 19).

With the proliferation of social media uses broadly, it should be of little surprise that social media is also more prevalent in legal contexts. Ironically, the internet is ripe with examples of social media use leading to legal trouble, from defamation suits to child custody disputes to murder. In *Vasquez-Santos v. Mathew* (2019), for example, the plaintiff was a semi-professional basketball player claiming physical disability resulting from a car accident. Defense presented Facebook posts "tagged" by friends of the plaintiff depicting him playing basketball and other activities; however, the plaintiff testified the photos were taken before the accident. Fortunately for the plaintiff, the court denied a defense motion to access private content on his devices to corroborate the timeline. In a far more sinister case, a 15-year-old from Texas shot and killed his family, posting gruesome pictures of their bodies on Discord (a social media app for gamers) and threatening to continue his violence spree at an unnamed school. He turned the gun on himself after police received a tip from an app user and tracked him down in an RV park (see Sharma, 2021). Some online resources even inform readers how social media use can be used against them in court (e.g., Arnold, 2018).

In 2014, the American Bar Association published guidance in their flagship journal on discovery of social media evidence, emphasising that "data residing on social media platforms is [sic] subject to the same duty to preserve as other types of electronically stored information (ESI)" (DiBianca, 2014). Failure to properly preserve social media data has led to court-sanctions. In the first known decision related to this issue (*Lester v. Allied Concrete Co.*, 2011), the court ruled the plaintiff and counsel engaged in spoliation of social media evidence by deleting photos and deactivating the plaintiff's Facebook account. Courts have also consistently agreed that social media users have no reasonable expectation of privacy and that "not public" does not necessarily mean "private" (DiBianca, 2014).

There is little doubt the social media waters can be murky. As online posting, streaming, scrolling, and messaging dominate our lives and increasingly seep into criminal and civil legal matters, forensic evaluators must consider how best to navigate these waters. Just as Bowie highlighted the duality of the internet – simultaneously producing good and bad outcomes – the challenges associated with using social media evidence in FMHA are countered by its potential benefits. Authenticated and admissible social media data, for example, can provide insight about immediate thought processes, estimate the proximity of a given data point to an event of interest, establish a pattern of behaviour over time (e.g., mapping the trajectory of psychiatric decompensation), or corroborating or discrediting other data sources (e.g., pictures of an individual golfing when they are claiming a serious arm injury).

As another type of collateral source, how can examiners access, select, and use these data as objectively as possible? The remainder of this chapter summarises existing research and commentary (albeit limited) regarding social media sources in forensic mental health assessment (FMHA) and offers practice recommendations aimed at (1) reducing skepticism toward social media evidence and (2) improving examiner competence when integrating such evidence into their forensic work. The chapter concludes with two practical exercises. With near-constant use of social media by so many people worldwide, this source of information cannot and should not be ignored in forensic psychological practice.

What We Know about Social Media Evidence in Clinical and Forensic Mental Health Practice

The integration of collateral data in clinical and forensic psychological assessment is widely encouraged and acknowledged as best practice (Heilbrun et al., 2015). As such, there is a substantial body of literature on types of collateral data and how experts should incorporate such data into professional practice (Otto et al., 2007; Knoll & Resnick, 2007). However, much of this work was disseminated without consideration for social media (in some cases because social media was not yet popularised or even in existence). To date, there remains little emphasis on newer forms of collateral data such as evidence obtained from internet sources. Even in general psychological practice, guidelines for the use and regulation of social media emerged only recently (ASPPB, 2020). As technology, and social media in particular, continue to advance and diversify, our professional understanding of what to do with these data is lagging. Yet, the use of social media data in both clinical (DiLillo & Gale, 2011; Kaslow et al., 2011) and psycho-legal contexts (Pirelli et al., 2018; Coffey et al., 2018) appears to be increasing. However, early survey and experimental research suggest examiners harbour skepticism towards social media data despite believing it could be useful in FMHA (Coffey et al., 2018; Batastini et al., 2020). What follows is a summary of extant research on social media data in FMHA that explores how professional perceptions and behaviours may introduce bias into the assessment process.

Estimates of Social Media Use

Coffey et al. (2018) investigated overall rates of social media evidence among forensic evaluators, what types of psycho-legal questions such evidence was used for, and legal and ethical concerns surrounding usage. Over half of the 102 professionals (63.7%) in their sample reported incorporating social media as collateral information in their FMHAs at least once. Common referral questions in both criminal (e.g., mental state at the time of offense [MSO], adjudicative competency, violence risk/threat assessment) and civil (e.g., child custody/parental fitness, disability, and personal injury) contexts were informed by social media data. In criminal cases, respondents who conducted MSO evaluations most frequently incorporated social media collateral information; in civil cases, the highest proportion of use was among those conducting family court (e.g., child custody or parental fitness) examinations. Examiners reported relying on social media for a variety of reasons, but most frequently did so to help determine an examinee's mental illness/mental state or extent of capabilities. As a qualitative example, one examiner noted that social media posts provided insight into an examinee's delusional or disordered thinking and showed potential changes in their psychological functioning over time. Others described using social media information to help validate an individual's story or provide insight into potential malingering, or determine an individual's true capabilities and skills, such as their ability to use language and other cognitive skills. In some cases, examiners reported that social media posts were directly related to the legal matter (e.g., an individual's harassment of others on Facebook) and were therefore essential to the evaluation. Examiners noted that social media posts provided helpful behavioural data such as the ways in which they interact with or portray themselves to others. Some examiners noted using social media information to help score psychological instruments such as risk-related tools used in violence or re-offense risk assessments.

Is There Evidence of a Social Media Bias?

There is a growing literature base highlighting the advantages, disadvantages, and ethical underpinnings to social media usage within therapeutic contexts. While some argue social media can provide helpful insight into a client's presenting issue, thereby enhancing clinical care (Hughs, 2009), others raise concerns surrounding potential boundary violations, client's expectations of privacy, trust, and confidentiality (Kaslow et al., 2011). But, how exactly do these concerns impact clinicians' attitudes and behaviours, and importantly, do these attitudes and behaviours include bias? In DiLillo and Gale (2011), most (76.8%) doctoral-level students surveyed believed conducting an independent search for clients via social media sites was generally unacceptable, even though an overwhelming majority (94.4%) had searched for at least one client themselves. While the authors suggest this apparent incongruence between action and belief may have resulted from the opportunity to reflect on the ethics behind conducting independent social media searches, this finding could also be explained by the common attributional bias known as the false-uniqueness effect; e.g., that "I'm different than everyone else" or "I'm an exception". In this study, perhaps students felt it was acceptable for them to search for clients because they believed they were uniquely (though falsely) capable of handling information ethically and/or were uniquely justified in their search. This effect explains the tendency noted earlier for forensic experts to view themselves as more objective than others.

However, among forensic examiners only 39% of respondents had searched online, most commonly conducting independent searches via Google (52%) or Facebook (20%), for information about a forensic examinee (Pirelli et al., 2018). Further, regardless of prior search behaviour, 41% supported the use of social media as evidence in FMHA. Interestingly, outcomes differed between graduate-level trainees and post-doctoral professionals, with the latter searching for forensic examinees more frequently and endorsing higher levels of support than trainees. In Coffey et al. (2018), while most examiners reported receiving social media information through discovery materials (53.3%), a similar number of professionals disclosed conducting their own search for the examinee (42.2%). Experience with social media data in FMHA was linked to increased acceptance of such information (Coffey et al., 2018). Together, these studies show that prior use of social media data may affect an examiner's decision to use these sources or not, which may ultimately influence how they answer a given referral question. What is less clear in this literature is whether general support for social media use in FMHA includes support for independent searches vs. sticking to material provided in court discovery. In other words, do examiners care how the information is obtained or comes to their attention? And could the method of selecting and accessing social media material be another way for bias to surface? Clearly, many examiners engage in this behaviour and searching for clients or examinees does not appear to be outright prohibited in existing guidelines for social media use, at least in general clinical contexts (ASPPB, 2020). In understanding the potential for bias, Pirelli et al. (2016) recommended forensic examiners consider internet searches on a case-by-case basis, paying particular attention to the utility versus prejudicial effects of such information. In their 2018 follow-up study, 90% of respondents supported this recommendation. Search procedures are discussed more explicitly later in this chapter under practice recommendations.

Beyond use and acceptability, Coffey et al. (2018) attempted to uncover perceptions of social media relative to other commonly used collateral sources (e.g., medical and criminal records, defendant self-report, third-party interviews, police reports). Among 11 different sources listed, clinicians ranked social media data as the lowest in utility, only above information gathered from other inmates. The proximity of social media evidence to inmate relayed information (which is typically viewed as unreliable) suggests examiners perceive considerable concerns with social media collateral data. Apprehensions towards social media data centred on questions of authenticity, truthfulness/reliability, relevance, and privacy/consent to access such data (Coffey et al., 2018). Based on the professional concerns articulated by respondents in Coffey et al. (2018), it stands to reason forensic examiners may perceive social media data as potentially biased for various reasons, and as such, may weigh this information less heavily, regardless of its ability to uniquely inform referral questions, which is an example of bias in and of itself. This assumption was supported by the first known experimental exploration of examiners' attitudes toward social media data. In this two-part study, respondents were randomly assigned to one of three conditions that contained virtually the same information (i.e., a physical altercation as reported by a hypothetical defendant), but presented in different formats (i.e., a Twitter post/tweet, a clinical note, forensic report excerpt) and told it was evidence in a criminal responsibility evaluation (Batastini et al., 2021). In the tweet condition, the information (a reported physical altercation) appeared as a post from the defendant's account; in the other two conditions, the information was presented as a direct quote from the defendant. Thus, in all three conditions, the information was assumed to be from the defendant's own words. Study 1 included a jury-eligible participants (a non-expert sample); results showed information presented as a tweet was viewed as less trustworthy, credible, and useful than both the clinical note and forensic report. Study 2 included participants who self-identified as having experience with FMHA (expert sample); likewise, the tweet was considered less trustworthy, credible, useful, and experts subsequently assigned less weight to the tweet as relevant evidence in forming their opinion about criminal responsibility. Similar findings were reported in study on the influence of social media evidence in parental fitness evaluations (Jones et al., 2020). In two separate studies of laypersons and experts, participants viewed nearly identical information that varied by source type (i.e., Instagram post, a medical note) and parent gender (i.e., mother, father). Both samples rated the Instagram post as less trustworthy and useful than the medical note regardless of which parent was the subject of the post/note. Notably, the effect size for the expert sample almost doubled that of the layperson sample, suggesting experts were significantly more wary of the social media post. Experts also believed the Instagram post should be given less weight than the medical note when determining parental fitness. Of course, these studies only serve as proxies of forensic examiners' and layperson perceptions given they were highly controlled. Real-world forensic cases are far more nuanced. In family court matters, for example, examiners are often inundated with emails, text exchanges, and social media data as one party's attempt to discredit or disgrace the other. However, despite several recognised benefits of social media, a general pattern of skepticism has no doubt emerged across both survey and experimental outcomes.

Underpinnings and Awareness of Bias

Given the hesitancy surrounding social media as collateral data, it is important to explore the underlying causes and build awareness so examiners can approach these data more objectively. One of the most common concerns raised by professionals relates to the authenticity of social media information, with many citing uncertainties about the veracity of information posted online, an inability to confirm authorship, and concern that social media posts do not always reflect an individual's true characteristics (Coffey et al., 2018). Although these concerns are valid, we argue they could (and should) be raised with all forms of collateral sources. For example, it would be erroneous to simply take self and other reports as fact without undertaking proper methods for uncovering the source's veracity, authenticity, and relevance to the referral question. The possibility of dishonesty is why tests of effort and impression management are common in forensic contexts. Similarly, while third-party reports from police, therapists, and even medical records are viewed as highly reliable (Coffey et al., 2018), they too offer an outside and potentially biased perspective that may not fully or accurately reflect the examinee and their presentation. Thus, while social media data may come with a unique set of challenges, there is currently no known evidence to suggest that information posted online is any more or less credible than information obtained from other sources or parties. In fact, recent recommendations for incorporating social media evidence as collateral information maintains that social media should be treated similarly to any other collateral source (Batastini et al., 2020). Ultimately, discounting evidence simply because it was posted to social media violates existing best practices for assessing the relevance and quality of collateral sources in FMHA (Heilbrun et al., 2015).

Although not specific to social media data, commentary by Neal and Grisso (2014) encourages efforts to further unpack cognitive biases and how they may play out in FMHA. While additional research is needed to confirm whether similar types of biases occur in the context of accessing or reviewing social media collateral, literature on decision-making processes and common mental shortcuts or heuristics (i.e., decision aids used to formulate conclusions when answers are not readily apparent; Tversky & Kahneman, 1974), suggests that all humans (forensic examiners included; Neal & Grisso, 2014) are susceptible to thinking errors. To improve awareness of biases, Table 16.1 offers several examples of common cognitive biases that could affect forensic examiners as they search for and interpret social media data sources. Importantly, this list is not exhaustive. Further, while this chapter has so far emphasised hesitancy and skepticism that may lead examiners to disregard the utility of social media in FMHA, some biases may conversely result in an undue overreliance on social media sources.

Where Do We Go from Here?

Despite a growing literature base on social media as collateral in FMHA, the availability of empirical work across subareas of FMHA is limited and, at the time this chapter was written, mostly lacking external validity. Table 16.2 provides suggestions for researchers to help expand our understanding about professional practices and needs, the extent to which biases exist, whether they directly impact psycho-legal opinions and outcomes, and how to minimise their impact. We hope researchers will use and build upon these ideas.

Recommendations for Using Social Media Data to Inform FMHA

Drawing on examiner's endorsed concerns about social media use in FMHA, this final section reviews and highlights best practice recommendations for accessing, managing, and evaluating social media sources in FMHA.

As noted by Coffey et al. (2018), the most common ethical concerns expressed by forensic evaluators when reviewing social media data were the ability to authenticate authorship of the source (e.g., determining if the examinee actually produced or uploaded the content) and its reliability (e.g., whether it was doctored or falsified in any way). Unlike official records, such as medical or academic, where examiners can more easily verify or clarify contents with the professional or agency, the verification of social media often must come from the examinee themselves. This creates an opportunity for error. Consider the potential consequences if a forensic examiner relied upon a long and rambling Facebook post to form the basis of their opinion about the presence of severe mental illness, only to later determine they were misled and someone else authored the post using the examinee's account. While these concerns are valid, social media information is not unique in that respect. Forensic evaluators should always consider the possibility that responses are being manipulated for secondary gain or that collateral contacts may have hidden agendas that influence their statements. In fact, there is no information suggesting social media is more

Table 16.1 Examples of common cognitive biases

Bias	Description	Examples in FMHA HA
Anchoring Bias	Placing too much emphasis or weight on one piece of information when making decisions (usually the first piece of evidence encountered on the subject).	An examiner completed most of his assessment, having come to a general conclusion about an examinee's mental state at the time of the offense. Based on the observed practices of his colleague, the examiner decided to do a quick search of the examinee's social media profiles, which uncovered information that appeared to conflict with his predetermined opinion. Instead of evaluating the merits of the social media data, he believed it to be inconsequential compared to the previously collected information.
		After receiving a referral for a threat assessment, an examiner immediately searched the defendant on Facebook. Exposure to posts showing the defendant celebrating at an LGBTQ+ Pride event subconsciously led the examiner to place less emphasis on other information encountered later in the assessment process, including the alleged victim's report.
Framing Effect	Drawing differing conclusions from the same information, depending on how the information is presented.	In a fitness for duty evaluation, the examiner receives bodycam footage of a physical altercation between a police officer and a citizen, a medical note detailing the citizen's alleged injuries by the officer, and a video shared via Snapchat by a bystander. Although all three sources detailed generally the same information, the examiner believed the Snapchat video to be less credible and disregarded it altogether. However, the bystander video was shot from a different angle and offered another perspective on the incident.
Mere Exposure Effect	Increased preference for things merely due to previous experience with them.	A child custody examiner is sorting through information pulled from both parents' social media profiles. The examiner personally enjoys Twitter and often scrolls through posts when not working. As a result, she inadvertently paid more attention to information pulled from Twitter, which was most often used by the mother in this dispute, than information from other sites like Facebook.

Confirmation
Bias

Searching for, focus on, and believe
information that confirms one's
previously held beliefs while
disregarding conflicting information.

In a disability case, a seasoned examiner with limited social media use (both
personally and professionally) sticks to her established method of relying
on medical records and collateral information from the examinee's
friends and family, even though she recently read about a case in which
social media data were used to discredit a plaintiff's claims.

An examiner is conducting an evaluation involving a workman's
compensation claim. Several data sources suggest the plaintiff is
suffering serious injury after a work-related accident; however, based
on results of psychological testing, the examiner suspects the plaintiff
may be exaggerating. After doing a cursory search of the plaintiff's
social media accounts, the examiner sees a post showing the plaintiff
doing a TikTok dance trend. Without confirming the date or
authenticity of the post, the examiner uses it to support his opinion the
plaintiff is feigning the extent of injuries.

Table 16.2 Suggestions for future research

Prevalence and professional consensus

- While there is evidence suggesting expert agreement on proposed recommendations (see Pirelli et al., 2018), the continued development of and agreement with developing best practice guidelines is needed.
- Exploring the potential mitigating impact of training and/or education on perceptions of social media data and professionals' willingness to integrate it more readily into forensic practice.
- Surveying opinions about the ways in which social media data are collected and should be reported. For example, is there more general support for social media use in FMHA when obtained via discovery materials versus an independent search by the evaluator?
- Mixed method designs should be used to obtain a richer understanding of layperson, expert, and legal personnel (e.g., attorneys) concerns regarding social media sources, particularly in psycho-legal contexts.

Types of biases

- Explorations into common types of biases underlying expert's decision-making regarding social media data are needed. For example, a study providing one group of experts with a social media post from a common source (e.g., Instagram, Facebook) and the other group with a more obscure internet source (e.g., discourse, Tumblr), all with virtually the same information, could provide insight into the mere exposure effect. Similar quantitative approaches could be implemented to cover the various biases likely at play in FMHA.
- Research exploring biases related to culture and diversity factors. For example, examiners may be more likely to misinterpret an examinee's religious posts as evidence of emotional instability if the examinee is from a community of colour or practices a religion unfamiliar to the examiner.
- Empirical studies focusing on ways to successfully reducing biases that may influence how social media data are used in FMHA across different forms of psycho-legal questions.
- Explorations of social media bias within specific types of psycho-legal questions (e.g., threat assessment, disability, criminal responsibility, police candidacy).

Impacts on examiner and legal decision making

- Experimental studies examining the weight relevant parties and legal personnel (e.g., potential jurors, attorneys, experts, judges) place on various collateral sources and the impact these sources have on subsequent psycho-legal decisions or related outcomes (e.g., competency, conditional release, violence risk estimates).

Impacts on expert witness credibility

- Studies examining whether an expert's reliance or inclusion of social media data impacts the credibility of their opinions.
- Examining impacts of cross-examination on experts who use social media data. For example, can cross-examination highlight concerns about social media that decrease the perceived credibility of an expert during testimony? What strategies might experts use on the stand to dismiss efforts to discredit their use of social media?

Review of case law and assessment practices

- Review of specific case law may be helpful to uncover how the use of social media has been challenged or upheld in court. This can help set precedent and inform experts and attorneys as they prepare for court. Systematic reviews of FMHA reports to provide further insight into current practices involving social media data and more specific estimates regarding the frequency of incorporating social media use in the assessment process. For example, researchers could code for specific types of referral questions, forms and platforms of internet data used, how the data were obtained (personal search, discovery materials, provided by a 3rd party), if social media access was explicitly discussed in the consent process with examinees, the opinion proffered by the evaluator, and if/how social media data are discussed in reports and testimony (e.g., are procedures for accessing, vetting, and weighing these data reported?).

(Continued)

Table 16.2 (Continued)

Methodological advances
- Current empirical studies provide only snapshots of the true assessment process or courtroom experience. Future empirical studies should develop methodologies to increase external validity by more closely mimicking FMHA procedures (e.g., exposing examiners to multiple types of sources at one time) and legal proceedings (e.g., including opinions from opposing experts in which one examiner used social media and the other did not; adding a jury deliberation component). Externally valid studies will help the field better understand the factors and circumstances that influence opinions when social media is involved in a forensic case.

Nuanced forms of social media
- Studies examining differences across various forms of social media. For example, varying the presentation of text-only and video content (e.g., Twitter posts and Instagram Reels). Images or videos may be more influential to forensic opinions and/or have the potential to include irrelevant or biasing information (e.g., objects in the background, facial expressions, symbols of political ideology) than text.
- Comparisons between social media sources to determine whether some are viewed as more trustworthy, credible, verifiable, and reliable than others. Importantly, these perceptions may change over time. At the time of this publication, for example, Facebook was being heavily scrutinised in the U.S. legal system for promoting divisive and false information; thus, data from Facebook and its affiliated companies may be seen as less valid than other sources.

---

at-risk for these types of distortions. Authentication and veracity of social media data may involve directly asking examinees or 3rd parties with personal knowledge about the data's origin and considering it in context with other available sources (e.g., does it fit a pattern of behaviour documented across sources; does it seem uncharacteristic based on other known information about the examinee or their circumstances). Examiners may also rely on the courts to determine authenticity through the evidence admissibility process, as attorneys wishing to have their client's social media data used must themselves demonstrate the evidence is what it is claimed to be (Federal Rules of Evidence 901(a)). All digital evidence is subject to the same admissibility standards as other types of evidence (Sozio, 2017).

Examiners also appear concerned about the relevance of social media data. In Coffey et al. (2018), one examiner was worried that the use of social media would "add to my biases while bringing minimal or ambiguous data value" (p. 352). While we argue social media can be relevant (even central in some cases), we also agree there is a very real possibility forensic evaluators will come across information online that is superfluous, and potentially biasing, to the psycho-legal issue at hand. Among others, examples include political ideologies, religious affiliations, sexual preferences, or cultural values. In other cases, normative behaviours could be misinterpreted as problematic; for example, assuming beer bottles in the background of a mother's Instagram post (shared by the father) mean she was intoxicated while supervising her young children. In a similar vein, Pirelli et al. (2016) warn that simply "liking" or "retweeting" a post should not be considered relevant unless it is directly related to the psycho-legal question.

Liking content from a known terrorist organisation, for example, could be relevant in a threat assessment case in which the examinee is believed to be engaged in radicalised activity. Importantly, biases regarding relevancy may also sway in the opposite direction: information encountered while reviewing social media could cause an evaluator to identify with the examinee (e.g., discovering similar interests or beliefs, sharing a marginalised identity), thereby making them more likely to render an opinion in favour of the examinee. As Zapf and Dror (2017) note, "It is naïve to think that a forensic evaluator can only collect and consider relevant information, especially since many times it is not clear what is relevant and what is irrelevant until all collected materials have been reviewed ..." (p. 233). Yet, forensic evaluators must be cognizant of the line between necessary information and not infringing on the liberties of their examinees. However, this issue is again not unique to social media, as examiners are often exposed to collateral sources that may be irrelevant or include irrelevant information (e.g., receiving discovery materials that include offense details when the question is about adjudicative competency). To mitigate potential biases, it is recommended examiners limit their exposure to erroneous information to the extent possible (perhaps having a third party weed out obviously irrelevant data first), systematically document what was reviewed and its impact on the examiner's conceptualisation of the examinee, and considering rival hypotheses before committing to a final opinion (see Zapf et al., 2018). Seeking consultation with a colleague to cross-check key decisions made at each stage of the process may also be helpful. Thus, relevancy issues should not necessarily deter examiners from considering social media sources.

Some examiners may fear courts will consider their reports less credible with this type of information. However, we could find no case law or research study indicating courts' reluctance to accept reports with social media as a collateral or viewing reports as less credible. Even the American Bar Association (ABA) has addressed and provided guidance on social media evidence in legal cases and courts have allowed this evidence numerous times. Thus, it seems safe to assume forensic examiners would not be unduly scrutinised for their use. However, as with any data sources used in FMHA, evaluators must have a clear rationale for consulting it and be able to explain its importance to addressing the referral question. This is consistent with initial recommendations outlined in Pirelli et al., (2016) in which the authors stated, "Forensic examiners should always be prepared to discuss with fact finders their methods and the data they considered, regardless of the weight they placed on it" (p. 15). This could be taken to include methods for not only identifying data, but also vetting it, determining its relevance to the evaluation, and any bias mitigation strategies used.

Finally, in response to examiners' reported concern about examinees' privacy and consent to access social media information (Coffey et al., 2018), courts have ruled that both public and private social media information can be admissible in litigation. Nonetheless, Pirelli et al. (2016) recommended discussing data found during any independent internet searches with the examinee and allowing them to address the information and provide context, if needed. Not only can this approach provide a sense of transparency, but consulting with an examinee about relevant social media information may also be particularly useful if there are unresolved questions or if the examiner believes they need more information that cannot be clarified through other means. This is like the treatment of other types of collateral information a forensic examiner may rely on when formulating their opinion.

Below is a summary of initial recommendations for appropriately using social media information in forensic cases that extends from cited research and ethical guidelines.

1   Forensic evaluators should be transparent in their use of social media data with examinees, courts, and/or retaining parties. All data sources used should be listed in the sources of information section of the report and evaluators must be specific in describing how the information was obtained and incorporated.

2   Evaluators are likely on safest ground when copies of social media information are included as part of the discovery packet provided by attorneys or the court. However, forensic evaluators may conduct their own search if they have a reasonable belief that social media information would be useful. In this case, evaluators are strongly advised against searching for the sake of curiosity and to take steps to avoid potentially biasing and useless information. One suggestion is to develop relevant search criteria at the outset and stay within these criteria to the extent possible, expanding the search only if there is clear justification to do so. Examiners who perform their own search are also advised to inform the courts about relevant data so it can be considered for inclusion in discovery. In situations where an examiner becomes aware of a potentially relevant social media source, they may consider asking the court to extract and authenticate it on their behalf.

3   Once information is obtained via social media, forensic evaluators have an ethical responsibility to determine its relevance to the psycholegal question. While we have already discussed this issue at length, we reiterate that most information uncovered in broadband social media searches is irrelevant to the psycho-legal question and should be approached with caution.

4   Relatedly, forensic evaluators have an ethical responsibility to determine the authenticity of the information. This may require a conversation with the examinee, consideration of other available information, or reliance on the court. Failure to properly authenticate collateral information can place the examiner in the precarious situation of having to retract their findings, or being embarrassed on the witness stand.

5   At all phases of interacting with social media data, forensic evaluators are encouraged to use effective strategies to minimise cognitive errors. In addition to strategies noted earlier, this may involve consultation/supervision with or peer-review by a trusted colleague who feels free to disagree and willing to check for biased and prejudicial information.

We recognise these recommendations are not comprehensive and ack professional consensus. We encourage the development of formal guidance that involves a multi-disciplinary team of experts in psychology and law with designated comment periods for general members of the profession. Guidance may vary depending on jurisdiction of practice.

Practical Case Exercises

We conclude by presenting two brief hypothetical cases that exemplify the challenges encountered by forensic examiners while evaluating information from social media. Interested readers are referred to Batastini and Vitacco (2020) – an edited volume that includes more extensive case examples across multiple types of criminal and civil forensic issues.

Scenario 1

A psychologist has been hired by the court to conduct a child custody evaluation. As part of that court order, the judge asked for an examination of which parent, if any, the child should be primarily placed while considering the best interests of the child. As part of the examination, the psychologist interviews both parents. After interviewing the child's father, the father hands the examiner a folder with copies of pictures from an Instagram account ostensibly belonging to his ex-wife (the mother in this case) where she is taking selfies at her child's eighth birthday party with an unknown male and they seem overly friendly. There are pictures of her child, other children, and the mother clearly touching the other man. The mother denies the man is a romantic partner or in any way involved with the children. Consider the following questions:

1 How might the psychologist handle the issue of authentication? In other words, what steps could be taken to ensure the Instagram post was authored by the mother and that the content was not doctored?
2 How should the psychologist document their acquisition of the Instagram post? Should the father's actions be reported to the court?
3 Using the suggestions earlier in the chapter, how could the psychologist ensure they are not allowing bias to influence their use of the evidence or opinion about custody?
4 If you were the psychologist in this case, what other information would you attempt to collect or consult?

Scenario 2

A psychiatrist is asked to complete a violence risk assessment on an individual who made some general threats at her workplace. On their own, the psychiatrist typed the examinee's name into a search engine and came across her Facebook page. The Facebook page primarily consisted of family photographs from vacations and pictures of two children's school events. There were also two noticeable posts from a Senate candidate who was clearly pro-Second Amendment that the examinee "liked". There was no apparent commentary from the examinee under these posts. Consider the following questions:

1   How might the psychiatrist's own political views or experiences with gun ownership impact their perceptions of the post's relevance or the examinee's risk of harm?
2   To what extent is Facebook information relevant in this case? Does it help support or discredit claims of workplace threats?
3   Using the suggestions earlier in the chapter, how could the psychiatrist ensure they are not allowing bias to influence their use of the evidence or forensic opinion?
4   If you were the psychiatrist in this case, what other information would you attempt to collect or consult?

Conclusion

Skepticism regarding the use of social media information in FMHA seems likely for the foreseeable future. A primary reason for mistrust surrounding the use of social media information in forensic evaluations may be a lack of education and clear direction from both the psychological and legal communities. Like many novel issues, the law and science take time to develop guidelines for navigating these challenging issues. However, increasing attention has been given to how forensic mental health practitioners should handle social media data and inherent biases associated with their use. Like most collateral information, information obtained from social media is not dispositive but can add nuance to a forensic evaluation and can certainly be an important part of the decision-making process.

Note

1 David Bowie was a musician, performer, actor, and cultural icon.

References

Allcott, H., Gentzkow, M., & Yu, C. (2019). Trends in the diffusion of misinformation on social media. *Research and Politics, 6*(2), 3. 10.1177/2053168019848554

Arnold, A. (2018, December 30). *Here's how social media can be used against you in court.* https://www.forbes.com/sites/andrewarnold/2018/12/30/heres-how-social-media-can-be-used-against-you-in-court/?sh=22e2fdc26344

Asay, P. A., & Lal, A. (2014). Who's Googled whom? Trainees' Internet and online social networking experiences, behaviors, and attitudes with clients and supervisors. *Training and Education in Professional Psychology, 8*(2), 105. 10.1037/tep0000035

Association of State and Provincial Psychology Boards. (2020, October 9). *Guidelines for the use of social media by psychologists in practice and by psychology regulatory bodies.* https://cdn.ymaws.com/www.asppb.net/resource/resmgr/guidelines/final_oct_9-2020_guidelines_pdf

Batastini, A. B., Vitacco, M. J., & Bozeman, A. R. (2020). General recommendations for integrating internet-based data in forensic mental health assessments and what we still need to know. In Batastini, A., & Vitacco, M. (Eds.), *Forensic mental health evaluations in the digital age: A practitioner's guide to using internet-based data*. New York: Springer International.

Batastini, A. B., Vitacco, M. J., Jones, A. C., & Davis, R. M. (2021). Perceived credibility of social media data as a collateral source in criminal responsibility evaluations using an experimental design. *International Journal of Forensic Mental Health*, 20(4)317–332. 10.1080/14999013.2021.1880504

Coffey, C. A., Batastini, A. B., & Vitacco, M. J. (2018). Clues from the digital world: A survey of clinicians' reliance on social media as collateral data in forensic evaluations. *Professional Psychology: Research and Practice*, 49(5–6), 345. 10.1037/pro0000206

DiLillo, D., & Gale, E. B. (2011). To Google or not to Google: Graduate students' use of the Internet to access personal information about clients. *Training and Education in Professional Psychology*, 5(3), 160. 10.1037/a0024441

DiBianca, M. (2014). Discovery and preservation of social media evidence. Bus. L. Today, 1.

Gearhart, S. , Moe, A. , & Zhang, B. (2020). Hostile media bias on social media: Testing the effect of user comments on perceptions of news bias and credibility. *Human Behavior & Emerging Technologies*, 2(2), 140–148.

Heilbrun, K., NeMoyer, A., King, C. M., & Galloway, M. (2015). Using third party information in forensic mental health assessment: A critical review. *Court Review*, 51(1), 16–35.

Hsieh-Yee, I. (2021). Can we trust social media? *Internet Reference Services Quarterly*, 25(1), 9–23. 10.1080/10875301.2021.1947433

Hughs, L. (2009). Ethics Corner: Is it ethical to Google patients? *Psychiatric News*, 44, 9 & 11. 10.1176/pn.44.9.0011

Jones, A. C. T., Davis, R. M., Batastini, A. B., & Vitacco, M. J. (2020, March). *Social media and gender bias in parental fitness evaluations: An empirical study of forensic expert and layperson perceptions*. Paper presented at the annual meeting of the American Psychology-Law Society, New Orleans, Louisiana.

Kaslow, F. W., Patterson, T., & Gottlieb, M. (2011). Ethical dilemmas in psychologists accessing Internet data: Is it justified?. *Professional Psychology: Research and Practice*, 42(2), 105. 10.1037/a0022002

Knoll, J. L., & Resnick, P. J. (2007). Insanity defense evaluations: Toward a model for evidence- based practice. *Brief Treatment and Crisis Intervention*, 8(1), 92–110. 10.1093/brief-treatment/mhm024

Kolmes, K., & Taube, D. O. (2014). Seeking and finding our clients on the Internet: Boundary considerations in cyberspace. *Professional Psychology: Research and Practice*, 45(1), 3. 10.1037/a0029958

Murrie, D. C., & Warren, J. I. (2005). Clinician Variation in Rates of Legal Sanity Opinions: Implications for Self-Monitoring. *Professional Psychology: Research and Practice*, 36(5), 519. 10.1037/0735-7028.36.5.519

Murrie, D. C., Boccaccini, M. T., Guarnera, L. A., & Rufino, K. A. (2013). Are forensic experts biased by the side that retained them? *Psychological Science*, 24(10), 1889–1897. 10.1177/0956797613481812

Neal, T. M. (2017). Identifying the forensic psychologist role. *The Ethical Practice of Forensic Psychology*, 1–31.

Neal, T. M. (2018). Discerning bias in forensic psychological reports in insanity cases. *Behavioral Sciences & the Law, 36*(3), 325–338. 10.1002/bsl.2346

Neal, T., & Brodsky, S. L. (2016). Forensic psychologists' perceptions of bias and potential correction strategies in forensic mental health evaluations. *Psychology, Public Policy, and Law, 22*(1), 58. 10.1037/law0000077

Neal, T., & Grisso, T. (2014). The cognitive underpinnings of bias in forensic mental health evaluations. *Psychology, Public Policy, and Law, 20*(2), 200. 10.1037/a0035824

Otto, R. K., Slobogin, C., & Greenberg, S. A. (2007). Legal and ethical issues in accessing and utilizing third-party information. In A. M. Goldstein (Ed.), *Forensic psychology: Emerging topics and expanding roles* (p. 190–205). Chichester: John Wiley & Sons Inc.

Pirelli, G., Hartigan, S., & Zapf, P. A. (2018). Using the internet for collateral information in forensic mental health evaluations. *Behavioral Sciences & the Law, 36*(2), 157–169. 10.1002/bsl.2334

Pirelli, G., Otto, R. K., & Estoup, A. (2016). Using internet and social media data as collateral sources of information in forensic evaluations. *Professional Psychology: Research and Practice, 47*(1), 12. 10.1037/pro0000061

Sharma, S. (2021, September 17). *Texas teen murders parents and sister, shares photos of dead family on social media before killing himself.* https://www.independent.co.uk/news/world/americas/crime/texas-teen-murder-social-media-b1921872.html

Sozio, M. B. (2017, April 27). *Authenticating digital evidence at trial.* https://www.americanbar.org/groups/business_law/publications/blt/2017/04/03_sozio/

Spence, P. R., Lachlan, K. A., Westerman, D. & Spates, S. A. (2013). Where the gates matter less: Ethnicity and perceived source credibility in social media health messages. *Howard Journal of Communications, 24*(1), 1–16. 10.1080/10646175.2013.748593

Tversky, A., & Kahneman, D. (1974). Judgment under uncertainty: Heuristics and biases. *Science, 185*, 1124–1131. 10.1126/science.185.4157.1124.

Zapf, P. A., & Dror, I. E. (2017). Understanding and mitigating bias in forensic evaluation: Lessons from forensic science. *The International Journal of Forensic Mental Health, 16*(3), 227–238. 10.1080/14999013.2017.1317302

Zapf, P. A., Kukucka, J., Kassin, S. M., & Dror, I. E. (2018). Cognitive bias in forensic mental health assessment: Evaluator beliefs about its nature and scope. *Psychology, Public Policy, and Law, 24*(1), 1–10. 10.1037/law0000153

Part III

Diversity and Forensic Populations: Theoretical and Practical Approaches

17 Gender-Sensitive Violence Risk Assessment

Vivienne de Vogel

Introduction

In the last two decades there has been increasing awareness of the unique needs of females who have offended, and substantially more theoretical and empirical research has been published on the assessment, management, and treatment of women in forensic services (see Brown & Gelsthorpe, 2021; de Vogel & Nicholls, 2016; Smith et al., 2021). Women and girls represent a minority in forensic mental health care and the criminal justice system (about 6% to 10%; Walmsley, 2017), however, a disproportionate growth of females entering forensic services has been observed in many countries (Nicholls et al., 2015). Still, most of the assessment tools and treatment programs currently being used in forensic services or the criminal justice system have mainly been developed and validated in male samples. This is worrying as the results can have a major impact on the future lives of these girls or women and their relatives, and we do not have sufficient evidence yet as to whether these tools and methods are also reliable for them. There is reason to assume that gender bias exists both in items of instruments as well as in assessment processes, especially for females from minority groups (Motz et al., 2021). In general, gender bias is still a detectable and powerful force in psychological practice which may lead to the inappropriate use and overuse of certain diagnoses in women, for instance the borderline personality disorder (American Psychological Association, Girls and Women Guidelines Group, 2018). Better assessment and more profound understanding of risks and mental health needs of females in forensic services is crucial to be able to provide the most adequate treatment. This is not only important for these females who have offended but also for preventing the intergenerational transmission of violence and crime and for the acknowledgement of their victims. Research has shown that children of antisocial or violent mothers have increased risks of developing serious mental health problems, including substance abuse, and delinquent, violence, or other risky behaviours (Kim et al., 2009).

One of the most relevant questions in forensic services is whether the use of commonly used risk assessment tools is reliable and valid for females and whether more gender-sensitive violence risk assessment is needed. Since the beginning of this century, the use of structured violence risk assessment tools has become

DOI: 10.4324/9781003230977-20

standard practice in most (forensic) mental health care and criminal justice set-tings (Douglas & Otto, 2021). A good violence risk assessment provides an insight into risk and protective factors and offers concrete guidelines for risk manage-ment and treatment and is thus of great importance. In the past two decades, major progress has been made in the area of structured violence risk assessment and multiple tools have become available to guide mental health professionals in the process of risk assessment and management. It is often assumed that these tools are "gender-neutral" (see for a discussion Yesberg et al., 2015), but the majority of risk assessment instruments have been developed based on vio-lence risk research conducted primarily in male samples. Some tools inherently include bias or unclarities in respect of gender, for instance, most instruments assessing risk of intimate partner violence seem to take the view of a male per-petrator and female victim. Another example is the widely-used *Psychopathy Checklist-Revised* (PCL-R; Hare, 2003) to assess psychopathy, an important risk factor for violence (Leistico et al., 2008). In the PCL-R, item 1 *Glibness/superficial charm* literally describes "macho men" as indicator for coding the item which is obviously difficult to code for women. Furthermore, research into the psycho-metric properties of these tools has been carried out mostly within male popu-lations. There are indications that the results of most commonly used assessment tools are less valid for female populations and that investment in gender-sensitive tools is necessary (e.g., Brennan et al., 2012; de Vogel et al., 2019; Salisbury et al., 2016). Belisle and Salisbury (2021) recently discussed the literature into risk/needs assessment for system-involved girls and concluded that none of the commonly used tools, some of which are marketed as gender-informed, are truly gender-neutral. Most tools tend to overclassify or misclassify risks in girls, as de-monstrated by empirical studies. Nonetheless, the use of these instruments with justice-involved females is common, and sometimes even mandated. The results of such assessments can have a strong impact on the future prospects of these females, particularly when they are used in pretrial assessments or in court to decide upon the necessity of (prolonged) mandatory treatment or incarceration. In fact, mis-classification may lead to violating the risk principle and may potentially increase likelihood of recidivism and failure to provide these females with the treatment they need (Belisle & Salisbury, 2021). To date, only a few risk assessment instruments are available that take gender-sensitive risks and needs into account.

In this chapter, the value of gender-sensitive violence risk assessment will be addressed. First, the literature into gender bias will be discussed, followed by a discussion of gender-specific risk and protective factors, followed by the value of commonly used risk assessment instruments for females. Finally, some re-commendations regarding gender-sensitive assessment and gender-responsive treatment will be provided.

Definition of Gender

It is first important to define the terms sex, gender, gender-sensitive and gender-responsive. The term sex refers to the biological aspects of being female or male whereas the term gender includes psychological, social, and cultural aspects associated with the biological aspects (see for a discussion Javdani et al., 2011a). This chapter mainly refers to the terms gender-sensitive (being aware of possible gender differences) and gender-responsive (responding to possible gender differences). By adopting these terms, gender is accounted for as a factor that works both ways. It should be noted that there is increasing awareness of multiple forms of gender identity, and society is becoming more sensitive to the needs of non-binary or transgender people, as well as for imprisoned populations (e.g., American Psychological Association, 2015; Hill et al., 2020; Sevelius & Jenness, 2017).

Gender Bias in Forensic Assessment

Gender bias is a construct that refers to beliefs, attitudes, and/or predispositions that involve preconceived and stereotypical ideas about the roles, abilities, and characteristics of women and men (American Psychological Association, Girls and Women Guidelines Group, 2018, p. 31). Gender bias is still considered to be a detectable and powerful factor in psychological practice which may lead to the inappropriate use and overuse of certain diagnoses in women, like the borderline personality disorder. This can be problematic, not only for females but also for males. For instance, symptoms of depressive and anxiety disorders are more easily reported, recognised, and diagnosed in women compared to men, possibly leading to underdiagnosing in males (Bekker & van Mens-Verhulst, 2007; Kuehner, 2017). Overall, more knowledge is needed about mental disorders with unequal prevalence rates between the sexes to provide the most effective treatment (Bekker & van Mens-Verhulst, 2007).

Gender bias is also a potential risk in forensic assessment processes, both in instrument items, and in the way these instruments are applied (see Brown & Gelsthorpe, 2021; Motz et al., 2021; Smith et al., 2021). Specific needs of females may be overlooked, and over or underdiagnosed because women are more likely than men to internalise problems (American Psychological Association, Girls and Women Guidelines Group, 2018). As forensic assessment is often focused on screening for externalising disorders, cluster B personality disorders, psychopathy and risk factors, internalising disorders like depression, anxiety, or PTSD may be missed. This has been reported to be particularly true for females from minority groups. In their recent book, Motz and colleagues (2021) describe the risks of gender bias and the vulnerabilities of marginalised women by virtue of their religion, cultural background, sexuality or past experiences. Especially BAME (Black Asian Ethnic Minority) women are often viewed through a lens of gender stereotyping that can blind those who encounter them to trauma and vulnerability (Motz et al., 2021, p. 195).

The use of reliable and validated gender-sensitive assessment tools is important to prevent gender bias and the misreporting of mental health problems and possible resulting stigmatisation in women in forensic services. The APA provides *Guidelines for Psychological Practice with Girls and Women* with the purpose to assist psychologists in the provision of gender-sensitive, culturally competent, and developmentally appropriate psychological practice with girls and women across the lifespan from all social classes, ethnic and racial groups, sexual orientations, abilities and disabilities, and other diversity statuses in the U.S. and globally.

Guideline 7 is important in this respect: Psychologists strive to assign diagnoses to girls and women only if and when diagnosis is necessary, use unbiased assessment tools, and bring to bear an understanding of the history of misuses and gender biases and diagnoses and assessment (American Psychological Association, Girls and Women Guidelines Group, 2018, p. 15).

Stereotypes with Respect to Offending

It should be noted that there may also be gender bias and stereotyping in society with respect to offending and in the criminal justice sentencing (Smith et al., 2021). To illustrate, it has been clearly demonstrated in intimate partner violence research that gender stereotypes play a role in reaction of society towards intimate partner violence. Overall, it is more difficult to see females as potential perpetrators, and males as potential victims, which may lead to secondary victimisation and inadequate interventions for both males and females (see for instance, Bates et al., 2019; Morgan & Wells, 2016; Stanziani et al., 2020). In general, there seems to be a tendency to treat females who have offended more leniently than their male counterparts, leading to shorter prison sentences, treatment instead of punishment, and to more insanity defences (Crocker et al., 2002; de Vogel & de Spa, 2018; Jeffries et al., 2003). Curry et al. (2004) discuss several theories explaining this phenomenon, for example, the blameworthiness attribution. This attribution asserts that judges make use of stereotypes; they see women as less to blame and put more emphasis on mental health problems. Females who demonstrate antisocial or violent behaviour deviates from standard social norm of "caring mothers" and, therefore, "must be insane or evil". The latter seems to be particularly true for sexual offenses (Wijkman et al., 2010) or terrorism offenses (Motz et al., 2021).

Gender Differences in Offending and Mental Health Needs

Empirical studies have found substantial gender differences in pathways to offending and nature of offending, and also in responses from the criminal justice system and society (see for a discussion of policies and societal factors Javdani et al. 2011b). Overall, research has demonstrated that the nature, severity, frequency, and victims of violent offending by women are significantly different from those committed by men, as well as the alleged motives for offending (for more elaborate discussions see de Vogel & de Spa, 2018). Female violence is more often reactive and relational and less often characterised as instrumental and sexual. Furthermore, violence by women less often results in serious injuries, is less visible and more subtle, for instance, in intimate partner violence and child abuse (Nicholls et al., 2015; Odgers et al., 2005).

Both men and women who enter forensic services have complex histories with high rates of victimisation and multiple mental health problems. However, several important gender differences have been found in empirical studies. Most importantly, women in forensic services compared to their male counterparts have: 1) more severe or complex trauma history, especially a higher prevalence of sexual abuse; 2) more comorbidity; 3) more internalising disorders like borderline personality disorder and posttraumatic stress disorder and less often antisocial personality disorder or narcissistic personality disorder; and 3) higher prevalence of self-harming behaviour (e.g., Coid et al., 2000; de Vogel et al., 2016; Zlotnick et al., 2008). Hence, females have different and usually more complex mental health needs than males. It should be noted that the above-described gender biases in diagnostic processes may also have played a role in these studies.

Risk Factors for Violence in Women

Most risk factors for violence, like previous violence, young age at first violence, and substance abuse, have been demonstrated to be valid for both men and women (Andrews et al., 2012; Brennan et al., 2012). However, there are some risk factors that are specifically valid for females or that have a different impact on women compared to men, such as pregnancy at a young age (Messer et al., 2004), prostitution (Morgan & Patton, 2002), and self-harm (Völlm & Dolan, 2009), although the predictive accuracy of these factors for violent recidivism needs to be demonstrated more firmly. A distinction can be made between risk factors to which women were exposed more often (e.g., sexual victimisation) and factors that have a stronger effect on later violent or criminal behaviour on women than men (e.g., disruptions in social relationships).

An example of a risk factor that manifests differently in females compared to males and may have a different impact on the risk of recidivism is psychopathy. Psychopathy has been found to be an important risk factor for (violent) re-cidivism in different populations and settings (Leistico et al., 2008). The PCL-R is a widely used tool to assess psychopathy, but the majority of studies into psy-chopathy and the PCL-R have been conducted in male samples and the as-sumption that the conceptualisation of psychopathy can be generalised to women has not been sufficiently proven. Although the PCL-R is assumed to have re-levance in female offenders (Nicholls, et al., 2005), concerns have been expressed about whether the PCL-R captures the construct of psychopathy satisfactorily in women (Beryl et al., 2014; de Vogel & Lancel, 2016; Forouzan & Cooke, 2005). It has been suggested that because women demonstrate fewer antisocial beha-viours, and generally have a later onset of antisocial behaviour than men, several of the PCL-R items are less suitable to assess the core traits of psychopathy in women (Dolan & Völlm, 2009). A recent study measuring invariance of the PCL-R for gender concluded that it seems reasonable to expect that specific scoring adjustments might go a long way in bringing about more equivalent assessment of psychopathic features in men and women (Klein Haneveld et al., 2021). Smith and colleagues (2021) developed the *Clinical and Forensic Interview Schedule for the PCL-R: Adapted for women*, which may be helpful for mental health practitioners.

Protective Factors for Violence in Women

Evidence has been found that females respond differently to protective factors compared to males. For example; close family ties, positive social relationships, sound finances, and being religious were found to have a stronger protective effect on females than on males (Hart et al., 2007). Another factor that is considered to have potentially strong protective influences in females is self-efficacy (van Voorhis et al., 2010). Rodermond and colleagues (2015) reviewed the literature into gender differences in desistance and suggested that the positive effects of family, social network, and community factors are particularly strong for women in combination with a willingness or motivation to change and a sense of agency.

The Value of Commonly Used Risk Assessment Instruments in Women

Research has demonstrated that unstructured clinical judgement of violence risk is sensitive to gender-biases. Both male and female mental health professionals tend to underestimate the risk for violence in females who have offended (Skeem et al., 2005) and the use of structured tools is recommended to diminish the chance of gender bias. The most commonly used structured risk assessment tools can be divided into actuarial tools, and tools which employ the Structured Professional Judgment (SPJ) method. An important distinction between actuarial and SPJ tools is how the final judgement is arrived at. In actuarial tools, the final judgement is obtained via an algorithm, whereas in SPJ tools information should be integrated, combined, and weighed by the assessor to come to a structured, individualised final judgement. An example of a widely used actuarial tool for general offending is the *Level of Service Inventory* (LSI, or revised versions, see Andrews & Bonta, 2000). Overall, research has demonstrated reasonably good predictive accuracy for the LSI in both male and female populations (Geraghty, & Woodhams, 2015; Marshall et al., 2021; Olver et al., 2014), although there are also some reported disadvantages on the use of the LSI in females (see Salisbury et al., 2016). With respect to females who have committed sexual offenses, it was recently concluded in a study into 739 females who had committed sexual offences that the commonly used actuarial tool, the STATIC-99R (Phenix et al., 2016) was not a valid predictor and thus not suitable for use in women (Marshall et al., 2020).

One of the most widely used SPJ risk assessment instruments for violence in forensic psychiatry is the *Historical Clinical Risk management-20* (HCR-20; Webster et al., 1997) or its revision, the *Historical, Clinical, Risk management-20 Version 3* (HCR-20^{V3}; Douglas et al., 2013). Several studies found lower predictive validity for the HCR-20 Version 2 for females than males (see the reviews of Garcia-Mansilla et al., 2009; McKeown, 2010). Yet, a meta-analysis showed that the HCR-20 had the best predictive efficacy among samples containing higher proportions of women, patients with Schizophrenia, and Caucasians (O'Shea et al., 2013). To date, there are only a few studies examining the predictive validity of the HCR-20^{V3} for women. Green and colleagues (2016) evaluated the HCR-20^{V3} with 24 female and 100 male insanity acquittals and found that women exhibited similar risk factors as men, although two items were rated higher for women (*Relationships* and *Traumatic experiences*). The relationship between scale scores and violence was higher among men than women, although gender was not a significant moderator in logistic regression analyses predicting likelihood of violence. In a Dutch multi-centre study with a sample of 78 discharged female forensic psychiatric patients, it was found that various risk assessment tools, including both Versions 2 and 3 of the HCR-20 and a gender-specific additional tool, the *Female Additional Manual* (FAM; de Vogel et al., 2014, for further *Gender-sensitive Violence Risk Assessment instruments*) had moderate predictive validity for general recidivism, but low predictive validity for violent recidivism (de Vogel et al., 2019). The FAM performed better than the HCR-20 but did not provide incremental predictive value to the HCR-20^{V3}.

The *Short-Term Assessment of Risk and Treatability* (START; Webster et al., 2009) is an SPJ tool for the short-term prediction of different forms of risk, including violence to others. There are several studies published into the value of the START in female populations which found good predictive accuracy (de Vogel et al., 2019; O'Shea & Dickens, 2015; Viljoen et al., 2011). Predictive accuracy of SPJ tools assessing protective factors was found to be lower in females compared to males (Viljoen et al., 2016). In the *Structured Assessment of Protective Factors for violence risk* (SAPROF; de Vogel et al., 2012) the most accurate predictors for abstention from violence differed. For men, the protective factors *Self-control, Work,* and *Attitudes towards authority* were the strongest predictors for not committing violent incidents during treatment, whereas for women, *Leisure activities, Coping* and *Intelligence* were the strongest (de Vries Robbé et al., 2016).

Summarising, it seems that most commonly used tools, like the LSI, HCR-20^{V3}, and START have some predictive value and can be used reliably in female populations. However, the assessor should be cognizant of the limited and sometimes ambivalent research results in females and exert caution in the interpretation of the results, especially when important decisions need to be made, for example, in pretrial assessments. Especially in female ethnic minority groups, practitioners should be cautious in their interpretation of risk assessment tools, as validity has not yet been tested. More in general, cross-cultural bias in risk assessment is an important topic that warrants further investigation (see for an overview Venner et al., 2020).

Gender-Sensitive Violence Risk Assessment Instruments

Only a few risk assessment tools have been developed or adapted for use with females. One of the earliest examples is the *Early Assessment Risk List for Girls* (EARL-21G; Levene et al., 2001) which was developed for assessing antisocial behaviour in girls between 6 and 12 years old. This tool contains risk factors valid for both boys and girls but also includes two items specific to girls: *Caregiver-daughter interaction* and *Sexual development*. The reliability, predictive validity and clinical applicability of the EARL-21G have been found to be reasonably good (Augimeri et al., 2021).

The LSI has been adapted for use in women to predict general recidivism (see Salisbury et al., 2009; van Voorhis et al., 2010). The results for this adapted LSI for women show that both gender-sensitive factors and gender-neutral factors were predictive of misconduct in prison and general recidivism after release (Salisbury et al., 2009; van Voorhis et al., 2010). Furthermore, a few actuarial instruments have been developed specifically for women who have offended. The *Women's Risk Needs Assessments* (van Voorhis et al., 2010; van Voorhis et al., 2013) are actuarial tools that assess both gender-neutral (e.g., substance abuse, criminal history, financial problems) and gender-responsive (e.g., sexual trauma, mental health issues, relationship conflict) factors in female prisoners. The *Security Reclassification Scale for Women* (SRSW: Blanchette & Taylor, 2007) was developed to anchor security level review decisions for federally sentenced female offenders in Canada.

The FAM is an SPJ tool that was developed in 2007 based on a literature review, interviews with mental health professionals, and a pilot study in a Dutch gender-mixed forensic psychiatric hospital. It was originally designed as an additional manual to the HCR-20 and in 2013 adapted for use with the HCR-20^{V3}. The FAM contains additional guidelines to two historical items of the HCR-20^{V3} (*Personality disorder* and *Traumatic experiences*) and eight new items with specific relevance to women (e.g., *Prostitution, Suicidal behaviour/self-harm*). Furthermore, the tool includes three extra risk final judgements: the risk for *Self-destructive behaviour, Victimisation,* and *Non-violent criminal behaviour*. These three judgements should be seen as experimental as there is currently limited empirical evidence supporting the assumption that the risk factors in the FAM are related to these risks. Still, the distinction between the different types of risk may be useful for clinical practice. To date, only a few studies have been published into the value of the FAM, and most of these studies included only small samples. These studies have shown good interrater reliability and moderate predictive validity for recidivism in females, but no incremental validity to the HCR-20^{V3} (see de Vogel et al., 2018; de Vogel et al., 2019; Green et al., 2016; Strand & Selenius, 2019). Much more research is needed into the FAM, as well as into other risk gender-sensitive assessment tools in different female populations, including consideration of not only psychometric properties but also potential clinical value of using these tools. In addition, future research may also take into account other outcomes like self-destructive behaviour and victimisation and pay more attention to female-specific protective factors.

Concluding Remarks and Recommendations for Clinical Practice

As described in this chapter, gender bias can be a major issue in both forensic and non-forensic psychological or risk assessments and practitioners should always be cognizant of possible gender bias and take steps to eliminate bias. In general, it is important, not only for practitioners but also for decision-makers to be aware of the possibility that bias may affect the reliability and validity of the assessment and potentially have serious consequences for defendants (Neal & Grisso, 2014). Therefore, it is essential that violence risk assessment instruments are relevant to the context and to the particular justice-involved person, and that they are employed by trained and experienced evaluators who take measures to limit potential biases (Neal et al., 2019). In the literature, several bias mitigation strategies are described, like consultation of colleagues and limiting exposure to irrelevant contextual information (see for example Croskerry et al., 2013; Neal & Brodsky, 2016).

The current body of knowledge leads to the conclusion that there are several notable differences between females compared to males in forensic services that assessors need to take into account. For instance, a substantially higher prevalence of internalising disorders and self-injury behaviours has been found, as well as more complex trauma history, especially sexual abuse. The routine use of reliable and validated gender-sensitive tools for risk assessment and for internalising and externalising disorders for both men and women is recommended. This corresponds to the *Guidelines for Psychological Practice with Girls and Women*, as formulated by the American Psychological Association, Girls and Women Guidelines Group (2018). The APA has also formulated guidelines for psychological practice with transgender and gender nonconforming people. For instance, Guideline 1: "Psychologists understand that gender is a nonbinary construct that allows for a range of gender identities and that a person's gender identity may not align with sex assigned at birth" (American Psychological Association, 2015, p. 834).

With respect to violence risk assessment, practitioners are currently advised to use the SPJ method, because it seems to be one of the most effective methods for both men and women (de Vogel et al., 2019; Garcia-Mansilla et al., 2009). Overall, commonly used SPJ tools like the START and HCR-20^{V3} and the FAM have some, but not very convincing, predictive value in adult female forensic psychiatric populations. The assessor should thus still exert caution in the interpretation of the results of risk assessments, especially when important decisions relating to the future prospects of clients, for instance, mandatory treatment or incarceration, need to be made. Furthermore, scholars may consider developing or adapting tools for gender-sensitive assessing risk of child abuse or intimate partner violence and risks in adolescent girls, as most of the currently used tools were developed and validated in predominantly male populations. In their recent review, Belisle and Salisbury (2021) provide several suggestions for more adequate assessment and treatment in justice-involved girls, especially emphasising the need for assessing protective factors and resilience.

Obviously, gender-sensitive risk assessment should lead to gender-responsive risk management and treatment. In the past decade, more knowledge and practical guidelines have become available regarding gender-responsive treatment interventions (see for example Bartlett et al., 2014; Logan, & Taylor, 2017).

Long et al., 2008). Generally, gender-responsive interventions should address criminogenic needs, include gender-responsive programs, and be trauma-informed (de Vogel & Nicholls, 2016). Prevention of (violent) offending is crucial, also for the next generations. Overall, the ultimate goal would be to prevent repeated violent behaviour in women and break the cycle of violence. Although advances have been made in the past decades, there remain substantial gaps in knowledge and debate regarding mental health needs of justice-involved females and more theoretical and empirical research is necessary to mitigate gender bias and provide the best possible treatment for both males and females. This seems to be particularly true for minority groups. For instance, Aiyegbusi (2021) discusses the vulnerability of black women in forensic mental health and criminal justice settings, also relating to the issue of transgenerational trauma, and emphasises the need for the voice of black women with lived experience in partnership with practitioners to educate and support staff working in these settings. Another minority group to pay more attention to is the group of transgender people, who relatively often suffer from stigmatisation, victimisation, and health risks within forensic and criminal settings (e.g., Van Hout et al., 2020).

References

Aiyegbusi, A. (2021). Caught in the racist gaze? The vulnerability of black women to forensic mental health and criminal justice settings. In A. Motz, M. Dennis, & A. Aiyegbusi (Eds.), *Invisible trauma. Women, difference and the criminal justice system* (pp. 54–68). Abingdon, Oxon: Routledge.

Andrews, D. A., & Bonta, J. (2000). *The level of service-inventory-revised.* Toronto: Multi-Health Systems.

Andrews, D. A., Guzzo, L., Raynor, P., Rowe, R. C., Rettinger, L. J., Brews, A., & Wormith, J. S. (2012). Are the major risk/need factors predictive of both female and male reoffending? A test with the eight domains of the Level of Service/Case Management Inventory. *International Journal of Offender Therapy and Comparative Criminology, 56,* 113–133. doi:10.1177/0306624X10395716

American Psychological Association (2015). Guidelines for psychological practice with transgender and gender nonconforming people. *American Psychologist, 70*(9), 832–864. Retrieved from https://www.apa.org/practice/guidelines/transgender.pdf

American Psychological Association, Girls and Women Guidelines Group (2018). *APA guidelines for psychological practice with girls and women.* Retrieved from http://www.apa.org/about/policy/psychological-practice-girls-women.pdf

Augimeri, L. K., Walsh, M., Enebrink, P., Jiang, D., Blackman, A., & Smaragdi, A. (2021). The Early Assessment Risk Lists for boys (EARL-20B) and girls (EARL-21G). In K. S. Douglas, & R. K. Otto (Eds.), *Handbook of violence risk assessment. Second edition* (pp. 227–252). Routledge.

Bartlett, A., Jhanjib, E., Whitec, S., & Harty, M. A. (2014). Interventions with women offenders: A systematic review and meta-analysis of mental health gain. *The Journal of Forensic Psychiatry & Psychology, 26,* 133–165. doi:10.1080/14789949.2014.981563

Bates, E. A., Kaye, L. K., Pennington, C. R., & Hamlin, I. (2019). What about the male victims? Exploring the impact of gender stereotyping on implicit attitudes and behavioural intentions associated with intimate partner violence. *Sex Roles, 81,* 1–15.

Bekker, M. H. & van Mens-Verhulst, J. (2007). Anxiety disorders: Sex differences in prevalence, degree, and background, but gender-neutral treatment. *Gender Medicine, 4*, S178–S193.

Belisle, L. A., & Salisbury, E. J. (2021). Starting with girls and their resilience in mind: Reconsidering risk/needs assessments for system-involved girls. *Criminal Justice and Behavior, 48*(5), 596–616. 10.1177/0093854820983859

Beryl, R., Chou, S., & Völlm, B. (2014). A systematic review of psychopathy in women within secure settings. *Personality and Individual Differences, 71*, 185–195. 10.1016/j.paid.2 014.07.033

Blanchette, K., & Taylor, K. N. (2007). Development and field test of a gender-informed security reclassification scale for female offenders. *Criminal Justice and Behavior, 34*, 362–379. doi: 10.1177/0093854806290162

Brennan, T., Breitenbach, M., Dieterich, W., Salisbury, E. J., & van Voorhis, P. (2012). Women's pathways to serious and habitual crime: A person-centered analysis incorporating gender responsive factors. *Criminal Justice and Behavior, 39*, 1481–1508. doi: 10.1177/0093854812456777

Brown, S., & Gelsthorpe, L. (Eds.) (2021). *The Wiley Handbook on what works with girls and women in conflict with the law: A critical review of theory, practice, and policy.* Wiley-Blackwell.

Coid, J., Kahtan, N., Gault, S., & Jarman, B. (2000). Women admitted to secure forensic psychiatry services: I. Comparison of women and men. *Journal of Forensic Psychiatry, 11*, 275–295. doi:10.1080/09585180050142525

Crocker, A. G., Eizner-Favreau, O., & Caulet, M. (2002). Gender and fitness to stand trial: A five-year review of remands in Quebec. *International Journal of Law and Psychiatry, 25*, 67–84. 10.1016/S0160-2527(01)00089-9

Croskerry, P., Singhal, G., & Mamede, S. (2013). Cognitive debiasing 2: Impediments to and strategies for change. *BMJ Quality & Safety, 22*(Suppl 2), ii65–ii72. 10.1136/bmjqs-2012-001713

Curry, T. R., Lee, G., & Rodriguez, S. F. (2004). Does victim gender increase sentence severity? Further explorations of gender dynamics and sentencing outcomes. *Crime & Delinquency, 50*, 319–343. doi:10.1177/0011128703256265

de Vogel, V., Bruggeman, M., & Lancel, M. (2019). Gender-sensitive violence risk assessment. Predictive validity of six tools in female forensic psychiatric patients. *Criminal Justice & Behavior, 46*(4), 528–549. doi:10.1177/0093854818824135.

de Vogel, V., de Ruiter, C., Bouman, Y., & de Vries Robbé, M. (2012). *SAPROF. Guidelines for the assessment of protective factors for violence risk* (2nd ed.). Utrecht, The Netherlands: Forum Educatief.

de Vogel, V., & de Spa, E. (2018). Gender differences in violent offending: Results from a multicentre comparison study in Dutch forensic psychiatry. *Psychology, Crime & Law, 25*(7), 739–751. doi:10.1080/1068316X.2018.1556267

de Vogel, V., & Lancel, M. (2016). Gender differences in the manifestation of psychopathy: Results from a multicentre study in forensic psychiatry. *International Journal of Forensic Mental Health, 15*, 97–110. doi:10.1080/14999013.2016.1138173

de Vogel, V., & Nicholls, T. L. (2016). Gender matters: An introduction to the special issue on women and girls. *International Journal of Forensic Mental Health, 15*, 1–25. doi:10.1 080/14999013.2016.1141439

de Vogel, V., Stam, J., Bouman, Y., ter Horst, P., & Lancel, M. (2016). Violent women: A multicentre study into gender differences in forensic psychiatric patients. *The Journal of Forensic Psychiatry & Psychology, 27*, 145–168. doi:10.1080/14789949.2015.1102312 de Vogel, V., de Vries Robbé, M., van Kalmthout, W., & Place, C. (2014). *Female Additional Manual (FAM): Additional guidelines to the HCR-20^V3 for assessing risk for violence in women*. Utrecht, The Netherlands: Van der Hoeven Kliniek.

de Vogel, V., Wijkman, M., & de Vries Robbé, M. (2018). Violence risk assessment in women: The value of the Female Additional Manual. In J. L. Ireland, C. A. Ireland, & P. Birch (Eds). *Violent and Sexual Offenders: Assessment, Treatment and Management* (2nd Edition) (pp. 182–200). London: Routledge.

de Vries Robbé, M., de Vogel, V., Wever, E., Douglas, K. S., & Nijman, H. L. I. (2016). Risk and protective factors for inpatient aggression. *Criminal Justice and Behavior, 43,* 1364–1385. doi: 10.1177/0093854816637889

Dolan, M., & Völlm, B. (2009). Antisocial personality disorder and psychopathy in women: A literature review on the reliability and validity of assessment instruments. *International Journal of Law and Psychiatry, 32,* 2–9. doi: 10.1016/j.ijlp.2008.11.002

Douglas, K. S., Hart, S. D., Webster, C. D., & Belfrage, H. (2013). *HCR-20^V3 : Assessing risk of violence – User guide*. Burnaby, Canada: Mental Health, Law, and Policy Institute, Simon Fraser University.

Douglas, K. S. & Otto, R. K. (Eds.) (2021). *Handbook of violence risk assessment*. 2nd edition. Routledge.

Forouzan, E., & Cooke, D. J. (2005). Figuring out la femme fatale: Conceptual and assessment issues concerning psychopathy in females. *Behavioral Sciences & the Law, 23,* 765–778. doi: 10.1002/bsl.669

Garcia-Mansilla, A., Rosenfeld, B., & Nicholls, T. L. (2009). Risk assessment: Are current methods applicable to women? *International Journal of Forensic Mental Health, 8,* 50–61. doi: 10.1080/14999010903014747

Geraghty, K. A., & Woodhams, J. (2015). The predictive validity of risk assessment tools for female offenders: A systematic review. *Aggression and Violent Behavior, 21,* 25–38. doi: 10.1016/j.avb.2015.01.002

Green, D., Schneider, M., Griswold, H., Belfi, B., Herrera, M., & DeBlasi, A. (2016). A comparison of the HCR-20^V3 among male and female insanity acquittees: A retrospective file study. *International Journal of Forensic Mental Health, 15,* 48–64. doi: 10.1080/14999013.2015.1134726

Hare, R. D. (2003). *Manual for the hare psychopathy checklist-revised*. Toronto, Ontario: Multi-Health Systems.

Hart, J. L., O'Toole, S. L., Price-Sharps, J. L., & Shaffer, T. W. (2007). The risk and protective factors of violent juvenile offending. An examination of gender differences. *Youth Violence and Juvenile Justice, 5,* 367–384. doi: 10.1177/1541204006297367

Hill, S. A., Thorpe, A., Petrauskaite, R., & Wilson, S. (2020). Characteristics of patients with gender dysphoria admitted to a secure forensic adolescent hospital. *The Journal of Forensic Psychiatry and Psychology, 31,* 854–867. DOI: 10.1080/14789949.2020.1807583

Javdani, S., Sadeh, N., & Verona, E. (2011a). Expanding our lens: Female pathways to antisocial behavior in adolescence and adulthood. *Clinical Psychology Review, 31,* 1324–1348. doi: 10.1016/j.cpr.2011.09.002

Javdani, S., Sadeh, N., & Verona, E. (2011b). Gendered social forces: A review of the impact of institutionalized factors on women and girls' criminal justice trajectories. *Psychology, Public Policy, and Law, 17,* 161–211. 10.1037/a0021957

Jeffries, S., Fletcher, G. J. O., & Newbold, G. (2003). Pathways to sex-based differentiation in criminal court sentencing. *Criminology, 41,* 329–354. 10.1111/j.1745-9125.2003.tb00990.x

Kim, H. K., Capaldi, D. M., Pears, K. C., Kerr, D. C. R., & Owen, L. D. (2009). Intergenerational transmission of internalising and externalising behaviours across three generations: Gender-specific pathways. *Criminal Behaviour and Mental Health*, *19*, 125–141. doi:10.1002/cbm.708

Klein Haneveld, E., Molenaar, D., de Vogel, V., Smid, W., & Kamphuis, J. H. (2021). Do we hold males and females to the same standard? A measurement invariance study on the Psychopathy Checklist-Revised. *Journal of Personality Assessment*, 1–12. 10.1080/00223891.2021.1947308

Kuehner, C. (2017). Why is depression more common among women than among men? *The Lancet Psychiatry*, *4*(2), 146–158.

Leistico, A. R., Salekin, R. T., DeCoster, J., & Rogers, R. (2008). A large-scale meta-analysis relating the Hare measures of psychopathy to antisocial conduct. *Law and Human Behavior*, *32*, 28–45. doi:10.1007/s10979-007-9096-6

Levene, K. S., Augimeri, L. K., Pepler, D. J., Walsh, M. M., Webster, C. D., & Koegl, C. J. (2001). *Early Assessment Risk List for Girls: EARL-21G. Version 1 - Consultation version*. Toronto: Earlscourt Child and Family Centre.

Logan, C., & Taylor, J. L. (2017). Working with personality disordered women in secure care: The challenge of gender-based service delivery. *The Journal of Forensic Psychiatry & Psychology*, *28*(2), 242–256. 10.1080/14789949.2017.1301531

Long, C. G., Fulton, B., & Hollin, C. R. (2008). The development of a 'best practice' service for women in a medium-secure psychiatric setting: Treatment components and evaluation. *Clinical Psychology and Psychotherapy*, *15*, 304–319. doi: 10.1002/cpp.591

Marshall, E., Miller, H. A., Cortoni, F., & Helmus, L. M. (2020). The Static-99R is not valid for women: predictive validity in 739 females who have sexually offended. *Sexual Abuse*, *33*(6), 631–653. 10.1177/1079063220940303.

Marshall, E. A., Miller, H. A., & Grubb, L. (2021). Examining the utility of the LSI-R in a sample of women who have sexually offended. *Criminal Justice and Behavior*, *49*(3), 311–329. 10.1177/00938548211054031.

McKeown, A. (2010). Female offenders: Assessment of risk in forensic settings. *Aggression and Violent Behavior*, *15*, 422–429. doi:10.1016/j.avb.2010.07.004

Messer, J., Maughan, B., Quinton, D., & Taylor, A. (2004). Precursors and correlates of criminal behaviour in women. *Criminal Behaviour and Mental Health*, *14*, 82–107. doi:10.1002/cbm.575

Morgan, M., & Patton, P. (2002). Gender-responsive programming in the justice system - Oregon's guidelines for effective programming for girls. *Federal Probation*, *66*, 57–65.

Morgan, W., & Wells, M. (2016). 'It's deemed unmanly': Men's experiences of intimate partner violence (IPV). *Journal of Forensic Psychiatry and Psychology*, *27*(3), 404–418. 10.1080/14789949.2015.1127986

Motz, A., Dennis, M., & Aiyegbusi, A. (2021). *Invisible trauma. Women, difference and the criminal justice system*. Routledge.

Neal, T. M. S., & Brodsky, S. (2016). Forensic psychologists' perceptions of bias and potential correction strategies in forensic mental health evaluations. *Psychology, Public Policy, and Law*, *22*(1), 58–76. 10.1037/law0000077

Neal, T. M. S., & Grisso, T. (2014). The cognitive underpinnings of bias in forensic mental health evaluations. *Psychology, Public Policy, and Law*, *20*(2), 200–211. 10.1037/a0035824

Neal, T. M. S., Slobogin, C., Saks, M. J., Faigman, D. L., & Geisinger, K. F. (2019). Psychological assessments in legal contexts: Are courts keeping "junk science" out of the courtroom? *Psychological Science in the Public Interest*, *20*(3), 135–164. 10.1177/1529100619888860

Nicholls, T. L., Cruise, K. R., Greig, D., & Hinz, H. (2015). Female offenders. In B. L. Cutler, & P. A. Zapf (Eds.), *APA handbook of forensic psychology: Vol. 2: Criminal investigation, adjudication, and sentencing outcomes* (pp. 79–123). Washington, DC: American Psychological Association. doi:10.1037/14462-004

Nicholls, T. L., Ogloff, J. P., Brink, J., & Spidel, A. (2005). Psychopathy in women: A review of its clinical usefulness for assessing risk for aggression and criminality. *Behavioral Sciences & the Law, 23*, 779–802. doi:10.1002/bsl.678

Odgers, C. L., Moretti, M. M., & Reppucci, N. D. (2005). Examining the science and practice of violence risk assessment with female adolescents. *Law and Human Behavior, 29*, 7–27. doi:10.1007/s10979-005-1397-z

Olver, M. E., Stockdale, K. C., & Wormith, J. S. (2014). Thirty years of research on the Level of Service Scales: A meta-analytic examination of predictive accuracy and sources of variability. *Psychological Assessment, 26*, 156. doi:10.1037/a0035080

O'Shea, L. E., & Dickens, G. L. (2015). Predictive validity of the Short-Term Assessment of Risk and Treatability (START) for aggression and self-harm in a secure mental health service: Gender differences. *International Journal of Forensic Mental Health, 14*, 132–146. doi:10.1080/14999013.2015.1033112

O'Shea, L. E., Mitchell, A. E., Picchioni, M. M., & Dickens, G. L. (2013). Moderators of the predictive efficacy of the Historical, Clinical and Risk Management-20 for aggression in psychiatric facilities: Systematic review and meta-analysis. *Aggression and Violent Behavior, 18*, 255–270. doi:10.1016/j.avb.2012.11.016

Phenix, A., Fernandez, Y., Harris, A. J. R., Helmus, M., Hanson, R. K., & Thornton, D. (2016). *Static-99R coding rules revised—2016.* Ottawa, Ontario: Public Safety Canada.

Rodermond, E., Kruttschnitt, C., Slotboom, A. M., & Bijleveld, C. C. (2015). Female desistance: A review of the literature. *European Journal of Criminology, 13*, 3–28. doi:10.1177/1477370815597251

Salisbury, E. J., van Voorhis, P., & Spiropoulos, G. V. (2009). The predictive validity of a gender-responsive needs assessment. *Crime & Delinquency, 55*, 550–585. 10.1177/0011128707308102

Salisbury, E. J., Boppre, B., & Kelly, B. (2016). Implications for the treatment of justice-involved women. In F. S. Taxman (Ed.), *Handbook on risk and need assessment: Theory and practice* (pp. 220–243). New York: Routledge.

Sevelius, J., & Jenness, V. (2017). Challenges and opportunities for gender-affirming healthcare for transgender women in prison. *International Journal of Prisoner Health, 13*(1), 32–40. 10.1108/IJPH-08-2016-0046

Skeem, J., Schubert, C., Stowman, S., Beeson, S., Mulvey, E., Gardner, W., & Lidz, C. (2005). Gender and risk assessment accuracy: Underestimating women's violence potential. *Law and Human Behavior, 29*, 173–186. doi:10.1007/s10979-005-3401-z

Smith, J. M., Gacono, C. B., & Cunliffe, T. B. (2021). *Understanding female offenders: Psychopathy, criminal behavior, assessment, and treatment.* Academic Press.

Stanziani, M., Newman, A. K., Cox, J., & Coffey, C. A. (2020). Role call: Sex, gender roles, and intimate partner violence. *Psychology, Crime & Law, 26*, 208–225. 10.1080/1068316X.2019.1652746

Strand, S. J., & Selenius, H. (2019). Assessing risk for inpatient physical violence in a female forensic psychiatric sample–comparing HCR-20v2 with the female additional manual to the HCR-20v2. *Nordic Journal of Psychiatry, 73*(4-5), 248–256.

Van Hout, M. C., Kewley, S., & Hillis, A. (2020). Contemporary transgender health experience and health situation in prisons: A scoping review of extant published literature (2000–2019). *International Journal of Transgender Health*, *21*(3), 258–306. 10.1 080/26895269.2020.1772937

van Voorhis, P., Bauman, A., & Brushett, R. (2013). *Revalidation of the women's risk needs assessment: Institutional results – Final report*. Cincinnati: Center for Criminal Justice Research.

van Voorhis, P., Wright, E. M., Salisbury, E., & Bauman, A. (2010). Women's risk factors and their contributions to existing risk/needs assessment. The current status of a gender-responsive supplement. *Criminal Justice and Behavior*, *37*, 261–288. doi:10.1177/0093854809357442

Venner, S., Sivasubramaniam, D., Luebbers, S., & Shepherd, S. M. (2020). Cross-cultural reliability and rater bias in forensic risk assessment: A review of the literature. *Psychology, Crime & Law*, *27*(2), 105–121. doi.org/10.1080/1068316X.2020.1775829

Viljoen, S., Nicholls, T. L., Greaves, C., de Ruiter, C., & Brink, J. (2011). Resilience and successful community reintegration among female forensic psychiatric patients: A preliminary investigation. *Behavioral Sciences and the Law*, *29*, 752–770. doi:10.1002/bsl.1001

Viljoen, S., Nicholls, T. L., Roesch, R., Gagnon, N., Douglas, K. S., & Brink, J. (2016). Exploring gender differences in the utility of strength based risk assessment measures. *International Journal of Forensic Mental Health*, *15*, 149–163. doi:10.1080/14999013.2016.1170739

Völlm, B. A., & Dolan, M. C. (2009). Self-harm among UK prisoners: A cross-sectional study. *Journal of Forensic Psychiatry & Psychology*, *20*, 741–751. doi:10.1080/1478994 0903174030

Walmsley, R. (2017). World Female Imprisonment List (fourth edition): Woman and girls in penal institutions, including pre-trail detainees/remand prisoners. Retrieved from: https://www.prisonstudies.org/sites/default/files/resources/downloads/world_female_ prison_4th_edn_v4_web.pdf

Webster, C. D., Douglas, K. S., Eaves, D., & Hart, S. D. (1997). *HCR-20: Assessing the risk of violence. Version 2*. Burnaby, British Columbia, Canada: Simon Fraser University and Forensic Psychiatric Services Commission of British Columbia.

Webster, C. D., Martin, M., Brink, J., Nicholls, T. L., & Desmarais, S. L. (2009). *Short-Term Assessment of Risk and Treatability (START). Clinical guide for evaluation risk and recovery. Version 1.1*. Ontario, Canada: St. Joseph's Healthcare Hamilton.

Wijkman, M., Bijleveld, C., & Hendriks, J. (2010). Women don't do such things! Characteristics of female sex offenders and offender types. *Sexual Abuse: A Journal of Research and Treatment*, *22*(2), 135–156. 10.1177/1079063210363826

Yesberg, J. A., Scanlan, J. M., Hanby, L. J., Serin, R. C., & Polaschek, D. L. L. (2015). Predicting women's recidivism: Validating a dynamic community-based 'gender-neutral' tool. *Probation Journal*, *62*, 33–48. doi:10.1177/0264550514562851

Zlotnick, C., Clarke, J. G., Friedmann, P. D., Roberts, M. B., Sacks, S., & Melnick, G. (2008). Gender differences in comorbid disorders among offenders in prison substance abuse treatment programs. *Behavioral Sciences & the Law*, *26*, 403–412.

18 Critical Reflection on Gender Identity Assessments with Trans and Gender Non-Binary Individuals: Challenges, Implications, and a Newly Proposed Approach in Forensic Psychology

Sören Henrich

Introduction

Psychological assessments are central to a lot of Trans individuals, especially when undergoing transition (i.e., accessing hormone treatment, gender-reaffirming surgeries, or other interventions aiming to establish bodily satisfaction). Assessments include the identification of treatment needs, therapy planning but also the review of service users' gender identity. This chapter outlines the issues regarding this assessment format, whilst navigating ethical arguments between safeguarding and gatekeeping. These reflections are also applied to the forensic setting and the challenges this brings. It is argued that undue pathologising of the Trans experience is preventing individuals from accessing care, thus, a new non-diagnostic approach to mental health is presented.

Trans as a Shifting Concept

Transgender refers to individuals who experience a mismatch between their assigned sex at birth and their gender (*trans* is the Latin prefix for "on the other side") and is used as an umbrella term for a variety of Gender Non-Conforming identities (GNC; e.g., Altilio & Otis-Green, 2011). If no mismatch is experienced, the appropriate label is *cisgender* (*cis* is the Latin prefix for "on the same side"; represents usually most of society). In this definition, *sex* commonly represents biological features, while *gender* refers to societal role expectations usually associated with either *male* or *female* (e.g., Udry, 1994). However, biological features, in the sciences are made up of six categories; chromosomes, hormones, internal sex organs, external sex organs, secondary sexual characteristics, general morphology, and are often misconstrued as ground truth (Fausto-Sterling, 1993). Biology scholars already recognise that these central features can all be considered on a spectrum, with past researchers only arbitrarily defining cut-offs to

DOI: 10.4324/9781003230977-21

fit into a binary male-female system. Depending on the individual's unique expression across all these categories, authors like Fausto-Sterling (1993) acknowledged that technically an infinite variety of sexes can exist and that shaping them into dichotomous categories is as much a cultural artefact as gender is itself. For example, the belief that X and Y chromosomes hold information pertaining to femininity and masculinity has been recently recognised as overly simplistic (Richardson, 2013; Steadman, 2015). Genomes hold other information as well, while the individual's biological expression of certain sex characteristics is also stored on entirely different genomes.

The historical and socio-political context is that the binary system was not part of Western society until after the 18th century (e.g., McLaren, 1993). Beforehand, a unary system was generally accepted, placing *male* on top of a ladder as the so-called purest human form, and *female* on the bottom of the ladder. The establishment of the two sexes as the only possible categories (no matter the unary or binary system) can be dated back to colonialist times and the missionary efforts by Christians (McLaren, 1993). Historians like Mogul et al. (2011) emphasise that other cultures previously embraced identities that would nowadays fall under the Trans umbrella. The reason for colonisers imposing a binary system and demonising other forms of gender expression and sexuality was rooted in their settlement strategy. It was easier to control a non-hierarchical community by dividing them along arbitrary lines that would destabilise those groups by pitting them against each other (e.g., Mogul et al., 2011; Buist et al., 2018). Furthermore, violence was possibly rooted in the colonialists' inability to understand these unfamiliar identities, instead presenting as a threat to their world views (Picq & Tikuna, 2019). Currently, examples can be found internationally in which a non-binary system has been the norm through the entirety of documented human history (e.g., Picq & Tikuna, 2019), such as in the indigenous Australian culture. They commonly hold a space for individuals that the Western perspective would label as GNC, but their community refers to them as *Sistergirls* and *Brotherboys* (e.g., Kerry, 2014).

The attempted eradication of those identities in the name of Christianity also links to the role of psychology and psychiatry and how diagnoses are used as social control (e.g., Brown, 1990). When reviewing historical developments in these fields with a focus on power imbalances, Dewey and Gesbeck (2017) noted that medicalisation is often used as a cultural instrument to address behaviours or traits that are deemed inappropriate or reprehensible in society. Medicalisation is defined to frame nonmedical issues as clinically relevant problems using biological models (Conrad, 1992), facilitating the dehumanisation of marginalised people and hence, allowing the control of such minorities through the medical system (e.g., Dewey & Gesbeck, 2017).

One of the most extreme examples was the complicity of psychiatrists during the genocide in the Third Reich (Vine, 2009), where empirical sciences were used to justify why certain groups in society (e.g., Jews, neurodivergent individuals, homosexuals) were considered to have a disorder and hence could be targeted (Stryker, 2008; Giles, 2010). As such, psychiatrists and psychologists actively contributed to and supported eugenics, developing strategies for diagnoses and medicalisation that would lay the methodological groundwork for modern psychiatry (Vine, 2009). The efforts by Nazis to eradicate those who they deemed unfit to be part of their society also resulted in the destruction of research related to Trans individuals (e.g., Lester, 2017). For example, studies and reports by the Berlin physician Magnus Hirschfeld, founder of the Institute for Sexual Science in 1928, were lost, subsequently stalling progress for the Trans community (Stryker, 2008; Vine, 2009). But even in the recent past it is possible to link the medicalisation of certain identities or behaviour to criminalisation as an effort to control social movements and establish conformity. For example, *transsexualism*, which became an official diagnostic term and medically defined problem in 1952 in the US (Ekins, 2005), was initially discussed in the context of sexual dysfunctions and paraphilic disorders (e.g., Dewey & Gesbeck, 2017). Not only did this enable psychiatrists and lawmakers across several Western legislations to section members of the Trans community, but it also allowed the punishment and imprisonment of those individuals, as science was seen as supporting the notion of those members of society being irredeemable, abnormal and even potentially corrupting (e.g., Dewey & Gesbeck, 2017).

Scholars like Bryant (2011) or Esposito and Perez (2014) even frame medical labelling as a form to create new patient categories to morally regulate society. The World Health Organisation (World Health Organization WHO, 2018) recently took steps to rectify some of this damage, technically declassifying Trans as a mental disorder and instead explicitly labelling it as an expression of identity. Hence, the American Psychology Association (APA) has also moved away from the term *gender identity disorder* introduced in the 1980s as a concept linked to the biomedical explanatory models (American Psychiatric Association, 2000). Instead, American Psychiatric Association (2013) is now focusing on *gender dysphoria*, which limits the diagnostic scope to distress instead of an entire identity, as explained in more detail below. This is also reflected in the guidance by the World Association of Transgender Health Professionals (WATHP; Coleman et al., 2012), an international association of practitioners and researchers working in the field and offering empirically supported guidance. Not only are the social sciences changing, focusing more on Trans advocacy (Henrich & Birch, 2020), but so is language (e.g., Lester, 2017). For example, instead of referring to transition-related surgeries as *gender re-assignment surgeries*, they are now labelled as *gender re-affirming surgeries*, highlighting the awareness that medical procedures do not re-assign a social construct such as gender but reinforce what is already expressed by the individual (Lester, 2017; Ahmad et al., 2019). Similarly, it was common in medical literature to refer to transitioning individuals as either *Male-to-Female* (MTF) or *Female-to-Male* (FTM), falsely implying that Trans individuals swap their genders, as opposed to reaffirming their gender by matching it to aspects of their biological features (Lester, 2017; Ahmad et al., 2019).

At the time of writing, the terms *transwoman* and *transman* are viewed as more appropriate. As a result, younger generations also refute the term *transsexual*, which was used to mark the medical difference between an individual starting transition-related treatment (i.e., *transgender*) and those that have finished that process (e.g., Lester, 2017). Nowadays, this language is viewed by some as assigning individuals different values depending on their access of treatment. As professional language is slowly catching up (Ahmad et al., 2019), it is likely that terminology will continue to shift as awareness around the previously mentioned issues grows. Furthermore, criticism around the psychological procedures that assign those labels through diagnosis – for example, by using gender identity assessments – remain (Henrich & Birch, 2020) and will be addressed next.

Gender Identity Assessments

As an extension of the previously outlined medicalisation process, gender identity assessment is a form of labelling approach in which an assessor utilises semi-structured, sometimes psychometric instruments to explore an individual's gender identity (Henrich, 2020). The purpose of these assessments can vary as demonstrated by Dewey and Gesbeck (2017) who interviewed 20 clinicians and 24 Trans individuals. Their findings suggest that these assessments are aiming to establish the authenticity with which individuals express their identity. As medical definitions about sex and gender remain arbitrary (e.g., Fausto-Sterling, 1993) interviewed practitioners state that they use individuals' willingness to adhere to stereotypically female or male expressions as an indication for such authenticity (Dewey & Gesbeck, 2017). However, the authors highlight that this ignores Gender Non-Binary (GNB) individuals, instead adhering to often outdated stereotypes that not even all Cis men and women would follow. Another identified purpose is the assessment of mental competence (Dewey & Gesbeck, 2017).

It appears that Trans individuals need to present as mentally stable to access services, while practitioners lack consensus of what constitutes mental competence. Hence, some practitioners may deny transition because of other diagnoses like depression, even though these could have lingered due to an inability to access treatment which is entirely unrelated to wishing to re-affirm their gender. Dewey and Gesbeck (2017) highlight that gender identity assessments are lacking standards and are highly contested. Furthermore, they appear procedurally problematic, as they require time and financial resources on the part of the Trans individual, while some professionals appear to view these assessments as "shams" (Dewey & Gesbeck, 2017, p. 64). Nevertheless, in some Western legal systems the legitimisation of gender through psychiatric diagnoses is a central requirement that Trans and GNC individuals must meet (Meadow, 2011).

Henrich (2020) conducted a systematic review of the available literature in respect of the empirical evidence regarding those assessments. The review demonstrated that despite international guidance, for example by the WATHP (Coleman et al., 2012), no assessment standard could be established. In fact, the 21 studies included in the review highlighted the lack of research in this area, with several suggested assessment instruments only offering preliminary evidence for their utility (Henrich, 2020). Furthermore, it became apparent that most instruments relied on the assumption of a binary system, therefore, being deemed inappropriate to be used with GNB individuals. Overall, the instruments appeared to address two main areas: (1) Instruments established for other populations assessing psychopathology and stereotypical binary gender expressions; and (2) Trans-specific instruments that are focusing on gender dysphoria.

The former category of instruments included tools like the Minnesota Multiphasic Personality Inventory-2 (MMPI-2), that have been well researched for clinical application but have only recently been applied to Trans individuals (Henrich, 2020). Whilst research such as by Langevin et al. (1977) or Caron and Archer (1997) highlight that there are no marked differences between the scores of Trans participants compared to Cis participants on the MMPI-2, it is unclear whether the assessment of gender identity is actually useful (Henrich, 2020). This is because most tools in category 1 rely on stereotypical gender expression (e.g., the MMPI-2 includes a Masculinity/Femininity-scale). However, it is questionable how such instruments portray individuals who refute classical gender roles, as they would not map accurately onto those scales, instead falsely locating them somewhere on the male-to-female spectrum. It appears that these instruments may not be entirely futile, possessing more utility in a research context (Henrich, 2020).

The latter category was more specific, focusing on gender dysphoria (Henrich, 2020). Put simply, this syndrome describes a persistent distress that is linked to the individual's experience of their gender (American Psychiatric Association, 2013). In several legislatures, this is a central requirement for becoming legally recognised and in turn access certain services (e.g., Meadow, 2011). However, it is also criticised for pathologising Trans identities (Schulz, 2018), and contributes to the argument made above that the medicalisation of an identity is viewed as stigmatising and contrasts it against the majority's experience as "other" (e.g., Lester, 2017). Furthermore, making gender dysphoria a central requirement of gender recognition assumes that all Trans and GNC individuals experience persistent distress linked to their body. However, research is showing that gender dysphoria is not as common in this population as previously assumed, with individuals often not meeting the criteria (e.g., Lester, 2017: Schulz, 2018). This is also reiterated in criticisms made by Trans individuals, who describe the assessment process as a catch-22 situation (e.g., Dewey & Gesbeck, 2017). On the one hand, they need to present with sufficient distress to be diagnosed with gender dysphoria. On the other hand, they need to present as sufficiently psychologically fit to be able to undergo transition-related treatment. Anecdotal reports describe how this can feel unjust, alienating, and potentially victimising.

It thus appears inappropriate to conduct gender identity assessments, at least in community settings. Instead, scholars and activists advocate for an informed consent approach, with practitioners merely providing guidance and empowering clients to choose their own treatment, subsequently shifting the discussed power imbalance (e.g., Lev, 2009). In some countries, this is already practiced in the form of legal self-identification (e.g., in France and Portugal; Lester, 2017). Here, individuals can change their legally recognised gender by submitting a form – either online or offline – but without any further assessments. Note that this is only in relation to gender identity assessments, not negating the importance of mental health assessments in other areas where it is appropriate to plan together with the individual their next treatment steps. While the solution in the community appears to be clear and easily applicable, psychologists often encounter a dilemma in secure forensic settings. This is described below.

The Psychologist's Predicament in Secure Forensic Settings

Having established the importance of being mindful of the approach used in the assessment of Trans and GNC individuals' identity, the focus for many psychologists then shifts to two other areas in secure forensic settings: cisgender offenders and mental health issues. The concern that is often shared in the media (Christina, 2018) is that (a) cisgender individuals claim to be Trans for ulterior motives (e.g., to gain access to other units); and that (b) some cisgender individuals present with mental health symptoms that make it unclear what their identity is (e.g., symptoms such as identity disturbance linked to the diagnosis of Borderline Personality Disorder). Both cases make it necessary that individuals are assessed to either safeguard others or safeguard the individuals themselves. While it appears now clear-cut who to assess and who not to assess, the reality is that in secure forensic settings this is not so simple. The distinction on who to assess would hinge on the assumption that who is Trans and who is Cis has already been established, before the assessment would even begin.

This presents psychologists with a predicament. They could choose to be lenient with their assessment approach. Hence, they will not scrutinise Trans individuals regarding their identity, instead expressing respect and honouring informed consent (as established in the previous section). However, in those instances, psychologists will be less likely to identify Cis individuals with ulterior motives or those with severe mental health issues impacting on their own understanding of identity. If psychologists counter this risk by taking a more scrutinising approach, the likelihood of identifying the aforementioned Cis individuals increases, thereby allowing them to safeguard others and allocate appropriate therapeutic interventions. However, in these circumstances, the assessor will risk causing severe distress to Trans individuals in their care, potentially (re-) victimising individuals through intrusive questioning.

This predicament is not to be taken lightly, as all assessment outcomes have a significant impact on individuals' care in secure forensic settings. The potential asymmetry between believing a genuine expression versus believing somebody who is not genuine is difficult to weigh against each other. Nowhere else is the balance between safeguarding and gatekeeping so urgent and so pronounced as here. It appears that current research does not offer any solutions. The review by Henrich (2020) only found one assessment instrument which claimed to distinguish Trans individuals who experience gender dysphoria from a general clinical sample, namely the Gender Identity/Gender Dysphoria Questionnaire for

Adolescents and Adults (GIDYQ-AA; Deogracias et al., 2007). This tool falls within the latter category established in the previous sections, namely instruments designed and tested with a Trans sample (Henrich, 2020). However, research in this area is in its infancy and more studies are needed to understand this tests' sensitivity and specificity. Furthermore, the methodology and the authors' way of establishing ground truth regarding the sample assignment is not explicitly stated in their paper. Lastly, this solution to the psychologist's predicament would again centre the gender dysphoria diagnosis, replicating the problems described above (Henrich, 2020).

It becomes apparent that more research is needed to establish best practice in this area. It must also be noted that conceptualisations by Dewey and Gesbeck (2017) suggest that the fear of sexualised violence in the context of Trans issues – even when discussed with cis offenders – is related to a longstanding history in psychiatry. For example, the previously described, now outdated diagnosis *gender identity disorder* was related to *Autogynephilia*, representing cis individuals who wanted to undergo transition-related surgeries due to alleged fetishistic obsession (e.g., Blanchard, 2005). This established the idea also in psychiatric circles that some Trans individuals are not genuinely expressing an identity, but instead attempting to fulfil sexual fantasies (Dewey & Gesbeck, 2017). Doubting Trans individuals' authenticity and stigmatising their lived experiences in such a manner resulted in limited medical access, for example, due to shame (Dewey & Gesbeck, 2017). As such, the fear that some individuals are cis with ulterior motives could also be an extension of the now overhauled diagnostic terms. Framing the psychologist's predicament in this context requires great care and reflection.

Next steps for research could include reviewing current assessment approaches amongst practitioners with the goal of establishing an international consensus. However, to not continue the power imbalance, this research must also involve Trans and GNC voices. The required discussions in this area must be open to appropriate scrutiny and criticism to work through the various predicaments and thus avoid creating new dilemmas. Furthermore, future research must move away from a pathologising approach and the diagnosis of gender dysphoria, instead exploring more empowering features which would support assessment and include a positive psychology element. This is particularly important as members of communities with a history of medicalisation and discrimination appear to be often viewed solely through the lens of traumagenic social consequences. This could further their experience of stigmatisation. Hence, new approaches could include a focus on resilience or *gender congruence*. The latter is a term introduced by Trans individuals to describe the feeling of euphoria and satisfaction, when the initially discussed mismatch between biological features and gender is resolved to a level that the individual feels comfortable with (e.g., Owen-Smith et al., 2018). The next section proposes a new perspective that could achieve a non-pathologising client-centred assessment approach, which potentially also accounts for the aforementioned positive aspects of the Trans experience.

The Power Threat Meaning Framework as Applied to Trans Care

This chapter has demonstrated the current paradigm shift in the field, moving towards a non-pathologising assessment that tries to counter the power imbalance between psychologist and interviewee. Johnstone and Boyle (2018a) offer an alternative approach to the diagnostic process, the so-called *Power Threat Meaning Framework* (PTMF). They introduced four concepts to support the understanding of mental health (Johnstone & Boyle, 2018a):

1   Power defined as interpersonal influences, as well as legal and societal control moderated by available resources;
2   threat which represents negative impacts of power resulting, for example, in emotional distress, mediated by biological factors;
3   meaning as making sense through beliefs, feelings and symbols based on social and cultural influences;
4   threat responses which are conceptualised as protection mechanisms shaped by early attachment styles.

Johnstone and Boyle (2018a; 2018b) see the advantages in the PTMF in its non-pathological approach that does not purely focus on biological explanations, instead favouring a holistic understanding that also accounts for culture and socio-political context, while offering the assessed individual agency in the process by creating their own narrative. All these aspects can be explored utilising the following questions (Johnstone & Boyle, 2018a, p. 8):

* "What has happened to you?" (How is power operating in your life?)
* "How did it affect you?" (What kind of threats does this pose?)
* "What sense did you make of it?" (What is the meaning of these situations and experiences to you?)
* "What did you have to do to survive?" (What kinds of threat response are you using?) […]
* "What are your strengths?" (What access to power resources do you have?)
* […] "What is your story?"

Applied to the work with the Trans community, each of these aspects could be utilised to understand distress in areas that are commonly pathologised, such as gender dysphoria. Hence, this chapter proposes the exploration of the following areas in line with the PTMF by Johnstone and Boyle (2018a):

* *Trans in the context of power.* Employing questions like the ones listed above allows the interviewee to reflect on the adversities in their lives. This is often conceptualised as *minority stress* (Meyer, 2003), highlighting that members of those groups do not only experience more stressors (e.g., Cole et al., 1997), but they also receive less support from the institutions systemically oppressing

them, resulting in chronic stress. While that can include discrimination, lower socio-economic status, and traumatic experiences (Johnstone & Boyle, 2018a), reflections during the interview can also focus on gender, the system of patriarchy, and the potential for mental health services to re-victimise the interviewee, amongst other aspects. This can even allow for a critical discourse about the assessment process itself. Discussions may also include the influences of overlapping powers, how they relate to an individual's multiple social roles, and how they put the individual at a disadvantage, as summarised under the term *intersectionality* (Crenshaw, 1989).

- *Threats linking to Trans needs*: Generally, physiological and psychological threats trigger individuals' need for security and safety (Johnstone & Boyle, 2018a). As such, clinicians working with Trans individuals should explore how aforementioned power influences (e.g., society's expectation to adhere to a binary gender system) result in the interviewee's distress. Furthermore, threats can be experienced, when potential or actual loss of these needs' fulfilments appears (Johnstone & Boyle, 2018a). For Trans individuals, this could mean the lack of bodily autonomy, the risk of physical harm when openly identifying as Trans, or the momentary inability to experience *gender congruence* (e.g., Owen-Smith et al., 2018). As such, it portrays a more positive outlook on the transition process and allows the exploration of what would feel satisfying relating to the Trans individual's own body. The term *gender euphoria* is sometimes used interchangeably (Lysenko, 2009).

- *Narratives that support the Trans experience*: As Johnstone and Boyle (2018a,b) describe, individuals make sense of the interplay of factors in the PTMF through narratives. While those feelings and beliefs can be positive and negative, the authors note that especially the occurrence of negative narratives (e.g., self-blame, shame, social avoidance) are linked to the experienced distress (Johnstone & Boyle, 2018a). Here, issues relate to *internalised transphobia*, a sub-clinical phenomenon refers to the internalisation of dismissive, discriminating and/or derogatory views held by outsiders about members of a certain group, in this case, about Trans individuals (Bockting, 2015). Due to their continued exposure to those discriminatory opinions, the individual might start believing some of those views, falsely assuming it must be true what others say about them, and integrating those attitudes into their self-concept (Bockting, 2015). In this context, it also becomes apparent again that a scrutinising assessment approach as outlined above could easily trigger those falsely held self-doubts and might have a detrimental effect on the individual's mental health (Bockting et al., 2020).

- *Trans individual's threat response*: Lastly, the adaptive and maladaptive responses of the interviewee must be explored in relation to all previously discussed facets. These can include reactive biological responses or complex behavioural patterns (Johnstone & Boyle, 2018a). This facilitates the understanding of a Trans individual's level of resilience and their specific coping strategies (e.g., binding breasts, padding the hips, or self-mutilation of genitals to counter negative perspectives regarding their own bodies). Johnstone and Boyle

(2018a) emphasise that this can also include reflections regarding the individual's resources (e.g., access to services, financial hurdles) and their social environment (e.g., support through family and friends). This is in line with the holistic care that is suggested by the WATHP (Coleman et al., 2012).

The above offers some initial considerations for applying an existing non-pathologising approach to working with Trans individuals for the instances where their distress must be further explored. It is important to note that this would not be suitable for an exclusive assessment of Trans individual's gender identity, but gender identity can be part of the exploration, as Johnstone and Boyle (2018ab) proposed the PTMF with mental health issues in mind. Other approaches relevant for the forensic context, such as risk assessments, are not discussed here due to the limited scope of the chapter. However, authors like Sahota (2020) provide further guidance. As the application of the PTMF approach to the Trans context is new and had not been discussed in the literature to date, future research will need to demonstrate its utility. Furthermore, the here proposed application must be open to elaboration and development by practitioners working in the field, as well as being critiqued criticism by professionals and Trans individuals alike in order to further improve the approach. The last section of this chapter will outline additional steps colleagues could adopt as part of developing their practice.

Final Practical Considerations

As research in this area is still in its infancy, it is recommended that psychologists remain vigilant. With more empirical data needed to fully understand how to resolve the psychologist's predicament, assessors need to be aware that consensus and guidance is currently lacking (Henrich, 2020). As such, not one assessment instrument is recommended and the tools discussed above appear to assist with the most pressing questions clinicians encounter in secure forensic settings (Henrich, 2020). Besides the outlined application of the PTMF to the Trans context, a few other practical considerations are considered here:

- *Demand training*: Several reviews link the lack of support for Trans individuals, the unacceptable low levels of good quality Trans care, the high rate of victimisation and discrimination against Trans individuals in the CJS and in mental health services, and the absence of professional education (e.g., European Union Agency for Fundamental Rights, 2014; James et al., 2016). In several legal systems courses are not readily available. A first step would be to voice the urgent need for appropriate guidance and for individuals to campaign in their organisations to access training. Raising awareness that practitioners have questions that are impacting Trans care can result in the broader availability of education.
- *Share experiences*: Linked to the previous point, colleagues must be encouraged to open up more in dialogue with each other (and with Trans and GNC

individuals), however exposing it might be. This will open up opportunities to discuss uncertainties and circumvent potential mistakes.

- *Use inclusive language*: As previously outlined, the medical field is currently becoming more aware of the use of more inclusive language that is affirming of individuals' gender (e.g., Ahmad et al., 2019). For example, an increasingly common practice is the use of personal pronouns (e.g., included in email signatures, presentation headings; Thoroughgood et al., 2020). This addresses long-held assumptions that it is appropriate or easy to assume someone's gender. Instead, explicitly discussing pronouns is an easily applied and quick way to show inclusivity and respect. Ideally, such behaviour becomes normalised, with individuals who hold higher positions in organisations modelling such language (e.g., using self-disclosing statements like "My pronouns are she/her. What are yours?").

- *Centring vs. avoiding gender identity:* Linked to the former point is the tendency of some clinicians to overemphasise the gender identity of the assessed individuals. Sahota (2020) published guidance on this and noted that similar to the salience bias an individual's feature that is viewed by others as central can impact the entire judgement regarding that individual. The opposite extreme is the avoidance of some clinicians to address gender identity, as they fear getting things wrong (Sahota, 2020). Professionals need to be mindful of both these tendencies so that balance is established.

- *Balancing risks and benefits*: When choosing an assessment approach to resolve the psychologist's predicament, clinicians are encouraged to be as explicit as possible about their reasoning in their planning and subsequent reports (e.g., Henrich, 2020). Not only should it be common practice to reflect on the lack of available empirical evidence, but psychologists should also explain their reasons for choosing to be either more lenient or more scrutinising in their approach. This will likely depend on the individual case but should be communicated explicitly to other professions and the clients in the write-ups to demonstrate transparency and accountability (e.g., Sahota, 2020).

Centre Trans voices: Lastly, but nonetheless equally important as the points above is the necessity for centring the experiences of Trans individuals (e.g., Wesp et al., 2019). This includes two aspects: (a) Centring the individual's experience who is the focus of the assessment, and (b) actively learning from the wider Trans community, as opposed to purely basing your knowledge on other cis professionals. The former point refers to the previously suggested informed consent approach that assumes that individuals accessing mental health services are their own expert of their own experiences (e.g., Swift & Dieppe, 2005). The second point reflects the wider issues around education and training regarding the Trans community. To fully comprehend issues relevant to members of this community, to remain updated (e.g., regarding the use of appropriate language) but also to meet a wide variety of authentic examples of Trans biographies, professionals need to seek out information by Trans individuals. This can include books, documentaries, trainings courses, podcasts, movies, and series. Seeking the exposure to those narratives and experiences allows professionals to become familiar with their clients, reduces biases, and supports the development of tolerance and respect

Overall, this chapter emphasises the complexity of issues and challenges that are interlinked in gender identity assessments. As research progresses, it is hoped that more guidance becomes available, aiding equally psychologists in their work and Trans individuals in receiving appropriate care. The current chapter is only viewed as a starting point in this endeavour, raising awareness, highlighting pitfalls and opportunities, and lending language to colleagues to communicate the predicaments they're facing in an appropriate and understandable manner. Additionally, it proposes a non-pathologising application of the PTMF to Trans care, expecting a refined understanding of Trans individuals' distress beyond stigmatisation. With a more widely shared understanding of these issues, it is likely that assessment approaches, guidance, and care can truly achieve their safeguarding purposes for individuals that need it, while leaving gatekeeping behind.

References

Ahmad, T., Lafreniere, A., & Grynspan, D. (2019). Incorporating transition-affirming language into anatomical pathology reporting for gender affirmation surgery. *Transgender Health*, *4*(1), 335–338.

American Medical Association House of Delegates. (2021, August 9). *Removing sex designation from the public portion of the birth certificate.* American Medical Association. https://www.ama-assn.org/system/files/2019-09/i19-005.pdf

American Psychiatric Association. (2000). *The diagnostic and statistical manual of mental disorders.* 4th ed. Washington, DC: American Psychiatric Association.

American Psychiatric Association. (2013). *The diagnostic and statistical manual of mental disorders.* 5th ed. Arlington, VA: American Psychiatric Association.

Altilio, T. & Otis-Green, S. (Eds.). (2011). *Oxford textbook of palliative social work.* Oxford University Press.

Bindel, J. (2021, August 3). *It's not an anti-trans crusade to be concerned about male sex offenders on female NHS wards.* The Telegraph. https://www.telegraph.co.uk/news/2021/08/03/not-anti-trans-crusade-concerned-male-sex-offenders-female-nhs/

Blanchard, R. (2005). Early history of the concept of autogynephilia. *Archives of Sexual Behavior*, *34*(4), 439–446.

Bockting, W. (2015). Internalized transphobia. *The international encyclopedia of human sexuality*, 583–625.

Bockting, W. O., Miner, M. H., Swinburne Romine, R. E., Dolezal, C., Robinson, B. B. E., Rosser, B. S., & Coleman, E. (2020). The Transgender Identity Survey: A measure of internalized transphobia. *LGBT Health*, *7*(1), 15–27.

Brown, P. (1990). The name game: Toward a sociology of diagnosis. *The Journal of Mind and Behavior*, SPECIAL ISSUE: Challenging the Therapeutic State: Critical Perspectives on Psychiatry and the Mental Health System, *11*(3/4), 385–406.

Brown, C., Frohard-Dourlent, H., Wood, B. A., Saewyc, E., Eisenberg, M. E., & Porta, C. M. (2020). "It makes such a difference": An examination of how LGBTQ youth talk about personal gender pronouns. *Journal of the American Association of Nurse Practitioners*, *32*(1), 70–80.

Buist, C. L., Lenning, E., & Ball, M. (2018). Queer criminology. In W. S. DeKeseredy & M. Dragiewicz (Eds.), *Routledge handbook of critical criminology* (pp. 96–106). Routledge.

Bryant, K. (2011). Diagnosis and medicalization. In *Sociology of diagnosis*. Emerald Group Publishing Limited.

Caron, G. R. & Archer, R. P. (1997). MMPI and Rorschach characteristics of individuals approved for gender reassignment surgery. *Assessment, 4*(3), 229–241.

Christina, M. (2018). The media, public opinion and sex offender policy in the US. In *Sexual offending* (pp. 116–137). Routledge.

Cole, C. M., O'boyle, M., Emory, L. E., & Meyer III, W. J. (1997). Comorbidity of gender dysphoria and other major psychiatric diagnoses. *Archives of Sexual Behavior, 26*(1), 13–26.

Coleman, E., Bockting, W., Botzer, M., Cohen-Kettenis, P., DeCuypere, G., Feldman, J., Fraser, L., Green, J., Knudson, G., Meyer, W. J. & Monstrey, S. (2012). Standards of care for the health of transsexual, transgender, and gender-nonconforming people, version 7. *International Journal of Transgenderism, 13*(4), 165–232.

Conrad, P. (1992). Medicalization and social control. *Annual Review of Sociology, 18*(1), 209–232.

Crenshaw, K. (1989). Demarginalizing the intersection of race and sex: A black feminist critique of antidiscrimination doctrine, feminist theory and antiracist politics. *u. Chi. Legal f.*, 139.

Deogracias, J. J., Johnson, L. L., Meyer-Bahlburg, H. F., Kessler, S. J., Schober, J. M. & Zucker, K. J. (2007). The Gender Identity/Gender Dysphoria Questionnaire for Adolescents and Adults. *Journal of Sex Research, 44*(4), 370–379.

Dewey, J. M., & Gesbeck, M. M. (2017). (Dys) functional diagnosing: Mental health diagnosis, medicalization, and the making of transgender patients. *Humanity & Society, 41*(1), 37–72.

Esposito, L., & Perez, F. M. (2014). Neoliberalism and the commodification of mental health. *Humanity & Society, 38*(4), 414–442.

Ekins, R. (2005). Science, politics and clinical intervention: Harry Benjamin, transsexualism and the problem of heteronormativity. *Sexualities, 8*(3), 306–328.

European Union Agency for Fundamental Rights (2014). Being Trans in the European Union Comparative Analysis of EU LGBT Survey Data, Publications Office of the European Union.

Fausto-Sterling, A. (1993). The five sexes: Why male and female are not enough. *The Sciences, 33*(2), 20–24.

Giles, G. J. (2010). The Persecution of Gay Men and Lesbians during the Third Reich. In *The Routledge history of the Holocaust* (pp. 405–416). Routledge.

Hale, C. J. (2007). Ethical problems with the mental health evaluation standards of care for adult gender variant prospective patients. *Perspectives in Biology and Medicine, 50*(4), 491–505.

Henrich, S. (2020). Gender identity assessment with trans individuals–findings of a systematic literature review of assessment instruments and ethical considerations. *Journal of Criminological Research, Policy and Practice, 6*(3), 203–216.

Henrich, S. & Birch, P. (2020). Guest editorial. *Journal of Criminological Research, Policy and Practice, 6*(3), 185–187.

James, S., Herman, J., Rankin, S., Keisling, M., Mottet, L., & Anafi, M. A. (2016). The Report of the 2015 U.S. Transgender Survey. Washington, DC: National Center for Transgender Equality.

Johnstone, L., & Boyle, M., with Cromby, J., Dillon, J., Harper, D., Kinderman, P., Longden, E., Pilgrim, D., & Read, J. (2018a). *The power threat meaning framework: Towards the identification of patterns in emotional distress, unusual experiences and troubled or troubling behavior, as an alternative to functional psychiatric diagnosis.* Leicester, England: British Psychological Society. Retrieved from www.bps.org.uk/PTM-Main

Johnstone, L., Boyle, M., Cromby, J., Dillon, J., Harper, D., Kinderman, P., Longden, E., Pilgrim, D., & Read, J. (2018b). The Power Threat Meaning Framework: Overview. Leicester, England:British Psychological Society. Retrieved from www.bps.org.uk/PTM-Overview

Judge, C., O'Donovan, C., Callaghan, G., Gaoatswe, G., & O'Shea, D. (2014). Gender dysphoria–prevalence and co-morbidities in an Irish adult population. *Frontiers in Endocrinology*, *5*, 87.

Kerry, S. C. (2014). Sistergirls/brotherboys: The status of indigenous transgender Australians. *International Journal of Transgenderism*, *15*(3–4), 173–186.

Langevin, R., Paitich, D. & Steiner, B. (1977). The clinical profile of male transsexuals living as females vs those living as males. *Archives of Sexual Behavior*, *6*(2), 143–154.

Lester, C. N. (2017). *Trans like me: A journey for all of us.* Hachette UK.

Lev, A. I. (2009). The ten tasks of the mental health provider: Recommendations for revision of the World Professional Association for Transgender Health's Standards of Care. *International Journal of Transgenderism*, *11*(2), 74–99.

Lysenko, N. (2009). Let's talk about trans: trans-positive'discourse, australian psychology and gender euphoria. *Gay & Lesbian Issues & Psychology Review*, *5*(3).

McLaren, A. (1993). *Thomas Laqueur. Making sex: Body and gender from the Greeks to Freud.* Cambridge: Harvard University Press.

Meadow, T. (2011). 'Deep down where the music plays': How parents account for childhood gender variance. *Sexualities*, *14*(6), 725–747.

Meyer, I. H. (2003). Prejudice, social stress, and mental health in lesbian, gay, and bi-sexual populations: Conceptual issues and research evidence. *Psychological Bulletin*, *129*(5), 674.

Meyer, I. H. (2015). Resilience in the study of minority stress and health of sexual and gender minorities. *Psychology of Sexual Orientation and Gender Diversity*, *2*(3), 209.

Mogul, J. L., Ritchie, A. J., & Whitlock, K. (2011). *Queer (in) justice: The criminalization of LGBT people in the United States* (Vol. 5). Beacon Press.

Owen-Smith, A. A., Gerth, J., Sineath, R. C., Barzilay, J., Becerra-Culqui, T. A., Getahun, D., … & Goodman, M. (2018). Association between gender confirmation treatments and perceived gender congruence, body image satisfaction, and mental health in a cohort of transgender individuals. *The Journal of Sexual Medicine*, *15*(4), 591–600.

Picq, M. L., & Tikuna, J. O. S. I. (2019). Indigenous sexualities: Resisting conquest and translation. *Sexuality and Translation in World Politics – E-International Relations (e-ir.info)*, *57*.

Pronouns: A How-To (n.D.). The Diversity Center of Northeast Ohio. https://www.diversitycenterneo.org/about-us/pronouns/

Richardson, S. S. (2013). *Sex itself.* University of Chicago Press.

Sahota, K. K. (2020). Transgender sex offenders: Gender dysphoria and sexual offending. *Journal of Criminological Research, Policy and Practice*, *6*(3), 255–267.

Schulz, S. L. (2018). The informed consent model of transgender care: an alternative to the diagnosis of gender dysphoria. *Journal of Humanistic Psychology*, *58*(1), 72–92.

Serano, J. (2020). Autogynephilia: A scientific review, feminist analysis, and alternative 'embodiment fantasies' model. *The Sociological Review*, *68*(4), 763–778.

Steadman, I. (2015). Sex Isn't Chromosomes: The Story of a Century of Misconceptions about X & Y. *New Statesman*.

Stryker, S. (2008). *Transgender history*. Seal Press.

Swift, T. L., & Dieppe, P. A. (2005). Using expert patients' narratives as an educational resource. *Patient Education and Counseling*, *57*(1), 115–121.

Thoroughgood, C., Sawyer, K., & Webster, J. R. (2020). Creating a trans-inclusive workplace. *Harvard Business Review*.

Udry, J. R. (1994). The nature of gender. *Demography*, *31*(4), 561–573.

Vine, C. N. (2009). Psychology under the Third Reich. *Psychology*.

Wesp, L. M., Malcoe, L. H., Elliott, A., & Poteat, T. (2019). Intersectionality research for transgender health justice: a theory-driven conceptual framework for structural analysis of transgender health inequities. *Transgender Health*, *4*(1), 287–296.

World Health Organization (WHO). (2018). ICD-11: classifying disease to map the way we live and die. www.who.int/news-room/spotlight/international-classification-of-diseases

Zimman, L. (2017). Transgender language reform: Some challenges and strategies for promoting trans-affirming, gender-inclusive language. *Journal of Language and Discrimination*, *1*(1), 83–104.

19 Neurodiversity

Nancy Doyle, Lorraine Hough, Karen Thorne, and Tanya Banfield

Neurodiversity Assessment in Forensic Contexts

In this chapter, authors will first present a whistle-stop tour of the "Neurodiversity Movement" and contemporary research, define the scope of neurodiversity and explore paradigm shifts occurring in what used to be known as Specific Learning Disabilities (SpLD) and Neurodevelopmental Disorders. Advice on terminology is included, as is conceptual critique of diagnostic boundaries, including comment on intersectional adverse impacts. Thirdly, we present discussion of neurominority conditions in forensic contexts, advice on using assessment and screening tools for Psychologists. Recommendations for support and embedding neurodiversity awareness into interventions, support, and education within the criminal justice system (CJS) conclude the chapter.

The New Paradigm of Neurodiversity, Its Definitions, and Terms

The term "Neurodiversity" was academically developed by the Australian, Autistic Sociologist Judy Singer, (Singer, 1998). Singer's intention was to give voice to the growing sense, amongst activists operating within the Social Model of Disability (Charlton, 1998), that there was nothing inherently disabling about Autism, and that diversity in neurological profiles should be considered a natural feature in the human species. There is no internationally agreed definition of neurodivergence, however, a recent UK Criminal Justice Joint Inspectorate Neurodiversity Review (CJJI, 2021) considered it an umbrella term referring to the group of conditions falling under the category of neurodevelopmental disorders (NDDs). These incorporate learning difficulties and disabilities (LDDs) generally including: Learning Disability, Dyslexia, Dyscalculia, and Dyspraxia (also known as developmental coordination disorder, DCD); clinical conditions, such as Attention Deficit Hyperactivity Disorder (ADHD, including ADD), Autism Spectrum Conditions (ASC), Developmental Language Disorder (DLD, including Speech and Language Difficulties), Tic Disorders (including Tourette's Syndrome and Chronic Tic Disorder) and cognitive impairments due to acquired brain injury

DOI: 10.4324/9781003230977-22

(ABI). Some definitions of neurodivergence incorporate disorders affecting executive functioning and cognition, whilst others reference Deafness and Sight Loss.

There is professional debate amongst Psychologists about current use, appropriateness, and relevance of the term neurodiversity and to which conditions it should be applied (see: Baron-Cohen, 2017; Kapp et al., 2013; Krcek, 2012; McLoughlin, 2021; Runswick-Cole, 2014). However, congruent to the British Psychological Society (BPS) Code of Ethics principle, "the right to self-determination" (BPS, 2018; p7), professionals should be aware of the many terms in use and offer service-users the opportunity to identify terms of their preference. In this chapter, we take our guide from neurodivergent researchers, activists, and self-advocates who assert rights to self-identify (Bottema-Beutel et al., 2020; Chapman, 2020a; Lorcan et al., 2016; Walker, 2012). We advise practitioners to invest time in staying abreast of changes to language as a signal of respect to individuals you are supporting, in the same way that you would want to adopt language preferred by other minoritized populations such as ethnicities and LGBTQIA2S+ people. Always also be respectful to clients by remaining open to changing your language, especially when working with an individual who may not follow current trends, (BPS, 2017, 2018). In this chapter, the following terms are used (see Appendix 1 for a glossary of terms):

> "Neurodiversity" – refers to the whole species, the concept that human cognition, emotions, behaviours and ways of being vary, and such variation is natural and evolutionarily purposeful.

> "Neurodivergent" or "neurodiverse" or "neurodifferent" – refers to the position of not having a typical cognitive ability profile or neurological presentation.

> "Neurotypical" – refers to those whose cognitive ability profiles or neurology are statistically normal or average.

> "Neurominority" – refers to a group or condition that is a-typical, a neurological subtype such as ADHD, Dyslexia etc.

The implication of the Neurodiversity model therefore is that there are essentially two types of people: "neurotypical", whose cognitive abilities and neurological functions fit within one or two standard deviations of the statistical "norm"; and a sizeable neurominority, estimated at 15–20%, whose profiles are neurodivergent from the norm, itself defined by the prevailing socio-historical context (Doyle, 2020). Also implied is that differences are natural variations in the human species, many entirely defined by complex adaptive social skills which would have been irrelevant prior to the industrial revolution, such as hyper-socialisation in large groups, literacy, or sitting still for prolonged periods (Chapman, 2020b; Riddick, 2001; Shelley-Tremblay & Rosen, 1996).

The neurotypical norm asserts dominance in education, work, and society, leading to pathologisation of difference and reduced agency for those with differences (Chapman, 2020a; Huijg, 2020). The Neurodiversity movement thus aligns itself with diversity and inclusion, seeking similar equity to race, gender, and LGBTQIA2S[1]+ movements, and has a relationship with other disability inclusion approaches; for example, the Deaf Community and corresponding Deaf Culture literature, (Davidson, 2008), (see also, chapter X). It enables recognition of the diversity of psychological cognitive characteristics and validation of uniqueness of patterns in cognitive strengths and weaknesses, with this juxtaposition termed a "Spiky Profile" (Pollack, 2009). It encourages a person-centred approach, focusing not on disability, but rather, focusing on ability. If, as Psychologists, we adopt this paradigm, then identifying/"playing to strengths", as well as recognising/respecting needs, we can both work responsively with individual needs and offer adaptive strategies/reasonable adjustment to individuals within the CJS.

General population prevalence rates of neurominorities (shown in parenthesis in Table 19.1) provide estimates for UK populations, and are taken from a chapter in the BPS 2017 publication "Psychology at Work" (Doyle, 2017), unless stated otherwise, along with summaries of functional traits associated with the conditions. Further details on prevalence within the CJS are provided in Table 19.4. Almost all studies exploring cooccurrence and overlap find this to be persistently high (see: Antshel & Russo, 2019; McGrath & Stoodley, 2019) and so listing prevalence individually can be misleading. Estimates of the whole population affected by one or more developmental neurominorities are around 15–20%; a substantial protected minority group (Doyle, 2020; Lollini, 2018) (Tables 19.2 and 19.3).

Table 19.1 Applied (task performance assessed) developmental neurominorities

Dyslexia (8–10%)	Individuals are often good at visual or spatial skills and at making connections (e.g., mind mapping), but may be less strong at literacy skills, (verbal capacity, writing, and reading). They are typically slower to read, less likely to read for pleasure and also display difficulties in processing or remembering new (verbally presented) information. Individuals can be gifted and reflect a higher-than-average level of (overall) intellectual capacity, (IQ). Dyslexia is differentiated in diagnosis from poor reading due to low educational engagement, which also affects those in custody. There are also individuals who will present with the mechanical skills of reading but without good comprehension of text.
Dyspraxia (1–6%)	Strengths might include perception of others (empathy), capacity to be innovative, verbal skills, with comparative weakness including organisation, balance, and motor coordination. Memory and speed of processing can be adversely impacted. Dyspraxia can affect the motor component of writing, also basic self-care tasks such as eating, dressing, and using equipment, particularly when it is new. Dyspraxic people can find map reading and spatial orientation difficult as they tend to have lower visuo-spatial reasoning skills.

(Continued)

Table 19.1 (Continued)

Dyscalculia (1–6%) (Butterworth et al., 2011)	Often individuals with stronger verbal skills but find working with numbers or mathematical concepts difficult, including estimation of size and speed, or where numeric information may be transposed, and maths errors not easily spotted. Dyscalculia is differentiated from a specific maths weakness arising from poor working memory and involves a more fundamental difficulty conceptualising numerosity.
Dysgraphia (<5%)	Relates to difficulties in expressive language and getting language-based thoughts onto paper, it may involve grammar, punctuation, and spelling/proof-reading limits, with speed of processing often being impacted. Those with Dyslexia may also be Dysgraphic, but it is differentiated from Dyspraxia

Table 19.2 Clinical (behaviourally-assessed) developmental neurominorities

Attention deficit hyperactivity disorder (ADHD) (2–6%)	ADHD is TYPICALLY thought to result from lower levels of dopamine and noradrenaline (Engert & Pruessner, 2009) which can impact upon concentration / attention and risk perception. Individuals may operate well in crisis, often reflect good verbal, visual, and abstract reasoning skills. Individuals may have good capacity for processing information, often being creative and novel thinkers, reflecting energy, passion, and drive. Working memory is significantly adversely affected, creating difficulties in concentration and the lack of dopamine creates restlessness, hyperactivity, and impulsiveness. Emotional dysregulation is also common.
Autism (1–2%)	Autistic individuals may find abstract reasoning difficult, with literal interpretation of information often being observed. Social interactional/ interpersonal skills can be impacted, for example limited eye contact, missed social cues, and communication style differences. Individuals may experience hypersensitivity to stimulation, (light, noise, smell, taste, temperature, touch) which can create extreme anxiety, pain and trauma when the environment is uncontrolled, leading to a strong preference for routine. Individuals often, however, demonstrate great attention to detail and levels of concentration. Autism may or may not be related to intellectual capacity, with some autistic individuals reflecting high IQ levels and others having cooccurring learning disability. Some Autistic people are considered "savants" with a particular expertise in one or more topics, and though this

(*Continued*)

Table 19.2 (Continued)

	stereotype does not reflect all Autistic people (Hughes et al., 2018) many Autists develop keen interests in specific areas such as art, historical events or technology.
Pathological demand avoidance (PDA)	A recently documented condition with no prevalence data as yet, thought to be a subset of Autism but also can co-occur with ADHD (Egan et al., 2019). Strengths can be similar to ADHD and Autism, but struggles tend to differ, as PDA leads to persistent "shutdowns" and avoidant behaviours in response to simple day-to-day demands. PDA is thought to be based mainly on an extreme level of anxiety, where every day routines create flight/fight/freeze responses.

Table 19.3 Neurological and sensory neurominorities

Visual stress	Prevalence data are not reliably available for general populations, but it is thought to be higher in dyslexic people. Visual stress, also sometimes known as Mearles-Irlen syndrome, or scotopic sensitivity syndrome, is not about functioning of an individual's eyes, rather, visual spatial/perceptual brain functioning implications and corresponding visual distortion, for example when reading. Reading/scanning written information can be tricky, with colours of print/contrasts being important. Many individuals can be supported by coloured lenses/filters, with type face, size, and font issues being important, as is the case for certain Dyslexic difficulties (Kriss & Evans, 2005).
Sensory processing disorder	There is some question as to prevalence of sensory processing disorder as a symptom of developmental neurominorities or actually as underlying neurological difference that leads to presentation of neurominority, however in general population prevalence is estimated between 5% and 23% (Gomez et al., 2021). Being hyper or hypo sensitive has clear evolutionary advantage to a community, within the theory of Complementary Cognition (Taylor et al., 2021) but can lead to difficulties acquiring language, concentrating, becoming overwhelmed and needing to withdraw. Hypersensitive people can have fear or startle responses to seemingly normal levels of noise, light, smell, temperature, colour and taste. Hyposensitive people risk serious injury due to failing to perceive pain and can present as

Table 19.3 (Continued)

	louder and more forceful than their peers. Sensory processing disorder is not listed on the DSM 5 (American Psychiatric Association, 2013) as an individual category but the symptoms are associated with Autism and ADHD, in particular.
Acquired neuro-cognitive disorders	Defined here as recognised, acquired medical reasons for changes to thinking/reasoning. Often affects memory/remembering; processing or speed of processing of information or concentration, and may result in cognitive deterioration, e.g., Dementia; Alzheimer's; Huntingdon's Chorea. Multiple Sclerosis can affect cognitive/brain functioning and nerves, as well as impacting physical and motor skills. Not all areas of cognition will be affected and therefore retained skills can be augmented and developed into strengths. Prevalence rates are reported per condition, each between 0.1% and 5% of the mature adult population, increasing with age.
Tic disorders (1%)	Development and presence of verbal and/or motor "tics", which can be as simple as just throat clearing and eye blinking, or complex including complex phrases and movements. Can also include coprolalia and copropraxia, which refer to rude or insulting words and gestures, though this is uncommon (around 10% of those with tic disorders). Where both verbal and motor tics occur with premonitory urges, this is known as Tourette Syndrome. Alongside, we typically find executive functions deficits, creative strengths, empathy and acquired cognitive control and high occurrence with ADHD.
Developmental disorders including learning/ intellectual disability (1.5%), (Public Health England, 2016).	Such implications can be pre-, peri- or post-natal due to a range of neurological (brain development) issues. They can affect development of a range of cognitive skills, (for example language acquisition, social skills, communication skills, motor/coordination skills). They also include neuro-genetic conditions, (e.g., Fragile X or Down's Syndrome – gene variation implications); birth trauma/infection during pregnancy/foetal alcohol syndrome or mother's use of substances. Includes also disorders such as Cerebral Palsy – where differing brain functioning areas can again be affected pre-/peri-birth or during brain development; whilst Deafness/Blindness can also be congenital and linked to brain functioning and have neurological implications. Strengths can include focused interests and specific skills, ability to work well in routine activities, as well as more socially relevant strengths such as loyalty and kindness. Some authors have also proposed "developmental language disorder" as a separate

(Continued)

Table 19.3 (Continued)

	category in which only language is affected, not co-occurring with learning disability, Autism or other conditions (Bishop et al., 2017).
Acquired brain injury (12 %) (Frost et al., 2013)	Damage to the brain can be acquired (ABI) as a result of stroke; brain haemorrhage; tumours; anoxia (lack of oxygen) or can arise from external and traumatic causes (TBI). Similarly, to acquired neurological conditions, ABI and TBI do not necessarily affect the whole brain and retained skills can be augmented and developed into strengths. Brain injury can cause Deafness/Hearing Loss, or Blindness/Sight Loss, or differing cognitive implications, such as executive functioning difficulties, language, or memory deficits. There can be a corresponding trauma implication or psychological transition/ adjustment requirement.

Table 19.4 Prevalence of neurominorities in forensic contexts

Study	Prevalence rates
(CJJI, 2021)	Over 50% of the prison UK population is dyslexic
(McNamara, 2012)	Up to 80% of people in a UK prison have some kind of speech, language, or communication difficulty
(Young et al., 2018)	Approximately one-quarter of people in prison in the UK would meet diagnostic criteria for ADHD
(CJJI, 2021)	Approximately 5–7% of those coming into contact with Liaison and Diversion services in the UK have Autistic traits, with around 16–19% of those in prison exhibiting indications of Autism
(Prison Reform Trust, 2021)	Approximately, 34% of people in custody in the UK have a Mild Intellectual Disability (MID) or Borderline Intellectual Functioning (BIF)
(Prison Reform Trust, 2021)	49% of women and 23% of men in custody in the UK have been diagnosed with anxiety or depression.
(Shiroma et al., 2010) (McMillan et al., 2019; Pitman et al., 2015)	Estimates of ABI and TBI in people in CJS vary significantly based on the jurisdiction / populations being studied and assessment approach adopted, but meta-analysis of international studies suggests that rates of TBI in convicted populations is approximately 60%. In Scotland and England, rates of ABI (in convicted populations) appear to be lower at 24% and 46% respectively. However, this is still higher than the general population at 12% (Table 19.3).
(Chester et al., 2018; Thorne, 2021)	In forensic settings in the UK, rates of ABI in individuals with MID or BIF are higher than general UK custodial populations. Chester et al. (2018) report 67% of individuals in the secure forensic hospital learning disabilities service. Thorne (2021) found 55% of males with MID-BIF in UK prisons reported a history of ABI.

Impact of Mental Health Conditions

MH distress or exposure to trauma impacts cognitive abilities, such as reducing working memory, for example (Otto et al., 2016; Solé et al., 2011) resulting in a "spiky profile", although this may be transient and return to neurotypical norms when health is recovered or effectively treated. People with lived experience of mental ill-health sometimes identify as neurodiverse, however poor MH is often a cooccurring condition within a primary diagnosis and wellbeing can lapse within a stressful prison environment.

Socio-Historic Influences on Neurominority Diagnosis

Two emerging issues in developmental neurominorities are construct validity and diagnostic unreliability. These arise from developments in neuropsychology which find evidence that contradicts existing diagnostic boundaries (Siugzdaite et al., 2020), as well as the socially defined nature of the conditions and the way they have evolved and changed over time. For example, changes to DSM means those diagnosed with ADHD today may not have been diagnosed 10 years ago (Sanders et al., 2019); Asperger's Syndrome has been classified, reclassified, and removed within a generation (Hosseini & Molla, 2021). There are geographic differences in diagnostic criteria (Ihori & Olvera, 2015). Some countries, for example, specify levels of statistical difference that should exist between cognitive tests to determine "weakness" (Grant, 2009; McLoughlin & Leather, 2013) while others recommend only scores lower than the 25th percentile would qualify (United States Department for Education's Office of Special Educational Needs, 2006). When considering the age of people in the CJS, practitioners should note probable under-diagnosis in older individuals and the cathartic improvements arising from exploring cognitive differences.

The way we conceptualise and measure neurodiversity is dependent on socially constructed norms of communication, tending towards white, middle class, male, cisgender, hetero presentation (Campbell, 2008; Mandell et al., 2009; Reyes et al., 2013; Young et al., 2020). Whilst no known studies (at time of writing) have systematically explored the role of sexuality in neurominority diagnosis, there are some exploratory studies. Below, we present a summary of current evidence concerning intersectional adverse impact.

Gender

Seemingly robust, persistent gender disparities between males and females with ASC or ADHD diagnoses are increasingly questioned in research due to the inherently gender-typed behavioural norms associated with levels of physical movement, expected social competence and expression of distress that form the DSM criteria (American Psychiatric Association, 2013), leading to systemic underdiagnosis of women and girls (Estrin, 2020; Young et al., 2020). One study examining the prevalence of Autism self-report symptoms between male-to-female and female-to-male transgender people (Heylens et al., 2018), suggested that when socialised gender traits are rejected, there are fewer differences. Incidence of Dyslexia, Dyscalculia, Dyspraxia also tends towards male presentation, but less dramatically so possibly because diagnosis is more reliant on objective skill assessment than socially coded behaviour. However, even in ability testing, there are significant psychosocial influences such as expectations of male abilities in maths and motor coordination, and gender stereotyping of literacy-based activities (OECD, 2015) which affect who presents for testing. Again, females are less likely to be identified as struggling.

Race / Ethnicity

Access to diagnosis is hampered by cultural norms affecting perceptions and have led to systemic underdiagnosis in non-white populations (CDC, 2011). It is, for example, considered polite in Afro-Caribbean cultures to avert eye contact when being spoken to by someone in authority (Akechi et al., 2013; Levine et al., 2006) and Asian cultures are known to place higher value on compliance and deference to authority than Anglo-white cultures, which contributes to lower diagnosis of ADHD in Japan, for example (Miyasaka et al., 2018). Black, Asian, Indigenous, People of Colour from the global ethnic majority (GEM) are more likely to have their behaviour misinterpreted and either under recognised or over pathologized by questionnaires/testing developed for Anglo-white populations (Hendren et al., 2018; Nicolaidis et al., 2020; Richardson & Wydell, 2003). This will affect clinical appraisal of social communication skills as defined for ADHD and Autism. Further and in general, concepts of "therapy" and "assessment" have been found to be white and westernised (Memon et al., 2016), having limited meaning or resonance for those not recognising such westernised norms, meaning that fewer neurominorities will seek support for difficulties before entering the CJS.

Socio-Economic status

Several studies have explored the effects of low economic status on neurominority diagnosis and consistently found higher rates of diagnosis in families living at or below poverty levels (CDC, 2011; Cree et al., 2018; Ellenberg et al., 2019). Similarly to GEM children, children living in poverty have higher rates of need and lower rates of support (Adak & Halder, 2017; Reyes et al., 2013). Families with means can provide scaffolding support in the form of additional tuition, help with remembering and completing homework and sufficient nutrition. In terms of presentation to the CJS, people living in poverty are less likely to be treated and supported for their neurodifferences or to develop strategies that assist them in navigating the system or advocating for needs; nor are they likely to acknowledge/accept support in terms of socio-economic anxiety.

Intersectionality

One recent UK-based Autism study (Roman-Urrestarazu et al., 2021) provides evidential insight when considering intersectional adverse impacts on diagnosis and support. Though male children are on average diagnosed at higher rates than females (4.39:1) they receive significantly higher levels of support, as measured by the presence of an Educational and Health Care Plan (ECHP) (4.94:1). Although Black children in this study were diagnosed more frequently than white children for the first time, they received less support. Chinese and Roma children were systematically underdiagnosed compared with white children. Children provided with free school meals were diagnosed at a rate of 1.61:1 compared with children without, however support was provided at a lower rate of 1.49:1. Lack of Special Educational Needs (SEN) support leads to isolation, exclusions, and educational failure, which affect occupational opportunities, leading to increased risk of criminality. This study highlighted the compound intersectional effect for Black girls living in poverty, for example, compared with white girls or Black boys UK-wide. Such detailed analysis is not available for all neurominorities but is likely to play out in a similar manner.

Identifying Neurodiversity in Forensic Contexts

There has been growing interest in understanding prevalence of neurodiversity in forensic settings. Data emerging from prevalence studies suggest that neurominorities are over-represented (see Table 19.4). Accurately estimating prevalence data in the CJS is, however, complicated by the presence of heterogenous populations (e.g., children and young people/adults, male/female) and variety of stages of these systems. Prevalence data is often drawn from populations in custodial settings, thereby failing to capture those arrested or charged with an offence but not sentenced to custody (e.g., Taylor & Lindsay, 2018). Furthermore, different CJS institutions have heterogenous assessment protocols and may not routinely screen for neurodivergence. Prevalence studies in CJS settings should be regarded as underestimates of true rates of neurodiversity.

Given the high prevalence of neurominorities in the CJS and the intersectional critique reflecting under-, over-, or incorrect diagnosis, it is not possible to assume diagnostic accuracy when an individual enters the CJS. Psychologists should not simply tick boxes and say, "Autism means this person will need XYZ" as ADHD, trauma or intellectual disabilities may have been missed. Nor should we say "no previous diagnosis of ADHD, therefore observations of distraction mid-sentence must indicate deceit, rather than cognitive processing".

In terms of legal frameworks outlined in the Equality Act (2010), diagnosis is not a requirement, only sustained difficulty in "normal day-to-day functioning" which can include memory and communication. To this end, a person presenting with sustained difficulties in communication or social skill, or erratic concentration and listening ability, should be presumed to have cognitive difference for which they require legal protection and reasonable adjustment until proven otherwise. Adopting this premise means Psychologists can move away from adopting a neurotypical approach and move towards a neuro responsive approach and take a more individualised, person-centred approach to working with those in the CJS. It is recommended that CJS practitioners pay less attention to diagnostic accuracy and more to individualised profiles of strengths and weaknesses, including consideration of cultural issues, which can lead to targeted support and goal setting. Assuming positive intention and an understanding of multiple barriers faced by those marginalised by their demographic will lead to trust and accurate signposting.

Catharsis and self-discovery can come from exploration of cognitive ability profiles and background history, with or without labelling at the end. In other words, take people at face value and help all individuals to understand their unique pattern of strengths and weaknesses, how these can lead to career opportunities, where technology and adjustments can make a difference to day-to-day functioning. This is the ultimate goal of all screening and cognitive testing; not seeking to limit people with labels that confer restrictions on ambitions, rather to understand how they can make the best use of innate abilities and signpost access to appropriate resources. If we consider cognitive challenges, respect strengths, and adapt/support, with the above in mind, we, as Psychologists, can make a significant difference. Evidence suggests that providing positive assessment of potential can lead to better outcomes for neurodivergent people (Armstrong, 2010; Doyle & McDowall, 2019; Pollack, 2009; Prevatt & Yelland, 2013). Screening and assessment should therefore be considered using a more widespread approach.

Assessment of Neurodiversity in Forensic Contexts

The Wechsler Adult Intelligence Scale, (WAIS: Weschler, 2008) or the Wechsler Intelligence Scale for Children (WISC: Wechsler, 2014) is the "Gold Standard" of assessment for spiky profiles. It provides reliable advice on abilities, strengths, weaknesses, and how these might be best considered to support need/decision-making. Both assessments require specialist training and administration/interpretation by a Registered Psychologist, or Trainee Psychologist under supervision. Though not considered as standard clinical assessment for some neurominorities, such as ADHD, Autism, and Tourettes, it is regularly used for assessment of Dyslexia, Dyspraxia, and other applied conditions (McLoughlin & Doyle, 2013; SASC, 2017). That is not to say that it, or some other measure of basic cognitive abilities, would not be useful for functional, formative assessment of strengths and identifying support needs. However, when this was used in a forensic setting, it became clear that, although positive, the WAIS cannot be deployed at scale as it is expensive, time-consuming, and only licensed to Applied Psychologists who have completed training.

There are many formal/standardised psychometrics, functional screening tools, and diagnostic questionnaires/behavioural checklists in current use. It is vital, however, that practitioners are aware of respective strengths, cautions, and caveats of each when assessing neurodifference (see Table 19.5).

Considerations in Terms of Test Use

Oakland (2016) signposts three broad aspects of testing that warrant consideration by the Test User, to maximise reliability/validity and minimise sources of bias or adverse impact potential.

1   **Test item/test construction issues:** The applicability, constitution, size, and utility of (forensic) norm groups available; robustness of technical data (reliability/validation studies) and availability of technical manual; test modifications needed and impact thereof on standardisation processes; all warrant consideration by the Test User.

    This focuses on nature and content of individual test items, including prerequisite knowledge, experiences, level, and nature of language skills needed by the test takers in order to understand, have equality of access to, and capacity to complete any given test. For example, literacy level and requirements for prolonged concentration and abstraction may affect the process of testing, not just the results. Equally, tendencies towards items that require experience of Anglo-centric middle-class education compromise validity. Completing questionnaires and psychometrics, validated on neurotypical populations, can lead to systemic barriers, where a test taker's true potential is masked by difficulty understanding test instructions or concentrating for prolonged periods.

2   **Personal qualities of person being tested:** Issues to be aware of focus on the wider biological-, behavioural-, social-, cognitive- and language-based skills of the individual, in terms of protected characteristics or intersectionality issues.

    In the case of neurodiversity, we need to consider issues such as processing speed; language weaknesses; impacts in terms of memory or cognitive demands; visual – perceptual skills, (e.g., colour vision, size, and type of font being used). Also relevant is exposure to social experiences; issues related to responsivity (such as need for concentration breaks) and ensuring that psychometrics use accessible language levels. Being mindful of social desirability; impression management; superficiality of understanding and not wanting to "appear stupid", with corresponding impacts on self-esteem for example, are also important to bear in mind.

    As Psychologists, it is important to ensure that assessment focuses on and signposts individual strengths as well as difficulty. Considering psychological well-being during testing and presenting results in the best possible light is an essential part of the intervention. When well-framed and psychologically

Table 19.5 Tools to support neurodiversity assessment

Tools to support neurodiversity assessment	Cautions; considerations; caveats around test use	Strengths of use	Limitations of use
Formal standardised psychometric measures, (such as the WAIS but also including other standardised assessment tools that might be more targeted such as specific literacy, numeracy, dexterity, and memory assessment tools) Peer-reviewed and standardised questionnaires that can support diagnostic processes/signpost evidence to support DSM 5 criteria	Standardisation can impact on individuals, e.g., speed of processing/cognitive overload. Items can be verbally loaded and reflect cultural/intersectional bias. Reading age requirements/implication in terms of functional literacy levels etc.	Good technical data; Special group data; standardised; norms wide-ranging and large, although may not be representational or up-to-date. Technical manual/professional literature base. Provides cognitive information to explore "spiky profiles" Requirement to be suitable qualified/trained in administration and interpretation. (Trainee Psychologists use under supervision.) Whilst not about diagnosing, can trigger access to specialist provision +/or diversion within CJS. May signpost previously undiagnosed neurodiversity, to inform ways of working with individuals to overcome barriers to progression or challenges experienced Correlational data, (reliability/validity)	Some items may systematically discriminate certain neurodiversity presentations, (e.g., use of metaphors; literal meaning; social opportunity limitations etc). Additionally, there are recognised cultural impacts on such formal assessment tools, such as white privilege/middle-class schooling, (see reliability/validity and other chapters), and unconscious bias issues; for example in terms of the test user. All of these require consideration and understanding of in order to correctly interpret any outcomes.
Self-Report measures/questionnaires	Dependent upon reading skills of test taker; exposure to language/social implications of test items.	Provides qualitative information which can be explored in the context of individual/case formulation processes.	Impression management; social desirability; requirement to read and understand information and experience social situations within items.

(Continued)

Table 19.5 (Continued)

Tools to support neurodiversity assessment	Cautions; considerations; caveats around test use	Strengths of use	Limitations of use
	Limited technical robustness/ literature base to support these.	May have "face validity" for the individuals we are working with. Limited reliability/validity information, but usually focuses more on behavioural/presentational aspects.	Where read to an individual via third party, this introduces other dynamics/ sensitivities
Non – Formal Measures, including a) Behavioural checklists; b) Screening Tools; c) Author developed/ non-standardised tools	Some literature/research base and inform case formulation. Behavioural checklists can inform Learning Disability/ Mental Capacity assessments. Can pick up on behavioural/ presentational information and reported symptomology. Author-developed tools are not necessarily peer-reviewed; have potential for bias; may not have supporting technical data or support standardisation of approach. May be supporting journal articles. Need caution to be applied and for professional judgement to be exercised, in terms of ethical and research considerations.	Multi-disciplinary and key worker insights gained; allow behavioural/ presentational consideration across "real life" contexts. Provide qualitative information to inform case formulation. May be grounded in theory/literature and informed by.	May be inter-personal differences between test taker so may be differences between and across different raters. Limited technical data/robustness in terms of psychometric properties.

safe, assessment can be the turning point for vulnerable, excluded people and can be used to recover self-esteem and hope around career potential. Badly conducted testing can reinforce low self-esteem and curtail ambition.

3   **Qualities of the test user:** Psychologists should consider it an important part of their continuing professional development to stay up-to-date with assessment practices and recommendations and to seek formal training in individual tests, their use and interpretation.

Psychologists should be competently able to critically appraise any potential tool in terms of its construction: validity, reliability, norm group sampling, cultural issues, and more. Practitioners should also be mindful of their own unconscious biases and undertake regular reflective practice. Issues such as dynamics and relational issues between the test taker and test user, (i.e., rapport building; responsivity to needs of the individual; establishing effective communication skills) also require consideration. Where the test user comes from a different ethnic background from the test taker, the impact of people reacting to this difference can affect testing outcomes. It is therefore important for test users to consider issues around positionality and white privilege, for example.

Further Testing Considerations for Neurodiversity and Forensic Contexts

Complexity in Causal Factors / Decision Making

If it seems confusing and ambiguous, that is because it is confusing and ambiguous! As professionals, we can't always ascertain what is "driving" something. The lack of validity and reliability in testing protocols for this population combine to make neurominority diagnosis an art rather than a science. Focusing on differential diagnosis is important, ensuring that there are no alternative explanations for symptoms that are unexplored, although this may require medical referral to confirm diagnosis. A detailed background history is essential, and testing should be used to confirm or refute hypotheses made during history taking, rather than as a basis for decision.

Functional Priorities

Despite complexity in diagnosis, there is urgent and practical need to conduct basic screening and assessment for most entrants to custody. Resources do not currently exist for full assessment for a range of possible conditions. Functional assessments in the form of screening tools exist within current practice and Psychologists should consider supporting and contributing to the development of this practice. Those which intend to replace or automatise diagnosis are risky; you cannot programme an algorithm to make reliable decisions when there is so much dispute around the concepts that we are assessing, and so many heterogenous reactions to testing protocols. For example, there is evidence of racism embedded in standardised forensic risk assessments (Woldgabreal et al., 2020), which shows the potential fallibility of seemingly robust measures. However, tools which focus on functional skills alone, such as memory, literacy, visual skills, communication, without attempting to "diagnose" can be used to signpost for support.

Case Formulation and Implications for Testing

Cognitive functioning patterns of neurodivergent individuals need consideration within the developmental history of the individual, alongside life, social, psychological/mental health functioning, and emotional experiences, that have shaped the individual. Using a bio-psycho-social approach, psychologists can hypothesise about causal factors, those that precipitate, influence or maintain an individual's behaviour and presentation, and the inter-relation of those in terms of offending behaviour in a holistic manner. Once wider understanding is gained, we can consider how best to support and work with facets of the individual that contribute to offending, including need for interventions, strategies, and managing risk. Forensic testing generally and neurodiversity assessment more specifically, support case formulation processes, offering insights into cognitive strengths and weaknesses or other aspects of the individual's functioning, in order to make sense of complex behaviours and presentations. Triangulating assessments and case information can help to support and refine the hypothesis process, complementing interviews, collateral reviews, and multi-disciplinary case discussion.

Providing Support

Implications of Unaddressed Needs

Limited consistent and systematic screening for neurominorities in many CJSs means that individuals with one or more cooccurring neurodifferences, can go undetected for much of a detention or probation period (e.g., CJJI, 2021). Many of those in CJS are likely to be living with these challenges with minimal support and without strengths being channelled towards intended to reducing reoffending (CJJI, 2021). Neurodivergence has cognitive, emotional, and behavioural implications, impacting on self-esteem, self-efficacy well-being, and sense of self, (agency) (Huijg, 2020; Nalavany et al., 2017). Where implications are not understood in the CJS, it can lead to frustration, shame, embarrassment, feeling isolated, angry, and aggression. Criminal justice staff are often working with, assessing, treating, and making recommendations for neurominorities but may be doing so without awareness of or regard to the impact of cognitive strengths and challenges. Service users (individuals within the CJS) raise concerns that they are misperceived as being intentionally lazy, arrogant, rude, or stupid especially where professionals have limited understanding or awareness. Research suggests that in the UK these concerns may be justified (O'Rourke et al., 2018; Yuhasz, 2013).

The structure, process, and regimes of CJS are neurotypical by design and have potential to exclude those who cannot fill in forms, read or process documents and in a timely fashion, respond effectively and understand or remember complexity of information within formal interviews (Prison Reform Trust, 2021). Challenges within a neurotypically designed system can impact on ability to adjust to the custodial environment and to engage with efforts to rehabilitate and reduce risk of re-offending.

Difficulties with concentration, reading comprehension, following instructions, distractibility, irritability, poor emotional regulation, and poor memory have been found to have significant impact on custodial behaviour and adaptation to prison life (Merbitz et al., 1995). This can contribute to more rule infractions, lower treatment completion rates (Piccolino & Solberg, 2014), and reduce success in applying for release on parole (e.g., Hawley & Maden, 2003). The impact of neurodivergence on service users does not just stop at the prison gate with many struggling with community re-entry on parole (Nagele et al., 2018). However, despite significant impacts of neurodivergence on an individual's functioning, their risk of offending, and ability to engage effectively with risk reduction and management activities, high levels of misconception about neurominorities exist amongst criminal justice staff (Ledingham & Mills, 2015; O'Rourke et al., 2018). Further, neurodivergence is not routinely considered in the management and treatment of those in custodial settings. We therefore encourage practitioners to consider how their general approach to promoting services, providing information, obtaining consent, undertaking interviews for the purposes of collaborating on a formulation or undertaking a risk assessment, or developing interventions can be adapted to be more neuro responsive for all.

Existing Resources for Support

Where there is a lack of, or limited, opportunities for specialised treatment/interventions, it is important for Psychologists to advise forensic contexts about how to take neurologically informed approaches to working with people in their care. Practitioners should consider opportunities to co-opt other colleagues to support individuals within their environment.

Prison or health care staff, for example, should receive psychoeducational training about different neurominorities, the lived experience of individuals with neurodifferences, and providing neuro-informed support to maximise strengths and help compensate for challenges. Tailoring assessment interviews to neurominorities would go some way to minimising disadvantage experienced by this group and enable individuals to communicate their understanding of risk and risk management skills more comprehensively to assessors.

Recommended Activities

Within Psychological reports, for the Parole Board for example, we can signpost the nature of support/intervention or provision that would best meet needs of neurodiverse individuals. Where not available, and potentially detrimental to an individual, this should be flagged, as should any lack of understanding in terms of unique/cultural background of a neurodivergent individual. Psychologists should advise personalised recommendations or bring in appropriate expertise. The list of potential support strategies below is not exhaustive, neither intended to replace appropriate referral to specialist treatment where needed. Whilst we have tried to signal issues across neurominority groups, in reality, strategies are applicable, supportive, and generalisable across different neurodifferences. Table 19.6 presents examples, though we caveat these recommendations with the need to consider adaptation for neurominorities of colour, LGBTQIA2S+, generational differences, and those with significant trauma histories. Some strategies will be culturally more familiar and therefore more relevant. Considered discussion with the individual and flexibility is always recommended.

Table 19.6 Summary of support

Functional difficulty	Recommendations for potential strategies and reasonable adjustments
Executive functions – working memory and processing speed	Memory aids /strategies – little and often; rehearsal; recency and primacy issues so structure key messages; mnemonics; visual imagery; internal aids; external memory aids – post-its, alarms, to-do lists, etc. Chunking. Concentration techniques such as anchoring, visualisation and hunger / time of day self-awareness. Useful resource – Effective Learning after Acquired Brain Injury: A practical guide to support adults with neurological conditions – (Lowings & Wick, 2016)
Executive functions – planning, time management, and organisation	Environmental aids such as signposts; labels; orientation boards; colour doors; wayfinding lines showing routes; use of daily routines. Errorless learning: break down tasks into smaller steps; build in opportunities for success; graded activities to ensure success. Teaching functionally equivalent or functionally related skills.
Language – verbal	Simplify complex instructions and avoid abstract tasks. Promote learning by doing. Repeat if needed. Practice role-play conversations that come up frequently; develop exercises to assist offenders during questioning. This might include supporting them to self-advocate with comments such as "sorry I can't process that all at once, can you ask me just one question at a time?" Develop packs of prompt cards for asking for help/ more detailed instructions to support people in daily interactions within the prison and through the gate, such as above or:

(Continued)

Table 19.6 (Continued)

Functional difficulty	Recommendations for potential strategies and reasonable adjustments
	"Can I stop you there? It would work for me if you allow me to practice while you talk, I remember better that way".
	"I'm sorry, I find it hard to process lots of words, could you possibly slow down?"
	PQRST – preview, question, read, study, test – this is a useful structure to support individuals with learning new information.
Language – written	Advocate for education departments to have access to assistive technology to meet demands of the modern world through the gate. Avoid temptation to replace 12 years of education with a 2-week literacy course, often not adapted for neurominorities. For example, phonic tuition alone may not correct spelling and reading difficulties; new strategies should be applied if these have failed repeatedly. Literacy support charities might offer a more specialised programme and can help with providing differentiated material that inspires engagement.
Motor control and balance	Train techniques for managing state and dealing with panic. Support individuals to avoid self-shame, slow down and take time with tasks that they find difficult.
	Advocate for education departments to have access to assistive technology – handwriting is reasonably obsolete in modern workplaces. Touch typing may be more appropriate to learn.
	Planning and practising movements and journeys before starting.
	Rehearsal of frequently required motor control tasks.
Sensory Sensitivity	Training awareness of sensory trigger and strategies for avoiding these within CJS. For example, planning days and wall chart reminders of which events happen in which order can help identify where sensory triggers are and how to avoid / reduce them.
	Advocate for adjustment of ear defenders wherever noise disruption is an issue; or wearing of sunglasses, reducing glare from strip lighting, as well as general notes on temperature, smell, touch, and taste sensitivities. Touch is particularly of relevance during shutdowns, when any attempt to physically approach a neurodivergent person may exacerbate defensive aggression rather than calm or control an outburst. Psychologists can strongly advocate for decompression time and space for those who are sensory sensitive.

(*Continued*)

Table 19.6 (Continued)

Functional difficulty	Recommendations for potential strategies and reasonable adjustments
Emotional dysregulation	Regular reflective, coaching-based sessions to increase self-awareness are essential for most neurominorities. Unhelpful or frightening behaviours can be supported by reinforcing positive behaviours; use of TOOTS, (Time Out On the Spot); structure sessions / session plans; anticipate hot spots. People frequently exhibit warning signs, such as knee jiggling or nail biting, or breath holding, which indicate a pre-meltdown. Developing self-awareness of triggers or premonitory activities can facilitate self-advocacy before a shutdown. Verbal communication is compromised during intense emotions. To counter, role-play short effective phrases to help attract support rather than control from staff. For example: "Can I self -isolate please, I am going into autistic meltdown?" "Help, fight or flight response happening". "Help, trauma flashback happening" Adopt a coaching response, predictability / stability; create consistency across staff groups; use planners; set goals; use checklists, enable individuals to plan and structure their day.

Future Considerations

Table 19.7 outlines a case study of a holistic intervention protocol, bringing identification and/or diagnosis into a pathway for neurodivergent individuals in which strengths are captured and utilised. It is noteworthy that this project was devised and delivered by an Autistic person (a co-author in this chapter). The case study demonstrates the value of including neurodivergent thinkers in the design of services. Indeed, all four authors in this chapter have lived experience of neurodiversity.

Considering the systemic level, we defer to the comprehensive *The HMIP Review* (CJJI, 2021) which identified a number of recommendations that add value in terms of psychologists working with neurominorities in CJS. To close this chapter, we draw specific attention to the following points of note:

- Data collection, consistency of approach, definition, tools, as well as consistent offers in terms of intervention support is key, as is raising colleagues' awareness. As Psychologists we are well-placed to advise on such issues.
- As Psychologists, we have potential roles in developing, supporting, and advising on culturally sensitive screening processes/assessment tools used for

Table 19.7 Case study

The Support Change Project – Tanya Banfield.

"The Support Change Project came about after I attended a meeting at the Ministry of Justice Head Quarters, London to talk about neurodiversity. They talked about finding a new operational way to rehabilitate and reduce offending by offenders from neurominority groups within a forensic setting.

Within the Support Change Project, offenders were screened when entering a CJS setting for neurominority symptom clusters, focusing on functional need as opposed to diagnosis. The screening produced an individual report which highlighted areas of strength and support needs. The reports make recommendations where appropriate for reasonable adjustments and strategies; these are practical, everyday suggestions such as organisation management strategies, modelling memory, visual spelling, improving self-confidence, and developing self-advocacy skills. A model of rehabilitation then followed which included one-to-one work, small group work, and attending larger groups, which developed the idea of self-directed strategies and the ability to request accommodation in certain circumstances such as education and work. The focus of these interventions was on understanding strengths and support needs in terms of cognitive ability and increasing self-awareness and self-regulation through a range of interactive group and one-to-one activity.

Offenders were screened within the first two weeks of entering the prison. This identified any potential areas of support. These findings were then shared in allocations meetings, with offender managers, wing staff, and probation. Having an idea of support needs of an individual offender ensured that appropriate decisions were made, and support put in place. From the strategy profiler, the project was able to determine who was likely to benefit from having a more in-depth cognitive assessment. This provided a further opportunity to understand that person's unique "spiky profile", defined as a significant gap between the scores of the four indices using the Weschler Adult Intelligence Scale, frequently used as the basis for diagnosing neurodevelopmental differences such as dyslexia (Grant, 2009; Doyle, 2017).

Findings indicated a positive effect from the 150 offenders that were identified from initial screening. Of the 150 offenders that took part in the study end-to-end (September 2017 to March 2020), only three were recalled to prison, but none reoffended. All of the offenders that took part in the project reached and sustained an exit outcome of either education, training, or employment. This is a significant effect, which has influenced ongoing practice in terms of the development of specialist neurodiversity prisons being built.

The implication of the project for supporting neurominorities in the prison are as follows:

1 Functional knowledge of day-to-day strengths and weaknesses may be a higher priority than labelling and diagnosis;
2 Working with offenders to develop self-knowledge and self-awareness leads to positive outcomes;
3 Offenders can confidently self-advocate their needs and adjustments to be at their best
4 Offenders all have an exit outcome into education, training, and employment which they can then sustain using acquired soft skills;
5 Reducing reoffending into the prison system;
6 Long-term access to community services to give focused ongoing support.

---

effective identification of neurodiverse service users, at relevant points and referring into specialist provision as needed. This would require upskilling the forensic psychology resource to respond to such challenge, and to support training of colleagues too.

- As Psychologists we have a potential role in offering guidance on responsivity needs and signposting internal and external cognitive and behavioural strategies to best support individuals, seeking also to communicate risk management/licence conditions to individuals themselves and CJS colleagues alike. We can also signpost specialist provision, literature, resources, and materials both internally within CJS and more widely, to those working with individuals in the community longer term.

Note

1 Lesbian, Gay, Bisexual, Transgender, Queer, Intersex, Asexual, Two-Spirit people and other terms which people may prefer, including pansexual.

References

Adak, B., & Halder, S. (2017). Systematic review on prevalence for autism spectrum disorder with respect to gender and socio-economic status. *Journal of Mental Disorders and Treatment, 03*(01), 1–9. 10.4172/2471-271x.1000133

Akechi, H., Senju, A., Uibo, H., Kikuchi, Y., Hasegawa, T., & Hietanen, J. K. (2013). Attention to eye contact in the West and East: Autonomic responses and evaluative ratings. *PLoS ONE, 8*(3), 1–10. 10.1371/journal.pone.0059312

American Psychiatric Association. (2013). *Diagnostic and Statistical Manual of Mental Disorders (DSM V)* (5th ed.). Arlington, VA: American Psychiatric Publishing.

Antshel, K. M., & Russo, N. (2019). Autism spectrum disorders and ADHD: Overlapping phenomenology, diagnostic issues, and treatment considerations. *Current Psychiatry Reports, 21*(5), 1–11. 10.1007/s11920-019-1020-5

Armstrong, T. (2010). *The power of neurodiversity*. Cambs, MA: De Capo Press.

Baron-Cohen, S. (2017). Editorial perspective: Neurodiversity – a revolutionary concept for autism and psychiatry. *Journal of Child Psychology and Psychiatry and Allied Disciplines, 58*(6), 744–747. 10.1111/jcpp.12703

Bishop, D. V. M., Snowling, M. J., Thompson, P. A., & Greenhalgh, T. (2017). Phase 2 of CATALISE: A multinational and multidisciplinary Delphi consensus study of problems with language development: Terminology. *Journal of Child Psychology and Psychiatry, 58*(10), 1068–1080. 10.1111/jcpp.12721

Bottema-Beutel, K., Kapp, S. K., Lester, J. N., Sasson, N. J., Hand, B. N., & Otr, L. (2020). Avoiding ableist language: Suggestions for autism researchers. *Autism in Adulthood, 00*(00), 1–12. 10.1089/aut.2020.0014

BPS. (2017). *Practice guidelines - Third Edition*. Leicester, UK: British Psychological Society. https://www.bps.org.uk/sites/bps.org.uk/files/Policy-Files/BPS Practice Guidelines (Third Edition).pdf, accessed 23rd January 2022

BPS. (2018). *Code of ethics and conduct*. Leicester, UK: The British Psychological Society. ISBN: 978-1-85433-759-7

Butterworth, B., Varma, S., & Laurillard, D. (2011). Dyscalculia: From brain to education. *Science, 332*(6033), 1049–1053. 10.1126/science.1201536

Campbell, F. A. K. (2008). Exploring internalized ableism using critical race theory. *Disability and Society, 23*(2), 151–162. 10.1080/09687590701841190

CDC. (2011). Percentage of Children aged 5-17 years ever receiving a diagnosis of Learning Disabiltiy by Race/ethnicity and family income group, United States, 2007-2009. *Morbidity and Mortality Weekly Report, 60*(25), 853. 10.1001/jama.296.11.1346

Chapman, R. (2020a). Defining neurodiversity for research and practice. In H. B. Rosqvist, N. Chown, & A. Stenning (Eds.), *Neurodiversity studies: A new critical paradigm* (pp. 218–220). Oxford: Routledge. 10.4324/9780429322297-21

Chapman, R. (2020b). Neurodiversity, disability, wellbeing. In H. B. Rosqvist, N. Chown, & A. Stenning (Eds.), *Neurodiversity studies: A new critical paradigm* (pp. 57–72). Oxford: Routledge. 10.4324/9780429322297-21

Charlton, J. (1998). *Nothing About Us Without Us: Disability Oppression and Empowerment.* Berkley, CA: University of California Press. http://www.jstor.org/stable/10.1525/j.ctt1pnqn9

Chester, V., Painter, G., Ryan, L., Popple, J., Chikodzi, K., & Alexander, R. T. (2018). Traumatic brain injury in a forensic intellectual disability population. *Psychology, Crime and Law, 24*(4), 400–413. 10.1080/1068316X.2017.1302583

CJJI. (2021). *Neurodiversity in the Criminal Justice System: a Review of Evidence.* https://www.justiceinspectorates.gov.uk/cjji/wp-content/uploads/sites/2/2021/07/Neurodiversity-evidence-review-web-2021.pdf, accessed January 23rd, 2022.

Cree, R. A., Bitsko, R. H., Robinson, L. R., Holbrook, J. R., Danielson, M. L., Smith, C., Kaminski, J. W., Kenney, M. K., & Peacock, G. (2018). Health care, family, and community factors associated with mental, behavioral, and developmental disorders and poverty among children aged 2–8 years — United States, 2016. *Morbidity and Mortality Weekly Report, 67*(50), 1377–1383. 10.15585/mmwr.mm6750a1

Davidson, J. (2008). Autistic culture online: Virtual communication and cultural expression on the spectrum. *Social & Cultural Geography, 9*(7), 791–806. https://www.tandfonline.com/doi/abs/10.1080/14649360802382586

Doyle, N. (2017). Neurodiversity at work. In BPS (Ed.), *Psychology at work: Improving wellbeing and productivity in the workplace* (pp. 44–62). British Psychological Society. https://doi.org/ISBN978-1-85433-754-2

Doyle, N. (2020). Neurodiversity at work: A biopsychosocial model and the impact on working adults. *British Medical Bulletin, 135*, 1–18. 10.1093/bmb/ldaa021

Doyle, N. E., & McDowall, A. (2019). Context matters: A review to formulate a conceptual framework for coaching as a disability accommodation. *PLoS ONE, 14*(8). 10.1371/journal.pone.0199408

Egan, V., Linenberg, O., & O'Nions, E. (2019). The measurement of adult pathological demand avoidance traits. *Journal of Autism and Developmental Disorders, 49*(2), 481–494. 10.1007/s10803-018-3722-7

Ellenberg, J., Paff, M., Harrison, A., & Long, K. (2019). Disparities based on race, ethnicity, and socio-economic status over the transition to adulthood among adolescents and young adults on the autistic spectrum: A systematic review. *Current Psychiatry Reports, 21*(32), 1–16. 10.1007/s11920-019-1016-1

Engert, V., & Pruessner, J. (2009). Dopaminergic and noradrenergic Contributions to functionality in ADHD: The role of methylphenidate. *Current Neuropharmacology, 6*(4), 322–328. 10.2174/157015908787386069

Estrin, G. L. (2020). Barriers to autism spectrum disorder diagnosis for young women and girls: A systematic review. *Review Journal of Autism and Developmental Disorders*, published online. 10.1007/s40489-020-00225-8

Frost, R. B., Farrer, T. J., Primosch, M., & Hedges, D. W. (2012). Prevalence of traumatic brain injury in the general adult population: A meta-analysis. *Neuroepidemiology, 40*, 154–159. 10.1159/000343275.

Gomez, I. N. B., Calsa, A. P., Esguerra, J. T., Joseph, P., Penetrante, H., Porlucas, K., Santos, M. E., Umali, C. B., & Lai, C. Y. Y. (2021). Psychometric properties of the sensory processing and self-regulation checklist: English version. *Occupational Therapy International*, 1–9. doi: 10.36413/pjahs.0501.002

Grant, D. (2009). The psychological assessment of neurodiversity. In D. Pollak (Ed.), *Neurodiversity in Higher Education* (pp. 33–62). Wiley-Blackwell.

Hawley, C. A., & Maden, A. (2003). Mentally disordered offenders with a history of previous head injury: are they more difficult to discharge? *Brain Injury*, *17*(9), 743–758. 10.1080/0269905031000089341

Hendren, R. L., Haft, S. L., Black, J. M., & White, N. C. (2018). Recognizing psychiatric comorbidity with reading disorders. *Frontiers in Psychiatry*, *9*(March). 10.3389/fpsyt.2018.00101

Heylens, G., Aspeslagh, L., Dierickx, J., Baetens, K., Van Hoorde, B., De Cuypere, G., & Elaut, E. (2018). The co-occurrence of gender dysphoria and autism spectrum disorder in adults: An analysis of cross-sectional and clinical chart data. *Journal of Autism and Developmental Disorders*, *48*(6), 2217–2223. 10.1007/s10803-018-3480-6

Hosseini, S., & Molla, M. (2021). Asperger syndrome. *National Library of Science*. https://pubmed.ncbi.nlm.nih.gov/32491480/

Hughes, J. E. A., Ward, J., Gruffydd, E., Baron-Cohen, S., Smith, P., Allison, C., & Simner, J. (2018). Savant syndrome has a distinct psychological profile in autism. *Molecular Autism*, *9*(1), 1–18. 10.1186/s13229-018-0237-1

Huijg, D. D. (2020). Neuronormativity in theorising agency. In H. B. Rosqvist, N. Chown, & A. Stenning (Eds.), *Neurodiversity studies: A new critical paradigm* (pp. 213–217). Oxford: Routledge. 10.4324/9780429322297-20

Ihori, D., & Olvera, P. (2015). Discrepancies, responses, and patterns: Selecting a method of assessment for specific learning disabilities. *Contemporary School Psychology*, *19*, 1–11. 10.1007/s40688-014-0042-6

Kapp, S. K., Gillespie-Lynch, K., Sherman, L. E., & Hutman, T. (2013). Deficit, difference, or both? Autism and neurodiversity. *Developmental Psychology*, *49*(1), 59–71. 10.1037/a0028353

Krcek, T. E. (2012). Deconstructing disability and neurodiversity: Controversial issues for autism and implications for social work. *Journal of Progressive Human Services*, *24*(1), 4–22. 10.1080/10428232.2013.740406

Kriss, I., & Evans, B. J. W. (2005). The relationship between dyslexia and Meares-Irlen Syndrome. *Journal of Research in Reading*, *28*(3), 350–364. 10.1111/j.1467-9817.2005.00274.x

Levine, T. R., Asada, K. J., & Park, H. S. (2006). The lying chicken and the gaze avoidant egg: Eye contact, deception, and causal order. *Southern Communication Journal Communication Journal*, published online, 401–411. 10.1080/10417940601000576

Ledingham, R ., & Mills, R. (2015).A preliminary study of autism and cybercrime in the context of international law enforcement. *Advances in Autism*, *1*(1), 2–11. https://doi.org/10.1108/AIA-05-2015-0003

Lollini, A. (2018). Brain equality: Legal implications of neurodiversity in a comparative perspective. *International Law and Politics*, *51*, 69–133.

Lorcan, K., Hattersley, C., Molins, B., Buckley, C., Povey, C., & Pellicano, E. (2016). Which terms should be used to describe autism? Perspectives from the UK autism community. *Autism*, *20*(4), 442–462. 10.1177/1362361315588200

Lowings, G., & Wick, B. (2016). *Effective learning after acquired brain injury*. London: Routledge. 10.4324/9781315746005

Mandell, D. S., Wiggins, L. D., Carpenter, L. A., Daniels, J., DiGuiseppi, C., Durkin, M. S., Giarelli, E., Morrier, M. J., Nicholas, J. S., Pinto-Martin, J. A., Shattuck, P. T., Thomas, K. C., Yeargin-Allsopp, M., & Kirby, R. S. (2009). Racial/ethnic disparities in the identification of children with autism spectrum disorders. *American Journal of Public Health, 99*(3), 493–498. 10.2105/AJPH.2007.131243

McGrath, L. M., & Stoodley, C. J. (2019). Are there shared neural correlates between dyslexia and ADHD? A meta-analysis of voxel-based morphometry studies. *Journal of Neurodevelopmental Disorders, 11*(1), 1–20. 10.1186/s11689-019-9287-8

McLoughlin, D. (2021). Neurodiversity and dyslexia: Paradigm shift of euphemism? *Assessment and Development Matters, 13*(2).

McLoughlin, D., & Doyle, N. (2013). *The psychological assessment of adults with specific performance difficulties at work.* Leicester: British Psychological Society. https://www.bps.org. uk/sites/bps.org.uk/files/Policy/Policy - Files/DOP Psychological Assessment of Adults with Specific Difficulties.pdf

McLoughlin, D., & Leather, C. (2013). *The dyslexic adult.* Chichester: John Wiley and Sons.

McMillan, T. M., Graham, L., Pell, J. P., McConnachie, A., & Mackay, D. F. (2019). The lifetime prevalence of hospitalised head injury in Scottish prisons: A population study. *PLOS ONE, 14*(1), 1–10. 10.1371/journal.pone.0210427

McNamara, N. (2012). Speech and language therapy within a forensic support service. *Journal of Learning Disabilities and Offending Behaviour, 3*(2), 111–117. 10.1108/2042 0921211280097

Memon, A., Taylor, K., Mohebati, L. M., Sundin, J., Cooper, M., Scanlon, T., & De Visser, R. (2016). Perceived barriers to accessing mental health services among black and minority ethnic (BME) communities: A qualitative study in Southeast England. *BMJ Open, 6*(11), 1–9. 10.1136/bmjopen-2016-012337

Merbitz, C., Jain, S., Good, G. L., & Jain, A. (1995). Reported head injury and disciplinary rule infractions in prison. *Journal of Offender Rehabilitation, 22*(3/4), 11–20. ISSN: 1050-9674

Miyasaka, M., Kajimura, S., & Nomura, M. (2018). Biases in understanding attention deficit hyperactivity disorder and autism spectrum disorder in Japan. *Frontiers in Psychology, 9*(FEB), 1–13. 10.3389/fpsyg.2018.00244

Nagele, D., Vaccaro, M., Schmidt, M. J., & Keating, D. (2018). Brain injury in an offender population: Implications for reentry and community transition. *Journal of Offender Rehabilitation, 57*(8), 562–585. 10.1080/10509674.2018.1549178

Nalavany, B. A., Logan, J. M., & Carawan, L. W. (2017). The relationship between emotional experience with dyslexia and work self-efficacy among adults with dyslexia. *Dyslexia, 24*(1), 1–16. 10.1002/dys.1575

Nicolaidis, C. C., Lopez, K., & Waisman, T. C. (2020). An expert discussion on structural racism in autism research and practice. *Autism in Adulthood, 2*(4), 273–281. 10.1089/aut.2020.29015.drj

O'Rourke, C., Linden, M. A., & Lohan, M. (2018). Misconceptions about traumatic brain injury among probation services. *Disability and Rehabilitation, 40*(10), 1119–1126. 10. 1080/09638288.2017.1288274

Oakland, T. (2016). Testing and assessment of immigrants and second-language learners. In F. T. L. Leong, D. Bartram, F. Cheung, K. F. Geisinger, & D. Iliescu (Eds.), *The ITC international handbook of testing and assessment* (pp. 318–332). Oxford: Oxford University Press. 10.1093/med:psych/9780199356942.003.0022

OECD. (2015). *The ABC of gender equality in education: Aptitude, behaviour, confidence.* Pisa, Italy: Organization for Economic Cooperation and Development. ISBN: 9789264229945

Otto, M. W., Eastman, A., Lo, S., Hearon, B. A., Bickel, W. K., Zvolensky, M., Smits, J. A. J., & Doan, S. N. (2016). Anxiety sensitivity and working memory capacity: Risk factors and targets for health behavior promotion. *Clinical Psychology Review, 49*, 67–78. 10.1016/j.cpr.2016.07.003

Piccolino, A. L., & Solberg, K. B. (2014). The impact of traumatic brain injury on prison health services and offender management. *Journal of Correctional Health Care: The Official Journal of the National Commission on Correctional Health Care, 20*(3), 203–212. 10.1177/1078345814530871

Pitman, I., Haddlesey, C., Ramos, S. D. S., Oddy, M., & Fortescue, D. (2015). The association between neuropsychological performance and self-reported traumatic brain injury in a sample of adult male prisoners in the UK. *Neuropsychological Rehabilitation, 25*(5), 763–779. 10.1080/09602011.2014.973887

Pollack, D. (Ed). (2009). *Neurodiversity in higher education*. Chichester: Wiley-Blackwell.

Prevatt, F., & Yelland, S. (2013). An empirical evaluation of ADHD coaching in college students. *Journal of Attention Disorders, 19*(8), 1–12. 10.1177/1087054713480036

Prison Reform Trust. (2021). *Bromley briefings prison factfile*. London: Prison Reform Trust. http://www.prisonreformtrust.org.uk/publications/factfile accessed November 15th 2020.

Public Health England. (2016). *Learning disabilities observatory people with learning disabilities in England 2015*. https://www.gov.uk/government/publications/people-with-learning-disabilities-in-england-2015 accessed 25th October 2020.

Reyes, N., Baumgardner, D. J., Simmons, D. H., & Buckingham, W. (2013). The potential for sociocultural factors in the diagnosis of ADHD in children. *Wisconsin Medical Journal, 112*(1), 13–17. ISSN: 10981861

Richardson, J. T., & Wydell, T. N. (2003). The representation and attainment of students with dyslexia in UK higher education. *Reading and Writing, 16*, 475. 10.1023/A:1024261927214

Riddick, B. (2001). Dyslexia and inclusion: Time for a social model of disability perspective? *International Studies in Sociology of Education, 11*(3), 37–41. 10.1080/09620210100200078

Roman-Urrestarazu, A., Van Kessel, R., Allison, C., Matthews, F. E., Brayne, C., & Baron-Cohen, S. (2021). Association of race/ethnicity and social disadvantage with autism prevalence in 7 million school children in England. *JAMA Pediatrics, 175*(6), 1–11. 10.1001/jamapediatrics.2021.0054

Runswick-Cole, K. (2014). "Us" and "them": The limits and possibilities of a "politics of neurodiversity" in neoliberal times. *Disability & Society, 29*(7), 1117–1129. 10.1080/09687599.2014.910107

Sanders, S., Thomas, R., Glasziou, P., & Doust, J. (2019). A review of changes to the attention deficit/hyperactivity disorder age of onset criterion using the checklist for modifying disease definitions. *BMC Psychiatry, 19*(1), 1–8. 10.1186/s12888-019-2337-7

SASC. (2017). *Guidance on the assessment of students with SpLD*. Student Assessment Standards Committee. http://www.sasc.org.uk/NewsItem.aspx?id=58 accessed 1st April 2018

Shelley-Tremblay, J. F., & Rosen, L. A. (1996). Attention deficit hyperactivity disorder: An evolutionary perspective. *Journal of Genetic Psychology, 157*(4), 443–453. 10.1080/00221325.1996.9914877

Shiroma, E. J., Ferguson, P. L., & Pickelsimer, E. E. (2010). Prevalence of traumatic brain injury in an offender population: A meta-analysis. *Journal of Correctional Health Care: The Official Journal of the National Commission on Correctional Health Care, 16*(2), 147–159. 10.1177/1078345809356538

Singer, J. (1998). *Odd People In: The Birth of Community Amongst People on the "Autistic Spectrum": a Personal Exploration of a New Social Movement based on Neurological Diversity.* Thesis, Sydney: University of Technology.

Singer, J. (1999). "Why can't you be normal for once in your life?" From a problem with no name to the emergence of a new category of difference. In M. Corker & S. French (Eds.), *Disability discourse* (pp. 59–67). Buckingham, UK: Open University Press.

Siugzdaite, R., Bathelt, J., Holmes, J., & Astle, D. E. (2020). Transdiagnostic brain mapping in developmental disorders. *Current Biology, 30*(7), 1245–1257.e4. 10.1016/j.cub.2020.01.078

Solé, B., Martínez-Arán, A., Torrent, C., Bonnin, C. M., Reinares, M., Popovic, D., Sánchez-Moreno, J., & Vieta, E. (2011). Are bipolar II patients cognitively impaired? A systematic review. *Psychological Medicine, 41*(9), 1791–1803. 10.1017/S0033291711000018

Taylor, J. L. & Lindsay, W.R. (2018). Offenders with intellectual and developmental disabilities: Future directions for research and practice. In *The Wiley handbook on offenders with intellectual and developmental disabilities: Research, training, and practice* (pp. 453–471). Wiley-Blackwell. https://doi.org/10.1002/9781118752982

Taylor, H., Fernandes, B., & Wraight, S. (2021). The evolution of complementary cognition: Humans cooperatively adapt and evolve through a system of collective cognitive search. *Cambridge Archaeological Journal, published online,* 1–17. 10.1017/s0959774321000329

Thorne, K. N. (2021). *Traumatic brain injury in men convicted of sexual offences.* PhD Thesis, University of Leicester. 10.25392/leicester.data.17099375.v1

UK Govt (2010). *The Equality Act.* http://www.legislation.gov.uk/ukpga/2010/15/introduction. Accessed 31st August 2020.

United States Department for Education's Office of Special Educational Needs (2006). *Individuals with Disabilities Education Act.* https://sites.ed.gov/idea/statuteregulations/ accessed 15th July 2019.

Walker, N. (2012). Throw away the master's tools: Liberating ourselves from the pathology paradigm. In J. Bascombe (Ed.), *Loud hands: Autistic people, speaking* (pp. 225–237). Autistic Self Advocacy Network.

Weschler, D. (2008). *Weschler adult intelligence scale IV.* Bloomington: Pearson.

Wechsler, D. (2014). *Wechsler intelligence scale for children V.* Bloomington: Pearson.

Woldgabreal, Y., Day, A., & Tamatea, A. (2020). Do risk assessments play a role in the enduring 'color line'? *Advancing Corrections, 10,* 18–28.

Young, S., Adamo, N., Ásgeirsdóttir, B. B., Branney, P., Beckett, M., Colley, W., Cubbin, S., Deeley, Q., Farrag, E., Gudjonsson, G., Hill, P., Hollingdale, J., Kilic, O., Lloyd, T., Mason, P., Paliokosta, E., Perecherla, S., Sedgwick, J., Skirrow, C., …Woodhouse, E. (2020). Females with ADHD: An expert consensus statement taking a lifespan approach providing guidance for the identification and treatment of attention-deficit/ hyperactivity disorder in girls and women. *BMC Psychiatry, 20*(1), 404. 10.1186/s12888-020-02707-9

Young, S., González, R. A., Fridman, M., Hodgkins, P., Kim, K., & Gudjonsson, G. H. (2018). The economic consequences of attention-deficit hyperactivity disorder in the Scottish prison system. *BMC Psychiatry, 18,* 1–11. 10.1186/s12888-018-1792-x

Yuhasz, J. E. (2013). Misconceptions about traumatic brain injury among correctional health care professionals. *Journal of Correctional Health Care, 19*(2), 135–143. 10.1177/1078345812474644

Appendix 1: Glossary of terms

Term	Current rationale – although note this will continue to evolve
Condition first language (i.e., disabled people rather than people with disabilities)	Though the person-first language, developed in the 80s and 90s was designed to draw attention to the humanity of disabled people, it is no longer in vogue for all. The current preference in this community elicits the social model, in that people are disabled by their environment, rather than a disability being something had at the individual level.
Condition or difference	As opposed to Disorder. Though many people experience their difference as disorder, we should avoid making assumptions of deficit and distress, mindful that our position as professional will be pivotal in framing the experience of those with whom we work. When we frame in the negative, this can be self-fulfilling for those who are in our care.
Autism/Autistic/Autists	As opposed to Autistic Spectrum Disorder, Asperger's, on the spectrum, or any other variation, this phrase is preferred though many people still identify as Asperger's or Aspie.
Dyslexic, Dyspraxic, Dyscalculic, Dysgraphic	As opposed to "person with dys*". The term Developmental Coordination Disorder (or DCD) is referred to as an alternative to Dypraxia, however, Dyspraxic people prefer the term Dyspraxia.
ADHDer/Touretter	These conditions are not easy to take out of person-first language, however people with lived experience use these adaptations.
Neurodiversity	A feature of the whole species and not a synonym for disability (Singer, 1999)
Neurominority/neurodifferences	An umbrella term. These are chosen in place of Specific Learning Disabilities (SpLD) or Neurodevelopmental Disorders for the same reason as the use of condition vs disorder, i.e., to infer neutrality and create space for a balanced narrative. Additionally, unpublished research conducted by the British Psychological Society's (BPS) Neurodiversity Working Group in 2015 and 2019 found that the older terms were preferred by less than 10% of those with lived experience (2015, N=115; 2019, N=267). This survey is currently being repeated and will be published.
Neurodiverse (/neurodifferent)	To refer to an individual, referring to the diversity at the individual level within the spiky profile. This term is not favoured by all, in particular

(Continued)

Term	Current rationale – although note this will continue to evolve
	the BPS survey indicated that Autistic people and those from USA/Australia do not identify with this term.
Neurodivergent (/neurodifferent)	To refer to an individual, noting the divergence from neurotypicality. This term is also sometimes contentious, potentially not favoured by ADHD/Dyslexic communities.
Person with learning disabilities	In learning disability communities those with lived experience still prefer the person-first language
Low/high/additional needs	Used instead of high/low functioning, a phrase has been used to separate Autistic people into two categories, typically those with or without cooccurring Learning Disability. The phrase has been widely criticised for framing "functioning" from the neuro-normative position and minimising the human value of those with lower IQs. Additionally, it does not account for the distress experienced by Autistics with high IQ who "mask" in order to pass for "functioning" and experience high rates of mental ill-health and suicide. Use of the word "need" centres the individual rather than the role they play and is therefore more respectful.
Capitalisation	Similarly, to the Deaf community and Black community, where the capitalisation denotes respect and acknowledgement of a group identity that has been marginalised, the capitalisation of Autism, Dyslexia, etc. serves to reinforce the autonomy and formal assertion of culture.

20 Forensic Risk Assessment in Learning Disability Populations

Emma Longfellow, Mark Callender, and Rachel Hicks

Introduction

The specialist needs of individuals with learning disability (LD) are becoming increasingly prominent in response to repeated failures in care; the catalyst for which was the exposure of physical and psychological abuse of people with LD at Winterbourne View (2011). The subsequent Transforming Care Agenda (Department of Health, 2012) placed emphasis on transitioning individuals with LD into the community. What this means in practice is that those caring for individuals with LD in forensic settings are required to evidence, to an Independent panel, that the current placement of an individual is the least restrictive intervention, proportionate to the level of risk. The emphasis is that all individuals with LD should be in the community unless in exceptional circumstances where risk cannot be managed. There has been some narrative that this is more difficult to navigate in forensic settings due to systemic failures in the physical availability of less secure beds or bespoke community services. There are further difficulties associated with disparity in specialism and skill to manage and assess forensic risks effectively in the community (Alexander et al., 2015; Lofthouse et al., 2020; Taylor et al., 2017) and how sociocultural differences in LD are accounted for. This adds further importance to forensic risk assessment with LD and in turn how we understand, manage, and reduce the likelihood of risk behaviour to ensure the level of security in the environment is proportionate (Chester et al., 2017).

Current Issues in Assessing Risk in LD

There are several foundational issues associated with the effective application of forensic risk assessment to LD populations which will be discussed below. One of the ongoing issues within the literature is dynamic nomenclature, with a range of terminology in use within research and clinical settings. Within this chapter, we have chosen to retain the LD terminology rather than adopt the Intellectual Disability (ID) or Intellectual Developmental Disability (IDD) term that is also used in the literature. This is considerate of Cluley's (2018) discussion around the meaning and drivers for semantic change in language and how this may be experienced. LD is used within this chapter as there has been minimal discussion

DOI: 10.4324/9781003230977-23

on the shift to ID in some contexts within the UK and it is the terminology in use within the National High Secure Service currently. What we prefer about the emphasis on "learning" rather than "intelligence" is the acknowledgement that there is a context to the difficulty beyond ability and it could be sociocultural including the opportunity to be taught. This also allows, although this remains limited in practice, consideration of the relationship between LD and ethnicity across contexts.

For clarity we would note the following definition as an overarching de-scription of the population we discuss in this chapter, whilst noting the substantial variation at an individual level and discourse around the impact of labels. A LD is principally defined by three core criteria: a significantly reduced ability to understand new or complex information in learning new skills, reduced ability to cope independently, and onset in childhood with a lasting effect on development (British Psychological Society, 2015). Individuals with LD are not a homo-geneous group, which is evident in varied cognitive, adaptive, social, and emo-tional functioning that is captured within the subcategories of mild, moderate, severe, and profound (Department of Health, 2001; Emerson & Hatton, 2007).

When there is clarity on population, there can be minimal consideration on diversity within this. For example, although LD populations are openly discussed as heterogenous requiring person-centred interventions, they are regularly grouped homogenously as people with LD. This negates the considerable variation in cognitive ability, adaptive functioning, and in turn agency and autonomy within the LD population. Furthermore, there is little consideration for the socio-cultural differences within the LD population, with ethnicity largely unreported in the forensic literature (Frize, 2015). For example, although the Bradley Commission Briefing (Saunders et al., 2013) commented on the varying ethnic groups at dif-ferent stages of the Criminal Justice System (CJS), they did not distinguish those with LD from those with Mental Health difficulties. The Bradley report (2009) and his report "Five Years On" (Durcan et al., 2014) note that issues remain with data collection with regards to LD and ethnicity in secure services (Lammy, 2017).

Progress has been made in recent years in extending the evidence base for risk assessment to the LD population. Empirical support for the validity and relia-bility of available measures enables clinicians to have more confidence in the use of assessment tools to support their decision making (Lofthouse et al., 2014). However, as a large proportion of "offending" in LD populations is unreported and those that are less likely to receive a conviction, it questions what prediction is being made when reconviction data is being used. Accordingly, it has been proposed that understanding dynamic risk factors is of higher importance and utility in LD populations, particularly in relation to context-specific risk (Boer et al., 2007; Lofthouse et al., 2014; Lofthouse et al., 2017; Matthews & Bell, 2020; Wheeler et al., 2014). Contributing to this is the suggestion that individuals with LD are more likely to have contact and reliance on support services, giving greater significance to the environmental factors, such as staff knowledge and the availability of activities, alongside individual factors (Boer et al., 2007; Lofthouse et al., 2013; Matthews & Bell, 2020).

Several risk assessments specifically for the LD population have been developed with the aim of enhancing the accuracy and utility of this process. This has included measures for sexual and general violence risk, such as the Assessment of Risk and Manageability for Individuals who Offend Sexually or Generally (ARMIDILO-S; Boer et al., 2004; ARMIDILO-G; Boer et al., 2012) and the Treatment Intervention and Progress Scale for Sexual Abusers with Intellectual Disability (TIPS-ID; McGrath et al., 2007), alongside numerous measures for physical violence. These are the Dynamic Risk Appraisal and Management System (DRAMS; Lindsay et al., 2004), Current Risk of Violence (CuRV; Lofthouse et al., 2014), and the Short Dynamic Risk Scale (SDRS; Quinsey, 2004) which all focus on dynamic risk factors. Additionally, a supplement has been developed for the HCR-20 which provides guidelines on the applicability and additional considerations when assessing an individual with LD with the aim of enhancing the efficacy of the tool for LD populations (Boer et al., 2010).

One study explicitly explored the effectiveness of the LD supplement for the HCR-20 in a sample of 59 individuals with LD who resided in the community and had a history of violent offending (Verbrugge et al., 2011). Of participants included, 15% were from culturally or linguistically diverse backgrounds and 25% were of Aboriginal or Torres Strait Islander background. This study found that participant characteristics, such as ethnicity, had no observable effect on risk assessment scores, although this was limited by insufficient data being available to conduct more in-depth analyses. They do not provide commentary on what others (Woldgabreal et al., 2020) have found to be an innate racial bias in risk assessment at the point of development. In comparison to the HCR-20 alone and the VRAG, it was found that the use of LD supplement resulted in a small improvement in the predictive validity, although this did not achieve statistical significance (Verbrugge et al., 2011). Similarly, O'Shea et al. (2015) explored the predictive ability of the HCR-20 for aggression in a secure psychiatric hospital, conducting a comparison for 109 individuals with LD and 504 without LD. The sample was predominantly white, with 45% of those with LD self-reporting Caucasian ethnicity, 11% non-Caucasian, and 44% unknown. Findings indicated that the predictive ability of HCR-20 total scores was comparable for both groups. The authors proposed that this may indicate that professionals working with individuals with LD are successfully considering the contribution of risk factors to their risk. As noted previously the relevance of predictive validity in LD populations is questionable considering the diversion from CJS. It was unclear whether the HCR-20 performed differently depending on ethnicity as no analyses of this sort were reported. Further research has also found that the HCR-20 is applicable and reliable for predicting institutional aggression in those with LD (Fitzgerald et al., 2013; Gray et al., 2007; Lindsay et al., 2008; Morrissey et al. 2007). What is likely critical to the effective use of the HCR-20 in practice is the expertise of the clinical team completing the assessment, their qualitative understanding of risk and contextual management, and its regular application to the population. What is less evident however is how socio-cultural aspects may be captured within this, if at all.

The CuRV and the SDRS have been found to have promising results in the prediction of verbal and physical aggression with greater than chance levels of accuracy in both secure forensic psychiatric settings and community LD settings (Lofthouse et al., 2014; Lofthouse et al., 2020). Further proposed strengths of the LD-specific dynamic risk measures include their ease of use as they can be completed by the multi-disciplinary members of an individual's support team, are efficient to complete, and do not require lengthy expensive training (Lofthouse et al., 2020). This would enable them to be completed regularly to provide current information on an individual's presenting risk and needs which would inform their care and treatment (Lofthouse et al., 2020). Similar to other evaluation studies the participant sample was predominantly Caucasian with 89% identifying as White British.

Although it has been suggested that dynamic measures that consider contextual and environmental factors will be more useful for understanding and managing risk for individuals with LD, meta-analysis and systematic reviews concluded that the LD-specific dynamic risk measures did not show superior predictive accuracy compared to tools from the general offending literature (Hounsome et al., 2018; Lofthouse et al., 2017; Matthews & Bell, 2020; Pouls & Jeandarme, 2015). Despite this, they were found to significantly predict risk of future aggression (Lofthouse et al., 2017). Professionals may find that they have practical utility for understanding treatment needs, determining the appropriate security level, and identifying environmental and individual support strategies which may be protective (Boer et al., 2007; Matthews & Bell, 2020). However, their generalisability to different socio-cultural groups remains to be explored.

Available research indicates that widely used risk assessment measures, both LD-specific and generic, can predict future aggression better than chance in individuals with LD (Camilleri & Quinsey, 2011; Hounsome et al., 2018; Lofthouse et al., 2017; Matthews & Bell, 2020; Pouls & Jeandarme, 2015). However, the evidence base for risk assessment in the LD population is still emerging and is sparse in comparison to the general population literature (Hounsome et al., 2018). Research conducted to date has also been limited by small sample sizes, little to no consideration of sociocultural differences, and the limited range of contexts in which they have been explored due to the unique population for whom they are applicable (Hounsome et al., 2018; Lofthouse et al., 2017; Matthews & Bell, 2020). The ability to generalise findings is also compounded by the inconsistency in outcome measure, variability in inclusion criteria (Lofthouse et al., 2017), and sample diversity. What is apparent is that any review of existing literature and validated assessment is going to be limited by the available research for this population. What this means is that clinicians may be reliant on being able to argue for the use of non-LD-specific risk assessments in the absence of a validated and developed alternative. Given the current impetus to ensure individuals with LD are in the least restrictive environment, being able to gain an accurate understanding of an individual's risk and the appropriate level of support and treatment needed to manage this is of high importance. Thus, further research is warranted to provide clarity on the most reliable and useful way to assess risk for those with LD.

Philosophical Differences in Assessing Risk in LD Services

Research within secure forensic psychiatric hospital settings has found that individuals with LD displayed more aggression and self-harm than service users without LD (Dickens et al., 2013; Fitzgerald et al., 2013; O'Shea et al., 2015), however, it is unclear whether consideration has been given to variation across minoritised ethnic groups. This potential higher display of agression suggests that accurate risk assessment within the LD population is important to ensure the safety and well-being of the individual and those that care for them (O'Shea et al., 2015). Within LD Clinical populations there are two primary areas of focus for risk assessment (Lofthouse et al., 2020):

1 To predict risk of offending and what may protect against this.
2 To predict and prevent *behaviour that challenges*.

This dual focus can result in a tension within services due to potentially competing philosophies at play. These directly influence descriptors of behaviour and in turn how it is interpreted and responded to. This can complicate the conceptualisation of risk and is driven by behaviour being viewed as either *behaviour that challenges* or offending behaviour, all of which usually cause harm to others (Douds & Bantwal, 2011). The pivotal issue appears to be accountability and agency of people with LD, with the population at times being viewed as less accountable, contributing to diversion from the CJS and an emphasis on enabling and pursuing community management (Boer et al., 2007; Steans & Duff, 2020).

Behaviour that challenges arises from a complex interaction between factors intrinsic to the individual, and factors intrinsic to the environment or context. For example, individual factors may include difficulties regulating anger (Chilvers & Thomas, 2011), difficulties with social problem-solving (Larkin et al., 2013), and communication difficulties (McNamara, 2012). Service factors might include exposure to excessive noise, disruption to routine, boredom, lack of clear communication by staff, and the excessive, unreasonable or inconsistent application of demands and rules (Department of Health, 2012). The term *behaviour that challenges* has been used as an attempt to avoid further stigmatising a population of individuals who are already marginalised. It is meant to demonstrate that the behaviour is an adaptive response to other factors or a means of communicating distress to others. Emphasis is placed on the function of the behaviour, meaning the relationship between the behaviour, the preceding events, and the consequences of the behaviour are explored. Treatment then focusses on altering preceding events or consequences to reduce the need for behaviour that can be harmful.

In contrast, when behaviour is viewed as offending or risk behaviour, emphasis is placed more on protecting others and preventing behavioural re-occurrence than its function. Individuals are expected to take responsibility for their behaviour and its consequences. These differing philosophies have implications for practice and research. For example, there can be a lack of formally pursued and recorded risk behaviour and/or variation in which narrative is applied across sociocultural groups (Lammy, 2017). This may impact upon the development and validation of the risk assessment, particularly when formally recorded offences are used as the outcome measure. What is apparent is that the boundaries between *behaviour that challenges* and offending are unclear. This can lead to a varied response in the CJS which is often reliant upon the clinical decision of the professional surrounding risk and culpability (Alexander et al., 2015). Therefore, the process of risk assessment for an LD population needs to balance the need for protection of others with the ethical consideration of avoiding inappropriate "forensicisation" (Douds & Bantwal, 2011) of *behaviour that challenges* that could lead to inappropriate deprivation of liberty (Alexander et al., 2015; Douds & Bantwal, 2011). This is pertinent for minoritised ethnic groups who often experience delays in LD diagnosis or are less likely to be identified on contact with the CJS (Lammy, 2017), meaning they may experience a disparity in the response to their behaviour.

Understanding Protective Factors

Alongside limitations in understanding risk and prediction in diverse LD populations, there is a paucity of research related to protective factors for people with LD or how this may vary across cultures. This is unsurprising considering its recency in research generally but represents further difficulties in assessing and moderating risk. Although relatively recent, there have been some validation studies on protective factors identified as part of the ARMIDILO-S which was the first LD-specific risk assessment to incorporate these. The protective scale is parallel but independent to the risk scale. For some items if the risk remains high, for example, high *sexual preoccupation*, but the protective factor is also high, for example, *constant supervision by experienced staff*, the protective factor counters the risk factor. These types of assessments provide a useful whole context consideration in assessment of risk. There have been discussions around progressing the assessment of protective factors in LD with the Structured Assessment of Protective Factors (SAPROF; de vogel, de Ruiter, Bouman & DeVries Robbe, 2011) looking to develop a specific measure, and the development of the ARMIDILO-G. However, the former has yet to be developed and the latter has yet to be validated or used consistently in practice.

What is also notable in the literature is the lack of identification of sociocultural factors that may be specifically protective to individual ethnic groups with LD. Additionally, the assessments which consider protective factors for LD do not make explicit reference to the ethnicity of the sample used in validation studies. It remains important to develop this area further in parallel to LD-specific risk assessment as it is increasingly accepted that a balanced risk assessment involves the evaluation of both risk and protective factors. Lindsay et al. (2018) noted in their paper that in at least two cases they evaluated, individuals were transferred out of services due to the identified protective factors. As such, the absence of culturally sensitive empirically identified protective factors for this population could lead to extended detention in restrictive environments beyond what is necessary (Hounsome et al., 2018).

Cultural Considerations and Risk Assessment

The "double discrimination" of minoritised ethnic groups and LD conceptualised as "double jeopardy" by O'Hara (2003) is evidently duplicated in risk assessment. There is little commentary on the issue in the literature and Frize (2015) suggested there was little consideration of ethnicity when evaluating risk assessment with LD populations. He noted in his review of risk assessments for LD that 70% of studies did not refer to ethnicity and of those that did, on average 78% of samples were Caucasian. Furthermore, Frize (2015) suggested that the infrequent reporting of ethnicity and limited geographical diversity of evaluations brings into question the generalisability of results given the importance of ethnicity and socio-culture. This is consistent with more recent narratives in the general risk assessment literature where it has been suggested that widely used risk assessment measures may fail to accurately capture the level of risk presented by people of non-white and non-westernised backgrounds (Shepherd & Lewis-Fernandez, 2016; Venner et al., 2021a; 2021b; Vincent & Viljoen, 2020; Woldgabreal et al., 2020). Research has indicated that some risk assessment tools are less accurate at predicting recidivism for black individuals and people of colour and that for these individuals, risk is more regularly misclassified (Chenane et al., 2015; Varela et al., 2013). This can have significant consequences, including exacerbating the overrepresentation of people of colour in correctional systems and placing individuals under unnecessary and prolonged restrictions (Woldgabreal et al., 2020).

One proposed mechanism for the possible reduced accuracy of risk assessment for people of colour and black ethnic backgrounds is rater bias (Shepherd & Lewis-Fernandez, 2016). Rater bias encapsulates the variation in ratings due to a clinician's perception of an individual who has offended (Hoyt, 2000). This may extend to culture and race whereby perceptions of an individual's background may impact upon the risk ratings assigned based on a clinician's own cognitive biases (Venner et al., 2021b). It is unclear how ethnic background interacts with LD diagnosis in rater bias, however, there is an acknowledged "double discrimination" commonly present generally. What is clear is there remains a paucity of research exploring rater bias and therefore further research is needed across cultures, contexts, and assessment tools to enable further understanding of the contribution of the rater's beliefs to risk classification (Venner et al., 2021a).

A further possibility is that the finding of differing risk classifications based on race and culture is reflective of systemic bias whereby risk items disparately impact people from certain ethnic and cultural backgrounds (Venner et al., 2021b). It has been proposed that risk assessment tools have an inherent bias in the psychometric properties and item content of the instruments because they have been normed on Western values, family arrangements, and behavioural expectations (Shepherd & Lewis-Fernandez, 2016; Venner et al., 2021a; Vincent & Viljoen, 2020). Therefore, the item content on widely used risk assessments may not sufficiently reflect the practices, belief systems, and experiences of people from non-Western cultures (Shepherd & Lewis-Fernandez, 2016). Furthermore, some of the included items may disproportionately disadvantage non-white and non-western individuals, such as those related to criminal history, as a result of increased arrest rates and contact with the CJS (Tonry, 2011; Venner et al., 2021a). For example, the Lammy (2017) found that young black people were nine times more likely to be in youth custody in the UK than young white people and that black people were more likely to be stopped and searched by the police. This is paradoxical to the diversion from the CJS seen with individuals with LD as those from minoritised ethnic groups are less likely to be identified as having LD or associated needs when they come into contact with CJS (Lammy, 2017). Clinicians having a lack of cultural awareness or failing to understand an individual from a different cultural background can impact upon the reliability of risk scores (Shepherd & Lewis-Fernandez, 2016). To support the completion of a culturally sensitive risk assessment, it has been recommended that clinicians should increase their knowledge of the individual's cultural norms, values, belief systems, and experiences including double discrimination (Shepherd & Lewis-Fernandez, 2016; Shepherd & Willis-Esqueda, 2018). Increased self-awareness of the possibility of their own bias and privilege has also been purported to minimise the power imbalance between the clinician and individual being assessed and reduce the impact of bias (Shepherd & Lewis-Fernandez, 2016). Importantly, assessors should be transparent in acknowledging the cross-cultural limitations when reporting risk assessment information (Shepherd & Lewis-Fernandez, 2016).

Considerations for Practice

One of the critical issues highlighted by the systematic abuse of people with LD in care and inpatient settings has been the service user-carer relationship. This is particularly pronounced in forensic services where there are power imbalances resulting in considerable restriction and influence over service users' lives. For example, removal of liberty, night-time confinement, restriction on items, contact with others. Co-production has been suggested as a way of relocating power whereby both professionals and service users are viewed as experts with different and complimenting knowledge (Morris et al., 2021). Co-production is commonplace within community LD populations but less evident in inpatient and secure services (Morris et al., 2021). Co-production has been identified as particularly important in empowering marginalised groups (Rycroft-Malone et al., 2016). Exploring the co-production of risk assessment to support reduction in restrictive practices is seen as a clinical priority (Morris et al., 2021). One of the critical issues in enabling co-production is the availability of accessible tools for the LD population. Although some specific LD risk assessment tools have been developed, these are few in number and there is a heavy reliance in forensic services on inaccessible non-LD-specific risk assessment such as the HCR-20. The use of non-LD-specific tools would significantly reduce the utility of co-produced risk assessments. Morris and colleagues (2021) explored the use of the SDRS for co-production and determined that co-production was feasible. What they did note is that further work developing effective co-production procedures for risk assessments for LD populations was needed, and this would be an important consideration in the emerging risk assessment research.

There are further unique considerations for this population that would need to be considered in understanding and preventing risk behaviour, such as their specific cognitive, social, and emotional needs. This includes increased potential for suggestibility, memory difficulties, communication difficulties, difficulty understanding complex concepts, and reading difficulties; all of which could contribute to responding inappropriately to questions if suitable adaptations are not utilised (Hounsome et al., 2018). Additionally, for many of the people with a LD in forensic settings, family and community systems can be part of the difficulties. As such, risk assessment and identification of protective factors for an individual requires consideration of the context and environment. For example, the external regulation and support that is required and afforded to them, and what would prompt or moderate behaviour that challenges and/or risk and criminogenic behaviour. Particular attention should be paid to the potential victimisation and discrimination that can be faced by individuals with LD in the community (Taylor et al., 2017) and how this could be a destabilising factor. In practice, inclusion of community services, parents, and caregivers earlier within risk assessment, review, planning and engagement can be particularly beneficial for this population. This not only allows the caregivers to be part of the support and change process but also allows them to be more aware of changes they may need to make and what may need to be understood about the environment and context for the individual. For example, caregivers can be supported to use strategies that do not inadvertently reinforce unhelpful attitudes/behaviours, retraumatise, or take away autonomy.

Lofthouse and colleagues (2020) discussed the issue of risk assessment across settings, noting that the physical and procedural security in secure services significantly moderated risk of offending. As a result, dynamic risk factors may present differently and at varying frequency in different settings. What is apparent within secure services is often the risk of initial concern (and reason for risk assessment) is then overtaken by the risk presented within the service itself (for example risk of specific sexual harm in the community to consistent verbal aggression or minor assault within forensic settings). Whilst not appropriate and having the potential to cause psychological and physical harm (Dusome & Melrose, 2015), this is often confused within the overall discussion of risk for the individual without sufficient emphasis on the contextual triggers. This can contribute to focus on the behaviour/s that warrant secure services being neglected because focus is on risk presented within the environment which may be context-specific (Lofthouse et al., 2020).

Concluding Thoughts

As discussed within this chapter, there are several pertinent issues to consider when assessing forensic risk within LD populations. Central to this is the heterogeneity of the LD population, not only cognitively but ethnically, and what this means for understanding, assessing, and moderating risk. What is clear is that although there are some advantages to the available structured risk assessments, these are limited for this group of individuals. There is a risk that focus is placed on developing risk assessment for LD as a homogenous group without considering the diversity of this group. As Frize (2015) notes, further forensic risk assessment research for LD would benefit from increased consideration of sociocultural differences and what this may mean for assessing both risk and protective factors for this population.

Enabling co-production in risk assessment is also an important process for empowering individuals with LD, which may enhance therapeutic relationships and increase engagement and motivation to develop coping strategies that reduce the need for harmful behaviour (Morris et al., 2021). Inaccessibility of widely used risk assessment tools presents a barrier to successful implementation of co-production, and therefore developing tools that are responsive to the needs of those with LD and person-centred formulation should be a core focus (Lofthouse et al., 2020; Morris et al., 2021).

References

Alexander, R., Devapriam, J., Michael, D., McCarthy, J., Chester, V., Rai, R., … & Roy, A. (2015). "Why can't they be in the community?" A policy and practice analysis of transforming care for offenders with intellectual disability. *Advances in Mental Health and Intellectual Disabilities*, *9*(3), 139–148. 10.1108/AMHID-02-2015-0011

Boer, D. P., Frize, M., Pappas, R., Morrissey, C., & Lindsay, W. R. (2010). Suggested adaptations to the HCR-20 for offenders with intellectual disabilities. In L. A. Craig, W. R. Lindsay, & K. D. Browne (Eds.), *Assessment and treatment of sexual offenders with intellectual disabilities: A handbook* (pp. 177–192). Chichester: Wiley, Blackwell.

Boer, D. P., Frize, M. C. J., Haaven, J., Lambrick, F., Lindsay, W. R., McVilly, K., Muddamage, G., & Sakdalan, J. (2012) The Assessment of Risk and Manageability of Intellectually Disabled Individuals who Offend (General Version) Scoring Manual. Retrieved from Frize, M. C. J. (2015). The Assessment of Risk of General Recidivism in Offenders with an Intellectual Disability. Thesis for the University of Sydney.

Boer, D. P., McVilly, K. R., & Lambrick, F. (2007). Contextualizing risk in the assessment of intellectually disabled individuals. *Sexual Offender Treatment*, *2*(2), 1–5.

Boer, D. P., Tough, S., & Haaven, J. (2004). Assessment of risk manageability of intellectually disabled sex offenders. *Journal of Applied Research in Intellectual Disabilities*, *17*(4), 275–283. 10.1111/j.1468-3148.2004.00214.x

Bradley, K. (2009). *The Bradley Report: Lord Bradley's review of people with mental health problems or learning disabilities in the criminal justice system*. London: Department of Health.

British Psychological Society (2015). *Guidance on the assessment and diagnosis of intellectual disabilities in adulthood*. Leicester: British Psychological Society.

Camilleri, J. A., & Quinsey, V. L. (2011). Appraising the risk of sexual and violent recidivism among intellectually disabled offenders. *Psychology, Crime & Law, 17*(1), 59–74. 10.1080/10683160903392350

Carr, N. (2017). The Lammy review and race and bias in the criminal justice system. *Probation Journal, 64*(4), 333–336. 10.1177/0264550517740461

Chenane, J. L., Brennan, P. K., Steiner, B., & Ellison, J. M. (2015). Racial and ethnic differences in the predictive validity of the level of service inventory – Revised among prison inmates. *Criminal Justice and Behavior, 42*(3), 286–303. 10.1177/0093854814548195

Chester, V., Brown, A. S., Devapriam, J., Axby, S., Hargreaves, C., & Shankkar, R. (2017). Discharging inpatients with intellectual disability from secure to community services: Risk assessment and management considerations. *Advances in Mental Health and Intellectual Disabilities, 11*(3), 98–109. 10.1108/AMHID-01-2017-0003

Chilvers, J., & Thomas, C. (2011). Do male and female forensic patients with learning disabilities differ on subscales of the Novaco Anger Scale and Provocation Inventory (NAS-PI)?. *Journal of Intellectual Disabilities and Offending Behaviour, 2*(2), 84–97. 10.1108/20420921111152469

Cluley, V. (2018). From "Learning disability to intellectual disability"—Perceptions of the increasing use of the term "intellectual disability" in learning disability policy, research and practice. *British Journal of Learning Disabilities, 46*(1), 24–32. 10.1111/bld.12209

Department of Health (2001). *Valuing people - A new strategy for learning disability for the 21st century*. London: Department of Health.

Department of Health (2012). *Transforming care: A national response to Winterbourne*. London: Department of Health.

Devapriam, J., Michael, D., McCarthy, J., Chester, V., Rai, R., Naseem, A., & Roy, A. (2015). "Why can't they be in the community?" A policy and practice analysis of transforming care for offenders with intellectual disability. *Advances in Mental Health and Intellectual Disabilities, 9*(3), 139–148. 10.1108/AMHID-02-2015-0011

de Vogel, V., de Vries Robbé, M., de Ruiter, C., & Bouman, Y. H. (2011). Assessing protective factors in forensic psychiatric practice: Introducing the SAPROF. *International journal of forensic mental health, 10*(3), 171–177. 10.1080/14999013.2011.600230

Dickens, G., Picchioni, M., & Long, C. (2013). Aggression in specialist secure and forensic inpatient mental health care: Incidence across care pathways. *Journal of Forensic Practice, 15*(3), 206–217. 10.1108/JFP-09-2012-0017

Douds, F., & Bantwal, A. (2011). The "forensicisation" of challenging behaviour: the perils of people with learning disabilities and severe challenging behaviours being viewed as "forensic" patients. *Journal of Learning Disabilities and Offending Behaviour, 2*(3), 110–113. 10.1108/20420921111186624

Durcan, G., Saunders, A., Gadsby, B., & Hazard, A. (2014). *The Bradley Report five years on: An independent review of progress to date and priorities for further development*. London: Centre for Mental Health.

Dusome, D., & Melrose, S. (2015). Sexuality: Promoting healthy sexual expression. In S. Melrose, D. Dusome, J. Simpson, C. Crocker, & E. Athens (Eds), *Supporting individuals with intellectual disabilities & mental illness: What caregivers need to know*. Canada: Vancouver, British Columbia.

Emerson, E., & Hatton, C. (2007). Mental health of children and adolescents with intellectual disabilities in Britain. *The British Journal of Psychiatry, 191*(6), 493–499. 10.1192/bjp.bp.107.038729

Fitzgerald, S., Gray, N. S., Alexander, R. T., Bagshaw, R., Chesterman, P., Huckle, P., ... & Snowden, R. J. (2013). Predicting institutional violence in offenders with intellectual disabilities: the predictive efficacy of the VRAG and the HCR-20. *Journal of Applied Research in Intellectual Disabilities, 26*(5), 384–393. 10.1111/jar.12032

Frize, M. (2015). *The assessment of risk of general recidivism in offenders with an intellectual disability* [Doctorate Thesis, University of Sydney]. University of Sydney Repository. https://ses.library.usyd.edu.au/handle/2123/13532

Gray, N. S., Fitzgerald, S., Taylor, J., MacCulloch, M. J., & Snowden, R. J. (2007). Predicting future reconviction in offenders with intellectual disabilities: The predictive efficacy of VRAG, PCL-SV, and the HCR-20. *Psychological Assessment, 19*(4), 474–479. 10.1037/1040-3590.19.4.474

Hastings, R. P., Gillespie, D., Flynn, S., McNamara, R., Taylor, Z., Knight, R., ... & Hunt, P. H. (2018). Who's challenging who training for staff empathy towards adults with challenging behaviour: Cluster randomised controlled trial. *Journal of Intellectual Disability Research, 62*(9), 798–813. 10.1111/jir.12536

Heyvaert, M., Maes, B., & Onghena, P. (2010). A meta-analysis of intervention effects on challenging behaviour among persons with intellectual disabilities. *Journal of Intellectual Disability Research, 54*(7), 634–649. 10.1111/j.1365-2788.2010.01291.x

Houlden, A. (2015). Building the right support: A national plan to develop community services and close inpatient facilities for people with a learning disability and/or autism who display behaviour that challenges, including those with a mental health condition. NHS England, the Local Government Association, and the Association of Directors of Adult Social Services.

Hounsome, J., Whittington, R., Brown, A., Greenhill, B., & McGuire, J. (2018). The structured assessment of violence risk in adults with intellectual disability: A systematic review. *Journal of Applied Research in Intellectual Disabilities, 31*(1), e1–e17. 10.1111/jar.12295

Hoyt, W. T. (2000). Rater bias in psychological research: When is it a problem and what can we do about it? *Psychological Methods, 5*(1), 64–86. 10.1037/1082-989X.5.1.64

Lammy, D. (2017). *The Lammy review: An independent review into the treatment of, and outcomes for, Black, Asian and Minority ethnic individuals in the criminal justice System.* London: Lammy Review.

Larkin, P., Jahoda, A., & MacMahon, K. (2013). The social information processing model as a framework for explaining frequent aggression in adults with mild to moderate intellectual disabilities: A systematic review of the evidence. *Journal of Applied Research in Intellectual Disabilities, 26*(5), 447–465. 10.1111/jar.12031

Lindsay, W. R., Hogue, T. E., Taylor, J. L., Steptoe, L., Mooney, P., O'Brien, G., ... & Smith, A. H. (2008). Risk assessment in offenders with intellectual disability: A comparison across three levels of security. *International Journal of Offender Therapy and Comparative Criminology, 52*(1), 90–111. 10.1177/0306624X07308111

Lindsay, W. R., Murphy, L., Smith, G., Murphy, D., Edwards, Z., Chittock, C., ... & Young, S. J. (2004). The dynamic risk assessment and management system: An assessment of immediate risk of violence for individuals with offending and challenging behaviour. *Journal of Applied Research in Intellectual Disabilities, 17*(4), 267–274. 10.1111/j.1468-3148.2004.00215.x

Lindsay, W. R., Steptoe, L.R., Haut, F., Miller, S., Macer, J., & McVicker, R. (2018). The protective scale of the Armidilo-S: The importance of forensic and clinical outcomes. *Journal of Applied Research in Intellectual Disabilities, 33*(4), 654–661 10.1111/jar.12456.

Lloyd, B. P., & Kennedy, C. H. (2014). Assessment and treatment of challenging behaviour for individuals with intellectual disability: A research review. *Journal of Applied Research in Intellectual Disabilities*, *27*(3), 187–199. 10.1111/jar.12089

Lofthouse, R., Golding, L., Totsika, V., Hastings, R., & Lindsay, W. (2017). How effective are risk assessments/measures for predicting future aggressive behaviour in adults with intellectual disabilities (ID): A systematic review and meta-analysis. *Clinical Psychology Review*, *58*, 76–85. 10.1016/j.cpr.2017.10.001

Lofthouse, R. E., Golding, L., Totsika, V., Hastings, R. P., & Lindsay, W. R. (2020). Predicting aggression in adults with intellectual disability: A pilot study of the predictive efficacy of the Current Risk of Violence and the Short Dynamic Risk Scale. *Journal of Applied Research in Intellectual Disabilities*, *33*(4), 702–710. 10.1111/jar.12665

Lofthouse, R. E., Lindsay, W. R., Totsika, V., Hastings, R. P., Boer, D. P., & Haaven, J. L. (2013). Prospective dynamic assessment of risk of sexual reoffending in individuals with an intellectual disability and a history of sexual offending behaviour. *Journal of Applied Research in Intellectual Disabilities*, *26*(5), 394–403. 10.1111/jar.12029

Lofthouse, R. E., Lindsay, W. R., Totsika, V., Hastings, R. P., & Roberts, D. (2014). Dynamic risk and violence in individuals with an intellectual disability: Tool development and initial validation. *The Journal of Forensic Psychiatry & Psychology*, *25*(3), 288–306. 10.1080/14789.949.2014.911946

Lofthouse, R. E., Totsika, V., Hastings, R. P., Lindsay, W. R., Hogue, T. E., & Taylor, J. L. (2014). How do static and dynamic risk factors work together to predict violent behaviour among offenders with an intellectual disability?. *Journal of Intellectual Disability Research*, *58*(2), 125–133. 10.1111/j.1365-2788.2012.01645.x

Lowder, E. M., Desmarais, S. L., Rade, C. B., Johnson, K. L., & Van Dorn, R. A. (2019). Reliability and validity of START and LSI-R assessments in mental health jail diversion clients. *Assessment*, *26*(7), 1347–1361. 10.1177/1073191117704505

Marshall-Tate, K., Chaplin, E., & McCarthy, J. (2017). Is "transforming care" failing people with autism?. *Advances in Autism*, *3*(2), 59–65. 10.1108/AIA-10-2016-0027

Matthews, M., & Bell, E. (2020). Assessment of risk of violent offending for adults with intellectual disability and/or autism spectrum disorder. *The Wiley handbook of what works in violence risk management: Theory, research and practice*, 349–366.

McGrath, R. J., Livingston, J. A., & Falk, G. (2007). A structured method of assessing dynamic risk factors among sexual abusers with intellectual disabilities. *American Journal on Mental Retardation*, *112*(3), 221–229. 10.1352/0895-8017(2007)112[221:ASMOAD]2.0.CO;2

McNamara, N. (2012). Speech and language therapy within a forensic support service. *Journal of Learning Disabilities and Offending Behaviour*, *3*(2), 111–117. 10.1108/2042 0921211280097

Morris, D. J., Webb, E. L., Stewart, I., Galsworthy, J., & Wallang, P. (2021). Comparing co-production approaches to dynamic risk assessments in a forensic intellectual disability population: Outcomes of a clinical pilot. *Journal of Intellectual Disabilities and Offending Behaviour*, *12*(1), 23–36. 10.1108/JIDOB-08-2020-0014

Morrissey, C., Hogue, T., Mooney, P., Allen, C., Johnston, S., Hollin, C., … & Taylor, J. L. (2007). Predictive validity of the PCL-R in offenders with intellectual disability in a high secure hospital setting: Institutional aggression. *The Journal of Forensic Psychiatry & Psychology*, *18*(1), 1–15. 10.1080/08990220601116345

Olver, M. E., Stockdale, K. C., & Wormith, J. S. (2014). Thirty years of research on the Level of Service Scales: A meta-analytic examination of predictive accuracy and sources of variability. *Psychological Assessment*, *26*(1), 156–176. DOI: 10.1037/a0035080

O'Shea, L. E., Picchioni, M. M., McCarthy, J., Mason, F. L., & Dickens, G. L. (2015). Predictive validity of the HCR-20 for inpatient aggression: The effect of intellectual disability on accuracy. *Journal of Intellectual Disability Research, 59*(11), 1042–1054. 10.1111/jir.12184

O'Hara, J. (2003). Learning disabilities and ethnicity: Achieving cultural competence. *Advances in Psychiatric Treatment,* 9(3),166–174. 10.1192/apt.9.3.166

Pouls, C., & Jeandarme, I. (2015). Risk assessment and risk management in offenders with intellectual disabilities: Are we there yet?. *Journal of Mental Health Research in Intellectual Disabilities, 8*(3-4), 213–236.

Quinsey, V. L. (2004). Risk assessment and management in community settings. In W. R. Lindsay, J. L. Taylor, & P. Sturmey (Eds.), *Offenders with developmental disabilities* (pp. 131–141). Chichester, UK: John Wiley & Sons Ltd.

Rycroft-Malone, J., Burton, C. R., Bucknall, T., Graham, I. D., Hutchinson, A. M., & Stacey, D. (2016). Collaboration and co-production of knowledge in healthcare: Opportunities and challenges. *International Journal of Health Policy and Management, 5*(4), 221–223. doi: 10.15171/ijhpm.2016.08

Saunders, A., Browne, D., & Durcan, G. (2013). *The Bradley Commission: Black and Minority Ethnic communities, mental health and criminal justice.* London: Centre for Mental Health.

Shepherd, S. M., & Lewis-Fernandez, R. (2016). Forensic risk assessment and cultural diversity: Contemporary challenges and future directions. *Psychology, Public Policy, and Law, 22*(4), 427–438. 10.1037/law0000102

Shepherd, S. M., & Spivak, B. L. (2021). Finding colour in conformity part II— Reflections on structured professional judgement and cross-cultural risk assessment. *International Journal of Offender Therapy and Comparative Criminology, 65*(1), 92–99. 10.1177/0306624X20928025

Shepherd, S. M., & Willis-Esqueda, C. (2018). Indigenous perspectives on violence risk assessment: A thematic analysis. *Punishment & Society, 20*(5), 599–627. 10.1177/1462474517721485

Steans, J., & Duff, S. (2020). Perceptions of sex offenders with intellectual disability: A comparison of forensic staff and the general public. *Journal of Applied Research in Intellectual Disabilities, 33*(4), 711–719. 10.1111/jar.12467

Taylor, J. L., McKinnon, I., Thorpe, I., & Gillmer, B. T. (2017). The impact of transforming care on the care and safety of patients with intellectual disabilities and forensic needs. *BJPsych Bulletin, 41*(4), 205–208.

The Lammy Review (2017). An independent review into the treatment of, and outcomes for, Black, Asian and Minority Ethnic individuals in the Criminal Justice System.

Tonry, M. H. (2011). *Punishing race: A continuing American dilemma.* Oxford University Press.

Varela, J. G., Boccaccini, M. T., Murrie, D. C., Caperton, J. D., & Gonzalez, E. (2013). Do the Static-99 and Static-99R perform similarly for white, black, and Latino sexual offenders? *International Journal of Forensic Mental Health, 12*(4), 231–243. 10.1080/14999013.2013.846950

Venner, S., Sivasubramaniam, D., Luebbers, S., & Shepherd, S. M. (2021a). Cross-cultural reliability and rater bias in forensic risk assessment: A review of the literature. *Psychology, Crime & Law, 27*(2), 105–121.

Venner, S., Sivasubramaniam, D., Luebbers, S., & Shepherd, S. M. (2021b). Exploring Rater Cultural Bias in Forensic Risk Assessment. *International Journal of Forensic Mental Health, 20,* 213–226.

Verbrugge, H. M., Goodman-Delahunty, J., & Frize, M. C. J. (2011). Risk assessment in intellectually disabled offenders: Validation of the suggested ID supplement to the HCR-20. *International Journal of Forensic Mental Health*, *10*(2), 83–91.

Vincent, G. M., & Viljoen, J. L. (2020). Racist algorithms or systemic problems? Risk assessments and racial disparities. *Criminal Justice and Behavior*, *47*(12), 1576–1584. 10.11 77/0093854820954501

Wheeler, J. R., Clare, I. C., & Holland, A. J. (2014). What can social and environmental factors tell us about the risk of offending by people with intellectual disabilities?. *Psychology, Crime & Law*, *20*(7), 635–658. 10.1080/1068316X.2013.854789

Wilson, H. A., & Gutierrez, L. (2014). Does one size fit all?: A meta-analysis examining the predictive ability of the level of service inventory (LSI) with aboriginal offenders. *Criminal Justice and Behavior*, *41*(2), 196–219. 10.1177/0093854813500958

Woldgabreal, Y., Day, A., & Tamatea, A. (2020). Do risk assessments play a role in the enduring 'color line'. *Advancing Corrections*, *10*, 18–28.

Yang, M., Wong, S. C. P., & Coid, J. (2010). The efficacy of violence prediction: A meta-analytic comparison of nine risk assessment tools. *Psychological Bulletin*, *136*(5), 740–767. 10.1037/a0020473

21 Challenging Bias in Forensic Psychological Assessment and Treatment for People with ADHD

Rachel Worthington

Introduction

ADHD is a disorder which appears across the lifespan with an estimated prevalence of 2.5% of adults meeting the criteria for a diagnosis (Simon et al., 2009). It is associated with early onset offending (Mohr-Jensen & Steinhausen, 2016) and higher rates of reoffending in adults (Young et al., 2011) with approximately 2.8 million prisoners worldwide meeting the diagnostic criteria for ADHD (Young et al., 2018). The purpose of this chapter is to highlight how bias may contribute to barriers in diagnosis/treatment of ADHD and provide practical suggestions for how these may be overcome.

What Is ADHD?

Attention Deficit Hyperactivity Disorder (ADHD) is a neurodevelopmental disorder characterised by a dysfunctional pattern of inattention, hyperactivity, or impulsivity, leading to negative outcomes in social, academic, and occupational contexts throughout an individual's life (Dalsgaard et al., 2015). ADHD may be distinguished into three types (Diagnostic and Statistical Manual of Mental Disorders – Version 5, 2015):

1   The predominantly inattentive type (IA),
2   The predominantly hyperactive/impulsive type (HI)
3   The combined type (C).

ADHD is known to extend into adulthood and old age (Emser et al., 2018) with approximately two-thirds of people diagnosed with ADHD in childhood continuing to have symptoms in adulthood (Bitter et al., 2019) with symptoms falling into the predominantly inattentive type (Kooij et al., 2010). In the UK, it is estimated that about 25% of prisoners have ADHD (Young et al., 2015).

What Causes ADHD?

ADHD is a genetic disorder with approximately 75–80% of ADHD variation being accounted for in human genes. As ADHD is a genetically influenced

DOI: 10.4324/9781003230977-24

neurochemical expression, medication has been shown to be an effective treatment for symptoms of ADHD in children, adolescents, and adults (Faraone et al., 2021) and surpasses the efficacy of medications used to treat non-psychiatric disorders (Leucht et al., 2012). Improvements with medication include reductions in: aggression (Young et al., 2011) vehicle accidents in males (Chang et al., 2014); suicide-related behaviours (Chen et al., 2014); criminality (33% for males and 40% for females) (Lichtenstein et al., 2012); and substance misuse (Chang et al., 2014). In addition, medication was not associated with any increases in: alcohol use; cocaine use; or cannabis abuse/dependence (Humphreys et al., 2013).

However, other factors may also contribute to gene expression such as exposure to: toxins; deprivation, stress, poverty, and trauma (Faraone et al., 2021); sexual abuse; physical neglect (Ouyang et al., 2008); and lower levels of family income (Larsson et al., 2014).

How Is ADHD Diagnosed?

ADHD can only be diagnosed by a licensed clinician (Faraone et al., 2021) and should rely on multiple sources of information such as clinical interviews, observations, ratings, and objective measures from multiple sources (Emser et al., 2018) to adhere to the DSM-5 classification systems. To overcome any lack of concordance in symptom reports information such as: educational history; family history; and asking about symptoms of ADHD in other family members (siblings and parents) should be obtained (Hamed et al., 2015). A wide range of assessment screening tools using ratings are available and it is not within the scope of this chapter to review them all. One example of a screening tool used to guide if further assessment would be of benefit is the Quantified Behavior Test [QbTest] which is a neuropsychological test with versions for children and those over the age of 12 (including adults).

Why Is ADHD Diagnosis Important in Forensic Settings?

ADHD in prisons far exceeds that of the general population with meta-analytic studies suggesting the prevalence to be approximately 25% for males (Baggio et al., 2018) and 40% in females (Farooq et al., 2016). Females diagnosed with ADHD have a seven times greater likelihood of being incarcerated than females without ADHD (Silva et al., 2014) in comparison to males who had two times the likelihood.

ADHD is associated with: earlier onset offending (Mohr-Jensen & Steinhausen, 2016); higher rates of reoffending in adults (Young et al., 2011); a greater risk of vehicle accidents/car crashes (Vaa, 2014); twice the rate of death by homicide (Chen et al., 2019); employment difficulties (Waite et al., 2013); family conflict and difficulties in parenting (Ginsberg et al., 2014).

Thus, untreated ADHD may have significant implications for the individual and their family as well as substantial economic burdens on society (Faraone et al., 2021). Dehaghani & Bath (2021) found deficits in the ability to identify people with ADHD in the UK CJS alongside a lack of interventions designed to meet their responsivity needs.

However, ADHD in itself does not cause offending behaviour but certain aspects of ADHD may contribute to both risk and resilience factors for offending (Al-Attar, 2021). These are conceptualised in the Framework for the Assessment of Risk and Protection in offenders with ADHD [FARAH, Al-Attar, 2021). Thus, given the literature on the benefits of identifying ADHD and accessing treatment this is something which is clearly of significance. However, access to diagnosis and treatment has considerable variability.

What Is Bias?

Bias is a personal judgement or prejudice in favour of or against a certain thing, person, or group that is considered to be unfair (Fitzgerald & Hurst, 2017). Bias may happen at an individual, group, or societal level (Fadus et al., 2020) and can be both conscious (explicit) or unconscious (implicit). Both can lead to differences in diagnostic decision making (Kahneman et al., 2021). Dror (2020) identifies six fallacies of bias and eight sources which may influence decision making contribute to bias.

Bias exists equally in healthcare professionals compared to the public (FitzGerald & Hurst, 2017) even when professionals state they are not biased and oppose this (Fadus et al., 2020) due to unconscious pejorative stereotypes (Devine et al., 2012). This can lead to a cycle of structural racism whereby society discriminates individuals through reinforcing systems such as housing, education, employment, healthcare, and criminal justice (Fadus et al., 2020). Schmengler et al (2021) note that divergence in diagnosis may occur due to differences in informant reporting based on cultural differences leading to differences in parent and teacher evaluations of behavioural difficulties (Sahuric et al., 2019). For example, in some cultures behavioural difficulties may be considered more of a social or spiritual problem rather than medical (Lawton et al., 2014).

What Is Diversity?

Discrimination is "the unjust or prejudicial treatment of different categories of people". It is against the law to discriminate against anyone because of a protected characteristic. These include age; gender; race; nationality; disability; ethnicity; religion; and/or sexual orientation (Equalities Act, 2010). Thus, diversity is the "action, practice, or policy of including any person in an activity, system, organisation, or process, irrespective of race, gender, religion, age, ability, etc." (Oxford English Dictionary, 2021). This will be considered in relation to ADHD subsequently.

Culture and Ethnic Diversity

Mental health practices in psychology and psychiatry have predominantly emerged from Western cultural traditions and perspectives which cause difficulties when they are applied in non-Western cultures (Gopalkrishnan, 2018). Hernandez et al. (2009, p. 1047) suggest "culture influences what gets defined as a problem, how the problem is understood and which solutions to the problem are acceptable". Thus, it is important that racial and cultural diversity is considered when exploring ADHD.

Significant racial disparities in the diagnosis of ADHD have been found in over 200,000 children whereby Asian, Black, Hispanic, and "migrant" children were significantly less likely to be diagnosed with ADHD compared with white children who were also more likely to receive treatment (Coker et al., 2016; Shi et al., 2021; Kazda et al., 2021). It has also been noted that people classed as "immigrants" or those who have had to flee their home country due to war or conflict may be at increased vulnerability for ADHD (Schmengler et al., 2021) although the overlap between trauma and ADHD symptoms has also been noted (Siegfried & Blackshear, 2016). Fadus et al. (2020) noted unconscious biases result in some children/adolescents behaviour being labelled as oppositional defiance disorder (ODD) or conduct disorder (CD) when there was contrary evidence indicating ADHD.

Slobodin & Masalha (2020) also found that certain biases associated with culture, race, and language resulted in some ethnic minority children being over-identified as having ADHD. Kazda et al (2021) found evidence in nine studies of diagnosis rates increasing rapidly in "Black youths" resulting in the rates of diagnosis overtaking the rates of white youth. It has been postulated this may be due to minority children having increased exposure to environmental risk factors and to cultural, linguistic, and racial biases leading to systemic forms of prejudice (Slobodin & Masalha, 2020).

In the UK prison system, ethnic disparities have been noted (Dehaghani & Bath, 2021) whereby prisoners who identified as being from black and minority ethnic backgrounds were less likely to be identified as having any learning difficulties.

Thus, cultural factors are to be taken into consideration in the diagnosis of ADHD as this appears to be linked with both over and under identification of ADHD.

Gender Diversity

Gender variations in ADHD diagnoses have been found in systematic reviews with females having lower diagnoses than males and females who had the same symptoms as males (Kazda et al., 2021). Whilst biological reasons may account for some differences in gender prevalence of ADHD (Huss et al., 2008) some variations exist due to the detection of symptoms in females compared to males (Hamed et al., 2015) who are likely to present with greater externalising symptoms, more hyperactivity and less impulse control which are seen as more problematic by parents than internalising symptoms and symptoms of inattention (Ginsberg et al., 2014).

Societal gender role expectations may also influence how teachers (Sciutto et al., 2004) and parents (Mowlem et al., 2019) respond to child ADHD resulting in females being undiagnosed. This is concerning given that females with ADHD are noted to: have greater difficulties with emotional dysregulation; are at greater risk of engaging in self-harm (Hollingdale et al., 2014); being admitted to psychiatric hospitals (Dalsgaard et al., 2015); have higher rates of alcohol and cannabis use; gang activity; and criminal behaviour (Young et al., 2020).

Internalising symptoms in females comprise of depression, anxiety, emotional difficulties, and borderline personality traits leading to misdiagnoses and delays in treatment for ADHD (Quinn & Madhoo, 2014). This is worsened by some assessment tools for ADHD using cut off scores from normative samples of males rather than females. Young et al. (2020) suggest that the SASI (Nadeau & Quinn, 2002) could be used to overcome some of these difficulties and where normative samples for females are not available in standardised tools then greater emphasis should be placed on the use of collateral information from parents/teachers/others/school reports, etc. Assessors should also be more attentive to symptoms such as excessive giggling (Young et al., 2020), excessive talking, fidgeting, interrupting, and blurting out the answers which are more common in women with ADHD (Quinn, 2011). In addition tools such as the DAWBA (Goodman et al., 2000) may also be useful for assessing adolescent females to assist in differentiating co-existing conditions. It is noted that both of the Conners scales (Epstein et al., 2001) for adults and adolescents/children have female norms (Young et al., 2020).

No differences exist in the efficacy of medication for females compared to males (both adults and children) but females are less likely to be prescribed medication (Dalsgaard et al., 2014). Thus it is recommended that people supporting females with ADHD should receive psycho-education on the benefits of ADHD medication (especially for inattention) (Young et al., 2020).

Religion/Spirituality

Research into ADHD and religion is sparse and hence few definitive conclusions can be drawn into this however there are a few studies which provide some insight into this.

In their study exploring Hindu mother's attitudes towards ADHD in India, Cadet et al. (2019) noted that regardless of a child's diagnosis, the child's behaviour is seen as a reflection of the mother's parenting (Viswanath & Chaturvedi, 2012). This may be because child-rearing in India is primarily undertaken by the mother which reflects cultural norms (Valk & Srinivasan, 2011). Thus, mothers may perceive seeking psychological help as stigmatising because it reflects badly on their parenting (Cadet et al., 2019).

Li (2013) found that evangelical Christians in the US were less likely to view ADHD as a disease and as being something that would improve with medication compared to participants who attended church (and were rated as being of non-evangelical denomination). The authors postulated that the difference in views may be related to how people of an evangelical faith conceptualised health and spirituality (Ellison & Levin, 1998) in that people should take responsibility for their behaviour (Emerson & Smith, 2001). However, further research in this area is recommended.

Kamaruddin et al. (2017) also found differences in the levels of stress reported by parents of children with ADHD whereby 62% of Muslims reported experiencing moderate levels of stress compared to 7.6% for Christian parents, 7.6% for Buddhist parents, and 32.7% for Hindu parents. This mirrored the findings of Gupta et al. (2012) who noted that religious coping is reported to reduce parenting stress and that high levels of stress are reported by mothers of children with disabilities in India but more than half of the respondents reported turning to God, mosques, and temples as a way of coping when they felt there was no other "cure" (Gupta et al., 2012).

Thus, religion is diverse and has individual meaning in terms of the impact this may have on beliefs about ADHD, seeking diagnoses, adhering to medication, and family support. Hence, it is imperative that clinicians are mindful of being culturally sensitive to the religious views of their clients and their families.

Age Diversity

As noted, adult ADHD symptoms are mainly inattentive which are associated with greater impairment than symptoms of hyperactivity and impulsivity. Whilst ADHD could have an adolescent or early adult-onset (Caye et al., 2016) it has been suspected this is more likely evidence of ADHD being undetected in childhood (Castellanos, 2015) especially where these are female (Vitola et al., 2017). Longitudinal research found no evidence for adult-onset ADHD when factors such as substance misuse and psychiatric history were accounted for (Sibley et al., 2017).

Rates of ADHD in people over the age of 55 are estimated to be between 2.8% and 3.3% with older adults having similar impairments to younger adults in terms of higher rates of: loneliness; depression; and divorce (Michielsen et al., 2015).

The relative age effect has also shown children born in the last month of the academic year were 1.6 times more likely to be diagnosed with ADHD and more likely to be prescribed medication. It is thought this is related to teacher perceptions of behaviour (Elder, 2010) given no age-related effects were noted based on parent self-report (Halldner et al., 2014).

Thus, it can be seen that accurate diagnoses of ADHD are important for all ages. See Young et al. (2018) for a comprehensive review of the range of tools which apply across adult and adolescent offender groups.

Comorbid Diagnoses

Estimating the prevalence of Intellectual Disabilities (ID) in people with ADHD (or vice versa) is complicated by differences in assessment tools, methodology, and levels of intellectual functioning across samples (Perera et al., 2021). Hence, it is recommended that objective assessment criteria and tools are used such as the Diagnostic Interview for ADHD in Adults with ID (McCarthy et al., 2017). In addition, recognising ADHD in clients with ID is important because this has been associated with a reduction in the overuse of psychotropic medication (Korb et al., 2019).

People with ID are overrepresented in prison settings (Perera et al., 2021) but little is known about the potential comorbidity of ADHD. Chaplin et al. (2017) found that of 240 prisoners, 7.5% were identified as likely having an ID, and of these 67% were considered likely to have ADHD compared not non-offender populations where this was 19.6% (La Malfa et al., 2008). Lindsay et al. (2013) also found that adults with ID and ADHD in a specialist forensic service had significantly higher rates of physical aggression and offending compared to the ID-only group. However, the exact role of ID and ADHD is largely understudied and further research is needed in this area.

People with ADHD may also be at a heightened risk of comorbid psychiatric diagnoses (Gerhand & Saville, 2021) with estimated prevalence ratings ranging from 19% to 34%. Comorbidity with ADHD has been identified in relation to: depression; bipolar disorder (Chen et al., 2018); autism spectrum disorders; eating disorders (Nazar et al., 2016); and substance misuse disorders. However, clients in psychiatric settings are often under-diagnosed and hence not treated for ADHD due to the overlap between ADHD and psychiatric symptoms (Katzman et al., 2017). For example, irritability, low mood, and poor concentration may also be markers for mood disorders as well as ADHD, creating both "false positives" (Youngstrom et al., 2010) as well as under-diagnoses.

Some studies have found gender differences in psychiatric comorbidity for ADHD between males and females whereby conduct disorder, substance use disorder (specifically alcohol), and antisocial personality disorder have all been found to be more prevalent in males with ADHD whilst mood disorders have been found to be more common in females (Bitter et al., 2019). Thus, Bitter et al. (2019) propose that clinicians should receive better training in understanding adult ADHD to inform the accuracy of their assessments.

Treatment

First line treatment for ADHD is medication. It is not within the scope of this chapter to review the entire medication literature base for ADHD, however, exploration of whether a person has been prescribed medication, their attitudes to this, and their adherence to such should be of importance to forensic practitioners. In addition to medication, it is recognised that non-pharmacological interventions for cognitive difficulties in ADHD may also play a role. These may be dependent on the age of the person as the efficacy of interventions and individual needs are likely to change across the lifespan (Young et al., 2020).

Psycho-education is considered a key component of treatment by adolescence and should include information on the purpose of medication and what benefits this may have (Young et al., 2020) as well as skills in relation to self-management, regulating emotions, low self-esteem, low mood, and managing anxiety. Given the risks in relation to impulsivity and risk-taking behaviours, it is also re-commended that psycho-education could attend to sexual behaviours (include online risks) and substance misuse. In adulthood psycho-education should con-tinue in addition to CBT-based interventions. For example, a systematic review of non-pharmacological interventions (Nimmo-Smith et al., 2020) found that CBT was associated with a reduction in the core behavioural symptoms of ADHD although the findings were mixed and more research is needed. The authors recommend that more research is needed to explore the efficacy of non-pharmacological interventions for adults with ADHD.

Lambez et al. (2020) provided a systematic review of the evidence in relation to improvement in cognitive functioning and ADHD. They found that physical ex-ercise interventions demonstrated the highest effect size followed by CBT and neurofeedback which demonstrated moderate effect sizes. Cognitive training in-terventions had the lowest effect. Furthermore, the findings were equally applicable to both participants who were medicated and those who were not on medication. The cognitive functions most impacted by treatment were inhibition and flexibility followed by attention and working memory (Lambez et al., 2020). They hy-pothesised this was due to the malleability of higher-order executive functions which was likely due to aerobic exercise causing neurotransmitter modifications and changes to blood flow in the prefrontal cortex (Pontifex et al., 2013).

Psycho-education is also imperative for people supporting someone with ADHD particularly in an institutional setting (Young et al., 2020) and/or when someone is transitioning from one setting to another (e.g., school to college, college to em-ployment, prison to the community, etc). The aim should be to provide education and regular reviews to share information on how best to support the person and to provide education to the receiving team on the person's needs.

Thus, in summary treatment should include the following in Table 21.1 and be adjusted so they are age-appropriate.

Recommendations

Fadus et al. (2020) note that few interventions have been longitudinally tested to reduce implicit bias, and some training has inadvertently increased bias in at-tendees who were not motivated to attend (Cooley et al., 2018). Hence, it is recommended that bias-reducing interventions should focus on the effects this can have on client outcomes (Forscher et al., 2017) to improve motivation and it is hoped this chapter has provided some insight into the detrimental effects of bias in relation to ADHD.

Tools such as the DSM-5 Cultural Formulation Interview (Aggarwal et al., 2016) could also be used which may assist practitioners to improve their cultural competence. Cultural formulations take into account cultural and ethnic differ-ences in reporting of behaviours and experiences and facilitate culturally in-formed interviewing. The Structural Vulnerability Assessment tool (Bourgois et al., 2017) can also be used to explore how the social structures around a person may act as protective or risk factors for their ADHD. Cultural formulations

Table 21.1 Summary of treatment aspects that should be included when working with
ADHD

[A] Psycho-education on:
1 What ADHD is and how someone "gets" ADHD.
2 The benefits of medication and the different types of medication.
3 How to find information on ADHD that is reliable.
4 Identification of which of the ADHD symptoms the person experiences and how
symptoms may have changed across the lifespan.
5 Acknowledgement of the positive aspects of ADHD for that person.
6 Understanding the ways in which ADHD impacts on the person's functioning and
their relationships, employment, social life, school, parenting, etc.
7 Self-management and self-monitoring.

[B] Interventions:
1 People with ADHD in forensic settings should have equal access to pharmacological
interventions and have a medication management plan (Young et al., 2018).
2 Direct interventions (group or individual CBT for adults/adolescents) such as the
Young-Bramham Programme for Adolescents and Adults (see Young et al., 2018).
See also Ramsay (2010) for ways in which CBT can be adapted.
3 Understanding the way in which ADHD may have contributed towards offending
could be enhanced by undertaking the FARAH (Al-Attar, 2021).
4 Offence focussed specific interventions should be of a shorter duration (less than 4
months) with access to a mentor and additional one-to-one skills-building sessions
outside of any group treatment (Young et al., 2018).
5 Interventions such as R&R2ADHD should be considered (Young et al., 2018).
6 For young people, treatment programmes should also include an education plan
informed by the CHAT screening tool (Young et al., 2018).
7 Adults in prisons should not have to access an academic course in order to be able to
participate in technical skills-building workshops (Young et al., 2018).
8 Where possible adults with ADHD should have access to Occupational Therapy
(OT) to assist them to identify strengths and needs in occupational functioning (e.g.,
health, self-care, finances, etc).
9 Adults/Adolescents in prison should have access to a Care Programme
Approach (CPA).
10 When contracting for interventions it is important to identify with the person what
challenges their ADHD may pose in therapy and how these will be overcome.
11 Direct psycho-education on ADHD should be provided to family members/carers/
staff.
12 Follow up sessions to evaluate the success of implementing any strategies should be
provided.
13 Sessions to share information at the point of key transitions in the person's life. If the
person is in prison/hospital this should include a transition care plan identifying the
designated person to support them into the community.

---

should also include information on how interventions could be adapted to take
into account individual cultural needs and expectations from therapy including
the five key areas identified by Hechanova and Waelde (2017).

Factors such as clinician burnout may also play a contributing role to both
implicit and explicit biases in decision making (Dyrbye et al., 2019) particularly

in relation to the volume of clients, hours working, and the chronicity of client difficulties. Randomised Control Trials (West et al., 2014) have found that reflection, mindfulness, and group discussions sharing experiences can help to reduce aspects of burnout such as depersonalisation. Supervision should also attend to reflecting on developing ethical autobiographies (Bashe et al., 2007) reflecting on personal ethics and acculturation and how this may impact on their decision making. As noted by Dror & Murrie (2018) practitioners should also familiarise themselves with the Hierarchy of Expert Performance (HEP) to understand the risk for biasilibility and how to adopt strength-based assessments to reduce the risk of bias.

Summary

ADHD may be exhibited in different ways across the lifespan. However, access to diagnosis and treatment can vary. Thus, clinicians are expected to provide specific and personalised formulations of a client's strengths and needs which are developed based on their own ability to consider bias. To achieve this, the following recommendations are made:

1   Screening for ADHD should be person-centred and take into consideration diversity factors such as culture, ethnicity, age, gender, and any other individual comorbid difficulties/disabilities.
2   Assessments should include culturally informed interviewing to develop cultural formulations.
3   Formulations should take into account the social history and structure surrounding the person.
4   Practitioners should be aware of their own risk of bias and seek regular supervision to reflect on these in their practice and to monitor for burnout and work overload.
5   Practitioners should develop their own ethical autobiography to provide a place to actively consider their potential for bias in decision making.

References

Act, E. (2010). UK government legislation. www.gov.co.uk
Aggarwal, N. K., Lam, P., Castillo, E. G., Weiss, M. G., Diaz, E., Alarcón, R. D., & Lewis-Fernández, R. (2016). How do clinicians prefer cultural competence training? Findings from the DSM-5 cultural formulation interview field trial. *Academic Psychiatry*, *40*(4), 584–591.
Al-Attar, Z. (2021). How can ADHD contextualise offending risk: The FARAH guidelines? Autism, learning disabilities, and the criminal justice system conference 2021.
American Psychiatric Association. (2015). *Neurodevelopmental disorders: DSM-5® selections*. American Psychiatric Pub, 2015.
Baggio, S., Fructuoso, A., Guimaraes, M., Fois, E., Golay, D., Heller, P., ... & Wolff, H. (2018). Prevalence of attention deficit hyperactivity disorder in detention settings: A systematic review and meta-analysis. *Frontiers in Psychiatry*, *9*, 331.

Bashe, A., Anderson, S. K., Handelsman, M. M., & Klevansky, R. (2007). An acculturation model for ethics training: The ethics autobiography and beyond. *Professional Psychology: Research and Practice, 38*(1), 60.

Bitter, I., Mohr, P., Balogh, L., Látalová, K., Kakuszi, B., Stopková, P., ... & Czobor, P. (2019). ADHD: A hidden comorbidity in adult psychiatric patients. *ADHD Attention Deficit and Hyperactivity Disorders, 11*(1), 83–89.

Bourgois, P., Holmes, S. M., Sue, K., & Quesada, J. (2017). Structural vulnerability: Operationalizing the concept to address health disparities in clinical care. *Academic Medicine: Journal of the Association of American Medical Colleges, 92*(3), 299.

Cadet, G. D., Adsul, P., Coudray, M. S., Siddaiah, A., Stephens, D. P., & Madhivanan, P. (2019). Knowledge, gender, and guidance: Factors influencing Indian mothers responses to Attention Deficit Hyperactivity Disorder (ADHD). *Indian Journal of Health and Wellbeing, 10*(7-9), 195–200.

Castellanos, F. X. (2015). Is adult-onset ADHD a distinct entity?, *American Journal of Psychiatry, 172*(10), 929–931.

Caye, A., Rocha, T. B. M., Anselmi, L., Murray, J., Menezes, A. M., Barros, F. C., ... & Rohde, L. A. (2016). Attention-deficit/hyperactivity disorder trajectories from childhood to young adulthood: Evidence from a birth cohort supporting a late-onset syndrome. *JAMA Psychiatry, 73*(7), 705–712.

Chang, Z., Lichtenstein, P., D'Onofrio, B. M., Sjölander, A., & Larsson, H. (2014). Serious transport accidents in adults with attention-deficit/hyperactivity disorder and the effect of medication: A population-based study. *JAMA Psychiatry, 71*(3), 319–325.

Chaplin, E., McCarthy, J., Underwood, L., Forrester, A., Hayward, H., Sabet, J., ... & Murphy, D. (2017). Characteristics of prisoners with intellectual disabilities. *Journal of Intellectual Disability Research, 61*(12), 1185–1195.

Chen, Q., Sjölander, A., Runeson, B., D'Onofrio, B. M., Lichtenstein, P., & Larsson, H. (2014). Drug treatment for attention-deficit/hyperactivity disorder and suicidal behaviour: Register based study. *Bmj, 348*, g3769.

Chen, Q., Hartman, C. A., Haavik, J., Harro, J., Klungsøyr, K., Hegvik, T. A., ... & Larsson, H. (2018). Common psychiatric and metabolic comorbidity of adult attention-deficit/hyperactivity disorder: A population-based cross-sectional study. *PLoS One, 13*(9), e0204516

Chen, V. C.-Hung, Chan, H.-Lin, Wu, S.-I, Lee, M., Lu, M.-L., Liang, H.-Y., Dewey, M. E., Stewart, R., & Lee, C. T.-C. (2019). Attention-deficit/hyperactivity disorder and mortality risk in Taiwan. *JAMA Network Open, 2*(8), 1–11.10.1001/jamanetworkopen.2019.8714

Coker, T. R., Elliott, M. N., Toomey, S. L., Schwebel, D. C., Cuccaro, P., Emery, S. T., ... & Schuster, M. A. (2016). Racial and ethnic disparities in ADHD diagnosis and treatment. *Pediatrics, 138*(3), e20160407.

Cooley, E., Lei, R. F., & Ellerkamp, T. (2018). The mixed outcomes of taking ownership for implicit racial biases. *Personality and Social Psychology Bulletin, 44*(10), 1424–1434. 10.1177/0146167218769646.

Dalsgaard, S., Leckman, J. F., Nielsen, H. S., & Simonsen, M. (2014). Gender and injuries predict stimulant medication use. *Journal of Child and Adolescent Psychopharmacology, 24*(5), 253–259.

Dalsgaard, S., Østergaard, S. D., Leckman, J. F., Mortensen, P. B., & Pedersen, M. G. (2015). Mortality in children, adolescents, and adults with attention deficit hyperactivity disorder: A nationwide cohort study. *The Lancet, 385*(9983), 2190–2196.

Dehaghani, R., & Bath, C. (2021). Neurodiversity and the appropriate adult safeguard: Evidence submitted to Ministry of Justice review into neurodiversity in the criminal justice system.

Devine, P. G., Forscher, P. S., Austin, A. J., & Cox, W. T. (2012). Long-term reduction in implicit race bias: A prejudice habit-breaking intervention. *Journal of Experimental Social Psychology*, *48*(6), 1267–1278.

Dror, I. E. (2020). Cognitive and human factors in expert decision making: Six fallacies and the eight sources of bias. *Analytical Chemistry*, *92*(12), 7998–8004.

Dror, I. E., & Murrie, D. C. (2018). A hierarchy of expert performance applied to forensic psychological assessments. *Psychology, Public Policy, and Law*, *24*(1), 11.

Dyrbye, L., Herrin, J., West, C. P., Wittlin, N. M., Dovidio, J. F., Hardeman, R., ... & Van Ryn, M. (2019). Association of racial bias with burnout among resident physicians. *JAMA Network Open*, *2*(7), e197457–e197457.

Elder, T. E. (2010). The importance of relative standards in ADHD diagnoses: Evidence based on exact birth dates. *Journal of Health Economics*, *29*(5), 641–656.

Ellison, C. G., & Levin, J. S. (1998). The religion-health connection: Evidence, theory, and future directions. *Health Education & Behavior*, *25*(6), 700–720.

Emerson, M. O., & Smith, C. (2001). *Divided by faith: Evangelical religion and the problem of race in America*. USA: Oxford University Press.

Emser, T. S., Johnston, B. A., Steele, J. D., Kooij, S., Thorell, L., & Christiansen, H. (2018). Assessing ADHD symptoms in children and adults: Evaluating the role of objective measures. *Behavioral and Brain Functions*, *14*(1), 1–14.

Epstein, J., Johnson, D. E., & Conners, C. K. (2001). Conners' Adult ADHD Diagnostic Interview for DSM-IV™. (CAADID™) [Database record]. APA PsycTest. https://doi.org/10.1037/t04960-000

Fadus, M. C., Ginsburg, K. R., Sobowale, K., Halliday-Boykins, C. A., Bryant, B. E., Gray, K. M., & Squeglia, L. M. (2020). Unconscious bias and the diagnosis of disruptive behavior disorders and ADHD in African American and Hispanic youth. *Academic Psychiatry*, *44*(1), 95–102.

Faraone, S. V., Banaschewski, T., Coghill, D., Zheng, Y., Biederman, J., Bellgrove, M. A., ... & Wang, Y. (2021). The world federation of ADHD international consensus statement: 208 evidence-based conclusions about the disorder. *Neuroscience & Biobehavioral Reviews*, *128*, 789–818.

Farooq, R., Emerson, L. M., Keoghan, S., & Adamou, M. (2016). Prevalence of adult ADHD in an all-female prison unit. *ADHD Attention Deficit and Hyperactivity Disorders*, *8*(2), 113–119.

Forscher, P. S., Mitamura, C., Dix, E. L., Cox, W. T., & Devine, P. G. (2017). Breaking the prejudice habit: Mechanisms, timecourse, and longevity. *Journal of Experimental Social Psychology*, *72*, 133–146.

Fitzgerald, C., & Hurst, S. (2017). Implicit bias in healthcare professionals: A systematic review. *BMC Medical Ethics*, *18*(1), 1–18.

Gerhand, S., & Saville, C. W. (2021). ADHD prevalence in the psychiatric population. *International Journal of Psychiatry in Clinical Practice*, 1–13.

Ginsberg, Y., Quintero, J., Anand, E., Casillas, M., & Upadhyaya, H. P. (2014). Underdiagnosis of attention-deficit/hyperactivity disorder in adult patients: A review of the literature. *The Primary Care Companion for CNS Disorders*, *16*(3), 23591.

Goodman, R., Ford, T., Richards, H., Gatward, R. & Meltzer, H. (2000) The Development and Well-Being Assessment: Description and initial validation of an integrated assessment of child and adolescent psychopathology. *Journal of Child Psychology and Psychiatry*, *41*, 645–655.

Gopalkrishnan, N. (2018). Cultural diversity and mental health: Considerations for policy and practice. *Frontiers in Public Health*, *6*, 179.

Gupta, V. B., Mehrotra, P., & Mehrotra, N. (2012). Parental stress in raising a child with disabilities in India. *Disability, CBR & Inclusive Development*, *23*(2), 41–52.

Halldner, L., Tillander, A., Lundholm, C., Boman, M., Långström, N., Larsson, H., & Lichtenstein, P. (2014). Relative immaturity and ADHD: Findings from nationwide registers, parent-and self-reports. *Journal of Child Psychology and Psychiatry*, *55*(8), 897–904.

Hamed, A. M., Kauer, A. J., & Stevens, H. E. (2015). Why the diagnosis of attention deficit hyperactivity disorder matters. *Frontiers in Psychiatry*, *6*, 168.

Hechanova R., & Waelde L. (2017). The influence of culture on disaster mental health and psychosocial support interventions in Southeast Asia. *Mental Health Religion Cult*, *20*, 31–44. doi: 10.1080/13674676.2017.1322048.

Hernandez, M., Nesman, T., Mowery, D., Acevedo-Polakovich, I. D., & Callejas, L. M. (2009). Cultural competence: A literature review and conceptual model for mental health services. *Psychiatric Services*, *60*(8), 1046–1050.

Hollingdale, J., Woodhouse, E., Asherson, P., Gudjonsson, G. H., & Young, S. (2014). A pilot study examining ADHD and Behavioural disturbance in female mentally disordered offenders. *AIMS Public Health*, *1*(2), 100.

Humphreys, K. L., Eng, T., & Lee, S. S. (2013). Stimulant medication and substance use outcomes: A meta-analysis. *JAMA Psychiatry*, *70*(7), 740–749.

Huss, M., Hölling, H., Kurth, B. M., & Schlack, R. (2008). How often are German children and adolescents diagnosed with ADHD? Prevalence based on the judgment of health care professionals: Results of the German health and examination survey (KiGGS). *European Child & Adolescent Psychiatry*, *17*(1), 52–58.

Kahneman, D., Sibony, O., Fusaro, R., & Sperling-Magro, J. (2021). Sounding the alarm on system noise. *The McKinsey Quarterly*, 18, 1–8.

Kamaruddin, K., Mamat, N., & Razalli, A. R. (2017). Parents' choices of preschool for their children: Issues and challenges. *International Journal of Contemporary Applied Researches*, *4*(8), 62–72.

Katzman, M. A., Bilkey, T. S., Chokka, P. R., Fallu, A., & Klassen, L. J. (2017). Adult ADHD and comorbid disorders: Clinical implications of a dimensional approach. *BMC Psychiatry*, *17*(1), 1–15.

Kazda, L., Bell, K., Thomas, R., McGeechan, K., Sims, R., & Barratt, A. (2021). Overdiagnosis of attention-deficit/hyperactivity disorder in children and adolescents: A systematic scoping review. *JAMA Network Open*, *4*(4), e215335–e215335.

Kooij, S. J., Bejerot, S., Blackwell, A., Caci, H., Casas-Brugué, M., Carpentier, P. J., … & Asherson, P. (2010). European consensus statement on diagnosis and treatment of adult ADHD: The European Network Adult ADHD. *BMC Psychiatry*, *10*(1), 1–24.

Kooij, J. S., Huss, M., Asherson, P., Akehurst, R., Beusterien, K., French, A., … & Hodgkins, P. (2012). Distinguishing comorbidity and successful management of adult ADHD. *Journal of Attention Disorders*, *16*(5_suppl), 3S–19S.

Korb, L., Perera, B., & Courtenay, K. (2019). Challenging behaviour or untreated ADHD?. *Advances in Mental Health and Intellectual Disabilities*, *13*(3/4), 152–157.

Lambez, B., Harwood-Gross, A., Golumbic, E. Z., & Rassovsky, Y. (2020). Non-pharmacological interventions for cognitive difficulties in ADHD: A systematic review and meta-analysis. *Journal of Psychiatric Research*, *120*, 40–55.

La Malfa, G., Lassi, S., Bertelli, M., Pallanti, S., & Albertini, G. (2008). Detecting attention-deficit/hyperactivity disorder (ADHD) in adults with intellectual disability: The use of Conners' Adult ADHD Rating Scales (CAARS). *Research in Developmental Disabilities, 29*(2), 158–164.

Larsson, H., Chang, Z., D'Onofrio, B. M., & Lichtenstein, P. (2014). The heritability of clinically diagnosed attention deficit hyperactivity disorder across the lifespan. *Psychological Medicine, 44*(10), 2223–2229.

Lawton, K. E., Gerdes, A. C., Haack, L. M., & Schneider, B. (2014). Acculturation, cultural values, and Latino parental beliefs about the etiology of ADHD. *Administration and Policy in Mental Health and Mental Health Services Research, 41*(2), 189–204.

Leucht, S., Hierl, S., Kissling, W., Dold, M., & Davis, J. M. (2012). Putting the efficacy of psychiatric and general medicine medication into perspective: review of meta-analyses. *British Journal of Psychiatry*, 200, 97–106. 10.1192/bjp.bp.111.096594.

Leucht, S., Helfer, B., Gartlehner, G., & Davis, J. M. (2015). How effective are common medications: A perspective based on meta-analyses of major drugs. *BMC Medicine, 13*(1), 1–5.

Li, K. (2013). Religion and medicalization: The case of ADHD. *Journal for the Scientific Study of Religion, 52*(2), 309–327.

Lichtenstein, P., Halldner, L., Zetterqvist, J., Sjölander, A., Serlachius, E., Fazel, S., ... & Larsson, H. (2012). Medication for attention deficit–hyperactivity disorder and criminality. *New England Journal of Medicine, 367*(21), 2006–2014.

Lindsay, W. R., Carson, D., Holland, A. J., Taylor, J. L., O'Brien, G., & Wheeler, J. R. (2013). The impact of known criminogenic factors on offenders with intellectual disability: Previous findings and new results on ADHD. *Journal of Applied Research in Intellectual Disabilities, 26*(1), 71–80.

McCarthy, J., Kooij, J. J. S., Francken, M. H., Bron, T. I., & Perera, B. D. (2017). Diagnostic interview for ADHD in adults with intellectual disability (DIVA-5-ID). *Journal of Mental Health Research in Intellectual Disabilities, 10*, 64–65.

Michielsen, M., Comijs, H. C., Aartsen, M. J., Semeijn, E. J., Beekman, A. T., Deeg, D. J., & Kooij, J. S. (2015). The relationships between ADHD and social functioning and participation in older adults in a population-based study. *Journal of Attention Disorders, 19*(5), 368–379.

Mohr-Jensen, C., & Steinhausen, H. C. (2016). A meta-analysis and systematic review of the risks associated with childhood attention-deficit hyperactivity disorder on long-term outcome of arrests, convictions, and incarcerations. *Clinical Psychology Review, 48*, 32–42.

Mowlem, F. D., Rosenqvist, M. A., Martin, J., Lichtenstein, P., Asherson, P., & Larsson, H. (2019). Sex differences in predicting ADHD clinical diagnosis and pharmacological treatment. *European Child & Adolescent Psychiatry, 28*(4), 481–489.

Nadeau, K., & Quinn, P. (2002). *Understanding women with AD/HD*. Silver Spring, MD: Advantage Books.

Nazar, B. P., de Sousa Pinna, C. M., Suwwan, R., Duchesne, M., Freitas, S. R., Sergeant, J., & Mattos, P. (2016). ADHD rate in obese women with binge eating and bulimic behaviors from a weight-loss clinic. *Journal of Attention Disorders, 20*(7), 610–616.

Nimmo-Smith, V., Merwood, A., Hank, D., Brandling, J., Greenwood, R., Skinner, L., ... & Rai, D. (2020). Non-pharmacological interventions for adult ADHD: A systematic review. *Psychological Medicine, 50*(4), 529–541.

Ouyang, L., Fang, X., Mercy, J., Perou, R., & Grosse, S. D. (2008). Attention-deficit/ hyperactivity disorder symptoms and child maltreatment: A population-based study. *The Journal of Pediatrics*, *153*(6), 851–856.

Perera, B., Korb, L., Courtenay, K., & Shankar, R. (2021). Attention deficit hyperactivity disorder (ADHD) in adults with intellectual disability, *Royal College of Psychiatry Report*, 1–46.

Pontifex, M. B., Saliba, B. J., Raine, L. B., Picchietti, D. L., & Hillman, C. H. (2013). Exercise improves behavioral, neurocognitive, and scholastic performance in children with attention-deficit/hyperactivity disorder. *The Journal of Pediatrics*, *162*(3), 543–551.

Quinn, P. O., & Madhoo, M. (2014). A review of attention-deficit/hyperactivity disorder in women and girls: Uncovering this hidden diagnosis. *The Primary Care Companion for CNS Disorders*, *16*(3), 27250.

Ramsay, J. R. (2010). CBT for adult ADHD: Adaptations and hypothesized mechanisms of change. *Journal of Cognitive Psychotherapy*, 24(1), 37–45. 10.1891/0889-8391.24.1.37

Ruiz-Goikoetxea, M., Cortese, S., Aznarez-Sanado, M., Magallón, S., Zallo, N. A., Luis, E. O., … &Arrondo, G. (2018). Risk of unintentional injuries in children and adolescents with ADHD and the impact of ADHD medications: A systematic review and meta-analysis. *Neuroscience & Biobehavioral Reviews*, *84*, 63–71.

Sahuric, A., Hohwü, L., Bang Madsen, K., Christensen, A. F., Snefstrup, M. V., Obel, C., & Plana-Ripoll, O. (2019). Differential parent and teacher reports of ADHD symptoms according to the child's country of origin: a quantitative study from Denmark exploring the implication for diagnosis. *Journal of Attention Disorders*, 1087054719895309.

Schmengler, H., Cohen, D., Tordjman, S., & Melchior, M. (2021). Autism Spectrum and Other Neurodevelopmental Disorders in Children of Immigrants: A Brief Review of Current Evidence and Implications for Clinical Practice. *Frontiers in Psychiatry*, *12*, 328.

Sciutto, M. J., Nolfi, C. J., & Bluhm, C. (2004). Effects of child gender and symptom type on referrals for ADHD by elementary school teachers. *Journal of Emotional and Behavioral Disorders*, *12*(4), 247–253.

Sibley, M. H., Swanson, J. M., Arnold, L. E., Hechtman, L. T., Owens, E. B., Stehli, A., … & Stern, K. (2017). Defining ADHD symptom persistence in adulthood: optimizing sensitivity and specificity. *Journal of Child Psychology and Psychiatry*, *58*(6), 655–662.

Siegfried, C. B., & Blackshear, K. (2016). Is it ADHD or child traumatic stress? A guide for clinicians. National Child Traumatic Stress Network. Los Angeles, CA & Durham, NC: National Center for Child Traumatic Stress.

Silva, D., Colvin, L., Glauert, R., & Bower, C. (2014). Contact with the juvenile justice system in children treated with stimulant medication for attention deficit hyperactivity disorder: A population study. *The Lancet Psychiatry*, *1*(4), 278–285.

Simon, V., Czobor, P., Bálint, S., Mészáros, A., & Bitter, I. (2009). Prevalence and correlates of adult attention-deficit hyperactivity disorder: Meta-analysis. *The British Journal of Psychiatry*, *194*(3), 204–211.

Shi, Y., Guevara, L. R. H., Dykhoff, H. J., Sangaralingham, L. R., Phelan, S., Zaccariello, M. J., & Warner, D. O. (2021). Racial Disparities in Diagnosis of Attention-Deficit/Hyperactivity Disorder in a US National Birth Cohort. *JAMA Network Open*, *4*(3), e210321–e210321.

Slobodin, O., & Masalha, R. (2020). Challenges in ADHD care for ethnic minority children: A review of the current literature. *Transcultural Psychiatry*, *57*(3), 468–483.

Vaa, T. (2014). ADHD and relative risk of accidents in road traffic: A meta-analysis. *Accident Analysis & Prevention*, *62*, 415–425.

Valk, R., & Srinivasan, V. (2011). Work–family balance of Indian women software professionals: A qualitative study. *IIMB Management Review*, *23*(1), 39–50.

Viswanath, B., & Chaturvedi, S. K. (2012). Cultural aspects of major mental disorders: A critical review from an Indian perspective. *Indian Journal of Psychological Medicine*, *34*(4), 306–312.

Vitola, E. S., Bau, C. H. D., Salum, G. A., Horta, B. L., Quevedo, L., Barros, F. C., … & Grevet, E. H. (2017). Exploring DSM-5 ADHD criteria beyond young adulthood: Phenomenology, psychometric properties and prevalence in a large three-decade birth cohort. *Psychological Medicine*, *47*(4), 744–754.

West, C. P., Dyrbye, L. N., Rabatin, J. T., Call, T. G., Davidson, J. H., Multari, A., Romanski, S. A., Hellyer, J. M. H., Sloan, J. A., & Shanafelt, T. D. (2014). Intervention to promote physician well-being, job satisfaction, and professionalism. *JAMA Internal Medicine*, *174*(4), 527–533. 10.1001/jamainternmed.2013.14387.

Waite, R., Vlam, R. C., Irrera-Newcomb, M., & Babcock, T. (2013). The diagnosis less traveled: NPs' role in recognizing adult ADHD. *Journal of the American Association of Nurse Practitioners*, *25*(6), 302–308.

Young, S., Adamo, N., Ásgeirsdóttir, B. B., Branney, P., Beckett, M., Colley, W., … & Woodhouse, E. (2020). Females with ADHD: An expert consensus statement taking a lifespan approach providing guidance for the identification and treatment of attention-deficit/hyperactivity disorder in girls and women. *BMC Psychiatry*, *20*(1), 1–27.

Young, S., Gudjonsson, G., Chitsabesan, P., Colley, B., Farrag, E., Forrester, A., … & Asherson, P. (2018). Identification and treatment of offenders with attention-deficit/hyperactivity disorder in the prison population: a practical approach based upon expert consensus. *Bmc Psychiatry*, *18*(1), 1–16.

Young, S., Moss, D., Sedgwick, O., Fridman, M., & Hodgkins, P. (2015). A meta-analysis of the prevalence of attention deficit hyperactivity disorder in incarcerated populations. *Psychological Medicine*, *45*(2), 247–258.

Young, S., Wells, J., & Gudjonsson, G. H. (2011). Predictors of offending among prisoners: The role of attention-deficit hyperactivity disorder and substance use. *Journal of Psychopharmacology*, *25*(11), 1524–1532.

Youngstrom, E. A., Arnold, L. E., & Frazier, T. W. (2010). Bipolar and ADHD comorbidity: Both artifact and outgrowth of shared mechanisms. *Clinical Psychology: Science and Practice*, *17*(4), 350.

22 Deaf People in Forensic Contexts

Mats Dernevik, Brendan Monteiro, Lorraine Hough, and Elizabeth Kimber

There are significant challenges associated with the assessment and treatment of profoundly deaf, British Sign Language (BSL) users with mental health problems. The challenges also apply and overlap for deaf people involved with the criminal justice system, (CJS). These problems can be associated with the mode of communication involving linguistic difficulties, i.e., BSL. Unfortunately, the availability of interpreters, in particular "Deaf relay interpreters" is still a problem in settings where deaf people come into contact with legal agencies and the CJS. There is often a lack of understanding of deafness and communication, particularly the effects of language deprivation in the CJS and forensic mental health services.

Furthermore, the availability of specialised expertise can be limited, and this chapter provides examples of the implications of this for deaf people. Deaf mental health is not a recognised specialism, and the pool of clinicians who specialise in deaf forensic mental health is limited in the UK and internationally. There is also a shortage of valid assessment and treatment methods, available also for clinicians with experience of deaf mental health, are compete in sign language and have "deaf awareness". The evidence-base for assessments and associated outcome data for deaf cohorts are limited. Epidemiological research is often hampered by limited demographic data, with very limited registration of level and type of hearing loss, making comparisons between deaf and hearing samples complicated. National information regarding the numbers of deaf patients admitted to adult, forensic or specialised mental health services is not available and consequently, there is a sparsity of reliable studies, describing residents in specialised, in-patient, and community services.

The aim of this chapter is to provide an overview and discuss if and how clinical and forensic assessment and treatment might differ for deaf people and biases that need to be considered while doing so. With this aim in mind, it is also important to consider the history of deaf people in the criminal justice system (CJS), models for understanding deafness and Deaf culture as well as deaf mental health and services. We will also discuss the fundamental issues of visual communication, information processing, and language deprivation for a wider understanding of issues and biases of assessing deaf individuals.

DOI: 10.4324/9781003230977-25

History of Deafness and the CJS

The concepts "deaf and dumb" or "deaf-mute" are both outdated and pejorative terms, but they have historically caused deaf people to experience major problems in contact with the law. Deaf people who could not "speak" could not enter a plea and were often denied access to justice. The Courts considered the lack of verbal statements and responses to charges as *"mute by malice"*, or *"mute by visitation of God"*. Having determined this to be the latter, the deaf person was invariably remanded into custody, until such time as he/she could speak and enter a plea, which rarely happened (Jackson, 1997). In the 15th Century, the English legal scholar, Sir Mathew Hale, stated,

> *A man who is surdus et mutus a nativiate (Deaf-mute from birth), is in the presumption of the law an idiot … But if it appears that he hath the use of understanding, by signs he may be tried and suffer judgement and execution, though great caution is to be used therein.* (Ibid).

More recently, the "deaf and dumb" bias appears to have persisted in the USA: *"A person who was born deaf and dumb, was considered to be an idiot"* (Myers, 1967). Deaf people who came into contact with the law, were regarded as mentally ill, or defective, because they could not speak, even though many could go about their daily lives using communication through sign language (Jackson, 1998). The case of R v Pritchard (1836) concerned a deaf man, Mr Pritchard, who was accused of bestiality. Criteria for determining if the defendant was fit to plead were set by Judge Alderson The "Pritchard criteria" have since been reframed and expanded in subsequent cases but still apply to all accused individuals, deaf and hearing (Young et al., 2001).

Mr Justice Delvin, put it succinctly in the case of R V Roberts in 1953;

> *If I find the accused unfit to plead, I have to make an order under the statute, as a result of which he would be determined as a criminal lunatic, and it would preclude any inquiry by the jury as to his guilt or not.* (Brown, 2019).

It was not until the Criminal Prosecutions Act in (1996) that process changed. The case of Glen Pearson, another deaf man, caused the position to be altered following a finding of Unfitness to Plead, and a trial of the facts was held with discretion for sentencing (White, 1992). The Courts now accept a plea expressed in sign language if qualified interpreters are used and the Pritchard criteria are met.

Specialised Forensic Services

In terms of provision, services specialising in deaf mental health are scattered throughout the UK and forensic services can be counted on the fingers of one hand. There is no national strategy or oversight of the provision although NHS

England is responsible for commissioning available beds, regardless of region in England (Young et al., 2001). There is an over representation of deaf patients in secure services, particularly in high secure services. The reasons for this are not well understood, it is possible that Deaf offenders get detained more often than their hearing counterparts because of insufficient acquirement of social understanding, but it may also be an artefact of biases in the CJS (Mitchell & Braham, 2011).

The concept of "Deaf mental health" has been suggested by researchers and clinicians as being different from "mental health services for deaf people" (Glickman & Hall, 2018). The distinction is more than semantic and indicates different approaches and qualities of services. While the latter indicates an approach where mainstream mental health assessment and treatment is made available to deaf individuals, deaf mental health indicates "a clinical speciality requiring the mastery of the complex interplay of cultural and disability considerations" (IBID, p.5). Services that provide for "Deaf mental health", usually embrace or consider a social or cultural model of deafness.

Models for Understanding Deafness

There are different viewpoints about how to understand "deafness". Disability models are widely used for all kinds of sensory and mobility loss. A deaf person is defined by their (in)ability to hear, and consequent inability to access aspects of the world around them. The concept of disability is widely used, ranging from parking permits to Disability Living Allowance (DLA). Health services define disability based on a medical model, aiming at correcting and compensating for the loss of ability, in diagnostic terms named as impairments, that affect a person's ability to function in society. The medical model also applies to forensic contexts and services, including mental health and secure services and the CJS, who are likely to understand the individual's problems and offending behaviour, in the context of a disability model; the inability to hear interferes with a person's ability to respond to environmental cues, to communicate effectively or join in mainstream life and culture. People who experience hearing loss after acquiring some degree of spoken language as well as those who are hard-of-hearing. often identify with this model, whereby the disability should be cured, or rehabilitated by all means possible.

In contrast to disability or medical models, many profoundly, pre-lingually deaf people prefer a socio-cultural model to understand deafness; some people prefer to use an established convention to spell Deaf with a capital **D** to emphasise that being Deaf can be understood as being part of a cultural and linguistic minority, parallel to other ethnic or diverse minorities, (for example, Davidson, 2008). This perspective places emphasis on the history, narratives, and culture of Deaf people, who view their condition as a linguistic and cultural hallmark, rather than a disability or impairment. Advocates of Deaf culture, distinguish cultural Deafness from deafness as a pathology. The inability to hear is not seen as a "loss" or having negative impacts on an individual's quality of life; instead, it should be regarded as assets in skills, knowledge, and fluency in sign language. The experience and perception of some Deaf people of being a linguistic minority, is comparable to other linguistic and ethnic minorities, where native languages are important for group and individual identification and for the preservation of a culture. In the past, day and residential schools for Deaf children have been important for the sharing of Deaf culture and sign language. These special schools are unfortunately decreasing in numbers, because of policies of educational integration but also weakening the cultural and identity aspects of being Deaf. The only Deaf university in the world, Gallaudet University in Washington DC has been central for the development of socio-cultural models.

In this text, the authors have chosen to use deaf rather than Deaf, and only use the capital letter when referring to cultural models and avoiding the cumbersome use of D/d that other authors prefer.

In the context of models for deafness, cochlear implants have been a controversial issue for some prelingually deaf people since their development in the 1990s. Implants work by turning sound into electrical signals in the cochlea, and on to the auditory cortex. Although widely accepted for individuals who lost hearing after the start of verbal language development, they are perceived as "giving in" to a disability model and not always accepted by profoundly Deaf people advocating the socio-cultural model of deafness (Szarkowsky, 2019).

Visual Communication

British Sign Language (BSL), used in the UK, has its own grammatical structure and syntax, independent of, and not significantly related to spoken English. BSL is used by 87.000 Deaf people and in total 151.000 people in the UK. (British Deaf association, 2021). Sign languages are no more universal than spoken languages, and different countries and regions have developed independent languages, influenced by local conditions, customs, and traditions. Despite this disparity, sign language always emphasises body language, facial expressions, and gestures, featured in visual languages.

BSL cannot be translated "word for sign" in a literal sense, but in fact, there are professional Deaf translators and Shakespeare has been translated, just not "word for word/sign". In the same Sign Supported English (SSE) is a form of Manually Coded English (MCE) and also known as conceptually accurate signed English. It is a variation of sign language that follows spoken and written English language and follows structure and syntax closely, often using fingerspelling. Expert hearing communicators in BSL are referred to as "interpreters" rather than 'translators. Most BSL users understand SSE, dependent on their knowledge and understanding of verbal language.

To understand the methods of communication preferred by deaf forensic service users, we need to consider the significant differences in means of language acquisition between those with pre-lingual/profound deafness, who use a visual-manual process, signing and/or lipreading, and individuals who become deaf later in life. There are clear differences in neural activity in the left hemisphere between visual-manual language users and auditory hearing or partially hearing individuals, for language reception and expression (Kuhl et al. 2005; Williams et al., 2015). The abilities of "readiness to listen" and "readiness to speak" are thought to develop between 6 and 24 months in children, but preparedness for language possibly starts to develop even before birth (Pinker, 1994). The profoundly deaf child depends on visual triggers to develop verbal language, even if residual hearing can be reinforced by hearing aids and cochlear implants. They find the acquisition of verbal language extremely difficult, without the foundation of auditory language on which to build an inner vocabulary they are dependent on sounds that they can hear, often incompletely, augmented by visual cues.

Expressively, most, but not all, do not develop proper speech because they cannot imitate the speech of others and are unable to monitor their own voice. Historically, this is the reason why many deaf people were also, incorrectly, considered "mute" or "dumb".

Some deaf people develop skills in lipreading, sometimes called speech reading. However, it is inexact, some sounds of speech are not accompanied by movements of the mouth or lips, and the movements are, sometimes, the same for different words. Lipreading also requires face to face line of sight, is compromised in conversations with more than one person and obstructions by facial hair. The use of facial masks during the Covid pandemic has proved to be problematic for lip reading, also when augmenting BSL. In an experiment with hearing students asked to repeat information from lipreading without sound, only 12.4% of words were correctly repeated. (Altieri et al., 2011). Estimations for even the best lip readers, who have been deaf for many years, are that only 30% of spoken English can be accurately lip read.

The deaf child goes through a prolonged pre-verbal developmental stage. The progress is usually slow also when language development starts. Deaf children can receive special education, but it is recognised that the majority of deaf school leavers, in spite of special help, have difficulty with speech production and limited verbal language. (Conrad, 1979). Units for partially hearing children (PHU) in mainstream schools, where oral/aural methods are preferred for communication, with little or no use of Sign Language can lead to deprivation and poor understanding of receptive and expressive language. Deaf children and adults invariably experience difficulties communicating with hearing people when reliance is placed on the written word and misunderstandings and confusion in the communication process often occurs.

Ninety per cent of deaf children are born to hearing parents (Mitchell & Karchmer, 2004). Most parents have little or no experience of deafness or knowledge of how to communicate with a deaf child. Consequently, deaf children may struggle to gain full access to the norms and shared experience of their family, and wider culture. Hearing parents are often given advice that causes them to view deafness as a disability, while correct in medical and physiological terms, it does the deaf child a great disservice, denying them proper access to tools for the development of language, which in turn can lead to stunted psychological, socio-moral development, and poor understanding of concepts, for example within the legal sphere.

Deaf children of Deaf parents typically acquire sign language as their mother tongue, and they develop a strong deaf identity. They form an integral part of the deaf community from an early age and do not express many of the difficulties encountered by deaf children of hearing parents who feel abandoned and lost when developing an identity.

Language Deprivation

Language deprivation is a dominant problem for many deaf people in forensic contexts, in parallel to the problems with the mode of communication or mental disorder. Early language deprivation can affect many pre-lingually deaf children, who are only exposed to oral/aural language during their formative years and are unlikely to have early access to visual-manual language. This type of language deprivation has several definitions and can even be considered a distinct diagnostic category: Language Deprivation Syndrome, LDS (Gulati, 2018). It is relevant to understand how LDS affects adults in clinical and forensic assessments as it is linked to deficiencies in "emotional, social and behavioural adjustment" (Glickman and Hall, 2018). A high percentage of people with prelingual and profound deafness will be deficient in spoken, written, and even signed languages and learn vocabulary at about half the rate of hearing children. As a result, their vocabulary in adulthood is roughly half that of people with normal hearing. (Paul, 1998).

LDS has its roots in the Deaf child growing up in a non-communicating environment and missing out on the "window of development" for language, particularly of higher-order and abstract constructs. In addition, there is a problem with the "fund of information", i.e., information that a person has stored about the world. Excluding auditory information in childhood, means missing out on incidental learning from overheard conversations (in the family, between peers, on the bus, etc.) and from media sources.

Apart from the problems with vocabulary, a poor fund of information and fluency in expressive language, there can also be emotional and behavioural problems associated with LDS. A communicating environment is essential for the development of attachment and well-being of the child (Kral & O'Donoghue, 2010). Attachment theory centres on emotional availability and parental sensitivity and have been associated with various problems in adult life (Bowlby, 1969), particularly in relationships (Simpson & Rholes, 1998) and dissocial behaviour and personality (Frodi et al., 2001). The relation between emotional availability and language development is more significant for Deaf children and their parents than for children with normal hearing. Stress levels in families, with Deaf children are affected by language delay and additional disabilities are higher and associated with socioemotional development (Gulati, 2018).

Poor language development contributes to behavioural problems and psychosocial difficulties in moderately to profoundly deaf children. Stevenson and colleagues (2010) found that the rate of psychosocial difficulties was equal for deaf children with high sign language ability compared to hearing children, suggesting that it is actually language deprivation, rather than deafness, that can be associated with psychosocial difficulties in adulthood.

The presentation of LDS may vary in clinical settings but is essential to clinical formulation for the individual's assessments and treatment plans. It is not an intellectual disability, although it can be considered as incomplete neurological/ cognitive development and correlates with IQ scores (see later in the chapter). It is not dissocial personality disorder, although social and behavioural problems can overlap. Although the concept of LDS is quite new, it has been phenomenologically described for 50 years, as specific to some deaf adults in contact with forensic and psychiatric services. Terje Basilier (Basilier, 1964) suggested the term "Surdophrenia" for *"the psychic consequences of congenital or early acquired deafness"*, i.e., for deaf people who came in contact with a psychiatrist. Basilier and others that observed the phenomenon did not suggest any aetiology of the problems they noted. A more recent literature study found some evidence for LDS as a neurodevelopmental disorder with sociocultural origins, although the area is not widely researched (Hall et al., 2017). Surdophrenia is an outdated and unfortunate term as it can be conflated with mental health conditions such as schizophrenia, which is incorrect.

There is no agreed measure or scale for LDS; Sanjay Gulati (2019) pointed out some central characteristics of LDS:

- Lack of fluency and linguistic deficits in expressive sign language or superficial use of signs. In a specialised psychiatric unit, 75% of a sample of deaf inpatients were not fluent communicators in either sign or spoken language (Black & Glickman, 2006).
- Problems with the concept of time, leading to problems with chronology and sequencing, also with own narratives, struggles to give an accurate life story, despite average cognitive abilities.
- Struggles with cause-and-effect, often related to problems with time, one thing happening before another, is usually seen as the "why" question. Problems with cause and effect are very significant for psychological treatments like CBT.
- Lack of awareness of the need for context when communicating with others. This is related to Theory of Mind, i.e., not appreciating reciprocity of communication.
- Problems with abstract concepts. This is a prevailing problem for clinicians who use abstract concepts in the line of treatment. Many basic concepts that we take for granted are actually quite abstract, e.g., diagnosis, insight, consent, risk and risk factors, etc.
- Difficulty learning new skills, Most language deprived Deaf people do not have a learning disability, using a diagnostic meaning, but they struggle to assimilate information, even in BSL.
- Problems with emotional regulation. Emotional regulation requires a person to be able to "step back" from feelings and distress, place it in context and name the feeling. Many people with LDS struggle to reflect and have limited

emotional vocabulary, beyond basic affect. They tend to act out feelings, rather than contain and use internal processes to regulate them.

•   Limited "fund of information" – but they may not be aware of this referring to a lack of information from missing out on incidental learning for basic knowledge of physical and mental health, norms for sexual behaviour, and deficits in learning and assimilating knowledge.

Deafness and Mental Health

Some causes of deafness are associated with other disabilities and mental health conditions and issues. Among these are genetic or syndromic conditions (Waardenburg and Ushers syndromes) and perinatal factors and infections (i.e., Rubella), (Nance, 2003). Deafness and comorbid disabilities can be acquired through post-natal infections (i.e., Meningitis). The causes of deafness, with or without association to other conditions, have been estimated to 39% for hereditary causes, 30% for post-natal or acquired causes, 24% with unknown causes and 7% with miscellaneous causes (Korver et al., 2011). The prevalence and rates of hearing impairment started declining in the 1990s.

Research about Deaf mental health, in particular, the comparability of population and demographic studies of deafness are hampered by different definitions of deafness. Diagnostically, classifications are rated solely on audiology levels of hearing loss, and ranges from mild to profound, the mild and moderate levels, sometimes referred to as hard-of-hearing. Other classifications refer to the developmental stage at which the hearing loss occurred, most importantly pre- or post-lingually, i.e., before or after the child's start of acquisition of language (CDC, 2019). However, as language acquisition is a process in childhood and into adulthood, making dichotomous classification such as "pre" and "post" an over-simplification and in poor correspondence to research on linguistics and cognitive and language development (Chomsky, 1987; Pinker, 1994).

Despite the problems with definitions and research focus, many studies have suggested that deafness is associated with increased rates of mental health difficulties. Data for children suggest a significant link between hearing impairment and neuro-developmental problems. A survey by the Gallaudet research institute (2008), found 27% of deaf children between 6 and 19 years, had additional disabilities, compared to rates in the general population, intellectual disabilities 9%, developmental delay 5%, specific learning difficulties 8%, and autism 2%. Despite the high prevalence of mental health problems, the degree of hearing loss does not appear to correlate with mental health (Stevenson et al., 2010).

Another US study found neurodevelopmental problems in 30% and intellectual disabilities in 26% of children with hearing impairments. (Van Naarden et al., 1999). A Danish study found the prevalence of psychosocial difficulties ratio 3:1 compared with hearing children. (Dammeyer, 2010).

Although no reports exist of incidence rates of specific mental illnesses in the adult Deaf population, a literature review (Fellinger et al., 2012), reviewing samples based on epidemiological methods and published work, suggested that deaf people do not have a specific psychopathology or mental health profile, but mental health problems were mostly the same as in hearing populations.

Deafness and the Law

There are few studies on the prevalence or characteristics of deaf offenders. Studies are hampered by methodological challenges; no registers exist that can enable the identification of deaf people in contact with the CJS. Deaf people are a small proportion of the people who come into contact with the CJS and there are problems with generalisability, baselines, and attrition with studies that investigate deaf offenders who pass through sections of the CJS, with or without mental disorders.

There are several challenges for deaf people who come into contact with complex legal systems. The challenges occur from the first arrest to the later understanding of roles and procedures in the justice process. Of particular interest is assessment of competency or "fitness to plead", where researchers have found a disproportionate lack of competence in deaf people, explained by deprivation or linguistic issues and lack of awareness of the CJS. (Young et al., 2001). BSL users are typically disadvantaged at the point of arrest. The Police and the "right to silence" in the UK (Police and Criminal Evidence, Act 1984, PACE) and the equivalent "Miranda Warning" in the USA, allows for all suspects to be informed that they have the right to remain silent and that anything they say can be given as evidence (Ventress et al., 2008). BSL Interpreters are essential at this stage, as, if the Deaf person does not understand this warning, any information subsequently obtained by the police, cannot be used as evidence. In preparation of psychiatric reports to the Criminal Courts, one of the authors, (BTM), found that deaf defendants, who did not have access to BSL Interpreters at the arrest, invariably informed him that the police *"said something"* but did not understand what had been said. The "Pritchard" criteria for fitness to plead are central to the court process, they include the ability/capacity to understand the charge, to enter a plea (guilty/not guilty), ability to instruct a solicitor, to follow evidence, and challenge a juror. The previous Criminal Procedure Justice Act from 1965, stated that a person found Unfit to Plead had to be admitted to a psychiatric hospital and Deaf people were often deprived of their liberty, unrelated to any mental disorder.

The act was changed in 1991 because of a case involving another deaf man, Glenn Pearson, who had been found Unfit to Plead, for a minor theft and was admitted to Rampton High Security Hospital (Phennell, 1992).

Young et al. (2001) studied forensic referrals to three specialist psychiatric services for deaf people in the U.K. In 46% of all cases, an opinion on Fitness to Plead was requested by a court. Of those cases, 63.7% were found Fit and 34.1% were found Unfit to Plead. The high percentage of deaf patients for whom an opinion on Fitness to Plead was sought, shows the courts considered deaf people's rights; the third that was Unfit, probably reflects the last Pritchard criteria; Unable to follow court procedures.

Psychological and Mental Health Assessments

There are several types of assessments required in forensic contexts for Deaf people:

- Communication
- Ability and Aptitude
- Knowledge and skills specific to Court
- Mental Health, including personality and personality disorders.
- Risk to others and self

There are some general considerations that apply to all types of assessments with Deaf people. The cultural implication and diversity issues are imperative in all types of assessments. The suitability of the tools used, need to be considered for potential language biases. Many tools, rating scales/self-report measures, and interviews are reliant on the understanding and expression of spoken language. The assessor also needs to consider issues of pre-or post-lingual deafness and preferred/first language of the client. Aspects of developmental progress of Deaf children, particularly language deprivation impacts on confidence, mental health, emotional well-being, and communication as well as on language competence.

There are few psychometric materials available specifically for pre-lingually profoundly deaf individuals. Likewise, any changes to the standardisation of any assessment, will affect reliability and validity. Consideration of the norm group (sample population) to whom individuals are being compared, as well as consideration generally of the meaning of outcomes and results are important.

Assessments of Communication

It is vital to assess the Deaf client's use of receptive and expressive language and level of communication before doing clinical formulations and adapt other assessments as well as treatment plans. Of particular interest is the level of LDS and how it influences understanding and fluency. There is no agreed assessment for LDS, but familiarity with the cognitive and linguistic characteristics of LDS is helpful (Gulati, 2018). "Communication Sunburst" is a structured clinical tool developed for assessing Deaf communication (Williams & Gagan, 2018). It maps communication in nine domains, such as concepts and vocabulary, understanding and retaining information, expressing self, etc. It requires significant BSL skills and awareness of LD from the clinician to be accurate and relevant and is best done by pairs of assessors.

Working with BSL interpreters is always recommended but particularly important when assessing communication abilities, both for individuals who prefer BSL and SSE apart from those clinicians who have high-level BSL fluency (rarely the case in reality).

Assessments and therapy working with an interpreter is a complex 3-way relationship. Prior discussions and preparation around concepts/language choices are vital, as is allowing time for debrief after the session to help the interpreter to work through reactions of potentially traumatic material in the session as well as acknowledge any sensitive information that may be sought/discussed in the session, and confidentiality aspects. Moreover, the development of rapport between the examiner and subject is likely to be affected by the indirect communication used when relying on an interpreter. It is also important for the clinician to have some skills in BSL or at least awareness as interpreters, although linguistically skilled, interpreters may not have the level of flexibility, adaptability, depth of language, and lexical choices to deal with clients with language deprivation. We have often experienced a mismatch between a client's basic expressive language and the eloquent language of the interpreter, leading to misunderstandings and overestimation of the client's communication ability. is that sensitive information may be sought/discussed in the session and confidentiality aspects of such an arrangement need acknowledgement.

BSL differs in dialects and signs used across the UK, and requires a shared understanding of different signs, by the interpreter and subject. Some words do not have equivalent signs, so the interpreter may need to fingerspell words, introducing additional cognitive processing for the subject. BSL interpretation may require the interpreter to use additional cues or clarifications, more or less information than comparable spoken presentation.

Ability and Aptitude Assessments

There is not any one complete and published test that can accurately and safely assess cognitive abilities of profoundly Deaf individuals. Some available tools have norms for Deaf people, the Raven's Progressive Matrices for adults (Conrad, 1979), and Leiter 3 for Deaf children (Alexander et al., 2015).

The use of any test that is heavily verbally loaded becomes highly questionable, particularly for those having experienced language deprivation. Verbal items or tools, in ability/aptitude tests, mental state examinations, or personality assessments are generally considered as not appropriate for Deaf people. Ability tests of non-verbal abilities generally provide better indicators for capacity. Consequently, performance scales of intellectual ability are widely used to provide estimates of overall level of intellectual ability (Braden, 1994). It is important to stress that any estimate of overall ability based on non-verbal performance only, cannot necessarily be extrapolated to a reliable IQ score.

Guidelines on use of (psychometric) tests with Deaf individuals, including consideration of competence levels of interpreters are available (Psychological Testing Centre, British Psychological Society, 2017). BSL is not comparable to spoken language and questions, instructions and administration is qualitatively different. The assessor is reliant on the perceptiveness of the interpreter and the "translation" of BSL into spoken language.

Deviations from standard process or procedure, like conducting an interview or giving instructions in BSL, have the potential to change the demand or nature of the task, (Braden, 1994; Maller, 2003), and the client's performance. We have previously discussed lip, or speech reading, and its limitations. Lip reading also requires increased concentration levels, which may lead to cognitive fatigue for the subject.

Whilst previous versions of the WAIS (Wechsler Adult Intelligence Scale) had capacity to calculate separate Verbal Intellectual Quotient (VIQ) and Performance IQ, (PIQ), the current version, WAIS-IV, does not. It includes two non-verbal indices that can be used, Perceptual Reasoning Index and Processing Speed Index. The subtests require verbal instructions but are performance-related and potentially better estimates of ability. (Grewer & O'Rourke, 2005). Working Memory Index, (WMI) is reliant upon verbal capacity.

Some memory tests cannot be relied upon as they are language-based and reliant upon ability to "think in English", but visual memory tasks, from neuropsychological tests such as Ray's Complex Figure (Osterrieth, 1944) or the visual parts of the Repeatable Battery for the Assessment of Neuropsychological Status, RBANS (Randolph, 1998). RBANS can be used to demonstrate visual memory skills also in profoundly Deaf people.

Cromwell (2005) provided a summary of considerations when using ability/aptitude tests with Deaf clients that the authors recommend.

1   Always use support from qualified BSL interpreters, even if you have some BSL skills.
2   Discuss the questions/test in advance with the interpreters.
3   Debrief with the interpreter. complex 3-way relationship and discuss any issues about responses and understanding from the client.
4   Consider which, if any, tests to use, nature of test items, adjustments in terms of test administration, and the need for appropriate reference/norm groups.
5   Interpret results with extreme caution, especially concerning some of the issues that arise in relation to communication. Make any such concerns explicit in the report.

Knowledge and Skills Specific to Court

One assessment of particular interest to the courts are "Fitness to Plead" and the "Pritchard criteria" In the UK, one-third of Deaf people committed to hospital were found to be unfit to plead (Young et al., 2001). Courts are also interested in assessments of vulnerability of defendants and witnesses, in terms of suggestibility, acquiescence, and compliance. Deaf people can be particularly vulnerable in interview situations and from how BSL affects the interview process (O'Rourke & Beail, 2004).

Mental Health and Personality Disorder Assessments

There is some anecdotal evidence that Deaf people who come in contact with mental health services risk attracting diagnoses that other patients don't. Two of the authors recently looked after a young man who came into a Deaf service with

14 distinct historical psychiatric diagnoses and left with 2. Deaf people may present differently to other patients and require assessment by practitioners with expertise in Deaf Mental Health (Glickman, 2007). The question of "hearing voices" can be hard to answer for Deaf people. Moreover, more severe LDS, complicates assessment procedures and in reality, excludes most language-based assessments, including mental state examinations and personality tools are considered as highly questionable (Grewer & O'Rourke, 2005).

Clinical assessments that look for abstract concepts, such as insight, empathy, or self-esteem are open to misunderstandings and interpretations if the assessor is not aware of language differences between BSL and spoken English as well as the effects of LDS. Clients sometimes pick up the signs for these types of concepts, repeating them without any deeper understanding of meaning. In ward-rounds patients sometimes states they have "improved" but struggle with the meaning of this concept. Recently, two of the authors (MD +BTM) had a patient in sex offender treatment for those who had committed sexual offences. He used the term "stalking" but did not understand the concept until a visual image of hunting and actual deerstalking was introduced and the "penny dropped". Deaf people with LDS are often called "poor historians" in psychiatric reports. Most Deaf people are not "poor historians" but struggle with chronology and prefer to think in a narrative way. In particular, it is difficult to use "open" and "why" questions, making Socratic questioning hard to achieve.

There is concern linked to Personality/Personality Disorder Assessments, as they are not only dependent upon verbal capacity, but the individual items assume exposure to social situations, experiences, or opportunities which may not apply to those of Deaf individuals.

In our experience, there are three major sources of mental health misdiagnosis with Deaf people. Firstly, LDS can be mistaken for intellectual impairment if assessments are not adapted and considers effects of language deprivation. Secondly, major mental disorders can remain undetected or wrongly attributed because of communication difficulties. Thirdly, mental disorders are often over-diagnosed and identified where none exist, particularly developmental disorders. There are several difficulties for assessing psychotic experiences in Deaf patients; do Deaf people hear voices? (Glickman, 2007). Subjective experiences of hallucinations, particularly any aural experiences, differ between deaf individuals and often complicated by tinnitus. (Critchley, 1983). It can also be hard to describe aural experiences as profoundly Deaf people might live in a silent world and have no reference point for "hearing voices" (Monteiro & Chritchley, 1994). Sacks (1989) elaborated on "phantasmal voices", a phenomenon that some post-lingually deaf people experience and this should not be mistaken as a psychotic symptom but is probably visual experiences that are being automatically translated into an aural correlate and probably has a neurological basis.

Visual and tactile hallucinations are indeed overrepresented in profoundly Deaf people with a diagnosis of schizophrenia compared to hearing patients with the same diagnosis. (Schonauer et al. 1998). Visual hallucinations in sign language represent "meaningful" perceptions corresponding to auditory hallu-cinations in hearing people and reflect the "Deaf way" of sensory processing. Chritchley and colleagues found that 10 out of 12 patients in an inpatient deaf unit experienced hallucinations in sign language, "*I can see the wipers on the car signing at me*" and "*I can hear voices, but someone is signing them to me*".

Two of the authors (BTM and MD) have found that elucidating these types of symptoms often require leading questions but is still the subject of mis-interpretation and misunderstanding, particularly with patients with limited command of BSL and conceptual understanding. We have also seen a patient who attributed his negative thoughts to royals and famous footballers and hearing their critical voices, causing him distress. However, with clarifications in BSL, he recognised that the voices are in "his head" and not real. However, they were persistent and formulated as 'pseudo hallucinations.

There is also the difficulty to differentiate poverty of language, which can be associated with language deprivation syndrome, as it can be misunderstood as a negative symptom of Schizophrenia and cause "over-diagnosing".

Another problem concerns "the nodding syndrome". Some Deaf people may often "nod" in conversations with clinicians, giving the impression of under-standing, while in fact they have not. This can obviously cause misunderstand-ings of hearing clinicians, who are not "Deaf aware".

Risk Assessment

The concept of risk is quite abstract, and most people struggle with understanding the concept. When clinicians talk about "risk-factors", the concept becomes even more abstract. BSL has a sign for risk, but it also translates to "hazard" and "bad outcome". Risk is often understood as a formula of the likelihood of an event occurring (probability), the consequence of the event happening (severity) and how it can be avoided or mitigated (controllability). The weighting of these elements is a complex process and difficult for most patients (Deaf and hearing) and almost impossible for people with LDS. Previous cautions and caveats when using tests with Deaf people, apply also to collaborative risk assessments.

There is no evidence that risk factors for violence or sexual offending are different for Deaf people. However, LDS tends to increase these risks as people with LDS have limited "fund of information" and struggle with cause and effect. They may not have concepts for consent, reciprocity, victim empathy, entitle-ment, etc. that are central to risk management, and language implications impact on understanding of concepts being assessed. Two of the authors (MD and BTM) have developed a group intervention to assess and address these conceptual problems for Deaf forensic patients with varying degrees of LDS, "*I'm a patient: Get Me Out of Here*", GMOP. The authors have found the HCR-20 to work well for the translation from "Englishness" of this Structured Professional Judgement Tool, as it divides factors into historical (past/before), Clinical (now), and Risk (future), all concepts can be discussed in BSL. It also works with a visual "5P model" (in boxes) for risk formulation:

1   Problem what?
2   Historical = problem before/predisposing,
3   Clinical = problem now/perpetuating
4   Clinical = problem now/triggers/precipitating
5   Risk = future/protective/do what?

Discussion about temporal sequences such as thought-feeling behaviour is particularly useful for people who struggle with sequencing and cause effect.

Norm Group Issues

Using a normative group which includes deaf individuals wherever possible is important, or at the very least, consideration of the constitution of a norm group and its corresponding utility or not, in terms of reliability and validity. Norms for deaf people are not common and there may be value in comparison of the individual with both hearing and deaf individuals when trying to draw any conclusions from psychometrics something to consider.

Acknowledgement

The authors would like to thank Gillian Jeffery for her invaluable input and comments on this text. Gillian is a Deaf Forensic Social Worker with unique expertise on Deaf people's experiences in forensic contexts.

References

Altieri, N. A., Pisoni, D. B., & Townsend, J. T. (2011). Some normative data on lip-reading skills (L). *The Journal of the Acoustical Society of America, 130*(1), 1–4.

Alexander, M. A., Matthews, D. J., & Murphy, K. P. (Eds.). (2015). *Paediatric rehabilitation: principles and practice.* 5th edition. Demos Medical Publishing.

Basilier, T. (1964). Surdophrenia. *Acta Psychiatrica Scandinavica, 39*, 363–372. doi: 10.1111/ j.1600-0447.1964.tb04948

Black, P. A., & Glickman, N. S. (2006). Demographics, psychiatric diagnoses, and other characteristics of North American deaf and hard-of-hearing inpatients. *Journal of Deaf Studies and Deaf Education, 11*(3), 303–321.

Bowlby, J. (1969). Attachment and loss v. 3 (Vol. 1).

Braden, J. P. (1994). *Deafness, deprivation, and IQ.* Springer Science & Business Media.

British Deaf Association (2021). *Sign Language Week.* 15-21 March 2021. http:// signlanguageweek.org.uk/bsl-statistics

British Psychological Society (2017). Hearing loss, deafness and psychometric testing. https://ptc.bps.org.uk/sites/ptc.bps.org.uk/files/guidance_documents/ptc25_ hearing_loss_and_deafness

Brown, P. (2019). Unfitness to plead in England and Wales: Historical development and contemporary dilemmas. *Medicine, Science and the Law, 59*(3), 187–196.

CDC. (2019 March 21). Types of Hearing Loss [Web page]. Retrieved from https:// www.cdc.gov/ncbddd/hearingloss/types.html

Chomsky, N. (1987). *Language and problems of knowledge: The Managua lectures* (Vol. 16). MIT press.

Conrad, R. (1979). *The deaf schoolchild.* London Harper & Row.

Chritchley, E. M. R., Denmark J. C., Warren & Wilson, K. A. (1981). Hallucinatory Experiences of Prelingually Profoundly Deaf Schizophrenics. *British Journal of Psychiatry, 138,* 30–32.

Critchley, E. M. R. (1983). Auditory experiences of deaf schizophrenics. *Journal of the Royal Society of Medicine, 76*(7), 542–544.

Cromwell, J. (2005). Deafness and the art of psychometric testing. *PSYCHOLOGIST-LEICESTER-, 18*(12), 738. Deafness and the art of psychometric testing | The Psychologist (bps.org.uk)

Dammeyer, J. (2010). Psychosocial development in a Danish population of children with cochlear implants and deaf and hard-of-hearing children. *Journal of Deaf Studies and Deaf Education, 15*(1), 50–58.

Davidson, J. (2008). Autistic culture online: virtual communication and cultural expression on the spectrum. *Social & Cultural Geography, 9*(7), 791–806. https://www.tandfonline.com/doi/abs/10.1080/14649360802382586

Emmins, C. (1986). Unfitness to Plead – Thoughts prompted by Pearson, Glenn case. *Criminal Law Review,* 604–618.

Equality and Human Rights Commission. Equality Act 2010 Employment Statutory Code of Practice. HMSO, 2010.

Fellinger, J., Holzinger, D., & Pollard, R. (2012). Mental health of deaf people. *The Lancet, 379*(9820), 1037–1044.

Frodi, A., Dernevik, M., Sepa, A., Philipson, J., & Bragesjö, M. (2001). Current attachment representations of incarcerated offenders varying in degree of psychopathy. *Attachment & Human Development, 3*(3), 269–283.

Gallaudet Research Institute. (2008). *Regional and national summary report of data from the 2007–08 annual survey of deaf and hard of hearing [Children and youth].* Washington, DC: GRI, Gallaudet University.

Glickman, N. (2007). *Do you hear voices? Problems in assessment of mental status in deaf persons with severe language deprivation.* Oxford University Press.

Glickman, N. S., & Hall, W. C. (Eds.) (2018). *Language deprivation and deaf mental health.* Routledge.

Grinker, R., Vernon, M., Mindel, E., Rothstein, D., Easton, H., Koh, S., et al (1969). *Psychiatric Diagnosis, Therapy and research on the psychotic Deaf* (No. Research Grant number RD-2407-S). Washington, DC: U.S. Department of Health, Education and Welfare.

Grewer, G., & O'Rourke, S. (2005). Assessment of deaf people in forensic mental health settings: A risky business! *The Journal of Forensic Psychiatry and Psychology, 16*(4), 671–684.

Gulati, S. (2018). Language deprivation syndrome. In Glickman, N. S., & Hall, W. C. (Eds.). (2018). *Language deprivation and deaf mental health.* Routledge.

Hall, W. C., Levin, L. L., & Anderson, M. L. (2017). Language deprivation syndrome: A possible neurodevelopmental disorder with sociocultural origins. *Social Psychiatry and Psychiatric Epidemiology, 52*(6), 761–776.

Jackson, P. (1997). *Deaf crime casebook.* Ipswich: Cox & Jackson.

Korver, A. M., Admiraal, R. J., Kant, S. G., Dekker, F. W., Wever, C. C., Kunst, H. P., … & DECIBEL-collaborative study group. (2011). Causes of permanent childhood hearing impairment. *The Laryngoscope, 121*(2), 409–416.

Kral, A., & O'Donoghue, G. M. (2010). Profound deafness in childhood. *New England Journal of Medicine, 363*(15), 1438–1450.

Kuhl, P. K., Conboy, B. T., Padden, D., Nelson, T., & Pruitt, J. (2005). Early speech perception and later language development: : Implications for the "critical period". *Language Learning and Development, 1*(3–4), 237–264.

Maller, S. J. (2003). Intellectual assessment of deaf people. In M. Marschark, & P. E. Spencer (Eds.) (2010). *The Oxford handbook of deaf studies, language, and education*, vol. 2. Oxford University Press.

Mitchell, R. E., Karchmer, M. A. (2004). Chasing the mythical ten percent: Parental hearing status of deaf and hard of hearing students in the United States. *Sign Language Studies, 4*(2), 138–163.

Mitchell, T. R., & Braham, L. G. (2011). The psychological treatment needs of deaf mental health patients in high-secure settings: A review of the literature. *International Journal of Forensic Mental Health, 10*(2), 92–106.

Monteiro, B. T. M. & Chritchley, E. M. R. (1994). Deafness and communication. In E. M. R. Critchley (Ed.) *Neurological boundaries of reality*. Farrand Press London.

Myers, L. J. (1967). *The law and the deaf.* US Department of Health, Education, and Welfare, Vocational Rehabilitation Administration.

Nance, W. E. (2003). The genetics of deafness. *Mental Retardation and Developmental Disabilities Research Reviews, 9*(2), 109–119.

Napier, J., & Holmes, B. (2021). Children with deaf parents. In *An introductory guide for professionals working with deaf and hard of hearing clients in clinical, legal, educational and social care settings*. Kindle Direct Publishing.

Newman, A. J., Supalla, T., Fernandez, N., Newport, E. L., & Bavelier, D. (2015). Neural systems supporting linguistic structure, linguistic experience, and symbolic communication in sign language and gesture. *PNAS* September 15, *112*(37), 11684.

O'Rourke, S. & Beail, N. (2004). Suggestibility and related concepts: Implications for clinical and forensic practice with deaf people. In S. Austen & S. Crocher (Eds.), *Deafness in mind*. London: Whurr.

Osterrieth, P. A. (1944). Le test de copie d'une figure complexe; contribution à l'étude de la perception et de la mémoire. Test of copying a complex figure; contribution to the study of perception and memory. *Arch Psychol, 30*, 206–356.

Paul, P. V. (1998). *Literacy and deafness: The development of reading, writing, and literate thought*. Pearson College Division.

Pinker, S. 1994. *The language instinct*. London: Penguin.

Phennell, P. (1992). The criminal procedure act 1991; Insanity and fitness to plead. *Criminal Law Review*.

"Police and Criminal Evidence Act 1984 (PACE) codes of practice". *Home Office*. GOV.UK. 26 March 2013. Retrieved 09 January 2022.

Pritchard, R. V. (1836). 173 E.R. 135.

Roberts, R. V. (1953). 3 WLR 178.

Randolph, C. (1998). *Repeatable battery for the assessment of neuropsychological status (RBANS) manual*. San Antonio, TX: The Psychological Corporation.

Sacks, O. (1989). *Seeing voices*. University of California Press. Picador.

Schonauer, K., Achtergarde, D., Gotthardt, U., & Folkerts, H. W. (1998). Hallucinatory modalities in prelingually deaf schizophrenic patients: a retrospective analysis of 67 cases. *Acta Psychiatrica Scandinavica, 98*(5), 377–383.

Schonauer, K., Achtergarde, D., Gotthardt, U. & Folkerts, H. W. (2007). Hallucinatory modalities in prelingually deaf schizophrenic patients: a retrospective analysis of 67 cases. *Acta Psychiatrica Scandinavia*.

Simpson, J. A., & Rholes, W. S. E. (1998). *Attachment theory and close relationships*. The Guilford Press.

Stevenson, J., McCann, D., Watkin, P., Worsfold, S., Kennedy, C., & Hearing Outcomes Study Team. (2010). The relationship between language development and behaviour problems in children with hearing loss. *Journal of Child Psychology and Psychiatry*, 51(1), 77–83.

Szarkowsky, A. (2019). Language development in children with cochlear implants: possibilities and challenges. In N. Glickman & W. Hall (Eds.). *Language deprivation and mental health*, Routledge, N.Y.

The King v Thomas Jones (1773). English Reports Citation. 168. E.R. 153.

Van Naarden, K., Decouflé, P., & Caldwell, K. (1999). Prevalence and characteristics of children with serious hearing impairment in metropolitan Atlanta, 1991–1993. *Paediatrics, 103*(3), 570–575.

Ventress, M. A., Rix, K. J., & Kent, J. H. (2008). Keeping PACE: fitness to be interviewed by the police. *Advances in Psychiatric Treatment, 14*(5), 369–381.

White, S. (1992). The Criminal Procedure (Insanity and Unfitness To Plead) Act. *Criminal Law Review*, 4–14.

Williams, J., Darcy, I., & Newman, S. (2015). Fingerspelling and print processing similarities in deaf and hearing readers. *Journal of Language and Literature, 6*(1), 56–65.

Williams, K. & Gagan, L. (2018). *Communication Sunburst*. John Denmark Unit, Greater Manchester NHS Foundation Trust.

Young, A., Howarth, P., Ridgeway, S., & Monteiro, B. (2001). Forensic referrals to the three specialist psychiatric units for deaf people in the UK. *Journal of Forensic Psychiatry, 12*(1), 19–35.

23 Criminally Diverse Offending

Phil Willmot

Introduction

There is a paradox at the heart of psychological approaches to the treatment of offending behaviour. On the one hand, the majority of people with multiple convictions for criminal offences, do not "specialise" in a single type of offence but offend in a variety of different ways. On the other hand, among those who commit the most serious offences the picture is more complex; while some individuals appear to specialise in a particular type of offence many do not, and their offending appears much more diverse and indiscriminate. However, treatment programmes for those who commit the most serious offences have tended not to recognise this diversity and focus instead on a single category of offending such as sexual offending, domestic violence or fire setting. This mismatch between the treatment needs of those who commit the most serious offences and the forensic treatments available to them creates a problem not only for these individuals but for those who are responsible for their care and management.

Criminal Versatility and Specialisation

A number of influential theories of crime such as Self-Control Theory (Gottfredson & Hirschi, 1990), and General Strain Theory (Agnew, 1992) present criminal behaviour as largely chaotic and opportunistic, and this view is supported by studies which show the majority of people who offend to be defined as criminally versatile, that is, to engage in a variety of different offences (Wiesner et al., 2018). However, a number of studies suggest that most people become less diverse in their range of offending as they get older (Nieuwbeerta et al., 2011), while DeLisi et al. (2019) found that once someone has committed a certain type of serious offence, they are more likely to do the same again.

Studies of people who have offended in specific ways show some groups to be highly specialised. These groups include those convicted of offences involving indecent images of children (Howard et al., 2013), sexual offences against children (Lussier et al., 2005), and subgroups of those convicted of fire setting (Lindberg et al., 2005) and domestic violence (Holtzworth-Munroe et al., 2000).

DOI: 10.4324/9781003230977-26

Versatility and Specialisation in Particular Offence Types

Sexual Offending

Men convicted of sexual offences have been the most studied group in relation to the question of offending specialisation. Harris, Smallbone et al. (2009) studied the offending histories of 572 adult males referred for civil commitment in the US for sexual offences. They compared a number of different definitions of offence specialisation based on the percentage of an individual's total previous arrests, charges, or sentencing occasions that involved a particular offence type. Harris, Smallbone et al. classed rape of an adult, child sexual abuse, and incest as separate offence types and compared the effects of setting the specialisation threshold at 50, 75, or 100%. With the specialisation threshold set at 50% (i.e., 50% of the individual's previous offences were for the same type of offence), 5% of those convicted of rape and 23% of those convicted of child sexual abuse were classified as specialists. When the specialisation threshold was set at 75%, 3% of those convicted of rape and 11% of those convicted of child sexual abuse were classified as specialists. With the specialisation threshold set at 100%, 1% of those convicted of rape and 5% of those convicted of child sexual abuse were classified as specialists.

Howard et al. (2013) investigated the degree of specialisation among a sample of 14,804 men convicted of sexual offences in England and Wales. Sexual offences were categorised into contact offences involving children, contact offences involving adults, offences involving indecent images, and paraphilias. Among individuals with a history of indecent images offending, 31% had convictions for non-sexual offences, compared to 81% of those with no history of indecent images offending. This group therefore appeared to be much more specialist than the others. Specialisation within sexual offending was observed for all four groups, but particularly for those convicted of paraphilic offences and those involving indecent images, whose offending behaviour is likely to be driven predominantly by their sexual interests.

Harris et al. (2009) studied the degree of specialisation and measures of antisocial traits and behaviour and sexual deviance among 374 men convicted of sexual offences referred for civil commitment in the US. They reported that versatile individuals showed higher levels of antisocial behaviour (substance misuse, adolescent antisocial behaviour, high levels of psychopathic traits) while specialist individuals showed higher levels of sexual deviance (emotional congruence with children, sexual preoccupation). Of their sample, 12% with offences against adults and 43% with offences against children were classified as specialists when the specialisation threshold was set at 50%. Similarly, Lussier et al. (2005) studied the criminal histories of 388 men convicted of sexual offences and found that the offending history of those who had offended sexually against women was usually part of a broader pattern of antisocial behaviour, while those offending against children tended to be less versatile in their pattern of offending.

Harris et al. (2011) studied the post-release offending patterns of 568 men convicted of sexual offences followed up for up to 10 years after discharge.

Individuals were classified as either versatile or specialist, depending on whether their previous offending was predominantly sexual offending or a mixture of offence types. Harris et al. found that versatile individuals were significantly more likely to reoffend overall or to reoffend violently but were no more likely to reoffend sexually than individuals with a specialist history. Overall, 85 out of 197 (43.1%) of those with a specialist sexual history reoffended, of whom 51 (60%) reoffended sexually. Harris et al used a relatively broad definition of specialisation (50% of previous offences were for a particular type of crime).

In summary, the literature on specialisation in sexual offending suggests that men who commit sexual offences vary in the degree to which they specialise in one particular type of offence. Men whose sexual offending is predominantly driven by paraphilic sexual interests or the use of pornography are more likely to offend in a narrow range of ways linked to those interests. Men who offend sexually against children are more likely to fit this specialist profile than those who offend against adults. Men whose sexual offending follows a more diverse trajectory are at greater risk of reoffending, and this may be explained in terms of the greater number of criminogenic factors associated with them, or because there is a much wider range of situations to which they might respond with criminal behaviour. It is not clear whether these patterns also apply to women who commit sexual offences.

Intimate Partner Violence

Holtzworth-Munroe and Stuart (1994) developed a typology of male perpetrators of intimate partner violence based on the severity and generality of violence and the level of psychopathology. They proposed three subtypes of intimate partner violence perpetrators. The first group, *family-only batterers*, tended only to offend against family members, their violence tended to be the least severe and they showed little evidence of other criminality or of personality disorder traits. *Borderline/ dysphoric batterers* offended primarily against family members but showed some intermediate levels of involvement in extra-familial violence and other criminality. They tended to be emotionally volatile and were often motivated by jealousy. Finally, *generally violent/antisocial batterers* were involved in psychological and sexual abuse as well as violent abuse, they were also involved in extra-familial violence and other crime, as well as substance misuse. Holtzworth-Munroe et al. (2000) tested this model on a sample of 102 men recruited from the community who admitted to a history of intimate partner violence. They identified four clusters of men, three of which resembled the predicted subtypes. The fourth group, labelled *low-level antisocial*, fell between the borderline/ dysphoric and generally violent/ antisocial groups on most measures.

Fire Setting

Lindberg et al. (2005) examined the pre-trial psychiatric assessments of 90 men with a history of repeat fire setting, of whom 43 (48%) had only arson in their previous criminal histories. The exclusive fire setting group included 15 out of 16 (94%) of individuals with an ICD-8 or 9 primary diagnosis of mental retardation and 15 out of 18 (83%) with a primary diagnosis of psychotic disorder, but only 12 out of 47 (26%) of with a primary diagnosis of personality disorder. Lindberg et al. reported that 35 out of 47 (74%) of their sample of individuals with repeat fire setting convictions who had a primary diagnosis of personality disorder had also committed other types of offence, though the nature of these offences was not specified. Of these 35 individuals, 20 were diagnosed with dissocial personality disorder, six immature, six emotionally unstable, two explosive, and one narcissistic.

Ducat et al. (2013) studied the offending and clinical characteristics of 207 consecutively sentenced Australian men and women convicted of fire setting offences. They reported that among those who had committed only fire setting offences, the prevalence of personality disorder was significantly lower than among criminally versatile fire setters (7.4% vs 31.4%), and that cluster B personality disorders were particularly common among the criminally versatile fire setter group. In contrast to Lindberg et al. (2005), the prevalence of psychotic illness did not differ between groups.

Violence

Lynam et al. (2004) investigated specialisation in violence among a cohort of young men in New Zealand. Individuals were classified as non-antisocial (5 or fewer self-reported offences), nonviolent specialists (6 or more offences, none of them violent), violent specialists (6 to 14 offences, 3 or more violent offences) and versatile offenders (6 or more offences, fewer than 3 violence). The two violent groups had higher levels of childhood conduct problems and negative emotionality. In this case, there was no difference between specialist "violent offenders" and the versatile offenders in terms of antisocial traits. However, the numbers of individuals in these groups were relatively small, and the results were based on self-report data rather than official records.

What Underlies Criminal Versatility?

Criminal versatility is associated with various indicators of risk, including early age of onset of offending, longer offending careers, greater number of offences and greater level of victim injury (Basto-Pereira & Farrington, 2020; Piquero et al., 1999; Vitacco et al., 2007). Most people who offend repeatedly are versatile in their offending. However, patterns of offending are not completely random, and there are also a number of clear patterns to specialisation. People are more likely to specialise in their range of offending as they age, and the focus of their offending may change in response to opportunities and life circumstances.

Among more serious offending a number of consistent themes emerge. Criminal versatility appears to vary on a spectrum with those at the versatile end of the spectrum more likely to be given a diagnosis of personality disorder, particularly dissocial or emotionally unstable personality disorders. What both those diagnoses have in common are traits of impulsivity and aggressiveness (Freestone et al., 2013; Howard et al., 2008). Other dissocial traits associated with criminal versatility include callousness and a coercive or manipulative interpersonal style (McCuish et al., 2021; Vitacco et al., 2007).

These findings are consistent with a trauma-based explanatory model. Levenson and Socia (2016) found that high rates of childhood adversity, particularly family dysfunction and a chaotic home environment were correlated with levels of adult criminal versatility, while Tsang (2018) found that greater exposure to violence among young people, either as a victim or a witness, was correlated with self-reported criminal versatility. Yoder and Precht (2020) found that justice-involved young people who had offended both sexually and non-sexually had experienced higher rates of physical and emotional abuse than those who had not offended sexually. Childhood maltreatment has been shown to be associated with later patterns of impulsivity (Hallowell et al., 2019), aggressiveness (Sarchiapone et al., 2009) and callousness (Kerig et al., 2012), the traits most commonly linked to criminal versatility.

van der Kolk (2003) has argued that chronic exposure to stress and threat in children affects the structure and organisation of their developing brains such that they are frequently either hyper-aroused and hypersensitive to threat or dissociated and emotionally numb in order to survive unbearable pain and distress. A common result of both hyperarousal and dissociation is to inhibit higher executive functions such as self-regulation, reasoning, and connection to others, leading to dysregulated and impulsive behaviour and to detachment from others.

An attachment-based model of development would suggest that children's ability to regulate themselves is shaped by repeated experiences of caregivers' sensitive regulation of their distress, which fosters a sense of security, and this ability is impaired by early experiences of abuse or neglect by caregivers (Scott et al., 2009). Children and young people who are unable to regulate the intensity of emotions and impulses may engage in a range of behaviours that can be understood as attempts to self-regulate, including aggression towards the self and others and substance misuse.

Aggressive behaviour is also understood to result from children's inability to regulate intense negative emotions, though social learning processes and hostile attribution styles of children exposed to violence also appear to be significant (Richey et al., 2016).

Freyd (1996) argued that maltreated children may learn to cope with distressing emotions through emotional numbing, which can develop into emotional detachment and callousness, and Kerig et al. (2012) found that the association between trauma exposure and callous-unemotional traits was mediated by emotional numbing.

In summary, there is evidence of a correlation between developmental adversity and subsequent criminally versatile behaviour. The links between adversity and criminal diversity may be mediated by neurodevelopmental, attachment, and social learning processes underlying the "antisocial" personality traits most commonly associated with criminally versatile behaviour.

Ethnicity and Criminal Versatility

There is very little research on the relationship between ethnicity and criminal versatility. Studies of psychopathy across different ethnic groups have found no significant differences in criminal versatility (Cooke et al., 2001; Sullivan et al., 2006). This is surprising, given that racially minoritized individuals are consistently found to be over-represented at every stage of the criminal justice system (Lammy, 2017). Black people are more likely to be arrested for robbery and Asian people more likely to be arrested for sexual offences (Phillips & Bowling, 2017). In the UK, Black and Asian men are over-represented among men convicted of sexual offences in prison (Cowburn et al., 2008), while the Crown Prosecution Service conceded that inter-group differences in prosecution rates could be due to their being "too reluctant to prosecute White defendants for rape or too quick to prosecute Chinese and Other or Black defendants" (Lammy, 2017; p.21).

Racism is recognised as a source of chronic and repetitive stress and trauma (Kirkinis et al., 2018; Wright et al., 2020). While there is evidence that people, particularly men, of colour engage in emotional numbing in response to chronic exposure to racism (Jackson, 2018; Unniver & Gabbidon, 2011), there has been little research into this or other potential mediating factors between racial trauma and offending behaviour. Clearly this is an under-researched area that requires further investigation.

Diagnosis Redux: The Dangers of "Specialism" and Silo Working

Offence categories are socially constructed and classified by legal systems that require precisely defined categories to determine whether or not an individual is guilty of a specific offence. However, psychological formulations of offending behaviour may not always be so clear. Take, for example, the case of somebody who derives sexual gratification from inflicting physical pain on others or from starting fires. The law would categorise such offences in terms of their behavioural outcomes, as "not sexual offences". On the other hand, if a person assaults a former partner whom they suspect of infidelity, inflicting injuries to the victim's genitals, that may be classified as a "sexual offence" even if the primary motivation was jealousy or rage, rather than a desire for sexual gratification. The legal system deals with the "symptoms", that is, the offending behaviour. It is not generally concerned with the underlying causes of that behaviour or the needs that it meets. In this respect, there are parallels with the medical approach to psychiatric diagnosis, which also focuses on surface symptoms rather than underlying causes. As Hart et al. (2011) point out, offences that appear on the surface to be very similar may be formulated in terms of very different risk factors and treatment needs.

As with psychiatric diagnosis, psychologists have perhaps been guilty at times of unquestioningly accepting the hegemonic approach to classification. In part, this may also be an artefact of the way in which correctional offending behaviour programmes have developed. Interventions for serious offending behaviour have traditionally developed in separate communities for different categories of offending. Psychologists have tended to specialise in treating those convicted of sexual, violent, fire setting, or intimate partner violence offences, with very little crossover between them. Despite extensive evidence to the contrary, this silo approach to programmes implicitly assumes that everyone who commits serious offences to be specialists. It has a number of drawbacks.

Firstly, not all serious offences will fit into the neat categories that these programmes suggest; consider the cases of somebody who commits a street robbery and also sexually assaults their victim; or who commits murder and sets the house on fire to hide the evidence; or who both physically and sexually assaults their partner. There is a danger that a specialist treatment programme will address the elements of an offence that fall within their remit but not fully address the other elements. Alternatively, it may be felt necessary to complete two, or even three, separate treatment programmes to address different aspects of the same offence, risking treatment fatigue or a reduction in engagement. There are therefore twin dangers, that aspects of risk "fall between the cracks" or that resources are wasted duplicating offence-specific treatment.

There is also a risk that silos become ghettoes. The separation of treatments perpetuates a toxic hierarchy in the criminal justice system that regards those convicted of non-sexual violence as being an "elite" and those convicted of sexual offences as an "underclass", a view that is unhelpful to both groups. On the other hand, a treatment approach that focuses on the underlying processes and unmet needs that both groups largely have in common would be more realistic and helpful for both groups. Such an approach has been adopted by the latest generation of correctional programmes in the UK, such as *Kaizen* and *Building New Me+* (Walton et al., 2017).

Most concerningly, categorical approaches to the treatment of offending appear to be based on flawed assumptions that specialisation is the norm among those who commit serious offences and that offences that appear similar will be driven by similar motivations and risk factors. This leads to the risk that such programmes will place undue emphasis on addressing treatment needs that are specific to one particular type of offending, such as deviant sexual interests or attitudes to fire, rather than to more global needs such as impulsivity or callous attitudes.

A Treatment Model for Criminally Diverse Individuals

In response to these concerns, the Men's Personality Disorder Service at Rampton Hospital developed the Offending Reduction Programme (ORP). We identified that a large proportion of the service's population is at the diverse end of the criminal diversity spectrum; most have established diagnoses of dissocial and/ or emotionally unstable personality disorders, patterns of impulsive behaviour and substance misuse and criminal records that included multiple types of serious offending. Figure 23.1 shows that 84% of patients (89 out of 107) in the

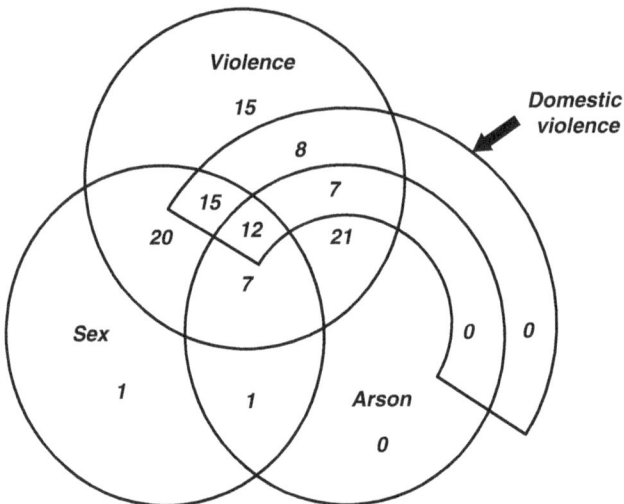

Figure 23.1 Conviction histories of patients in the men's personality disorder service.

service had a diverse history of serious criminal convictions. Based on the offence categories from the criminal versatility item of the Psychopathy Checklist (Hare, 2003), the mean number of offence types committed by patients in the Men's Personality Disorder Service was 6.74. In contrast, among a sample of male patients from the same hospital with a primary diagnosis of mental illness, only 19% (13 out of 67) had a history of diverse serious offending and the mean number of offence types committed was 2.51.

The Offending Reduction Programme (ORP) is based on the Violence Reduction Programme (VRP: Wong & Gordon, 2013), an established treatment programme originally designed for the treatment of individuals with a history of violent offending. Like the VRP, the ORP is based on the principles of effective correctional programming (Andrews et al., 1990) and designed to meet the needs of those who present a medium- to high-risk of reoffending including those with significant antisocial personality or psychopathic traits (Wong & Gordon, 2013).

Within the Men's Personality Disorder Service, the VRP/ORP sits within a wider treatment pathway. This is described by Evershed (2011) and is similar to the framework described by Livesley (2012). Treatment progresses through stages that address needs for *safety and containment, control and self-regulation, exploration and change* and *integration and synthesis*. Safety and containment are initially achieved through therapeutic relationships providing support, empathy, and structure, supplemented with medication as needed. The first stage of treatment (self-regulation) generally consists of dialectical behaviour therapy (DBT: Linehan, 1993), which targets life-threatening behaviours and equips participants with self-regulation skills. More recently, radically open dialectical behaviour therapy (RO-DBT, Lynch, 2018) has been introduced as a first-stage therapy for over-controlled patients. During the exploration and change phase, most patients undertake schema therapy (Young et al., 2003), to explore and change ineffective or harmful patterns of behaviour and relationship. Depending on the strengths and needs of the patient, trauma-specific therapies such as Eye-Movement Desensitisation Reprocessing (EMDR: Korn, 2009) can be integrated into this stage of treatment or can take place later, following offence-focused treatment.

The ORP is based on the schema therapy principle that unhelpful and problematic behaviours are best understood in terms of the core emotional needs that they meet or are intended to meet (Young et al., 2003), and on the formulation of "personality disorder" proposed by Willmot and Evershed (2018) as "a set of learned responses to perceived threat, or … survival strategies for keeping physically and psychologically safe in interpersonal environments that are seen by the individual as dangerous, hostile, abusive, or neglectful" (p. 340). The ORP applies these principles to offending lifestyles and behaviours so that offending behaviour is understood as an extreme means of meeting core emotional needs. The emotional needs most often described by group participants as related to offending include the need for physical or emotional safety, attachment to others (often described as a need for respect or group belonging), self-expression (often described as a need to communicate distress to others or to "feel heard") and autonomy (described as a need to feel in control).

The VRP/ORP is delivered in three phases. Phase one focuses on developing group cohesion and working alliance in order to create a therapeutic "safe space", developing participant's understanding of the origins and maintenance of offending behaviour and collaboratively identifying individual treatment targets.

Phase two introduces the idea of offending behaviour cycles and focuses on the acquisition of relevant skills to effectively manage internal risk factors (perceptions, thoughts, and feelings) and external risk and protective factors (relationships, antisocial peers, mental health and medication, substance misuse, weapon use, employment/activity, weapon use, and supervision) that make up these cycles. The modular format of phase two makes it particularly easy to adapt its order or content to meet the needs of participants. For example, not all participants' offending will have involved a history of weapon use or offence-related violent fantasising, and these issues may therefore be addressed in individual therapy sessions rather than in the group. At the end of phase 2 each participant presents a detailed formulation of their offending behaviour to the group. This formulation focuses on the unmet needs and the sequence of events leading up to offending, rather than on a detailed analysis of the offence itself.

Phase three involves group members formulating a good lives/relapse prevention plan, and practising the skills learned from phase two.

A key element of the programme is the use of behaviour cycle logs, which participants use to record any episodes where they experience elements of their behaviour cycles, along with how they responded. These are then reviewed in group sessions.

Group and Individual Processes

An important adaptation from Wong and Gordon's original programme is the inclusion of parallel-group and individual therapy sessions. Each group participant has their own individual therapist. Individual therapy sessions provide additional support and coaching. They also provide an opportunity for the participant to discuss issues they feel unable to discuss in the group, such as their own victimisation, family dynamics or offence details. This is particularly important when it comes to the offence formulation at the end of phase 2 which is done in two stages. In the first stage the participant, their individual therapist, and another group facilitator work together, usually over several weeks, to develop a detailed offence formulation. During this process the details of offences will be discussed, as well as other sensitive issues such as childhood abuse. Once this is complete the participant will present a summary of the formulation to the rest of the group, which omits these sensitive issues and focuses on the broad patterns on their offending cycle. This approach contributes to participants' sense of safety and avoids the potentially iatrogenic effects that discussing details of serious offending or of abuse could have either on the participant or on other group members (Jones, 2007).

Individual therapy sessions also provide a safe space in which to explore the impact of diversity issues that patients may not have reflected on previously, and to rehearse these before discussing them in the wider group setting. For example, one group member from the Traveller community was able to explore not only his experiences of exclusion and discrimination as a Traveller, but also the intense stigma he felt within the Traveller community in response to his mental health difficulties, and that community's suspiciousness towards mental health services which prevented him from accessing professional care. Exploring these issues in individual sessions enabled him to articulate issues that he had not previously explored, and to work through his sense of being disloyal to his family, before discussing it in the group.

Another key aspect of individual and group elements of the ORP is that they provide a structure for participants to develop their abilities to meet their core emotional needs in less self-defeating ways. For example, participants who derive a sense of safety by being aloof and hostile in order to keep others at a distance can explore how this strategy tends to perpetuate a sense of threat and test out alternative approaches of being more open and connected to others, first in individual sessions, then within the group where they are supported to practise this approach outside the group. Similarly, participants who derive their sense of connection and belonging by demonstrating antisocial attitudes and behaviours to their peers can explore and test out a more empathic and considerate approach within the ORP. Individual and group therapy sessions therefore provide a safe and containing graded structure for participants to explore and test out new behavioural strategies.

Sexual Offending and Toxic Shame

Of the ten patients with a history of sexual violence who have started the ORP so far, seven have shared a similar pattern in their diverse offending. All seven of these participants reported an increase in the frequency, severity, and/or diversity of their offending after committing a sexual offence. In all these cases, this sexual offence appears to have triggered intense feelings of shame and distress, arguably more so that for patients with an established pattern of sexual offending. Often for these individuals, their sexual offence has occurred impulsively at a time of extreme crisis, intense distress, or altered state of consciousness (see Jones, in press) and so feels "out of character" and impossible to understand. Often, these patients had themselves been the victim of a childhood sexual abuse that they found extremely distressing, and this caused them to feel intense confusion and shame that they had become "just like their own abuser". This reaction often appears to drive an increase in risk, not only of suicide and self-harm, but also of harm to others who trigger feelings of shame. This pattern reflects the findings of Butler et al. (2021), that an index sexual offence and pattern of self-harming behaviour were among the strongest predictors of institutional violence and disruptive behaviour in incarcerated young men. All the patients with this pattern of escalating risk following a sexual offence identified as white British, so it is not possible to draw any conclusions about the impact of race. However, we might expect toxic shame to be particularly relevant as a driver of offending in communities with strongest taboos against sexual violence.

What we have often observed in the histories of these patients is a pattern of relatively minor offending and a single sexual offence followed by a pattern of escalating non-sexually violent offending. The escalation tends to intensify in prisons where the pressure to keep physically and emotionally safe given their "sex offender" label becomes even stronger. Ironically, for clinicians and decision makers in the criminal justice system, the original sexual offence often becomes the focus of treatment and of decision making about risk, precisely because it appears "out of character" and difficult to formulate, thus inadvertently increasing shame and shame-driven risk behaviours. Therefore, for many of these patients, addressing their sexual offending - both developing a compassionate understanding of why it happened and helping them to manage toxic shame safely – become the central task of the ORP.

Summary and Conclusions

There is growing evidence of a link between developmental adversity and criminal versatility. In particular, there is evidence that the psychological correlates of criminally diverse behaviour – impulsivity, callousness, and hostility – can all be understood as responses to developmental adversity.

In common with other recent offence-related correctional programmes such as *Kaizen* and *Becoming New Me+*, the focus of the ORP is not on the details of offending behaviour, but on underlying criminogenic developmental processes. Within this framework, offending lifestyles and behaviours are understood as extreme means of meeting core emotional needs such as the need for connection to others, validation and, above all, safety.

We cannot conclude at this stage that developmental adversity is relevant in every case of serious or diverse offending. Indeed, we should be mistrustful of any model that purports to explain every case of something as complex and heterogeneous as criminal versatility. As various authors have argued (e.g., Butler, 1998; Johnstone, 2018), rather than focusing on the "truth" of a formulation, it is better to consider its usefulness. This approach is most likely to prove useful for working with service users with a history of repeated or pervasive developmental adversity, or whose offending appears to be a response to adversity. Adversity here covers a wide range of developmental experiences; not just abuse and neglect, but also deprivation, exclusion, racism, and other forms of discrimination. It may therefore be particularly relevant for racially minoritized people given the evidence that these groups are less likely to access correctional programmes because of concerns that programmes will not understand their needs or cultural identity (Brookes et al., 2012; Hunter et al., 2019).

The observation that, among our participants, the seriousness and range of offending often appears to increase following a sexual offence is a reminder that offence formulation should not simply consider offences in isolation but should reflect the links between offending and how offending develops over time.

When offence-related treatment takes place in environments that feel unsafe, participants are likely to revert to their learned protective strategy of callous unemotionality in order to reduce their vulnerability to emotional harm. We have found, without exception, that creating a safe space in the ORP allows participants to express and start to process the feelings of shame they feel about their offending. It is a reminder of the importance of addressing shame with people who have offended (Taylor & Hocken, 2021), and of the critical importance of creating safety in therapy.

There are important considerations for programme developers and policy makers involved in the development of new treatments. Continuing to develop separate treatment programmes based on offence characteristics perpetuates the silo approach to programme development and risks wasting scarce resources on individuals whose needs do not exactly match the programme goals.

Finally, this review of criminal diversity should serve as a reminder to forensic practitioners to be cautious about the language we use. Widely used categories such as "violent offending", "sexual offending", or even "criminal diversity", do not necessarily reflect any common underlying causal processes or treatment needs. Moreover, such terms, when used carelessly, can obscure a range of personal, social, and cultural factors that should be addressed on an individual formulation-led basis.

References

Agnew, R. A. (1992). Foundations for a general strain theory of crime and delinquency. *Criminology*, *30*, 47–88. 10.1111/j.1745-9125.1992.tb01093.x

Andrews, D. A., Bonta, J., & Hoge, R. D. (1990). Classification for effective rehabilitation: Rediscovering psychology. *Criminal Justice and Behavior*, *17*(1), 19–52. 10.1177/0093854 890017001004

Basto-Pereira, M., & Farrington, D. P. (2020). Lifelong conviction pathways and self-reported offending: Towards a deeper comprehension of criminal career development. *The British Journal of Criminology*, *60*(2), 285–302. 10.1093/bjc/azz037

Brookes, M., Glynn, M., & Wilson, D. (2012). Black men, therapeutic communities and HMP Grendon. *Therapeutic Communities: The International Journal of Therapeutic Communities*, *33*(1), 16–26. 10.1108/09641861211286294

Butler, G. (1998). Clinical formulation. In A. S. Bellack & M. Hersen (Eds.), *Comprehensive clinical psychology* (pp. 1–23). Pergamon: Oxford.

Butler, H. D., Caudill, J. W., Craig, J. M., DeLisi, M., & Trulson, C. R. (2021). 99 percenters: An examination of the misconduct careers of the most violent and disruptive incarcerated delinquents. *Aggression and Violent Behavior*, *60*, 101520. 10.1016/j.avb.2020.101520

Cooke, D. J., Kosson, D. S., & Michie, C. (2001). Psychopathy and ethnicity: Structural, item, and test generalizability of the Psychopathy Checklist—Revised (PCL-R) in Caucasian and African American participants. *Psychological Assessment*, *13*(4), 531–542. 10.1037111040-3590.13.4.531

Cowburn, M., Lavis, V. & Walker, T. (2008). Black and minority ethnic sex offenders. *Prison Service Journal*, *178*, 44–49.

DeLisi, M., Bunga, R., Heirigs, M. H., Erickson, J. H., & Hochstetler, A. (2019). The past is prologue: Criminal specialization continuity in the delinquent career. *Youth Violence and Juvenile Justice*, *17*(4), 335–353. 10.1177/1541204018809839

Ducat, L., McEwan, T., & Ogloff, J. R. (2013). Comparing the characteristics of fire-setting and non-firesetting offenders: are firesetters a special case? *The Journal of Forensic Psychiatry & Psychology*, *24*, 549–569. 10.1080/14789949.2013.821514

Evershed, S. (2011). A treatment pathway for high security offenders with a personality disorder. In P. Willmot & N. Gordon (Eds.) *Working positively with personality disorder in secure settings* (pp. 66–90). Wiley-Blackwell.

Freestone, M., Howard, R., Coid, J. W., & Ullrich, S. (2013). Adult antisocial syndrome co-morbid with borderline personality disorder is associated with severe conduct disorder, substance dependence and violent antisociality. *Personality and Mental Health*, *7*(1), 11–21. 10.1002/pmh.1203

Freyd, J. J. (1996). *Betrayal trauma: The logic of forgetting childhood abuse.* Harvard University Press.

Gottfredson, M. R., & Hirschi, T. (1990). *A general theory of crime.* Stanford, CA: Stanford University Press.

Hallowell, E. S., Oshri, A., Liebel, S. W., Liu, S., Duda, B., Clark, U. S., & Sweet, L. H. (2019). The mediating role of neural activity on the relationship between childhood maltreatment and impulsivity. *Child Maltreatment*, *24*(4), 389–399. 10.1177/107755951 9835975

Hare, R. D. (2003). *The Hare psychopathy checklist-revised* (2nd Edition). Multi-Health Systems.

Harris, D. A., Knight, R. A., Smallbone, S. W., & Dennison, S. (2011). Postrelease specialisation and versatility in sexual offenders referred for civil commitment. *Sexual Abuse: A Journal of Research and Treatment*, *23*, 243–259.

Harris, D. A., Mazerolle, P., & Knight, R. A. (2009). Understanding male sexual offending a comparison of general and specialist theories. *Criminal Justice and Behavior*, *36*, 1051–1069. 10.1177/1079063210384276

Harris, D. A., Smallbone, S., Dennison, S., & Knight, R. A. (2009). Specialization and versatility in sexual offenders referred for civil commitment. *Journal of Criminal Justice*, *37*(1), 37–44. 10.1016/j.jcrimjus.2008.12.002

Hart, A., Gresswell, M. & Braham, L. (2011). Formulation of serious violent offending using multiple sequential functional analysis. In P. Sturmey & M. McMurran (Eds.) *Forensic case formulation* (pp. 129–152). John Wiley & Sons.

Holtzworth-Munroe, A., Meehan, J. C., Herron, K., Rehman, U., & Stuart, G. L. (2000). Testing the Holtzworth-Munroe and Stuart (1994) batterer typology. *Journal of Consulting and Clinical Psychology, 68*, 1000–1019. 10.1037/0022-006X.68.6.1000

Holtzworth-Munroe, A., & Stuart, G. L. (1994). Typologies of mate batterers: Three subtypes and the differences among them. *Psychological Bulletin, 116*, 476–497. 10.1037/0033-2909.116.3.476

Howard, P. D., Barnett, G., & Mann, R. E. (2013). Specialization in and within sexual offending in England and Wales. *Sexual Abuse: A Journal of Research and Treatment.* 1079063213486934

Howard, R. C., Huband, N., Duggan, C., & Mannion, A. (2008). Exploring the link between personality disorder and criminality in a community sample. *Journal of Personality Disorders, 22*(6), 589–603. 10.1521/pedi.2008.22.6.589

Hunter, S., Craig, E., & Shaw, J. (2019). "Give it a Try": experiences of black, Asian and minority ethnic young men in a prison-based offender personality disorder service. *Journal of Forensic Practice, 21*(1), 14–26. 10.1108/JFP-07-2018-0026

Jackson, B. A. (2018). Beyond the cool pose: Black men and emotion management strategies. *Sociology Compass, 12*(4), e12569. 10.1111/soc4.12569

Johnstone, L. (2018). Psychological formulation as an alternative to psychiatric diagnosis. *Journal of Humanistic Psychology, 58*(1), 30–46. 10.1177/0022167817722230

Jones, L. F. (2007). Iatrogenic interventions with personality disordered offenders. *Psychology, Crime & Law, 13*(1), 69–79. 10.1080/10683160600869809

Jones, L. F. (In press). Trauma-Informed Risk Assessment and Intervention: Understanding the Role of Triggering Contexts and Offence-Related Altered States of Consciousness (ORASC). In P. Willmot & L. Jones, (Eds.) *Trauma-informed forensic practice.* Routledge.

Kerig, P. K., Bennett, D. C., Thompson, M., & Becker, S. P. (2012). "Nothing really matters": Emotional numbing as a link between trauma exposure and callousness in delinquent youth. *Journal of Traumatic Stress, 25*(3), 272–279. 10.1002/jts.21700

Kirkinis, K., Pieterse, A. L., Martin, C., Agiliga, A., & Brownell, A. (2018). Racism, racial discrimination, and trauma: A systematic review of the social science literature. *Ethnicity & Health*, 1–21. 10.1080/13557858.2018.1514453

Korn, D. L. (2009). EMDR and the treatment of complex PTSD: A review. *Journal of EMDR Practice and Research, 3*(4), 264–278. 10.1891/1933-3196.3.4.264

Lammy, D. (2017). The Lammy Review: An independent review into the treatment of, and outcomes for, Black, Asian and Minority Ethnic individuals in the Criminal Justice System.

Levenson, J. S., & Grady, M. D. (2016). The influence of childhood trauma on sexual violence and sexual deviance in adulthood. *Traumatology, 22*(2), 94–103. 10.1037/trm0000067

Levenson, J. S., & Socia, K. M. (2015). Adverse childhood experiences and arrest patterns in a sample of sexual offenders. *Journal of Interpersonal Violence, 31*(10), 1883–1911. 10.1177/0886260515570751

Lindberg, N., Holi, M., Tani, P., & Virkkunen, M. (2005). Looking for pyromania: Characteristics of a consecutive sample of Finnish male criminals with histories of recidivist fire-setting between 1973 and 1993. *BMC Psychiatry, 5*, 1–5. 10.1186/1471-244X-5-47

Linehan, M. M. (1993). *Cognitive-behavioral treatment of borderline personality disorder.* Guilford Press.

Livesley, W. J. (2012). Integrated treatment: A conceptual framework for an evidence-based approach to the treatment of personality disorder. *Journal of Personality Disorders, 26*(1), 17–42. 10.1521/pedi.2012.26.1.17

Lussier, P., LeBlanc, M., & Proulx, J. (2005). The generality of criminal behavior: A confirmatory factor analysis of the criminal activity of sex offenders in adulthood. *Journal of Criminal Justice, 33*, 177–189. 10.1016/j.jcrimjus.2004.12.009

Lynam, D. R., Piquero, A. R., & Moffitt, T. E. (2004). Specialization and the Propensity to Violence Support from Self-Reports but Not Official Records. *Journal of Contemporary Criminal Justice, 20*, 215–228. 10.1177/1043986204263781

Lynch, T. R. (2018). *Radically open dialectical behavior therapy: Theory and practice for treating disorder of overcontrol.* New Harbinger Publications.

McCuish, E., Bouchard, M., & Beauregard, E. (2021). A network-based examination of the longitudinal association between psychopathy and offending versatility. *Journal of Quantitative Criminology, 37*(3), 693–714. 10.1007/s10940-020-09462-w

Nieuwbeerta, P., Blokland, A. A., Piquero, A. R., & Sweeten, G. (2011). A life-course analysis of offense specialization across age: Introducing a new method for studying individual specialization over the life course. *Crime & Delinquency, 57*(1), 3–28. 10.1177/0011128710376336

Phillips, C. & Bowling, B. (2017). Ethnicities, racism, crime and criminal justice. In A. Liebling, S. Maruna & L. McAra (Eds.), *Oxford handbook of criminology,* (pp. 190–212). Oxford: Oxford University Press.

Piquero, A., Paternoster, R., Mazerolle, P., Brame, R., & Dean, C. W. (1999). Onset age and offense specialization. *Journal of Research in Crime and Delinquency, 36*(3), 275–299. 10.1177/0022427899036003002

Richey, A., Brown, S., Fite, P. J., & Bortolato, M. (2016). The role of hostile attributions in the associations between child maltreatment and reactive and proactive aggression. *Journal of Aggression, Maltreatment & Trauma, 25*(10), 1043–1057. 10.1080/10926771.2016.1231148

Sarchiapone, M., Carli, V., Cuomo, C., Marchetti, M., & Roy, A. (2009). Association between childhood trauma and aggression in male prisoners. *Psychiatry Research, 165*(1–2), 187–192. 10.1016/j.psychres.2008.04.026

Scott, L. N., Levy, K. N., & Pincus, A. L. (2009). Adult attachment, personality traits, and borderline personality disorder features in young adults. *Journal of Personality Disorders, 23*(3), 258–280. 10.1521/pedi.2009.23.3.258

Sullivan, E. A., Abramowitz, C. S., Lopez, M., & Kosson, D. S. (2006). Reliability and construct validity of the psychopathy checklist-revised for Latino, European American, and African American male inmates. *Psychological Assessment, 18*(4), 382–392. 10.1037/1040-3590.18.4.382

Taylor, J., & Hocken, K. (2021). People hurt people: Reconceptualising criminogenic need to promote trauma sensitive and compassion focussed practice. *The Journal of Forensic Practice, 23*(3), 201–212. 10.1108/JFP-04-2021-0015

Tsang, S. (2018). Troubled or traumatized youth? The relations between psychopathy, violence exposure, posttraumatic stress disorder, and antisocial behavior among juvenile offenders. *Journal of Aggression, Maltreatment & Trauma, 27*(2), 164–178. 10.1080/10926771.2017.1372541

Unniver, J. D. & Gabbidon, S. L. (2011). *A theory of African American offending: Race, racism, and crime.* Routledge.

van der Kolk, B. A. (2003). The neurobiology of childhood trauma and abuse. *Child and Adolescent Psychiatric Clinics, 12*(2), 293–317. 10.1016/S1056-4993(03)00003-8

Vitacco, M. J., Caldwell, M. F., Van Rybroek, G. J., & Gabel, J. (2007). Psychopathy and behavioral correlates of victim injury in serious juvenile offenders. *Aggressive Behavior: Official Journal of the International Society for Research on Aggression, 33*(6), 537–544. 10.1002/ab.20211

Walton, J. S., Ramsay, L., Cunningham, C., & Henfrey, S. (2017). New directions: Integrating a biopsychosocial approach in the design and delivery of programs for high risk services users in Her Majesty's Prison and Probation Service. *Advancing Corrections: Journal of the International Corrections and Prison Association, 3*, 21–47.

Wiesner, M., Yoerger, K., & Capaldi, D. M. (2018). Patterns and correlates of offender versatility and specialization across a 23-year span for at-risk young men. *Victims and Offenders, 13*(1), 28–47. 10.1080/15564886.2016.1250691

Willmot, P., & Evershed, S. (2018). Interviewing people given a diagnosis of personality disorder in forensic settings. *International Journal of Forensic Mental Health, 17*(4), 338–350. 10.1080/14999013.2018.1508097

Wong, S. C., & Gordon, A. (2013). The violence reduction programme: A treatment programme for violence-prone forensic clients. *Psychology, Crime & Law, 19*(5–6), 461–475. 10.1080/1068316X.2013.758981

Wright, J. L., Jarvis, J. N., Pachter, L. M., & Walker-Harding, L. R. (2020). "Racism as a public health issue" APS racism series: At the intersection of equity, science, and social justice. *Pediatric Research, 88*(5), 696–698. 10.1038/s41390-020-01141-7

Yoder, J., & Precht, M. (2020). Victimization experiences and executive dysfunction as discriminating risk indicators for youth offender typologies. *International Journal of Offender Therapy and Comparative Criminology, 64*(1), 63–82. 10.1177/0306624X19865185

Young, J. E., Klosko, J. S., & Weishaar, M. E. (2003). *Schema therapy*. Guilford Press.

24 Challenging Bias in the Assessment of Extremist Offending

Christopher Dean and Monica Lloyd

Introduction

Perhaps more so than any other form of offending, extremist offending in the form of terrorist attacks elicits a strong emotional response from the public. The clue is the word "terror" and its impact. Those responsible for making risk decisions do not want to be the ones who miss or underestimate a risk of harm that manifests in a high-profile loss of life. Risk aversion is therefore an understandable "default" position of those responsible for assessing and managing risk. This context alone provides fertile ground for assessment bias, compounded by additional ethical, methodological, and assessor issues which may directly or indirectly contribute to bias. This chapter outlines the emergence of the role of forensic psychologists working with those convicted of terrorist-related offences in the UK in response to the wave of Islamist extremist offending that broke at the turn of the millennium and placed extremist offending firmly on the map for those working in correctional contexts. It describes the development of psychological risk assessment and its susceptibility to bias, given the scale of terrorism's potential for harm and its sensitivity to political context, and discusses how these may be mitigated.

This chapter sets the scene for this sea change in correctional practice and then examines the contextual issues that are unique to extremist offending in more depth. The implicit bias of the terminology used to describe terrorist offending is explored and how words reflect power, perspective, and privilege. The counter-terrorism challenge of intervening before an offence is committed is also discussed, and the methodological issues concerning the assessment of low base rate violence, of which terrorist violence is a pertinent example. Here the risk of identifying false positives is high and provides scope for implicit bias and risk aversion to do their worst. The current risk assessment frameworks are discussed in the context of their respective strengths and utility, given the importance of understanding the geo-political context of extremist offending, and the final section of the chapter addresses different forms of assessor bias directly. The importance of self-awareness, peer supervision, and ethical practice is stressed throughout to build reflexivity and awareness of the complexity of working across potential political, cultural, race, and gender divides to achieve best practice in the assessment of extremist offending.

DOI: 10.4324/9781003230977-27

Setting the Scene

Forensic psychology in the west has developed largely from correctional practice with those convicted of sexual and violent offences. Extremist offending has typically been viewed as the product of rational political choice and not the rightful province of psychologists. In the UK this remained the case throughout the Troubles in Northern Ireland that spanned the early 1970s to the Good Friday Peace Agreement in 1998, during which psychologists had little direct contact with paramilitary prisoners. The attacks on the London transport system in July 2005 changed this fundamentally. These demonstrated that British and American foreign policy in the Middle East, and support for authoritarian regimes in Arabic lands were able to activate deep-seated grievances that could mobilise Muslims in the West to carry out terrorist attacks in their home countries. The London attacks were perpetrated by four British Muslims of black and minority ethnic heritage on their fellow citizens in acts of self-martyrdom, and two weeks later a second attack on the underground was attempted. Although these bombs failed to detonate, Londoners feared that such attacks would become a regular threat to their security, and the whole country became sensitised to its vulnerability.

The legislation that followed criminalised various activities that were considered to be preparatory to, or glorifying of terrorism in an attempt to disrupt potential terrorist plotting[1], and brought into custody a cohort of individuals who varied in terms of their risk of harm to the public. Their crimes ranged from the possession of information that could be used for terrorism purposes to large-scale plotting of civilian attacks, and their sentences ranged from short, fixed terms to indeterminate terms with lengthy tariffs. Initially, they were treated as a homogenous group who were deemed to be inherently "high-risk", effectively formalising a systemic bias against them. This was due in part to the lack of an evidence base to make sense of their offence pathways, motivations, and intentions that would be able to inform risk decisions. Understanding these therefore became a matter of urgency to meet their sentence planning needs, manage them proportionately and protect the public. "Extremist" offending was defined as *"any offense associated with a group, cause or ideology that propagates extremist views and actions and justifies the use of violence and other illegal conduct in pursuit of its objectives"*. This definition supported a focus on the offending behaviour rather than ideology as the target for change, and avoided criminalising beliefs. The reasoning was that in a liberal democracy where there are legitimate ways to express political dissent the use of violence is not acceptable.

Contextual Issues in the Assessment of Extremist Offending

Terminology

This new area of work brought significant ethical challenges to the UK as a democratic, pluralist, and secular society. It was important not only to avoid criminalising beliefs but also to avoid being drawn into debates about the legitimacy of political violence when the UK's involvement in wars in the Middle East was a prime source of grievance. Those who commit extremist offences typically harbour feelings of grievance against their governments, which makes it potentially difficult for them to work with those they may see as representing the authority they oppose. There is also a reciprocal risk that staff may be implicitly biased against these individuals because of their apparent willingness to harm fellow civilians in the pursuit of their cause. Words also reflect power, perspective, and privilege. The term "terrorist" is particularly problematic as it reflects the perspective of the user in relation to the perpetrator and can be used to delegitimise them. Oppressive states can label their own citizens as terrorists when, as non-state actors, they use violence to progress what might be widely viewed as a legitimate cause. Such a homogenising label is therefore resisted by those who believe they are pursuing a noble cause and whose offending focuses on government targets, the military, or fighting as an insurgent abroad, rather than perpetrating random civilian attacks.

Another problematic term is "radicalisation". It implies that it is necessary to be radicalised to commit extremist offences, and that all those who carry out extremist offences hold "radical" beliefs. In reality only a small number of those who are apparently "radicalised" go on to carry out a terrorist offence (Hafez & Mullins, 2015) and of those who do, many have only a superficial engagement with ideology (McCauley & Moskalenko, 2014). Assessing the degree of engagement separately to an intent to cause harm is therefore central to assessing risk, for which the term radicalisation lacks precision. The concepts of "equifinality" and "multifinality" capture this complexity (Borum, 2011). The former refers to the empirical finding that there are many individual pathways to the same destination, and that not all those who complete a pathway to offending are radicalised. Mulitifinality refers to the reality that there are many possible outcomes for those on an apparently common path, and not all those who embark on a "radicalisation" pathway complete it. The dynamic push and pull factors that underlie engagement and disengagement are in constant tension, and individuals can disengage at any point along their pathway and for many reasons, including disillusionment with group members or ideology, or the pull of the previous life that was abandoned (Bjørgo & Horgan, 2009; Altier et al., 2017). The assessment process itself therefore acts as a means through which individual pathways are explored, which if undertaken with awareness and insight can mitigate against homogenisation and implicit bias.

Race, Power, and Privilege

A significant challenge for those working with those who commit such offences is that they often have specific and different racial and cultural profiles to those who assess them, manage their lives, and make decisions about them, and differential experiences of the "post" colonial world in which asymmetries of power continue to resonate. The Islamist extremist narrative, simply put, is that a morally decadent West has persecuted Muslims over their entire history and continues to shore-up un-Islamic regimes in Muslim lands for its own ends; and likewise, the Far-Right extremist narrative is that white people are being displaced by immigrants in their home countries and robbed of their birth-right to jobs and a good life, despite their natural superiority. Both reflect a distribution of power and privilege that is experienced by some as unjust to the extent that it perpetuates their disadvantage, and by others to the extent that it robs them of their previous advantage. There remains a dynamic tension be-tween these two perspectives. The threat of Islamist extremism has fuelled white nationalists' belief in the "Great Replacement" conspiracy[2] that proposes that Muslim migration into Europe at a time when the European birth rate is dropping and the Muslim birth rate is rising, will eventually culminate in the replacement of white European culture by a non-white Muslim culture; as-sisted by complicit "replacist" elites in government. Such narratives both re-flect and respond to ongoing geo-political change. It follows that a level of political awareness and sensitivity is required by those working in this area to understand the issues of power, privilege, culture, race, and threat that provide its context. Specifically, psychologists need to be aware of their privilege, mindful that inter-generational trauma continues to resonate at a personal level with those who engage in extremist violence (Volkan, 2006), and that race and privilege continue to divide us from our clients. In this context the Power, Threat, Meaning framework (Boyle & Johnstone, 2020) can be a helpful way to identify sources of disempowerment and threat at the macro level that may resonate with personal experiences that can be framed by ideology and imbued with political meaning at the micro-level.

When this work began in 2008 the numbers of those convicted for terrorism-related offences who were willing to work with psychologists grew slowly from a handful to a sizable cohort as individuals responded to an approach that helped them make sense of their pathways and choices through a shared un-derstanding without judgement. This was supported by robust peer supervision and ongoing reflective practice by those involved in this work, together with oversight from an international expert steering group to monitor its legitimacy and rigour. By 2011 this project had produced a methodology for assessing risk and needs, and interventions to develop dialogue and create opportunities for reflection about past and future choices. It has also, subsequently, informed BPS ethical guidance for psychologists working with extremism in the UK[3] and for mental health practitioners working to prevent violent extremism in Europe[4], under the BPS headings of Respect, Responsibility, Competence, and Integrity. These include the importance of practitioner psychologists being aware of their own cultural perspective and the unconscious biases embedded in the science and language of western psychology; remaining mindful about how their practice may be viewed by the communities from which their clients are drawn; avoiding labels that may be experienced as stigmatising and alar-mist; ensuring regular supervision to reflect on how current geo-political events may be affecting attitudes towards their clients (including their own); and if necessary avoiding working with those whose causes they strongly oppose, and where they cannot remain objective and non-judgmental.

Assessing Potential Extremist Risk Before a Crime Has Been Committed

A particularly problematic area of work is in Prevent/Countering Violent Extremism (P/CVE), where SPJ frameworks may be employed by law enforcement or intelligence analysts who lack the psychological expertise to understand the significance of mental health when it is co-morbid with potential extremist interest. A survey of mental health practitioners was carried out by the Radical Awareness Network (RAN) of the concerns of mental health practitioners working in P/CVE in Europe to inform guidelines to support their practice (referenced in footnote 4). This confirmed that most P/CVE assessment hubs in the UK and Europe are assisted by mental health practitioners who provide this expertise, but that not all feel competent to do so. Neither do some feel comfortable working in a multi-agency setting where client information is shared with other agencies, and full medical confidentiality is not possible. Psychiatrists have also expressed specific concerns about the danger of pathologising beliefs, especially in young people for whom embracing idealistic beliefs can be a normal part of their development (Royal College of Psychiatrists, 2017).

The above RAN report specifically addresses these concerns and the ethics of intervening before a crime has been committed, when mental health assessment cannot be compelled by law. It clarifies the role of mental health practitioners in these circumstances and the boundaries of ethical practice. It acknowledges that although medical confidentiality is the norm, in no European member state is this considered to be absolute where this would prejudice the prevention, detection, or prosecution of serious crime. It stresses that the key task of mental health professionals is not to predict risk but to prevent it. As with any co-morbidity between mental health and violence, this involves identifying mental health symptoms that may, either directly or indirectly, account for an apparent interest in extremist ideology or violence, such that treating or managing the mental health issue, or providing support, might prevent a violent outcome. A direct link between mental health and the risk of harm might be a command hallucination to attack a specific target, where treating the psychosis will directly reduce the risk of harm. An indirect link might be the presence of psychological distress where treatment may increase resilience against radicalisation, but where there is no link between the two, addressing a mental health concern will not in itself mitigate engagement in extremist ideology or violence. This is important to clarify to law enforcers and is arguably crucial to ensuring that the response of the authorities to concerns about the co-morbidity of extremist interest and mental health is properly informed and proportionate to the low base rate of extremist violence. Clearly, disinformation, misinformation, and misunderstanding about mental health, extremist offending, and their relationship leaves significant space for bias and prejudice to influence decision making.

Methodological Issues in Assessing Extremist Offending

Low Rate of Offending and Recidivism

The biggest challenge in assessing the likelihood of any form of violence is its low base rate in the general population, and this applies even more so to terrorist-related violence. Sageman (2021) reports that the base rate for those involved in Islamist-related terrorist violence in the West (between 2000 and 2019) is a thousand times smaller than the annual homicide base rate in the West (p. 303). This is equivalent to 3 new individuals per year, per 100 million people. The annual base rate is also 10 times lower than the annual homicide rates for European countries categorised as having (relatively) low homicide rates (Sageman, 2021 p. 303). Similarly, the recidivism rate of those convicted for terrorist-related offences is also relatively low compared to other forms of criminal recidivism.[5] Between 2013 and 2019, out of 196 individuals released from custody in England and Wales, only six were reconvicted of a further terrorist offence, equivalent to a 3% recidivism rate.[6] In Northern Ireland, of the 453 paramilitary prisoners released in 1998 as part of the Good Friday Peace Agreement, only 10 have been recalled to custody for involvement in terrorist activities, equivalent to a 2.2% recidivism rate (Silke & Morrison, 2020). These UK figures are similar to terrorist-related recidivism rates of 4.2% in the Netherlands (Van der Heide & Schuurman, 2018), 2.3% in Belgium (Renard, 2020), and 1.6% (for any form of recidivism) in the USA (Hodwitz, 2021). Whilst this may in part reflect the use of restrictive licence conditions and ready recall of those who breach them, it is nevertheless apparent that this group currently present a relatively low risk of recidivism (see Silke & Morrison, 2020).

These relatively low rates of offending and recidivism rule out actuarial assessment of the risk of re-offending. Though helpful in identifying the risk of disease in medical epidemiology where it has been widely deployed, actuarial assessment has proved less effective in identifying the risk of general violence for which the base rate is low and discrete "symptomatology" lacking (Harris & Rice, 2015). Based on probability theory it relies on high rates of recidivism and the presence of distinctive characteristics that are able to act as predictors (Hart & Cooke, 2013; Cooke & Michie 2014). Like individuals convicted for other violent offences the consensus is that those who have committed extremist offences are characterised by their normality and heterogeneity (Crenshaw, 1981; Silke, 2008), and there is no single pathway or propensity that distinguishes them from each other. Assumptions that dangerousness is dispositional, static, and dichotomous, and that risk factors contribute to risk in a summative and linear fashion, do not apply. Dangerousness is now understood to be an emerging construct that is contextual, dynamic, and distributed along a continuum of probability (Borum, 2015; Fein et al., 1995). Structured Professional Judgment (SPJ) has become the favoured approach to assessing the risk of low base rate violence and recommended as the most appropriate methodology for the assessment of extremist offending (Borum, 2011;

Monahan, 2012; 2015; Sarma, 2017). Given the scope this affords for professional judgement, specific attention needs to be given to how assessor subjectivity is managed in or out of assessment (Dean & Pettet, 2017. p. 95).

Frameworks for Assessing Extremist Offending

Several SPJ frameworks have been developed in this field (see Lloyd, 2019), including the ERG22+ in the UK correctional service (Lloyd & Dean, 2015) and the VERA-2R developed in Canada and deployed widely in Europe (Pressman & Flockton, 2012). These structure the professional judgement of already experienced risk assessors and are based on similar principles, methodologies, and administrative approaches as those used to assess other forms of offending. The ERG22+ was derived from the empirical accounts of true positives in the UK, informed by the academic literature and the testimony of those formerly engaged with extremist groups; the VERA-2R was derived from the academic literature triangulated against the experience of law enforcement officers and intelligence analysts. The risk factors in these frameworks do not apply to all those who commit extremist offences because of their heterogeneity and cannot therefore be summed, and they apply differentially to leaders, followers, and criminal opportunists, so are not evidenced in every case. Neither can such individualised formulations be easily aggregated for statistical analysis. They are designed to identify individual drivers and discriminate between those with and without a mind-set of intent (readiness to commit extremist offences, including violence) or with greater or lesser capability to carry out an extremist offence in specific scenarios. In many western countries a range of relatively benign behaviours that correspond with curiosity or sympathy for an extremist cause have been criminalised (see Sageman, 2021), such that without a transparent methodology for identifying a mind-set of intent, appropriate risk discriminations may not be made. As multi-finality affirms, not all those who show an interest in extremist groups, causes, or ideologies commit extremist offences.

Such frameworks are not without criticism, including that they are implicitly vulnerable to bias in their design and construction (Dean & Pettet, 2017, p. 92). Reasons for this include the limited empirical evidence for their putative risk and protective factors and an absence of published reliability studies at the time of their development. However, it is important that this narrative is reviewed as their provenance is progressively endorsed (Logan & Lloyd, 2018) and evidence grows for their validity and utility (Corner et al., 2021; Gill et al; Knight et al., 2017; Wolfowicz et al., 2019; 2021). These frameworks conform to good psychological practice to the extent that they strive to be:

1   *Evidence-based*, to mitigate the tendency to reach conclusions based on opinion, heuristics, or prejudice.
2   *Transparent, systematic, and consistent* to prevent the intrusion of idiosyncratic or esoteric approaches.

3   *Reflexive* and *clear* regarding the parameters of their use so that they are not misapplied or their findings taken out of context.
4   *Responsive and sensitive* to the individual, avoiding group characteristics that can be influenced by stereotyping, prejudice, and discrimination.

Assessor Bias

Professional judgement is based on tacit knowledge made up of several elements, such as a disciplinary perspective, work experience, ongoing professional training, and personality variables, as well as clinical insight, gut feelings, hunches, "cognitive heuristics" (see Kahneman, 2011), potential cognitive distortions and "the socio-cultural organisational context in which a terrorism risk assessment is completed" (Dean & Pettet, 2017 p. 95). However, empirical research on assessor bias is almost non-existent, as is research on how to mitigate it. The following are associated with assessor bias in this field.

Assessor Antipathy and Reputational Risk

Extremist offences are typically high profile and newsworthy, attracting significant and arguably disproportionate media attention. Exposure to national and social media coverage can reinforce "mainstream" beliefs, opinions, and norms about perpetrators, the threat they pose, their impact on victims and what the consequences should be for their actions. Assessment therefore carries significant political, organisational and reputational risks that can contribute to conformity with mainstream opinion, (See Baron et al., 1996; Darley, 1966; Deutsch & Gerard, 1955) and to risk aversion (Lerner et al., 2003). The importance of the task and the consequences of getting it wrong can disproportionately impact those who are sensitive to normative social influences, averse to social disapproval and/or less confident in their own knowledge and expertise. Allied to this is the possibility of assessors over-identifying with victims. Indirect "assessor victimisation" is poorly understood but may also contribute to distorted pre-conceptions and confirmation bias (Mynatt et al., 1977), as well as defensive attribution bias or "blaming" (see Grubb & Harrower, 2008). Such attitudes on the part of the assessor are likely to affect the quality of the information obtained in interview and contribute to an over-emphasis on risk and an under-emphasis on protective influences, and a potential bias towards recommending monitoring and supervision over treatment and intervention.

To mitigate this, assessors need to be mindful about the impact of media reporting. They need to be informed about the context of the offence, but they also need to ensure that their judgements remain proportionate and objective. Peer support or supervision are recommended to ensure that professionalism and proportionality is sustained. Assessors may need to deselect themselves from cases where they or their professional peers consider that the impact on them may be affecting their objectivity and judgement. Alternatively, assessors can choose to acknowledge the possibility of bias in their reports by making explicit the circumstances and context of the assessment and the potential that these may have prejudiced its conclusions.

In assessing the risk of re-offending, including mitigating the influence of availability bias in which recent, unusual and/or emotionally charged memories are more available than others because of their saliency, which can result in overestimating the likelihood of a similar event occurring again (See Schwarz et al., 1991), assessors might benefit from reminding themselves about the rarity of extremist offending and recidivism (especially offences resulting in significant harm). "Comparative framing" provides an alternative way of assessing the risk of harm. If, for example, we accept recidivism rate of 3% for committing further terrorist-related offences in England and Wales (as identified between 2013 and 2019)[7] assessors may ask themselves whether the individual being assessed appears (based on all the evidence available, including presence of dynamic risk factors and proposed/current risk management strategies) more or less likely to be that 1 in 33 individuals who will commit a further extremist offence in the future. This can challenge rigid assumptions about the likelihood of future offending and directs attention to the more appropriate task of advising how risk can be managed effectively and proportionately in different scenarios. Interestingly, recent research has reported that *conscientiousness* is the most important personality trait, and *objectivity* the second most important intellectual ability of a good assessor of terrorism risk (Salman & Gill, 2021).

Assessor Sympathy

In the opposite direction, assessor sympathy may also detract from the quality of assessment of offences that purport to defend individual rights, the climate or animal rights, or that address social injustice. There is broad public consensus about what should be classified as a crime, but the designation of crimes against the state can be contentious, not least because they appear to serve the interests of government. A consequence of this is that some assessors – as with some members of the public - may have a measure of sympathy for these types of offences or for the individuals who commit them, (Bhui et al., 2016; 2019). This is more likely if assessors identify with the motives or cause, or with the perpetrators themselves. Where their causes resonate with the assessor's own values, in-group bias may produce a more appreciative assessment (see Tajfel, 1974; Yamagishi & Mifune, 2009). Assessors may believe that "I'm not risky, therefore they can't be risky", or the end is seen as justifying the means and the seriousness of their offences is discounted (e.g., posting messages on the internet which may incite others to commit violence).

To mitigate this, it is suggested that assessors monitor their perspective and their feelings, or lack of feelings, towards such individuals, their motives, objectives, and ideology. One practical method of doing this is to run through a checklist of self-reflective questions such as "to what extent do I sympathise or identify with the same cause or share ideas with this individual?"; "to what extent is my background similar or different to theirs?"; "to what extent do I believe what they did was ok or not ok?" This type of issue could also be mitigated by a newly emerging approach which explicitly seeks to control assessor bias and subjectivity by comparing and triangulating "in-the-head" knowledge (tacit knowledge based on experience, intuition, gut feelings) with "disciplinary" knowledge (the professional evidence base) and "analytical" knowledge (based on quantitative data). Discrepancies between these sources may expose a need for further evidence that will mitigate subjectivity and enhance professional judgement (Dean & Pettet, 2017).

Deception and the Absence of Behavioural Manifestations of Risk

The issue of deception is important because it has been argued that those who commit extremist offences are not as honest and open as those who commit other offences, and that their true risk may not be revealed in their outward behaviour, though this has not been empirically evidenced. But this does raises questions about how well assessors are able to detect and assess deception. It is argued that more emphasis should be placed on the ability to forensically probe, explore and investigate cognitions that include ideological beliefs and associated thinking. This raises questions about whether psychologists are competent to do this, or whether assessing beliefs requires nuanced theological or ideological knowledge.

Most assessors will be familiar with those who, in legal settings present in socially desirable ways but are deceptive, evasive, or fail to disclose information. For some of those who commit extremist offences, deception may be used as a specific tactic (some would say a military tactic) to avoid detection. Some will have received training or be self-educated in counter-surveillance and/or counter-interrogation techniques to deceive assessors and the authorities. This will degrade the amount, integrity, and quality of the information available to inform the assessment, potentially compromising its validity. However, such assumptions about deception on the part of the assessor in those known to be associated with a militarised group who adopt these tactics might also result, unfairly, in group attribution bias and risk aversion (Corneille et al., 2001).

Suggested mitigation can include the need for the assessor to thoroughly probe responses, be vigilant about inconsistencies in self-reported information, not over-rely on self-disclosure that cannot be independently evidenced, and specifically evaluate the individual's possible awareness of or training in counter-surveillance or interrogation techniques. Triangulation of information across different sources, contexts, and domains will be particularly important with these individuals, and the results of assessment should be reported tentatively in-light of the possibility of deception. It is of note that legislation was approved by HM government in 2021 authorising the use of polygraph assessments with those convicted of terrorist-related offences assessed as high or very high risk of causing serious harm, and who will be on licence in the community.

Expertise Regarding Social and Political Context

Another area of expertise associated with the assessment of extremist offending is an appreciation of its political and social context. Professionally, practitioner psychologists focus on the individual, and without due regard for the context of extremist offending can potentially overlook the role of ideology, group, or cause that is embedded in a wider geo-political forum. The Multi-Level Guidelines (MLG) are structured to ensure an appropriate focus on contextual issues by including risk factors at the individual, individual-group, group and group-societal level, in a nested ecological model (Cook et al., 2013). It includes the role of group dynamics such as violent leadership, violent group norms and group cohesion at the individual-group level, inter-group threat at the group level and the local and national context of conflicts abroad and government policies at the group-societal level. As previously mentioned, a full assessment requires a level of political awareness, sensitivity, and understanding of the issues of power, privilege, culture, race, and threat that provide the context to these offences and their assessment. Ignorance of contextual circumstances, misinterpreting them, or over-emphasising the role of individual pathology or personality may all contribute to attribution bias (Jones & Harris, 1967) and a less appreciative and complete assessment that lacks clarity about how future risk may be managed.

To mitigate this, assessors may need to develop their understanding of groups and their influence on behaviour, including the role of obedience to leadership and compliance with the violence norms of the group. In addition, it stresses the importance of collaborative assessment with those who have fuller intelligence about how the group operated and funded itself in the community, its structure, leadership and international links, its internal dynamics and methods of control. Whilst such an approach may not always be practical in some settings (Webster et al., 2017), it exemplifies how assessment can more systematically consider the impact of contextual factors on individual behaviour. Again, the Power, Threat, Meaning framework is well suited to identifying how individuals' engagement with ideologies, groups, or causes may be a survival response to cope with abuses of power within the context of their own lives. Likewise, its focus on working with individuals to help them negotiate their responses to context and agencies of power - without harming others – may also provide inspiration to those working in this field.

Assessor/Assessee Dynamics

As outlined previously, many of those who commit extremist offences are racially and culturally different to those who assess them, and are often of a different gender. This has the capacity to exacerbate in-group and outgroup thinking and reinforce outgroup homogeneity bias, in which individuals see members of groups to which they don't belong as being more like each other and different to their own group (Quattrone & Jones, 1980), though it also has the capacity to challenge stereotyped thinking if handled with insight (Lloyd & Dean, 2015). The danger is that all those who are convicted of terrorism-related offences are assumed to be the same, which can translate into perceiving their risk as the same regardless of the diversity of their offences. Where individual characteristics are judged to be different or "abnormal" they can also be seen as risky, or a cultural reticence about disclosing information or simply a lack of trust may unfairly impact on perceptions of riskiness, with non-disclosure being interpreted as possible deception.

To mitigate this, assessors need to be mindful and vigilant about actual and perceived similarities and differences between themselves and those they assess. They need to explicitly acknowledge these differences and focus on their clients as individuals, albeit also as members of a group. They should also consider very carefully whether and how the appearance, practices, activities, or beliefs of their clients are relevant to the assessment. This may mean explicitly asking them to clarify or explain these in their own words so their significance for engagement or intent can be evaluated. It might also involve assessors being culturally and/or racially matched to those being assessed, though in reality this degree of choice is rarely available. Assessors should be prepared from the outset to discuss openly the differences between them, and the individual being assessed, to build trust and prevent this negatively impacting their relationship and the assessment process.

Conclusion

A global wave of extremism, from Islamist to the Far Right, reflecting international asymmetries of power has been exposed by advances in communication technology that have created easy worldwide communication. As well as conferring advantage for some, these advances have also created grievance in others who perceive themselves as disadvantaged, disrespected, and victimised by the current world order, of whom a relatively small number have sought to advance their cause through violence. In this post-colonial world, issues of race and worth have risen to the surface, catalysed by recent events. These require greater awareness on the part of the West about issues that concern race, privilege, and power, not least in relation to understanding, assessing, and managing the risk of extremist offending.

This chapter has described how psychological assessment of extremist offending is particularly susceptible to bias, and specifically to issues associated with race and privilege that are intrinsic to extremist offending. Bias can influence the assessment process through terminology and the use of language, through the level of risk aversion created by large-scale terrorist attacks, by overlooking the role of context, and through subtle biases that demonise and homogenise this group. Assessment frameworks have been developed to assist in the task of making basic risk discriminations, but they are only as good as the skills and mind-set of the assessor. Significant progress remains to be made, and by making the role of implicit bias explicit and suggesting how it may be mitigated, we hope to contribute to this progress.

Notes

1 See Terrorism Act (2006).
2 https://www.adl.org/resources/backgrounders/the-great-replacement-an-explainer, accessed 2.9.21.
3 https://www.bps.org.uk/news-and-policy/ethical-guidelines-applied-psychological-practice-field-extremism-violent-extremism
4 https://ec.europa.eu/home-affairs/orphan-pages/page/ethical-guidelines-working-pcve-mental-health-care-2021_en
5 Other forms of criminal recidivism are estimated to be between 40% and 60% worldwide (Fazel & Wolf, 2015).
6 "Terrorism: Prisoners' release: written question – HL782, Answer by Lord Keen of Elie", U.K. House of Lords, February 11, 2020. https://www.parliament.uk/business/publications/written-questions-answers-statements/written-question/Lords/2020-01-27/HL782/
7 "Terrorism: Prisoners' release: written question – HL782, Answer by Lord Keen of Elie", U.K. House of Lords, February 11, 2020. https://www.parliament.uk/business/publications/written-questions-answers-statements/written-question/Lords/2020-01-27/HL782/

References

Altier, M. B., Boyle, E. L., Shortland, N. D., & Horgan, J. G. (2017). Why they leave: An analysis of terrorist disengagement events from eighty-seven autobiographical accounts. *Security Studies, 26*(2), 305–332. 10.1080/09636412.2017.1280307

Baron, R. S., Vandello, J. A. & Brunsman, B. (1996). The forgotten variable in conformity research: Impact of task importance on social influence. *Journal of Personality and Social Psychology 1996, 71*(5), 915–927. 10.1037/0022-3514.71.5.915

Bhui, K., Silva, M. J., Topciu, R. A., & Jones, E. (2016). Pathways to sympathies for violent protest and terrorism. *The British Journal of Psychiatry, 209*(6), 483–490. 10.1192/bjp.bp.116.185173

Bhui, K., Otis, M., Silva, M. J., Halvorsrud, K., Freestone, M., & Jones, E. (2019). Extremism and common mental illness: Cross-sectional community survey of White British and Pakistani men and women living in England. *The British Journal of Psychiatry, 217*(4), 1–8. https://psycnet.apa.org/doi/10.1192/bjp.2019.14

Bjørgo, T., & Horgan, J. (2009). *Leaving terrorism behind: Individual and collective disengagement.* Oxon, United Kingdom: Routledge. ISBN 9780415776684

Borum, R. (2011). Radicalization into violent extremism II: A review of conceptual models and empirical research. *Journal of Strategic Security, 4*(4), 37–62. 10.5038/1944-0472.4.4.2

Borum, R. (2015). Assessing risk for terrorism involvement. *Journal of Threat Assessment and Management, 2*(2), 63–87. https://psycnet.apa.org/doi/10.1037/tam0000043

Boyle, M., & Johnstone, L. (2020). *The power threat meaning framework: An alternative to psychiatric diagnosis.* Monmouth: PCCS Books. ISBN 9781910919712

Cook, A., Hart, S. D., & Kropp, P. R. (2013). *Multi level guidelines.* User Manual. Simon Fraser University & ProActive ReSolutions.

Cooke, D., & Michie, C. (2014). Violence risk assessment: Challenging the illusion of certainty. In B. McSherry & P. Keyser (Eds). *Managing high risk offenders: Policy and practice.* London: Routledge. ISBN 9781583911587

Corner, E., Taylor, H., Van Der Vegt, I., Salman, N., Rottweiler, B., Hetzel, F., Clemmow, C., Schulten, N., & Gill, P. (2021). Reviewing the links between violent extremism and personality, personality disorders, and psychopathy. *The Journal of Forensic Psychiatry & Psychology, 32*(3), 378–407. 10.1080/14789949.2021.1884736

Corneille, O., Yzerbyt, V. Y., Rogier, A., & Buidin, G. (2001). Threat and the group attribution error: When threat elicits judgments of extremity and homogeneity. *Personality and Social Psychology Bulletin, 27*(4), 437–446. 10.1177/0146167201274005. S2CID 17149379.

Crenshaw, M. (1981). The causes of terrorism. *Comparative Politics, 13*, 379–399. https://www.jstor.org/stable/i217462

Darley, J. M. (1966). Fear and social comparison as determinants of conformity behavior. *Journal of Personality and Social Psychology, 4*, 73–78. 10.1037/h0023508

Deutsch, M., & Gerard, H. B. (1955). A study of normative and informational social influences upon individual judgment. *Journal of Abnormal and Social Psychology, 51*, 629–636. https://psycnet.apa.org/doi/10.1037/h0046408

Dean, G., & Pettet, G. (2017). The 3 R's of risk assessment for violent extremism. *Journal of Forensic Practice, 19*(2), 91–101. 10.1108/JFP-07-2016-0029

Fein, R., Vossekuil, B., & Holden, G. (1995). *Threat assessment: An approach to prevent targeted violence.* Washington, DC: U.S. Department of Justice, Office of Justice Programs, National Institute of Justice, Publication NCJ 155000.

Fazel, S., & Wolf, A. (2015). A systematic review of criminal recidivism rates worldwide: Current difficulties and recommendations for best practices. *PLoS One, 10*(6), 1–8. 10.1371/journal.pone.0130390

Gill, P., Clemmow, C., Hetzel, F., Rottweiler, B., Salman, N., Van Der Vegt, I., Marchment, Z., Schumann, S., Zolghadriha, S., Schulten, N., Taylor, H., & Corner, E. (2021). Systematic review of mental health problems and violent extremism. *The Journal of Forensic Psychiatry & Psychology, 32*(1), 51–78. 10.1080/14789949.2020.1820067

Grubb, A., & Harrower, J. (2008). Attribution of blame in cases of rape: An analysis of participant gender, type of rape and perceived similarity to the victim. *Aggression and Violent Behavior, 13*(5), 396–405. doi:10.1016/j.avb.2008.06.006.

Hafez, M., & Mullins, C. (2015). The radicalization puzzle: A theoretical synthesis of empirical approaches to homegrown extremism. *Studies in Conflict & Terrorism, 38*(11), 958–975. 10.1080/1057610X.2015.1051375

Harris, G. T., & Rice, M. E. (2015). Progress in violence risk assessment and communication: Hypothesis versus evidence. *Behaviour Science and Law, 33*(1), 128–145. 10.1002/bsl.2157

Hart, S. D., & Cooke, D. J. (2013). Another look at the (im-)precision of individual risk estimates made using actuarial risk assessment instruments. *Behavioral Sciences and the Law, 31*, 81–102. 10.1002/bsl.2049

Hodwitz, O. (2021). The Terrorism Recidivism Study (TRS): Examining Recidivism Rates for Post-9/11 Offenders. *Perspectives on Terrorism, 13*(2), 54–64. ISSN 2334-3745

Jones, E. E., & Harris, V. A. (1967). The attribution of attitudes. *Journal of Experimental Social Psychology, 3*(1), 1–24. https://psycnet.apa.org/doi/10.1016/0022-1031(67)90034-0

Kahneman, D. (2011). *Thinking, Fast and Slow*, Straus and Giroux, Farrar, MO. ISBN 9780374533557

Knight, S., Woodward, K., & Lancaster, G. (2017). Violent versus nonviolent actors: An empirical study of different types of extremism. *Journal of Threat Assessment and Management, 4*(4), 230–248. https://psycnet.apa.org/doi/10.1037/tam0000086

Lerner, J. S., Gonzalez, R. M., Small, D. A., & Fischhoff, B. (2003). Effects of fear and anger on perceived risks of terrorism: A national field experiment. *Psychological Science, 14*(2), 144–150. 10.1111%2F1467-9280.01433

Logan, C., & Lloyd, M. (2018). Violent extremism: A comparison of approaches to assessing and managing risk. *Journal of Legal and Criminological Psychology*. 10.1111/lcrp.12140

Lloyd, M., & Dean, C. (2015). The development of structured guidelines for assessing risk in extremist offenders. *Journal of Threat Assessment and Management*, *2*(1), 40–52. https://psycnet.apa.org/doi/10.1037/tam0000035

Lloyd, M. (2019). Extremist risk assessments: A directory. *Centre for Research and Evidence in Security Threats*. https://crestresearch.ac.uk/resources/extremism-risk-assessment-directory/

McCauley, C., & Moskalenko, S. (2014). Towards a profile of lone wolf terrorists: What moves an individual from radical opinion to radical action. *Terrorism and Political Violence*, *26*, 69–85. 10.1080/09546553.2014.849916

Monahan, J. (2012). The individual risk assessment of terrorism. *Psychology, Public Policy, and Law*, *18*, 167–205. 10.1037/a0025792

Monahan, J. (2015). The individual risk assessment of terrorism: Recent developments. *Virginia Public Law and Legal Theory Research Paper*, *57*, 520–534.

Mynatt, C. R., Doherty, M. E., & Tweney, R. D. (1977). Confirmation bias in a simulated research environment: An experimental study of scientific inference. *Quarterly Journal of Experimental Psychology*, *29*(1), 85–95. https://psycnet.apa.org/doi/10.1080/00335557743000053

Pressman, E. D., & Flockton, J. (2012). Calibrating risk for violent political extremists and terrorists: The VERA 2 structured assessment. *The British Journal of Forensic Practice*, *14*, 237–251. 10.1108/14636641211283057

Quattrone, G. A., & Jones, E. E. (1980). The perception of variability within in-groups and out-groups: Implications for the law of small numbers. *Journal of Personality and Social Psychology*, *38*(1), 141–152. 10.1037/0022-3514.38.1.141

Renard (2020). Overblown: Exploring the Gap Between the Fear of Terrorist Recidivism and the Evidence. *CTC Sentinel*, *13*(4), 19–29.

Royal College of Psychiatrists. (2017). *Ethical considerations arising from the government's counter-terrorism strategy*. Position Statement PS04/16S. http://www.rcpsych.ac.uk/pdf/PS04_16S.pdf

Sageman, M. (2021). The Implication of Terrorism's Extremely Low Base Rate, *Terrorism and Political Violence*, *33*(2), 302–311. 10.1080/09546553.2021.1880226

Salman, N., & Gill, P. (2021). Terrorism risk assessment: What makes a good assessor? *CREST Security Review. Summer 2021* (Issue 11), 14–15.

Sarma, K. M. (2017). Risk assessment and the prevention of radicalization from non-violence into terrorism. *American Psychologist*, *72*(3), 278–288. https://psycnet.apa.org/doi/10.1037/amp0000121

Schwarz, N., Bless, H., Strack, F., Klumpp, G., Rittenauer-Schatka, H., & Simons, A. (1991). Ease of Retrieval as Information: Another Look at the Availability Heuristic. *Journal of Personality and Social Psychology*, *61*(2), 195–202. 10.1037/0022-3514.61.2.195

Silke, A. (2008). Cheshire-cat logic: The recurring theme of terrorist abnormality in psychological research. *Psychology, Crime, and Law*, *4*, 51–69. 10.1080/10683169808401747

Silke, A., & Morrison, J. (2020). Re-Offending by Released Terrorist Prisoners: Separating Hype from Reality. *International Centre for Counter-Terrorism – The Hague (ICCT)*. Policy Brief. https://icct.nl/publication/re-offending-by-released-terrorist-prisoners-separating-hype-from-reality/

Tajfel, H. (1974). Social identity and intergroup behaviour. *Social Science Information*, *13*, 65–93. 10.1177/053901847401300204

Van der Heide, L., & Schuurman, B. (2018). Reintegrating terrorists in the Netherlands: Evaluating the Dutch approach. *Journal for Deradicalization, 17,* 196–239.

Volkan, V. (2006). *Killing in the name of identity: A study of bloody conflicts.* Charlottesville, Virginia: Pitchstone Publishing. ISBN 0972887571

Webster, S., Kerr, J., & Tompkins, C. (2017). *A process evaluation of the structured risk guidance for extremist offenders.* Ministry of Justice Analytic Series. https://assets.publishing.service. gov.uk/government/uploads/system/uploads/attachment_data/file/661787/process-evaluation-srg-extremist-offender-report.pdf

Wolfowicz, M., Litmanovitz, Y., Weisburd, D., & Hasisi, B. (2019). A field-wide systematic review and meta-analysis of putative risk and protective factors for radicalization outcomes. *Journal of Quantitative Criminology.* https://psycnet.apa.org/doi/10. 1007/s10940-019-09439-4

Wolfowicz, M., Litmanovitz, Y., Weisburd, D., & Hasisi, B. (2021). Cognitive and behavioural radicalization: A systematic review of the putative risk and protective factors. *Campbell Collaboration Wiley.* 10.1002/cl2.1174

Yamagishi, T., & Mifune, N. (2009). Social exchange and solidarity: In-group love or out-group hate? *Evolution Human Behaviour, 30,* 229–237. 10.1016/j.evolhumbehav.2009.02.004

25 The Assessment of Psychopathy

Jenny Tew and Jacob Seaward

The idea of "the psychopath" has attracted much attention over many decades and across continents. It is viewed as important for criminal justice through links with a range of relevant outcomes, including increased risk of re-offending (e.g., Singh & Fazel, 2010) and problematic institutional behaviour (e.g., Langton et al., 2011). It also impacts the therapeutic climate of groups (Harkins et al., 2013) and the ability to complete and benefit from treatment (Olver et al., 2011). Although the relationships between psychopathy and these areas is variable and still debated (Larsen et al., 2020), understanding the nature of someone's traits can inform sentence management and treatment design (Tew et al., 2013). It therefore remains a relevant concept for forensic practice and one where effective assessment is beneficial.

A great deal has been written about psychopathy and it is not possible or necessary to cover all of this here, although it can be difficult to separate out the various challenges and debates. This chapter provides an overview of the theoretical and practical areas that have impact on assessment with the aim of furthering debate and promoting more informed practice.

It is worth noting some of the issues around the use of language in relation to psychopathy. We consider the use of "psychopath" to be unhelpfully stigmatising, and associated with extreme representations in popular culture and the media. Given the substantial evidence for the heterogeneity of the construct (Burt et al., 2016), the term is reductive, artificially suggesting a single presentation. Although not without issue, we use the term "psychopathy" to capture the concept in question, but consider this to encompass a range of actual presentations (McCallum et al., 2021).

The Concept of Psychopathy

To be able to operationalise and assess a concept, we must first have a coherent understanding and description of it. This is something that for psychopathy, despite the attention it receives, remains sadly lacking. Defining psychopathy has been described as one of the most fundamental questions for psychological science (Skeem et al. 2011). Indeed, there are puzzling contradictions; individuals are described as hostile and aggressive but also as having superficial emotions,

DOI: 10.4324/9781003230977-28

they are impulsive and reckless but also capable of elaborate scheming and manipulation (Skeem et al., 2011).

Although not the first person to write about psychopathy, Cleckley is often cited as the first person to systematically study it. He collated information on patients with similar presentations that engendered conflicting professional views. He identified 16 common traits which he felt described psychopathy. His work has shaped, directly or indirectly, several assessment measures (Lilienfeld et al., 2018).

Psychopathy is often spoken about in the language of the most commonly used tool directly derived from Cleckley's work; the Psychopathy Checklist Revised (PCL-R, Hare, 2003). It is, however, important to unpick the concept from this assessment. Psychopathy continues to be typically described in terms of a collection of cognitive, emotional, interpersonal, and behavioural characteristics that have impact on relationships and everyday functioning (Kiehl & Hoffman, 2011).

One model of psychopathy receiving increased attention over recent years is the Triarchic model (Patrick et al., 2009). This proposes three trait domains: boldness, meanness, and disinhibition. Within this model the boldness domain attracts most debate with it not being considered maladaptive or leading to impairment. This forms part of a wider discussion within the literature on the relevance or inclusion of adaptive traits to psychopathy. Several models of psychopathy have included elements that consistently exhibit positive correlations with markers of adaptive functioning (Hanniball et al., 2019).

Some have suggested that Triarchic model's boldness may actually mitigate against some of the negative outcomes associated with the meanness and disinhibition domains. It has also been suggested that interpersonal traits of psychopathy may protect against negative outcomes when antisocial strategies, such as instrumental violence, are reappraised as ineffective and the traits redirected towards pro-social goals (Burt et al., 2016). A related debate has been about whether criminality is part of the concept of psychopathy or whether it is an outcome, with a growing view that criminality is an outcome (e.g., Corrado et al., 2015).

There remains a counter view, however, that adaptive psychopathy is oxymoronic (Benning et al., 2018), given an inherent capacity to cause harm. The relevance of these potentially adaptive traits has been suggested to be through their interaction with other traits, with them combining with more problematic traits to provide the surface level charm and confidence (Cleckley's (1988) "mask"), potentially intensifying any negative outcomes. More research is therefore needed into if and how any seemingly positive aspects of psychopathy interact with other elements and contribute to the concept. It is possible that prevailing views of psychopathy may be impacting this debate, with people questioning the relevance of adaptive or successful traits to " … .. one of the more severe and dangerous personality disorders" (Hanniball et al., 2019, p. 349). Although clearly relevant, if researchers overly focus on dangerousness, there is an ongoing risk that any model, and therefore assessment, will not consider the concept holistically.

As with many conditions, the development of traits relevant to psychopathy appears to be multicausal, reflecting nature and nurture (Ribeiro da Silva et al.,

2020). Recent reviews indicate the effect of heritability may be moderate to high (e.g., Johanson et al., 2020). This is likely to be mediated by the environment, with some suggesting that psychopathy may be, at root, a developmental disorder (Ribeiro da Silva et al., 2020). Harsh child rearing, abuse, neglect, or the absence of warmth are significant risk factors for the development of psychopathic traits (Ribeiro da Silva et al., 2020); equally, positive parenting appears to moderate this (Lee & Kim, 2021). Adaptive traits (e.g., fearlessness) may develop towards less healthy alternatives (e.g., meanness) when functional attachment and socialisation are disrupted (Tuvblad et al., 2019). Hence, psychopathic traits may develop to protect individuals from emotions that would otherwise overwhelm them, enabling them to project an outward sense of invulnerability, fearlessness, and dominance (Ribeiro da Silva et al., 2020).

Assessing Psychopathy

Using any measure when the concept is still debated may be questionable, but assessment can also help develop our understanding of the concept. There are an increasing number of tools used to assess psychopathy, influenced by different perspectives on appropriate models and we touch on some of these below.

The Psychopathy Checklist Family of Assessments

Despite ongoing debates around the presence and definition of psychopathy, this is an area where one assessment tool has dominated practice and research. The PCL-R (second edition: Hare, 2003) is the most well-known and well-researched assessment of psychopathy. Reviewing information across a lifespan from collateral sources and an interview, this tool reviews functioning relative to 20 items believed by the authors to define psychopathy.

There has been debate in the literature regarding the factor structure of the PCL-R (Cooke & Michie, 2001; Hare, 1991, 2003), influenced by whether criminality is part or an outcome of psychopathy. The PCL-R's focus on criminality has led to the suggestion that tools cannot be used in the same way with forensic and non-forensic populations, contributing to why psychopathy may be seen as more common in forensic populations than non-forensic ones (Debowska et al., 2018).

In addition to the PCL-R there is a Psychopathy Checklist Screening version (PCL:SV; Hart et al., 1995). This is made up of 12 PCL-R items and was designed to identify individuals for further assessment with the PCL-R. However, given the PCL:SV still requires an interview and a review of records, little time is saved, particularly when a PCL-R is then recommended.

There is a youth version of the assessment, the PCL:YV (Forth et al., 2003) developed specifically for use with people aged 12 to 18. Items were adapted from the PCL-R to better capture how the traits and behaviours would be expressed in this population. There is much ongoing controversy around the assessment of personality in youths (Lee & Kim, 2021) which is relevant to the use of this tool but which cannot be covered in detail here. The PCL:YV aims to help understand and identify precursors to psychopathy in adulthood, identify potential risk and resilience factors, and promotes research and the early application of effective treatment approaches (Brazil & Forth, 2016).

Historically, PCL-R cut-off scores distinguished between "psychopaths" and "non-psychopaths" and research considered appropriate scores for different populations (Cooke & Michie, 1999; Cooke et al., 2005a; Hare, 2003). This could be viewed as a start to diversity considerations within the assessment of psychopathy. However, psychopathy is now viewed as being a continuum rather than a discrete taxon (e.g., Guay et al., 2007). This is in line with developments in wider psychiatric practice moving away from discrete diagnosis to focus on traits (Anckarsäter, 2010). Although cutoff scores may be less relevant to clinical practice this does not mean that issues of diversity are not relevant, and these are discussed later.

The Self-Report Psychopathy Scale (SRP-4; Paulhus et al., 2016) is a self-report measure analogous to the PCL-R. It comprises 64 items loading onto four subscales of interpersonal manipulation: callous affect, erratic lifestyle, and criminal tendencies. The SRP-4 is considered a good reflection of the PCL-R model of psychopathy and so has potential utility as an assessment where the PCL-R is not possible. Alternatively, the Levenson Self-report Psychopathy Scale (Levenson et al., 1995) and the Expanded Levenson Self-report Psychopathy Scale (ELSRP; Christian & Selbom, 2016) conceptually mirror the three-factor PCL-R structure proposed by Cooke and Michie (2001). There is also a Youth Psychopathic Traits Inventory (YPI; Andershed et al., 2002) which is a self-report measure also mirroring Cooke and Michie's three factor model.

CAPP

Although a PCL-R can be repeated in certain circumstances, it is not designed to measure change over time. Consequently, Cooke et al. (2012) developed the Comprehensive Assessment of Psychopathic Personality (CAPP). The CAPP aims to provide a comprehensive conceptual model of psychopathy independent of criminal behaviour. The authors provide a psychopathy concept map split into six domains: the self, attachment, emotional, behavioural, dominance, and cognitive domains and that aims to guide clinical formulation. This was designed to be over-inclusive to guide further research into the core components of psychopathy (Sellbom et al., 2021). There is a practitioner-led institutional rating scale comprising an interview and collateral information to assess 33 symptoms and more recently a self-report measure comprising 99 items (CAPP-SR; Sellbom & Cooke, 2020). As a tool rationally developed from theoretical, clinical, and research literature, the domains have not been confirmed through statistical methods (Sellbom et al., 2021).

DSM-5

The Diagnostic and Statistical Manual of Mental Disorders, Fifth Edition (DSM-5; American Psychiatric Association, 2013) Section III provides an alternative model for maladaptive personality with the intention of encouraging further research. This trait dimensional system considers maladaptive personality as impairments in self and interpersonal functioning (Criterion A) and then five broad domains of dimensional traits considered relevant to pathological personality (negative affect, disinhibition, antagonism, detachment, and psychoticism) structured into 25 facets. Within this model, Antisocial Personality Disorder (ASPD) has an increased focus on interpersonal and affective features and a psychopathy specifier. This specifier includes traits of attention seeking, low anxiousness, and low withdrawal and follows work emphasising fearlessness, boldness, and invulnerability within the construct (Dunne et al., 2019). This is operationalised using the Personality Inventory for DSM-5 (PID-5; Krueger et al., 2012). Although both the psychopathy specifier and PID-5 have attracted some criticism, they are as intended, contributing to the widening consideration of the construct and its measurement, including work looking at the DSM-5 characterisation of psychopathy through the triarchic model (Drislane et al., 2019).

Additional Self-Report Measures

The Triarchic Psychopathy Measure (TriPM; Patrick, 2010) is a 58-item self-report measure that considers the three domains of the Triarchic model. However, some have raised concerns about the extent to which the measure accords with the model (Roy et al., 2020).

Additionally, the Elemental Psychopathy Assessment (EPA, Lynam et al., 2011) is organised across 18 scales, from the perspective of the Five-Factor Model (FFM) of personality. A short form and super short form have also been developed (Lynam et al., 2013 and Collison et al., 2016, respectively).

The Psychopathic Personality Inventory Revised (PPI-R; Lilienfeld & Widows, 2005), measures 154 items across eight subscales. Developed with students this does not include explicit criminological items but includes some adaptive characteristics and considers more of the interpersonal traits. The PPI-R looks at features relating to "boldness", rather than "meanness" which the PCL-R is thought to measure. Researchers have consistently concluded that the PPI-R measures a different construct of psychopathy to the PCL-R (e.g., Copestake et al., 2011).

The Method of Assessment

Regardless of the model of psychopathy adopted and its impact on the content of any assessment, the actual method of assessment needs to be considered. Broadly speaking there are two options: practitioner-rated and self-report measures. Practitioner-rated assessments usually encompass a range of information sources including clinical interviews, observations, and collateral information and so are often considered the superior approach. This said, they are not without problems.

Research often reports high levels of inter-rater agreement in PCL-R scores (Hare, 2003). However, studies looking at PCL-R assessments completed in practice rather than research, found evidence partisan alliance influences outcomes (e.g., Blias & Forth, 2014) with prosecution assessments being routinely higher than defense ones. This has led to the suggestion that the strong predictive validity of the PCL-R in research may not represent what is happening in practice (Hare et al., 2018). Hare suggests that it is not the tool (in this case the PCL-R) at fault but the adversarial nature of legal proceedings and poor practice. He cites limited training and experience and improper use of the tool including not considering measurement error, not relating practice to current research and an inability or unwillingness to adhere to professional and ethical standards as the cause of differences (Hare, 2016).

Practitioner-rated assessments can be completed without interview and so do not necessitate individual cooperation, although this can impact outcomes (Serin, 1993). However, sufficient good quality collateral information is not always available, meaning they are not always feasible. In addition, practitioner-rated assessments are completed on an individual basis by highly trained assessors. They are therefore necessarily resource intensive to complete with need often outweighing the resources available.

In contrast, self-report measures are quick and easy to complete, with minimal training required and no need for extensive collateral information. Self-report assessments also do not require assessors to make subjective judgments about aspects of the individual that are not readily observable (e.g., having a lack of empathy; Lilienfeld & Fowler, 2006). They do, however, require individual co-operation which is not always granted.

Practitioners may intuitively avoid using self-report assessments when considering psychopathy given traits such as deceitfulness. Indeed, some have explicitly advised against their use in forensic settings (Ray et al., 2013) due to the particular vested interest in manipulation. However, several such measures exist and research has shown that individuals with high levels of relevant traits can have good insight into their personality and report traits accurately, relative to informant reports, particularly when there are no personal consequences (Miller et al., 2011). This suggests that the timing of self-report assessments should be considered. Also, how any findings can best support individual need should be clearly communicated at the outset.

It is promising, despite the stark difference between the two approaches, that some researchers have found high levels of convergence between them (e.g., Kelley et al., 2017). Circumstances may well then determine which approach to assessment is taken, although some have suggested that self-report assessments may be an efficient supplement to practitioner assessments (Ray et al., 2013).

Individual Factors Impacting Assessment

To better understand individual presentations of psychopathy, a number of additional factors should be considered by the practitioner. These include gender, cognitive functioning, culture, and ethnicity. Other potentially relevant variables either await further research (e.g., sexual and gender identity), or may be best understood within a developmental framework (e.g., age) and are outside the scope of this chapter.

Gender

The existing research into gender does not routinely distinguish between gender as a socio-cultural construction, and sex as a marker for biological and genetic inheritance (Nicholls & Petrila, 2005); similarly, the impact of fluid, non-binary identities on the expression of psychopathy, as well as their developmental interaction, is likely to be an important topic for future understanding.

Research into gender and psychopathy has shown that, although degrees of heritability and environmental influence are similar across genders, prevalence rates are markedly lower in females across all populations and age ranges (Tuvblad et al., 2019). Part of the explanation appears to be that psychopathy expresses itself differently in women (Forouzan & Cooke, 2005), reflecting both biological variation and gendered socialisation (Kreis & Cooke, 2011). A greater preference for relational aggression has been observed in women (Kreis & Cooke, 2011) as well as the use of indirect strategies to achieve goals (e.g., flirtation and sexuality; Kreis & Cooke, 2012). There is a particular relationship in females between the interpersonal aspects of psychopathy and use of indirect aggression, and between the affective aspects and the use of physical aggression (Thomson et al., 2020). The pathway for the latter appears to be the experience of traumatic abuse, with affective traits associated with physical aggression specifically in women with histories of lifetime physical abuse (Thomson 2019). It has been suggested that highly traumatised women develop a disposition that superficially resembles psychopathy in its affective aspects but is not linked to the wider construct (Odgers et al., 2005); others consider psychopathy has a more common emotionally unstable presentation in females than in males (Verona & Vitale, 2018).

These different possibilities must be considered within assessments. It should be carefully evaluated whether particular presentational differences reflect the gendered aspects of psychopathy, are comorbidities with other disorders, or have different origins entirely. An implicit bias in the available tools must also be considered, and whether lower incidence of psychopathy is an artefact of assessments mainly developed using male samples. Practitioners should therefore take due care when assessing female presentations of psychopathy.

Cognitive Functioning

Although Cleckley considered intact intelligence to be characteristic of psychopathy and its "mask", a relationship between the two variables has either not been found (Boccio & Beaver, 2018), or has been shown to be mildly negative (de Ribera et al., 2019). As reduced volume and connectivity in the prefrontal cortex is associated with higher assessed levels of psychopathy and lower scores on intelligence tests, this may provide an explanation (Kavish et al., 2018).

Specific relationships have been found between particular aspects of psychopathy and domains of cognitive functioning. Overall cognitive ability shows a small positive relationship with interpersonal aspects of psychopathy, and a weak negative relationship with affective aspects (de Ribera et al., 2019). It has further been shown that some deficits typically attributed to the affective aspects (e.g., emotional perception ability) may actually be related to overall cognitive ability, which is often left untested (Olderbak et al., 2018). The impulsive lifestyle aspects of psychopathy have consistently been related to lower levels of overall cognitive ability (Kavish et al., 2021). Although there have been fewer studies, the pattern in women has essentially been similar (Thomson et al., 2020).

Current research therefore highlights a potential confound between elements of psychopathy and cognitive ability, and it is unclear whether relationships are primarily correlational. This could mean that cognitive impairments (or strengths) might sometimes be interpreted through the frame of psychopathy. Moreover, in cases where psychopathy corresponds with above average cognitive ability, it is important to consider whether this operates like Cleckley's mask in concealing and enabling any harmful aspects, or may instead work adaptively (Lillienfeld et al., 2015). Overall, this raises questions around assessing psychopathy in isolation from cognitive ability.

Culture

Culture is important in forensic personality assessment. Although sometimes conflated with concepts of "race" and "ethnicity", "culture" is generally considered a more sensitive term as it has a broad, flexible application to all humans and their histories (Strauss-Hughes et al., 2019), while still being inclusive of the significant diversity involved.

In a series of early studies, Cooke and colleagues (e.g., Cooke et al., 2004; Cooke et al., 2005a, 2005b) attempted to quantify this variation, albeit between relatively homogenised cultures of Western Europe and North America. Interpersonal aspects of psychopathy showed most cultural variation and were most evident at higher levels of traits, suggesting these were particularly culturally determined. The impulsive lifestyle aspects showed a lower degree of cultural variation, and discriminated well only at low levels of psychopathy, suggesting cultural influence but one not necessarily distinct to psychopathy. Finally, the aspects reflecting impaired emotional experience showed fewest cross-cultural differences and were suggested to be psychopathy's "pan-cultural core" (Cooke et al., 2005b, p. 292). Recently a different methodology (Verschuere et al. 2018) has again demonstrated the centrality of affective traits across several US samples. However this was different in a Dutch sample, which instead emphasised the centrality of items reflecting deviations from societal obligation, illustrating the impact of differences in cultural and behavioural norms.

Culture is an important factor to consider regardless of the assessment used, and practitioners should interpret someone's presentation within their own context of cultural norms and influences. Individuals are often nested within multiple cultural systems (Schmidt et al., 2021), and these influences are likely to be multi-facetted, diverse, and conflicting. Determining whether differences on personality measures equate to actual cultural differences in behaviour is therefore challenging, requiring other hypotheses to first be excluded.

These differences also impact the practitioner. Schmidt et al. (2021, section 4.1.1) highlight that an individual's "cultural traits" will "direct [their] attention towards certain kinds of cues, encourage the experience of culturally normative emotions, promote certain kinds of goals, and highlight certain behavioural regulation systems", and so provide an interpretative optic. This is particularly germane to those who use interviews, where close attention is paid to interpersonal style, emotional display, and behavioural norms.

Emotional display provides one example. Rules for emotional display are culturally defined (e.g., Safdar et al., 2009), as are other non-verbal behaviours such as body language, eye contact, and facial expressivity; to consider these through the norms of a different culture can therefore lead to misinterpretations (Weiss & Rosenfeld, 2012). Although the cultural traits of the client influence what they "display", the assessor's characteristics also influence what they perceive and understand about that display. As the practitioner is already primed to understand the client's emotional responses in terms of psychopathy, any deviations from their own norms may be understood in terms of this and alternative explanations not considered.

In the end, it is impossible to step outside of culture. It is therefore critical for practitioners to be reflexive about their own cultural heritage and learning, seek alternative hypotheses for unusual presentations, and examine assumptions behind interpretations.

Ethnicity

Although culture is considered a more helpful focus than ethnicity there are some specific ethnicity considerations worth noting. Research generally shows few differences among Caucasian, Hispanic, or Aboriginal individuals in the measurement of psychopathy. However, ethnicity does seem to moderate the relationship among psychopathy, antisocial outcomes, impulsivity, and cognitive processing (for a summary see Gatner et al., 2018). There is some indication this is particularly the case for African Americans, who have sometimes shown slightly higher levels of psychopathy (e.g., Cooke et al., 2001). Some have therefore argued for ethnic differences in psychopathy (DeLisi, 2018), but as this argument has relied on other antisocial indicators as indexes for psychopathy, there are likely to be other explanations, not least environmental factors (Threadcraft-Walker & Henderson, 2018), and there is a growing interest in the intersection of ethnicity with other relevant demographic variables in the presentation of psychopathy (e.g., Anestis et al., 2019). It should be noted that much research in this area uses assessments from the PCL-R family. Although there have been similar findings across other measures (e.g., PPI), the PCL-R was found to produce the fewest ethnicity-based differences (Gatner et al., 2018).

Some research, using the Triarchic model, while again finding slightly higher psychopathy levels and increased adverse outcomes for the African American group, notes that the "boldness" factor, often seen as adaptive or as reflecting Cleckley's "mask", appeared to show reduced impact in this group (Anestis et al., 2019), suggesting it may have been interpreted more negatively. This all suggests that ethnicity may have some impact on the presentation of psychopathy but the nature of this and its relevance to specific assessment tools and approaches requires further investigation.

Implications for Practice

As psychologists must base their practice on scientific evidence the debates surrounding psychopathy and the range of models presents some challenges. Ultimately, the most appropriate method of assessment and model of psychopathy may determine the best tool to use. Although the range of available assessments continues to increase, the evidence base for any tool, particularly in relation to reliability and validity remains critical to consider, including the availability of suitable normative groups.

Any assessment of psychopathy, using psychometric measurement, may on its own be insufficient, as quantification is not explanation. This is not to disregard the substantial evidence base for measures such as the PCL-R, but to argue that they provide a start rather than end point. It has been increasingly recognised that the next step is one of formulation, including the development of individual personality functioning and specifying the nature of the link between this and the outcomes of concern (Cooke et al., 2012). The goal should ultimately be to understand how and why the individual developed relevant traits, the factors that have a bearing on their manifestation and the relationship with functional impairment. More adaptive characteristics should also be considered. Within the forensic setting this is considered in the context of understanding risk and relevant responsivity factors; it is therefore to understand psychopathy as one factor informing a broader, but individually specific risk.

Some tools naturally lend themselves to this, for example, the CAPP. This enables concerns about the differential "topography" of traits according to factors such as culture, gender, age, and cognitive functioning to be accounted for through flexible and sensitive application of relevant indicators (Cooke & Logan, 2015). However, other tools, such as the PCL-R require more effort to achieve this. The dominance of the PCL-R in the field has contributed to an ongoing negative focus for psychopathy in forensic practice given its emphasis on negative traits and negative indicators of them. This requires practitioners to make a conscious effort to formulate findings constructively to support engagement in subsequent risk management or treatment plans.

Psychopathy could be considered unique amongst psychological disorders in that individuals are not considered to "suffer" from psychopathy. The disorder itself often does not directly cause distress to the individual, although the individual may cause significant distress to others. This may affect attitudes towards those assessed, for whom it may be hard to feel empathy. Practitioners should consider the role of early adversity and the possibility that psychopathy, particularly affective and interpersonal aspects, develops as a result of the self-overcoming of traumas. It may be that the Power Threat Meaning Framework (Johnstone & Boyle, 2018, see chapter 12), offers a relevant supplementary approach here.

It is also important to be mindful of the potential negative impacts of psychopathy assessment. Although there is a risk of stigmatisation associated with personality disorder in general, this is particularly true for psychopathy given how it is often portrayed and its connection to criminality. Berryessa and Wohlstetter (2019) found the label of "Psychopathy" brought support for more punitive legal sanctions, increased perceptions of dangerousness and therapeutic pessimism, although effect sizes were small and mediated by factors such as age. Such a label impacts how individuals are treated within the criminal-justice system, both at court and by those administering resulting sentences.

Although this response was when a label was applied, it is possible that the knowledge an individual has even had a psychopathy assessment impacts on how they are viewed and treated. Given assessments are often only completed when a concept is thought relevant, then the consideration of psychopathy may itself contribute to negative perceptions. It is therefore critical that practitioners are aware of the relevant issues and debates and communicate findings appropriately, with a focus on an individual's relevant traits likely to be most effective.

Conclusion

It is clear that different purposes for psychopathy assessment impact the different aspects of the concept and model focused on and therefore, the choice of tools used. Although there is ongoing debate around psychopathy there are also some elements of consistency within the literature. It is positive that the research field is widening its perspective when considering psychopathy and that this, along with other research into areas such as personality, assessment, and desistance from crime, is starting to influence forensic practice. This brings a welcomed increased focus on diversity in both theory and practice. It is hoped that this continues, and forensic practice becomes better; able to unpick the concept of psychopathy and the assessments chosen to assess it. As part of this, it is important for practitioners to remain aware of the potential for the assessment of psychopathy itself to lead to bias and to retain a constructive and holistic approach to formulate and report any assessment findings. This includes taking into account individual factors considered in this chapter, such as culture, gender, and cognitive ability, to better understand the differences in and diversity of psychopathy presentations.

References

American Psychiatric Association. (2013). *Diagnostic and statistical manual of mental disorders* (5th ed.) Arlington, VA: American Psychiatric Publishing.

Anckarsäter, H. (2010). Beyond categorical diagnostics in psychiatry: scientific and methodological implications. *International Journal of Law and Psychiatry, 33*, 59–65.

Andershed, H., Kerr, M., Stattin, H., & Levander, S. (2002). Psychopathic traits in non-referred youths: a new assessment tool. In E. Blau & L. Sheridan (Eds.), *Psychopaths: Current international perspectives* (pp. 131–158). Amsterdam, Netherlands: Elsevier.

Anestis, J. C., Prestona, O. C., Harropa, T. M., & Sellbom, M. (2019). The intersection of sociodemographic characteristics within the nomological network of the triarchic psychopathy model in a forensic sample. *Journal of Criminal Justice, 61*, 13–25.

Benning, S. D., Venables, N. C., & Hall, J. R. (2018). Successful psychopathy. In C. J. Patrick (Ed.), *Handbook of psychopathy* (2nd ed, pp. 585–608). The Guilford Press.

Berryessa, C. M., & Wohlstetter, B. (2019). The Psychopathic "label" and effects on punishment outcomes: a meta-analysis. *Law and Human Behavior, 43*, 9–25.

Blias, J., & Forth, A. E. (2014). Prosecution-retained versus court-appointed experts: comparing and contrasting risk assessment reports in preventative detention hearings. *Law and Human Behaviour, 38*, 531–543.

Blais, J., Forth, A. E., & Hare, R. D. (2017). Examining the Interrater Reliability of the Hare Psychopathy Checklist—Revised across a large sample of trained raters. *Psychological Assessment, 29*(6), 762–775.

Brazil, K., & Forth, A. (2016). Psychopathy Checklist: Youth Version (PCL:YV). In V. Zeigler-Hill & T. K. Shackelford (Eds.), *Encyclopedia of Personality and Individual Differences?*. Springer International Publishing.

Boccio, C. M., & Beaver, K. M. (2018). Psychopathic personality traits and the successful criminal. *International Journal of Offender Therapy and Comparative Criminology, 62*(15), 4834–4853.

Burt, G. N., Olver, M. E., & Wong, S. C. P. (2016). Investigating characteristics of the nonrecidivating psychopathic offender. *Criminal Justice and Behavior, 43* (120), 1741–1760.

Christian, E., & Sellbom, M. (2016). Development and validation of an expanded version of the three-factor Levenson Self-Report Psychopathy Scale. *Journal of Personality Assessment, 98*(2), 155–168.

Cleckley, H. (1988). *The mask of sanity.* (5th Ed.). St Louis: Mosby.

Collison, K. L., Miller, J. D., Gaughan, E. T., Widiger, T. A., & Lynam, D. R. (2016). Development and validation of the super-short form of the elemental psychopathy assessment. *Journal of Criminal Justice, 47*, 143–150.

Cooke, D. J., Hart, S. D., Logan, C., & Michie, C. (2012). Explicating the construct of psychopathy: development and validation of a Conceptual Model, the Comprehensive Assessment of Psychopathic Personality (CAPP). *International Journal of Forensic Mental Health, 11*(4), 242–252.

Cooke, D. J., Hart, S. D., & Michie, C. (2004). Cross-national differences in the assessment of psychopathy: do they reflect variations in raters' perceptions of symptoms? *Psychological Assessment, 16*(3), 335–339.

Cooke, D. J., Kosson, D. S., & Michie, C. (2001). Psychopathy and ethnicity: Structural, item, and test generalisability of the Psychopathy Checklist – Revised (PCL—R) in Caucasian and African American participants. *Psychological Assessment, 13*(4), 531–542.

Cooke, D. J., & Logan, C. (2015). Capturing clinical complexity: towards a personality-oriented measure of psychopathy. *Journal of Criminal Justice, 43*(4), 262–273.

Cooke, D. J., & Michie, C. (1999). Psychopathy across cultures: North America and Scotland compared. *Journal of Abnormal Psychology, 108*, 58–68. DOI:10.1037//0021-843X.108.1.58

Cooke, D. J., & Michie, C. (2001). Refining the construct of psychopathy: toward a hierarchical model. *Psychological Assessment, 13*, 171–188. DOI: 10.1037/1040-3590.13.2.171

Cooke, D. J., Michie, C., Hart, S. D., & Clark, D. (2005a). Assessing psychopathy in the UK: concerns about cross-cultural generalisability. *British Journal of Psychiatry, 186*, 335–341.

Cooke, D. J., Michie, C., Hart, S. D., & Clark, D. (2005b). Searching for the pan-cultural core of psychopathic personality disorder. *Personality and Individual Differences, 39*, 283–295.

Copestake, S., Gray, N. S., & Snowden, R. J. (2011). A comparison of a self report measure of psychopathy with the Psychopathy Checklist-Revised in a UK sample of offenders. *The Journal of Forensic Psychiatry and Psychology, 22*, 169–182.

Corrado, R. R., DeLisi, M., Hart, S. D., & McCuish, C. (2015). Can the causal mechanisms underlying chronic, serious and violent offending trajectories be elucidated using the psychopathy construct? *Journal of Criminal Justice, 43*, 251–261.

Debowska, A., Boduszek, D., Dhingra, K., Sherretts, N., Willmott, D., & DeLisi, M. (2018). Can we use Hare's psychopathy model within forensic and non-forensic populations? An Empirical investigation. *Deviant Behavior, 39*(2), 224–242.

DeLisi, M. (2018). Race and (antisocial) personality. *Journal of Criminal Justice, 59*, 32–37.

de Ribera, O. S., Kavish, N., Katz, I. M., & Boutwell, B. B. (2019). Untangling intelligence, psychopathy, antisocial personality disorder, and conduct problems: a meta-analytic review. *European Journal of Personality, 33*(5), 529–564.

Drislane, L. E., Sellbom, M., Brislin, S. J., Strickland, C. M., Christian, E., Wygant, D. B., Krueger, R. F., & Patrick, C. J. (2019). Improving characterization of psychopathy within the Diagnostic and Statistical Manual of Metal Disroders, fifth edition (DSM-5), alternative model for personality disorder: creation and validation of Personality Inventory for DSM-5 Triarchic Scales. *Persoality Disorders: Theory, Research and Treatment, 10*(6), 511–523.

Dunne, A. L., Lloyd, C., Lee, S., & Daffern, M. (2019). Associations between the Diagnostic and Statistical Manual of Mental Disorders, fifth edition, alternative model of antisocial personality disorder, psychopathic specifier and psychopathy related facets with aggression in a sample of incarcerated males. *Personality Disorder: Theory, Research and Treatment, 11*(2), 108–118.

Forouzan, E., & Cooke, D. J. (2005). Figuring out la femme fatale: conceptual and assessment issues concerning psychopathy in females. *Behavioral Sciences and the Law, 23*(6), 765–778.

Forth, A. E., Kosson, D. S., & Hare, D. (2003). *The hare psychopathy checklist: youth version.* Toronto: Multi-Health Systems.

Gatner, D. T., Blanchard, A. J. E., Douglas, K. S., Lilienfeld, S. O., & Edens, J. F. (2018). Psychopathy in a multiethnic world: imnvestigating multiple measures of psychopathy in Hispanic, African American, and Caucasian Offenders. *Assessment, 25*(2), 206–221.

Guay, J., Ruscio, J., Knight, R. A., & Hare, R. D. (2007). A taxometric analysis of the latent structure of psychopathy: evidence for dimensionality. *Journal of Abnormal Psychology, 116*, 701–716.

Hanniball, K. B., Gatner, D. T., Douglas, K. S., Viljoen, J. L., & Aknin, L. B. (2019). Examining the Triarchic psychopathy measure and comprehensive assessment of psychopathic personality in self-identified offender populations. *Persoality Disorders: Theory, Research and Treatment, 10*(4), 340–353.

Hare, R. D. (1991). *Hare Psychopathy Checklist-Revised (PCL-R).* Toronto, Ontario, Canada: Multi-Health Systems.

Hare, R. D. (2003). *Hare Psychopathy Checklist-Revised (PCL-R): 2nd edition.* Canada, Toronto: Multi-Health Systems Inc.

Hare, R. D. (2016). Psychopathy, the PCL-R and criminal justice: some new findings and current issues. *Canadian Psychology, 57*(1), 21–34.

Hare, R. D., Neumann, C. S., & Mokros, A. (2018). The PCL-R assessment of psychopathy: development, properties, debates, and new directions. In C. J. Patrick (Ed.), *Handbook of psychopathy* (2nd ed, pp. 39–79). The Guilford Press.

Harkins, L., Beech, A. R., & Thornton, D. (2013). The influence of risk and psychopathy on the therapeutic climate in sex offender treatment. *Sexual Abuse: A Journal of Research and Treatment, 25,* 103–122. DOI: 10.1177/1079063212443384

Hart, S. D., Cox, D. N., & Hare, R. D. (1995). *Manual for the Hare Psychopathy Checklist: Screening Version.* Toronto, Ontario, Canada: Multi-Health Systems Inc.

Johanson M., Vaurio O., Tiihonen J., & Lähteenvuo M. (2020). A systematic literature review of neuroimaging of psychopathic traits. *Frontiers in Psychiatry, 10,* 1027.

Johnstone, L., & Boyle, M. (2018). The power threat meaning framework: an alternative nondiagnostic conceptual system. *Journal of Humanistic Psychology.* 10.1177/002216781 8793289

Kavish, N., Bailey, C., Sharp, C., & Venta, A. (2018). On the relation between general intelligence and psychopathic traits: an examination of inpatient adolescents. *Child Psychiatry & Human Development, 49,* 341–351.

Kavish, N., Bergstrøm, H., Narvey, C., Piquero, A. R., Farrington, D. P., & Boutwell, B. B. (2021). Examining the association between childhood cognitive ability and psychopathic traits at Age 48. *Personality Disorders: Theory, Research, and Treatment, 12*(1), 81–85.

Kelley, S. E., Edens, S. E., Donnellan, J. F., Mowle, M. B., & Sorman, K. (2017). Self and informant perceptions of psychopathic traits in relation to the triarchic model. *Journal of Personality, 86,* 738–751.

Kiehl, K. A., & Hoffman, M. B. (2011). The criminal psychopath: history, neuroscience, treatment, and economics. *Jurimetrics, Journal of Law, Science, and Technology, 51,* 355–397.

Kreis, M. K. F., & Cooke, D. J. (2011). Capturing the psychopathic female: a prototypicality analysis of the Comprehensive Assessment of Psychopathic Personality (CAPP) across gender. *Behavioral Sciences and the Law, 29*(5), 634–648.

Kreis, M. K. F., & Cooke, D. J. (2012). The manifestation of psychopathic traits in women: an exploration using case examples. *International Journal of Forensic Mental Health, 11*(4), 267–279.

Krueger, R. F., Derringer, J., Markon, K. E., Watson, D., & Skodol, A. E. (2012). Initial construction of a maladaptive personality trait model and inventory for DSM-5. *Psychological Medicine, 42,* 1879–1890.

Langton, C. M., Hogue, T. E., Daffern, M., Mannion, & Howells, K. (2011). Personality traits as predictors of inpatient aggression in a high-security forensic psychiatric setting: prospective evaluation of the PCL-R and IPDE dimension rating. *International Journal of Offender Therapy and Comparative Criminology, 55*(3), 392–415.

Larsen, R. R., Jalava, J., & Griffiths, S. (2020). Are Psychopathy Checklist (PCL) psychopaths dangerous, untreatable and without conscience? A systematic review of the empirical Evidence. *Psychology, Public Policy and Law, 26*(3), 297–311.

Lee, Y., & Kim, J. (2021). Psychopathic traits among serious juvenile offenders: developmental pathways, multidimensionality, and stability. *Crime & Delinquency, 67*(1), 82–110.

Levenson, M. R., Kiehl, K. A., & Fitzpatrick, C. M. (1995). Assessing psychopathic attributes in a noninstitutionalized population. *Journal of Personality and Social Psychology, 68,* 151–158.

Lilienfeld, S. O., & Fowler, K. A. (2006). The self-report assessment of psychopathy: problems, pitfalls and promises. In C. J. Patrick (Ed.), *Handbook of psychopathy*. (pp. 107–132). London: The Guilford Press.

Lilienfeld, S.O., Watts, A. L., & Smith, S. F. (2015). Successful psychopathy. *Current Directions in Psychological Science*, 24, 298–303. 10.1177/0963721415580297

Lilienfeld, S. O., Watts, A. L., Smith, S. F., Patrick, C. J., & Hare, R. D. (2018). Hervey Cleckley (1903-1984): Contributions to the study of psychopathy. *Personality Disorders: Theory, Research and Treatment, 9*(6), 510–520.

Lilienfeld, S. O., & Widows, M. (2005). *Psychopathic Personality Inventory – Revised: Professional Manual*. Lutz, Florida: Psychological Assessment Resources Inc.

Lynam, D. R., Gaughan, E. T., Miller, J. D., Miller, D. J., Mullins-Sweatt, S., & Widiger, T. A. (2011). Assessing the basic traits associated with psychopathy: development and validation of the Elemental Psychopathy Assessment. *Psychological Assessment, 23*(1), 108–124.

Lynam, D. R., Sherman, E. D., Samuel, D., Miller, J. D., Few, L. R., & Widiger, T. A. (2013). Development of a short form of the Elemental Psychopathy Assessment. *Assessment, 20*(6), 659–669.

McCallum, K. E., Boccaccini, M. T., Varela, J. G., & Turner, D. B. (2021). Psychopathy profiles and personality assessment inventory scores in a sex offender risk assessment field setting. *Assessment*, 10.1177/10731911211015312

Miller, J. D., Jones, S. E., & Lynam, D. R. (2011). Psychopathic traits from the persepctive of self and informant reports: is there evidence for a lack of insight? *Journal of Abnormal Psychology, 3*, 758–764.

Nicholls, T. L., & Petrila, J. (2005). Gender and psychopathy: an overview of important issues and introduction to the special issue. *Behavioral Sciences and the Law, 23*(6), 729–741.

Odgers, C. L., Reppucci, N. D., & Moretti, M. M. (2005). Nipping psychopathy in the bud: an examination of the convergent, predictive, and theoretical utility of the PCL-YV among adolescent girls. *Behavioral Sciences and the Law, 23*(6), 743–763.

Olderbak, S. G., Mokros, A., Nitschke, J., Habermeyer, E., & Wilhelm, O. (2018). Psychopathic men: deficits in general mental ability, not emotion perception. *Journal of Abnormal Psychology, 127*(3), 294–304.

Olver, M. E., Neumann, C. S., Sewall, L. A., Lewis, K., Hare, R. D., & Wong, S. C. P. (2018). A comprehensive examination of the psychometric properties of the Hare Psychopathy Checklist-Revised in a Canadian multisite sample of indigenous and non-indigenous offenders. *Psychological Assessment*, 30(6), 779–792.

Olver, M. E., Stockdale, K. C., & Wormith, J. S. (2011). A meta-analysis of predictors of offender treatment attrition and its relationship to recidivism. *Journal of Consulting and Clinical Psychology, 79*, 6–21.

Patrick, C. J. (2010). Triarchic psychopathy measure (TriPM). Retrieved from https://patrickcnslab.psy.fsu.edu/wiki/index.php/Triarchic_Psychopathy_Measure

Patrick, C. J., Fowles, D. C., & Krueger, R. F. (2009). Triarchic conceptualization of psychopathy: developmental origins of disinhibition, boldness and meanness. *Development and Psychopathology, 21*, 913–938.

Paulhus, D. L., Neumann, C. S., & Hare, R. D. (2016). *Manual for the Self-report Psychopathy Scale*. Toronto: Multi-Health Systems.

Ray, J. V., Hall, J., Rivera-Hudson, N., Poythress, N. G., Lilienfeld, S. O., & Morano, M. (2013). The relation between self-reported psychopathic traits and distorted response styles: a meta-analytic review. *Personality Disorders: Theory, Research, and Treatment, 4*, 1–14.

Ribeiro da Silva, D., Rijo, D., & Salekin, R. T. (2020). Psychopathic traits in children and youth: the state-of-the-art after 30 years of research. *Aggression and Violent Behavior, 55,* Article 101454. 10.1016/j.avb.2020.101454

Roy, S., Vize, C., Uzieblo, K., van Dongen, J. D. M., Miller, J., Lynam, D., Brazil, I., Yoon, D., Mokros, A., Gray, N. S., Snowdon, R., & Neumann, C. S. (2020). Triarchic or Septarchic? Uncovering the Triarchic Psychopathy Measure's (TriPM) structure. *Personality Disorders: Theory, Research and Treatment, 12*(1), 1–15.

Safdar, S., Friedlmeier, W., Matsumoto, D., Yoo, S. H., Kwantes, C. T., Kakai, H., & Shigemasu, E. (2009). Variations of emotional display rules within and across cultures: a comparison between Canada, USA, and Japan. *Canadian Journal of Behavioural Science, 41*(1), 1–10.

Schmidt, S., Heffernan, R., & Ward, T. (2021). The cultural agency-model of criminal behavior. *Aggression and Violent Behavior, 58,* 101554.

Sellbom, M., & Cooke, D. J. (2020). *Manual for the Comprehensive Assessment of Psychopathic Personality – Self-report (CAP-SR).* Unpublished manual. Dunedin, New Zealand.

Sellbom, M., Liggins, C., Laurinaityte, I., & Cooke, D. J. (2021). Factor structure of the Comprehensive Assessment of Psychopathic Personality Self-Report (CAPP-SR) in community and offender samples. *Psychological Assessment.* Advanced online publication. 10.1037/pas0001029.

Serin, R. C. (1993). Diagnosis of psychopathy with and without an interview. *Journal of Clinical Psychology, 49*(3), 367–372.

Singh, J. P., & Fazel, S. (2010). Forensic risk assessment: a metareview. *Criminal Justice and Behavior, 37,* 965–988.

Skeem, J. L., Polascheck, D. L. L., Patrick, C. J., & Lilienfeld, S. O. (2011). Psychopathic personality: bridging the gap between scientific evidence and public policy. *Psychological Science in the Public Interest, 12*(3), 95–162.

Strauss-Hughes, A., Heffernan, R., & Ward, T. (2019). A cultural–ecological perspective on agency and offending behaviour. *Psychiatry, Psychology and Law, 26*(6), 938–958.

Tew, J., Harkins, L., & Dixon, L. (2013). What works in reducing violent reoffending in psychopathic offenders. In L. A. Craig, L. Dixon, & T. A. Gannon (Eds.) *What Works in Offender Rehabilitation: An Evidenced Based Approach to Assessment and Treatment* (pp. 129–141). Chichester: Wiley-Blackwell.

Thomson, N. D., Bozgunov, K., Psederska, E., Aboutanos, M., Vasilev, G., & Vassileva, J. (2019). Physical abuse explains sex differences in the link between psychopathy and aggression. *Journal of Interpersonal Violence.* 10.1177/0886260519865956

Thomson, N. D., Kevorkian, S., Bozgunov, K., Psederska, E., Aboutanos, M., Vasilev, G., & Vassileva, J. (2020). Fluid intelligence moderates the link between psychopathy and aggression differently for men and women. *Journal of Interpersonal Violence.* 10.1177/0886260520943718

Threadcraft-Walker, W., & Henderson, H. (2018). Reflections on race, personality, and crime. *Journal of Criminal Justice, 59,* 38–41.

Tuvblad, C., Wang, P., Patrick, C. J., Berntsen, L., Raine, A., & Baker, L. A. (2019). Genetic and environmental influences on disinhibition, boldness, and meanness as assessed by the triarchic psychopathy measure in 19–20-year-old twins. *Psychological Medicine, 49,* 1500–1509.

Verona, E., & Vitale, J. (2018). Psychopathy in women: assessment, manifestations, and etiology. In C. J. Patrick (Ed.), *Handbook of psychopathy* (2nd ed, pp. 509–528). The Guilford Press.

Verschuere, B., van Ghesel Grothe, S., Waldorp, L., Watts, A. L., Lilienfeld, S. O., Edens, J. F., Skeem, J. L., & Noordhof, A. (2018). What features of psychopathy might be central? A network analysis of the Psychopathy Checklist-Revised (PCL-R) in three large samples. *Journal of Abnormal Psychology*, *127*(1), 51–65.

Weiss, R. A., & Rosenfeld, B. (2012). Navigating cross-cultural issues in forensic assessment: recommendations for practice. *Professional Psychology: Research and Practice*, *43*(3), 234–240.

26 Technological Assessment Methods: New Directions in the Assessment of Sexual Offending and Sexualised Violence

Derek Perkins and Ignazio Puzzo

Introduction

This chapter will set out some developments in the use of technological assessments in forensic psychological practice with a focus on sexual offending and sexualised violence. It will describe the empirical underpinnings of these assessments and discuss some of the challenges and potential benefits of these methods.

Technological assessments, in the context of this chapter, concern some aspects of the functioning of the individual being assessed and technological, equipment-based measurements of that functioning. In physical medicine, for example, the electrocardiograph (ECG) measures heart functioning in ways that enable health risks to be identified and appropriate treatments to be established and monitored. Similarly, the use of technological methods to assess psychological traits or states of the individual has the potential to assist understanding, enhance risk assessments, and guide relevant interventions.

Assessment Purposes

Forensic psychological assessments address a range of objectives, including risk assessment, identification of treatment needs, evaluations of interventions, and sometimes formal diagnostic assessments for the purposes of, for example, accessing specialised mental health services or commenting on capacity and diminished responsibility within Court proceedings. The danger in carrying out a variety of assessments is that of ending up with a list of assessment outcomes, that might be difficult to integrate into a whole. It is now generally accepted that doing so through a case formulation approach is an important and overarching task. These issues will be addressed next.

Case Formulation

This might be summarised as developing a working hypothesis about the causes and maintenance of behaviours of concern, which can be then explored and tested with the individual in question (Johnstone & Dallos, 2014). Within forensic

DOI: 10.4324/9781003230977-29

services, case formulation typically includes: (a) the individual's history: early life attachments, social and intimate partner relationships, educational and occupational history, mental health and forensic history, etc; (b) a functional analysis of antisocial behaviours of concern: interpersonal violence, sexual offending, property offences, etc; (c) potential future risks and related treatment needs; and (d) any related or coexistent mental health issues: typically, mental illness, personality disorder, developmental disorders, and substance use. The use of multimodal methods of assessment is particularly important in forensic case formulation – notably, interviews with the individual and relevant others, observed behaviours, psychometric and psychophysiological assessments, and structured professional judgement tools – thereby enabling the triangulation of different types of assessments.

Risk of Future Harm

This comprises an estimation of the *probability* of future specified harmful behaviour (e.g., 10% probability of committing a contact sexual offence over the following four years), its *imminence* (e.g., within days of being at liberty vs developing over several years), and the *circumstances* in which the offending is most likely to occur (e.g., when unemployed and socially alienated vs within a gradually deteriorating intimate partner relationship). As Hart et al. (2016) observe, the main purpose of risk assessments is not just to predict the occurrence of harmful behaviours but to mitigate these identified risks by applying interventions such as monitoring, therapy, and support.

Intervention Planning

Interventions can target criminogenic factors, including those that have an empirically determined association with reoffending, as well as factors that are likely to enhance the overall effect of the intervention, (e.g., low self-esteem or low motivation to change), which could otherwise adversely affect the criminogenic interventions. Such intervention plans are ideally guided by the above-mentioned case formulation. They should identify both the nature and sequencing of appropriate interventions – for both the criminogenic factors (offence-predictive) and the other factors (such as mental health issues) – as not all relevant interventions can be delivered simultaneously. The case formulation will aim to guide the implementation of the treatment/risk management plan. Such interventions can range from specific psychological therapies (e.g., EMDR to address past traumatic experiences linked to current offending (Shapiro, 1995; 2001; Wright & Warner 2019) through to situational risk management strategies (e.g., polygraph-assisted risk management compliance (Collins, 2020)).

Assessing Change

Within forensic services, therapeutic progress is rarely linear and uninterrupted, often fluctuating between progress and lapses that ought to be understood and managed. Wherever possible, measures of change should include different classes and modalities of information – e.g., *interviews* with the individual and others able to comment on the individual's behaviour and progress; *behavioural observations* within the community or a residential setting (e.g., Chart of Interpersonal Reactions in Closed Living Environments (CIRCLE; Blackburn & Renwick, 1996)); *structured professional judgement (SPJ)* tools (e.g., HCR-20, SVR-20); *psychometric assessments* of general personality and mental health functioning (e.g., MCMI-IV, Millon et al., 2015); or specific traits such as impression management (e.g., Paulus Deception Scales (PDS; Paulhus, 1999, 2002); or interpersonal violence potential (e.g., Maudsley Violence Questionnaire (MVQ), Walker, 2005; Walker, 2006). These have been increasingly complemented by technological assessments that are explored later.

Diagnosis

This may be particularly relevant where alleged offences come before the Courts (e.g., regarding consideration of the diminished responsibility defence in alleged murder cases) and/or where mental disorder(s) may have contributed to offending or may be sequalae to the offending (with implications for prison vs hospital placement). These considerations may relate to a single disorder, e.g., paranoid schizophrenia, or may involve complex interactions between, e.g., mental illness, personality disorder (Blackburn et al., 2003), and /or substance use disorders (Cappai et al., 2017).

Technological Assessments

Technological assessments can improve the accuracy of assessments, enhance the relevance of interventions, and remove biases which are present in the development of psychometric measures (notably lack of diversity in norm groups), in the assessment process and in clinicians themselves. These assessments include analogues of impulsiveness, risky decision-making, reactive aggression, and sexual interests/paraphilias, by the use of VR, penile plethysmography, polygraphy, and implicit measures, such as time viewing, eye-tracking, and implicit association tests. The use and potential value of such methods are discussed throughout the chapter.

Using technological assessments/computerized tasks to either replace or complement other forms of assessment can be advantageous for several reasons.

Technological assessments are generally more engaging and interactive (e.g., VR) compared to filling out paper-based questionnaires and this could potentially facilitate the participant's effort and interest in the task. This can be helpful when trying to engage across the age spectrum, i.e., with young people/adolescents, when working with those with neurodiverse conditions, and in engaging with those for whom the default language and couture of other assessments can be a barrier to accurate assessment.

Another benefit linked to computerized tasks is that, based on behavioural performance (e.g., missed responses, excessively slow response times), the assessor can easily establish if the participant shows low effort during the assessment. This is not easy to establish whilst the participant is completing a self-report.

Importantly because computerized tasks measure behavioural performance directly, they are less influenced by demand characteristics (i.e., it is difficult for participants to give misleading or false information based on their beliefs concerning the purpose of the task or the aim of the assessor in conducting the assessment); and are therefore often more objective than self-report questionnaires.

Regarding objectivity, computerized tasks are also quite effective in preventing potential negative effects of unconscious biases and stereotypes in relation to various aspects (e.g., gender, age, ethnicity, religion, etc.) that the assessor might exert during the assessment, such as semi-structured interviews/or paper-based assessments (Reynolds & Suzuki, 2012). For optimal utility, such methodologies should be readily accessible in the contexts in which they are needed, e.g., penile plethysmograph (PPG) assessments (see below) require laboratory facilities that will not be readily accessible to those working with individuals requiring assessments of their sexual preferences as part of their treatment and case management.

Finally, technological assessments/computerized measures are effective in promoting diversity and equality in the sense that these assessments can be customized/tailored based on specific situations and demands. For example, these assessments are often not contingent on reading ability, allowing participants with different literacy abilities to complete the same tasks. That said, care needs to be taken to ensure that potential biases inherent to other assessments are also addressed within technological assessments. These include, for example: *construct bias* (differences in the appropriate of an assessed construct within different cultures), *item bias* (in which specific items or elements of a test might be incorrectly translated from one system to another), and *method bias* (e.g., ambiguous directions or participants being unfamiliar with the technology; Reynolds & Suzuki, 2012).

Although a number of these methods have been utilised in forensic settings for many decades, there are also more recently developed methods that will be described and discussed. This will be done in the sections that follow under the headings of the forensic problem areas of concern.

Sexual Interests and Sexual Violent Offending

Scale of the Problem

Violent sexual offences are devastating crimes. They include crimes such as rape and sexual assault, and in its extreme, can take the form of sexual homicide. According to the Crime Survey for England and Wales (CSEW) https://www.ons.gov.uk/peoplepopulationandcommunity/crimeandjustice/articles/natureofsexualassaultbyrapeorpenetrationenglandandwales/yearendingmarch2020) in the year ending March 2020 it was estimated that 3.8% of adults aged 16–74 years (1.6 million) had experienced sexual assault by rape or penetration since the age of 16 years, with female victims being more prevalent (7.1%) than male victims

(0.5%). In 2020, the International Watch Foundation (IWF) identified 153,383 instances of child sexual abuse imagery or UK-hosted non-photographic child sexual abuse imagery, a 16% increase from 2019. The total estimate economical cost of rape and sexual assaults in England and Wales in 2015/16 was £12.2 billion. Yet these staggering figures may be an underestimate of the real size of the problem as shown by the CSEW data which suggest that, for the years ending March 2017 and March 2020 combined, fewer than one in six victims (16%) had reported the assault to the police. Despite the significant negative impact of sex offending on society, both its sexual (paraphilic/hypersexual) and personality (antisocial/violent/psychopathic) aspects have been understudied and deserve further scrutiny. In the following sections, we will describe potential ways in which these aspects can be assessed and how such assessment could directly inform risk assessment, clinical formulations, and interventions.

Types of sexual offending range from non-contact offences (e.g., indecent exposure and voyeurism, as well as the rapidly expanding offence of possessing child sexual exploitation material (CSEM; Babchishin et al., 2018) to contact offences such as rape and indecent assault, to culminate in the extreme manifestation of sexual homicide (e.g., Carter & Perkins, 2018). Typologies of sexual offending typically highlight the importance of two major dynamic risk factors: *deviant sexual interest* and *antisocial/psychopathic traits* (Hanson & Bussiere, 1998; Hanson & Morton-Bourgon, 2004, 2005, 2007, 2009). Research on sexual homicide similarity highlights the role of both sexual paraphilias, such as sexual sadism, and grievance-based motives, typically related to previous negative experiences with women (e.g., Stefanska et al., 2015). The personality profiles of sexual killers tend to cluster around either psychopathic/narcissistic traits or schizoid/avoidant traits (Carter & Perkins, 2018), each with their own assessment challenges. The question next arises: Can technological methods help in assessment of sexual offending behaviours – risks, needs, and outcomes?

We now consider a range of technological assessment developments related to, (1) the assessment of sexual arousal/interests, such as PPG (Murphy et al., 2020) and polygraph assessments (Collins, 2020), the Explicit and Implicit Sexual Interest Profile (EISIP; Banse et al., 2010) and VR.; (2) The assessment of various aspects linked to violent sexual offending, such as: reactive and proactive aggression, impulse control/impulsivity, response inhibition, and risky decision-making.

Psychophysiological Assessments of Offence-Sexual Interests

Offence-related sexual interests are one of the major stable dynamic predictors of sexual offending, especially when combined with antisocial and aggressive traits, which will be considered later.

For many decades, psychophysiological assessments of sexual arousal/interests have been demonstrated to make useful contributions to case formulations, risk assessment, treatment planning, and treatment evaluation. Notable amongst these are PPG (Murphy et al., 2020) and polygraph assessments (Collins, 2020). Used, respectively, for assessing differential sexual interests and assessing accuracy of self-reporting/treatment compliance, these methods provide a useful complementary data source to other modalities of assessment.

The PPG is used to assess the sexual preferences/arousability of male subjects by the direct measurement of penile tumescence during the presentation of sexual stimuli that depict illegal sexual targets (e.g., children) and/or acts (e.g., rape) in comparison with their responses to alternative "legal" sexual targets. The stimuli in these assessments can be visual (still or moving) or auditory (descriptions of different types of sexual behaviours) and must comply with professional guidelines for their ethical and appropriate use (e.g., British Psychological Society, 2008). PPG findings can assist with case formulation, risk management, treatment planning, and treatment evaluation and can facilitate disclosure of offence-related sexual interests by those taking part (Dean & Perkins, 2008; Murphy et al., 2020).

Polygraph assessment is used to facilitate disclosure of information relevant to (usually sexual) offending behaviour and related treatment planning. It involves measurement of the subject's heart rate, blood pressure, respiration, and galvanic skin responses by a trained operator. Agreed questions are presented by the operator, e.g., about nature and extent of previous offending or cooperation with risk management plans, such as avoiding certain locations at certain times of day.

With technological and computing developments over recent years, several tests have been developed from research into, e.g., implicit measurements of traits such as anger, distorted thinking, and sexual preferences (Snowden et al., 2008; Babchishin et al., 2013), as well as use of choice reaction time methodology (Santtila et al., 2009), eye tracking procedures (Hogue et al., 2016), and latency responding (Harper et al., 2016).

In the area of sexual offending, The Explicit and Implicit Sexual Interest Profile (EISIP; Banse et al., 2010) combines two self-report measures of sexual interest (past behaviours/fantasies and ratings of adult, pubescent, and child images) with two empirically validated objective measures (viewing time and an implicit association test). This computerised assessment, which typically takes 20–30 minutes to administer, uses the so-called "not real images" stimulus set developed by Laws and Gress (Pacific Psychological Assessment Cooperation, 2004). The images are categorised in the five Tanner (T) age groups of males and female – adult (T5), adolescent (T4), pubescent (T3) pre-pubescent, aged about 8 (T2) and about 4 (T1). The EISIP has been used in research, as well as has been contributing to clinical case formulation, risk assessment, and treatment planning (Schmidt & Perkins, 2020).

Assessments such as this in which images of white people are used raises issues of transferability to cultures in which people of colour predominate. The first author has at the time of writing been working with colleagues in the Far East on the possibility of developing and researching stimulus sets more appropriate to that context. A similar, albeit imperfect, attempt was made to balance images of white, black, and Asian characters in the production of PPG stimuli for the assessment of assault sexual violence (see Hogue et al., 2018).

Caution in terms of using the tool in isolation is recommended as highlighted by Schmidt & Perkins (2020, page 73–74), "On its own, it is unable to, and is therefore inappropriate for, explaining past sexual offending or assessing risks of future offending. However, given that paedophilic sexual interest is one of two major risk factors for sexual recidivism (Hanson & Morton-Bourgon, 2005; Stephens et al., 2019) – the second being general antisociality - the EISIP, when combined with measures of other relevant factors, such as antisocial attitudes, patterns of socio-sexual behaviour, opportunities to offend and the absence of barriers to offending, can have a useful part to play within Court or similar proceedings".

Technological Assessment of Deviant Sexual Interest Using VR

VR refers to all technological components that are necessary to facilitate interactions between an individual and an artificially generated environment (Riener & Harders, 2012). The aim of VR is to generate/induce sensory experiences, feelings, and interaction (between an individual and a computer-generated environment) which cannot be distinguished from reality (Parsons et al., 2017). Similar caveats apply as those mentioned earlier about trying to ensure that these methodologies are as free as possible from cultural and ethnicity biases.

The subjective feeling of being present in the virtual environments (virtual presence) depends on the technological basis of a VR system (e.g., extent of the field of view), which will determine the level of immersion (Fromberger et al., 2015). Although the subjective feeling that a virtual character in fact exists in the virtual environment is referred as social presence (Parsons et al., 2017). Virtual presence and social presence induced by VR environments enable individuals to experience emotions (like the ones experienced in real life), and consequently, trigger behaviours that are comparable to the ones experienced in real life (Alsina-Jurnet et al., 2011). Therefore, in contrast to non-VR environments, more ecologically valid environments provided by VR offer the opportunity to simulate and induce behaviour comparable to real-life situations.

VR as a clinical tool has been implemented for over 20 years in general psychiatry and psychology and its potential advantages have also been realised for patients within forensic mental health patients. These include the crucial possibility to expose those who have offended to situations that elicit disorder-relevant behaviour – without endangering others (Fromberger et al., 2014). For example, VR can easily allow the assessment of participants' self-regulation abilities by exposing them to highly salient realistic physical, social, and emotional stimuli in virtual environments; especially with child abusers (Fromberger et al., 2014; 2018). Few studies have explored the efficacy of VR for the assessment of deviant sexual interests. For instance, Renaud et al. (2014) showed that compared to auditory stimuli, highly immersive visual stimuli were significantly more effective in inducing sexual arousal assessed with penile plethysmography (PPG) and consequently more precise in classifying child abusers from healthy controls. These findings replicated earlier findings from the same lab (Renaud et al., 2013) strongly suggesting that VR in combination with psychophysiological measures seem to be a powerful tool for the assessment of deviant sexual interests. VR could also be very useful from a risk assessment/ management of future offending point of view. This is because current actuarial and structural professional judgement risk assessment tools do not provide enough information about the behaviour of child abusers in concrete situations (Logan, 2016). For instance, clinicians at some point face the very difficult decision to grant unsupervised privileges on the basis that the child abuser will be able to use his/her necessary coping skills learned within controlled environment outside during unsupervised privileges. One-way VR could help in this context is to examine whether behavioral monitoring of child abusers in highly immersive virtual risk situations provides additional information for risk management. To achieve that Meyer et al. (2017) carried out a pilot study whereby six child abusers and seven non-child-abusers walked through three virtual risk situations, confronting them with a virtual child character. When confronted with the virtual child character both child abusers and non-child-abusers had to choose between predefined answers reflecting approach (e.g., interact with the children) or avoidance behaviour (e.g., avoiding interaction with the child). According to what child abusers learned in therapy – in real risk situations – they should avoid approaching behaviour to decrease the risk of reoffending (McGrath et al., 2010). However, only in 50% of all cases the child abusers behaved consistently with the coping skills that therapists stated that they had focused on during therapy; and in most cases, child abusers showed a behaviour that did not reflect their own belief about adequate behaviour in comparable risk situations. This study – despite the small sample size – demonstrate the potential of VR applications for the risk assessment of child abusers.

Technological Assessments of Reactive and Proactive Aggression

The role of reactive and proactive aggression in violent and sexual offending has recently been considered to potentially provide new insights into pathways to offending that may increase our understanding of the factors predisposing an individual to act with reactive or proactive aggression in the context of a sexual or violent offence.

Reactive aggression refers to an unplanned and/or impulsive, defensive re-action paired with anger and a loss of control that leads to an act of violence in response to some form of provocation, threat, or danger. The reactive aggression response is usually accompanied by high, uncontrolled autonomic arousal such as increased heart rate (Berkowitz, 1963, 1993; Dollard et al., 1939; Houston et al., 2003). This response serves the function of self-defence or retribution with the aim of harming the source of the negative stimuli.

By contrast proactive aggression refers to an act of violence that is goal-directed and therefore planned and executed in a predetermined manner to achieve a reward which may be external/material (e.g., money or drugs) or internal/psychological (e.g., coercion) in nature. This type of aggression refers to a response learned through positive reinforcement (Bandura, 1973, 1983) rather than preceded by autonomic arousal.

Recently James and colleagues (2020) investigated whether the reactive/proactive aggression distinction might be useful in characterising those who have committed violent sexual offences. They tested the role of adverse childhood experiences (ACEs) as well as psychopathology relevant to physical and sexual violence (psychopathy and sexual sadism) in predicting the type of aggression (reactive/proactive) expressed within a sample of individuals who had committed a sexual homicide. They classified those who had committed sexual homicide in two ways: as "reactive" (SHO-R) when the sexual homicide was committed with no evidence of premeditation and in an impulsive or circumstantial manner; as "proactive" (SHO-P) when a rigorously planned sexual homicide was committed and contained elements such as, e.g., the choice of a targeted victim or the presence of an identified location for the offense. The two groups, SHO-R and SHO-P were compared in terms of ACEs and psychometric measures of psychopathy (PCL: SV) and sexual sadism (SeSaS). Their findings revealed that ACEs and PCL: SV Factor 2 were associated with reactive aggression in the context of sexual homicide, whereas PCL: SV Factor 1 and sexual sadism were associated to proactive aggression.

Technological Assessment of Impulse Control/Impulsivity

As described above, reactive aggression in those who have committed severe violent sex offences including sexual homicides has been linked with Factor 2 items of the PCLR-SV such as impulsivity and poor behavioural control (James et al., 2020). The link between reactive aggression and poor impulse control has been extensively documented in various samples of participants who have offended. For example, a meta-analysis of 21 studies reported that across age, gender, race, and offence status low self-control was one of the strongest predictors of criminal behaviour (Pratt & Cullen, 2000). Furthermore, poor impulse control (high impulsivity) has been found to be an important contributing risk factor for increased engagement in other unhealthy behaviours such as drug misuse, reckless driving, excessive drinking, and gambling that are in turn linked to risk of offending and recidivism (for reviews, see DeWit 2000; Longshore, 1998; Perry & Carroll, 2008). Impulse control deficits have been proposed amongst the core components contributing to the development of sexually aggressive behaviour. Specifically, in the Integrated Theory of Sexual Offending (ITSO), Ward and Beech (2006, 2016) describe the functioning of the action selection and control system as playing a dual functioning role: (i) being responsible for planning, implementing, and evaluating action plans; and for (ii) controlling behaviour, thoughts, and emotions in service of higher level goals (Ward & Beech, 2006). Abnormal functioning of the action selection and control system could lead to general problems with self-regulation including increased impulsivity (Ward & Beech, 2016). Behaving impulsively, in turn, could facilitate sexual offending (Krasowska et al., 2013). It is generally accepted that impulsivity is a multidimensional construct comprising several domains (Caswell et al., 2015; Stahl et al., 2014) such as response inhibition and impulsive decision-making.

Response inhibition is defined as the ability to suppress an activated or already ongoing action. Successful inhibition involves three inter-related processes: (i) inhibition of the initial prepotent or automatic response to an event; (ii) stopping of an ongoing response allowing to make the decision to respond; and (iii) preventing competing events and responses from interfering with self-directed responses (i.e., interference control). Empirical evidence suggests that those who have committed offences have a reduced ability to stop themselves from responding to targets or other cues that signal withholding of a response (Chen et al., 2008; Chen et al., 2005). This reduced ability to suppress a response is often associated with negative outcomes such as the impulse to react with violence following a negative confrontation. If assessment participants have underlying deficits in their ability to inhibit their responses and behaviour, they may be more likely to engage in disruptive behaviour that contributes to initial arrest, disciplinary problems while in prison, and re-arrest after release.

Another domain of impulsivity which is often displayed by those who have committed offences is impulsive or risky decision-making. Impulsive-risky decisions are often characterized by choices that are ill-judged, imprudent, and lacking in judgment of consequences (De Wit, 2009). One example of impulsive decision-making, known as temporal discounting is the drive to obtain immediate smaller rewards in place of larger future ones. Evidence suggests that those who have committed offences find it difficult to delay gratification on temporal discounting tasks (Åkerlund et al., 2016; Carroll et al., 2006; Lee et al., 2017; Mishra & Lalumière, 2016). Specifically, giving less value to temporally delayed rewards has been found to be a reliable predictor of future engagement in criminal behaviour (Lee et al., 2017). Impaired decision-making has clear relevance to maintaining long-term patterns of non-criminal behaviour and avoiding re-arrest. In the context of sexual offending, poor response inhibition could lead to an inability to inhibit an impulse to have sexual contact with a victim. Furthermore, impulsive decision-making could represent the tendency to satisfy one's sexual desire by abusing an individual, while ignoring the future negative consequences that act is likely to give rise to the abuser (i.e., conviction, imprisonment, or feelings of shame and guilt) and the long-term trauma caused to the victim. For these reasons, it is important to reliably assess these two domains.

Methodological advances in experimental psychology have led to the development of validated, computerized measures of response inhibition and impulsive decision-making that are going to be described in turn below.

Technological Measures of Response Inhibition

Several behavioural tasks have been developed to measure response inhibition, including the go/no-go paradigm, stop-signal task, and continuous performance test (CPT).

GO/NO-GO TASK

In a typical go/no-go paradigm (e.g., Kamarajan et al., 2005; Simmonds et al., 2008), participants are presented with a frequent visual cue that indicates they should respond (a "go" stimulus) and an infrequent visual cue that indicates they should withhold their response (a "no-go" stimulus). Performance on this task is measured by the number of responses made to a no-go stimulus (i.e., commission errors) and the number of times a response is not made to a go stimulus (i.e., omission errors).

STOP-SIGNAL TASK

The stop-signal tasks (Logan, 1994; Verbruggen & Logan, 2008) is a test of inhibition of prepotent responses. Stop-signal tasks measure how quickly a participant can stop an initiated key press response when they are presented with a stop signal shortly after (within hundreds of milliseconds) the go signal is presented. Performance on this task is measured by the speed of responding to go signals, and the probability of suppressing the response or the time needed to suppress the response (stop-signal reaction time). Shorter times indicate better reactive inhibition skills.

CPT

The CPT (Connors & Staff, 2000) requires a participant to pay sustained attention to a frequently presented target stimulus and to inhibit a response to infrequent target stimuli. Participants are asked to respond to a target stimulus (e.g., blue dot) when it is preceded by a specified pre-target stimulus (e.g., A). Thus, participants must only respond when presented with A – blue dot in succession and withhold the response otherwise. Like the go/no-go task, performance on these tasks is measured by omission errors (i.e., target stimuli missed) and commission errors (i.e., responses to non-target stimuli).

Technological Measures of Impulsive or Risky Decision-Making

Several computerised behavioural tasks have been developed to measure impulsive/risky decision-making. These include: delay and probability discounting tasks and computerized gambling decision-making tasks such as the Iowa Gambling Task (IGT) and the BART.

DELAY AND PROBABILITY DISCOUNTING

In delay discounting tasks (Stein & Madden, 2013) participants are required to choose between smaller sooner and larger later rewards. Monetary rewards are typically used (e.g., "Would you rather have £40 today or £100 in 1 month"?), however other rewards (e.g., drugs of abuse, food, health outcomes) have also been used. Independently of the reward used these tasks involve systematically varying the magnitude of the immediate reward and delay for the future reward to estimate indifference points corresponding to equal preference for immediate and delayed alternatives. Similarly, in probability discounting tasks individuals are asked to make choices between a smaller certain reward and a larger uncertain reward (e.g., "Would you rather have £25 for sure or a 50% chance to have £100"?). The size of the certain reward and the probability are systematically varied across trials to estimate the participant's indifference point corresponding to equal preference for certain and probabilistic rewards. In these tasks the primary depended variable is the rate of delay or probability discounting which indicate the rate at which rewards lose their value as a function of delay or probability.

THE IGT

Bechara et al., 1994) presents participants with four virtual decks of cards and requires them to select one card at a time to maximize monetary gains and minimize losses. Two of the decks result in large gains (e.g., win £250) but larger losses (e.g., lose £250; "disadvantageous decks"), whereas two other decks result in smaller gains (e.g., win £50) but smaller losses (e.g., lose £50; "advantageous decks"). Adaptive performance requires that participants avoid disadvantageous decks with large immediate rewards to avoid larger losses. The IGT can examine emotion-based learning effects on decision-making, as individuals who choose from the advantageous decks with smaller rewards (associated with even smaller penalties) end up gaining money on the task. The dependent variable is the net overall score, computed as the number of cards drawn from the advantageous decks minus the number drawn from the disadvantageous decks.

THE BALLOON ANALOGUE RISK TASK (BART)

Lejuez et al. (2002) is a computerised task in which participants are asked to blow up a virtual balloon by clicking a button. With every click, the balloon inflates and the participant obtains a small amount of money (£0.05). At any time during the task, the balloon can burst, resulting in the participant losing the accumulated money. The participant can, at any point, decide to collect the money gained during that round or continue clicking. After the participant has collected the money or the balloon has exploded, another balloon appears. The primary dependent variable for the BART is the adjusted average number of pumps on unexploded balloons, with higher scores indicative of greater risk-taking propensity.

Evidence has shown the potential utility of some of the computerised tasks described above in the context of sexual offending against children (see Turner & Rettenberger, 2020, for a review). For example, Turner and colleagues (2018) compared response inhibition abilities and the degree of impulsive decision-making between child sexual abusers and non-offending controls. For the first time, they used modified versions of the Go/No-Go task and the IGT which included pictures of the Not Real People-Set depicting nude adults and children. Their findings indicated that child sexual abusers showed more deficits in response inhibition in the Go/No-Go task compared to non-offending controls. They also found that in child sexual abusers decision-making was impaired by the presence of child images with more intense pedophilic sexual interests, whereas in the non-offending controls the presence of preferred sexual cues (pictures of women) improved decision-making performance.

As discussed earlier in the chapter, there is evidence supporting the idea that perhaps the assessment of factors predisposing individuals to display reactive aggression might be useful in the context of violent sexual offending. Reactive aggression is particularly relevant in violent sex offending as there is established evidence supporting the link between the feeling of being rejected by a potential sexual partner and violent sex offending. For example, a survey by the Australia Institute found that one-quarter (25%) of women in their sample (n = 1426) had been threatened after rejecting the sexual advances of a stranger (Johnson & Bennett, 2015). Hostile/aggressive behaviours in response to sexual rejection are much more frequent in men than women. A recent study carried out in the United States indicated that even though both men and women reported feelings of rejection, only men responded with hostility (Andrighetto et al., 2019). In line with these findings, Woerner and colleagues (2018) used a two-dimensional VR simulation dating laboratory task to investigate how sexual dominance motivation and casual sex attitudes interacted with hostile perceptions of a woman (virtual agent) rejecting sexual advances; and how this predicted the likelihood of an aggressive response. They found that men with high scores on sexual dominance motivation and positive attitudes about casual sex were more likely to respond aggressively when they formed extremely hostile perceptions of the woman who rejected them.

Conclusions

In this chapter, we have described a range of technological assessment methods that might be used to complement more conventional forensic psychological assessments that use interview, psychometry, and SPJ tools. Some of these technological methods are in their early stages of development and we have attempted to set out some of the potential challenges and benefits of using these.

A key issue within forensic psychological practice is that of unconscious bias. This may relate to the assessor's own personal beliefs and emotional responses to different types of cases being dealt with or to contextual factors to the assessment. For example, it has been shown that significant variations can occur in the completion of even standardised tools such as the PCL-R (Hare, 2003) and HCR-20 (Webster et al., 1997), with stringent completion guidance criteria, depending on whether psychologists are instructed by the defence or prosecution in Court proceedings cases (see Hogue and Dernevik chapter for more details).

Where the results of technological assessments run counter to those from other forms of assessment, the question arises of how these differences should be interpreted or reconciled. The approach adopted in the application of the EISIP, which incorporates both self-report and technological methods, is to seek to resolve this through hypothesis development and testing in collaboration with the client (see Schmidt & Perkins, 2020).

In developing the use of technological assessments, a number of issues need to be kept in mind. Although some of these methods may be easier to deliver than some conventional assessments, and their automated nature can make them cost-effective in terms of clinician time, it is important not to separate them from the holistic process of formulation-based forensic clinical assessments, as set out earlier in the chapter. Dean and Perkins (2008), for example, set out why PPG findings, which emerge as graphical representations of sexual interests should never simply be interpreted in this way but should be integrated with other information, a point also stressed in the relevant BPS Guidelines (2008) on PPG use.

It is hoped that some of the technological assessments we have described, or which could be developed from the research described in this chapter, may go some way towards minimising biases that can occur in other forms of assessment and complement interview, psychometric, or structured professional judgement tool assessments.

References

Andrighetto, L., Riva, P., & Gabbiadini, A. (2019). Lonely hearts and angry minds: online dating rejection increases male (but not female) hostility. *Aggressive Behavior*, *45*(5), 571–581.

Alsina-Jurnet, I., Gutiérrez-Maldonado, J., & Rangel-Gómez, M.-V. (2011). The role of presence in the level of anxiety experienced in clinical virtual environments. *Computers in Human Behavior*, 27, 504–512 10.1016/j.chb.2010.09.018.

Åkerlund, D., Golsteyn, B.H. H., Grönqvist, H., & Lindahl, L. (2016). Time discounting and criminal behavior. *Proceedings of the National Academy of Sciences*, *113*(22), 6160–6165. 10.1073/pnas.1522445113.

Babchishin, K. M., Nunes, K. L., Hermann, C. A. (2013). The validity of Implicit Association Test (IAT) measures of sexual attraction to children: A meta-analysis. *Archives of Sexual Behavior*, *42*(3), 487–499.

Babchishin, K. M., Merdian, H. L., Bartels, R. M., & Perkins, D. E. (2018). 'Child sexual exploitation materials offenders: a review. *European Psychologist (2018)*, *23*(2), 130–143. 10.1027/1016-9040/a000326

Bandura, A. (1983). Psychological mechanisms of aggression. *Aggression: Theoretical And empirical Reviews*, 1, 1–40.

Berkowitz, L. (1963).*Aggression: A social learning analysis.*New York: McGraw-Hill.

Bechara, A., Damasio, A. R., Damasio, H., & Anderson, S. W. (1994). Insensitivity to future consequences following damage to human prefrontal cortex. *Cognition*, 50(1-3), 7–15. 10.1016/0010-0277(94)90018-3.

Banse, R., Schmidt, A. F., & Clarbour, J. (2010). Indirect measures of sexual interest in child sex offenders a multimethod approach. *Criminal Justice and Behavior*, *37*, 319–335. doi:10.1177/0093854809357598

Blackburn, R., & Renwick, S. J. (1996). Rating scales for measuring the interpersonal circle in forensic psychiatric patients. *Psychological Assessment*, *8*(1), 76.

Blackburn, R., Logan, C., Donnelly, J., & Renwick, S. (2003). Personality disorders, psychopathy and other mental disorders: co-morbidity among patients at English and Scottish high-security hospitals. *The Journal of Forensic Psychiatry & Psychology*, 14, 111–137. 10.1080/1478994031000077925.

British Psychological Society. (2008). *Penile Plethysmography Professional Guidelines*. Retrieved from https://www1.bps.org.uk/content/penile-plethysmography-guidance-psychologists-1

Carter, A. & Perkins, D. (2018). The assessment of perpetrators of sexual homicide for the purposes of risk reduction in secure psychiatric hospital and prison settings. In J. Proulx, E. Beauregard, A. J. Carter, A. Mokros, R. Darjee & J. James (Eds.) *Routledge International Handbook of Sexual Homicide Studies*. Abingdon: Routledge.

Chen, C, Muggleton, N, Juan, C, Tzeng, O, & Hung, D (2008). Time pressure leads to inhibitory control deficits in impulsive violent offenders. *Behavioural Brain Research*, 187(2), 483–488. 10.1016/j.bbr.2007.10.011

Chen, C.-Y., Tien, Y.-M., Juan, C.-H., Tzeng, O. J. L., & Hung, D. L. (2005). Neural correlates of impulsive-violent behavior: an event-related potential study. *Neuroreport*, 16(11), 1213–121610.1097/00001756-200508010-00016

Collins, N. (2020). The use of polygraph test in clinical forensic psychiatry setting. In Artemis Igoumenou (Ed.). *Ethical Issues in Clinical Forensic Psychiatry* (pp. 85–96). Springer.

Conners, C. K., & Staff, M. H. S. (2000). Conners' continuous performance test (CPT II). NorthTonawanda, NY: Multi-Health Systems Inc.

Cappai, A., Wells, J., Tapp, J., Perkins, D., Manners, A., Ferrito, M., Gupta, N., & Das, M. (2017). Substance misuse in personality disorder and schizophrenia: findings and clinical implications from a high secure hospital. *Journal of Forensic Practice*, 19, 217–226. 10.1108/jfp-07-2016-0035

Caswell, A. J., Bond, R., Duka, T., & Morgan, M. J. (2015). Further evidence of the heterogeneous nature of impulsivity. *Personality and Individual Differences*, 76, 68–74. 10.1016/j.paid.2014.11.059

Carroll, A., Hemingway, F., Bower, J., Ashman, A., Houghton, S., & Durkin, K. (2006). Impulsivity in juvenile delinquency: Differences among early-onset, late-onset, and non-offenders. *Journal of Youth and Adolescence* 35(4), 517–527.

Dean, C. & Perkins, D. (2008). Penile plethysmography. *Prison Service Journal*, *178*(July), 20–25.

DeWit, D. J. (2000). Age at first alcohol use: A risk factor for the development of alcohol disorders. *American Journal of Psychiatry*, 157(5),745–75010.1176/appi.ajp.157.5.745

Dollard, J., Doob, L. W., Miller, N. E., Mowrer, O. H., & Sears, R. R. (1939). *Frustration and aggression*. New Haven, CT: Yale University Press.

Fromberger, P., Meyer, S., Kempf, C., Jordan, K., & Müller, J. L. (2015). Virtual viewing time: The relationship between presence and sexual interest in Androphilic and Gynephilic Men. *PLOS ONE*, 10, e0127156. 10.1371/journal.pone.0127156

Fromberger, P., Jordan, K., & Müller, J. L. (2014). Anwendung virtueller Realitäten in der forensischen Psychiatrie. Der Nervenarzt, 85, 298–303. 10.1007/s00115-013-3904-7

Fromberger, P., Meyer, S., Jordan, K., & Müller, J. L. (2018). Behavioral monitoring of sexual offenders against children in virtual risk situations: A feasibility study. *Frontiers in Psychology*, 9, 224. 10.3389/fpsyg.2018.00224.

Hanson, R. K., & Morton-Bourgon, K. E. (2005). The characteristics of persistent sexual offenders: a meta-analysis of recidivism studies. *The Journal of Consulting and Clinical Psychology*, *73*(6), 1154–1163.

Hanson, R. K., & Bussiere, M. T. (1998). Predicting relapse: a meta-analysis of sexual offender recidivism studies. *Journal of Consulting and Clinical Psychology*, *60*, 348–362.

Hanson, R. K., & Morton-Bourgon, K. E. (2004). *Predictors of sexual recidivism: an updated meta-analysis (User Report 2004-02).* Ottawa, ON: Public Safety and Emergency Preparedness.

Hanson, R. K., & Morton-Bourgon, K. E. (2007). *The accuracy of recidivism risk assessments for sexual offenders: a meta-analysis 2007-01.* Ottawa, Ontario: Public Safety and Emergency Preparedness Canada.

Hanson, R. K., & Morton-Bourgon, K. E. (2009). The accuracy of recidivism risk assessments for sexual offenders: a meta-analysis of 118 prediction studies. *Psychological Assessment, 21,* 1–21.

Hare, R. D. (2003). *Hare Psychopathy Checklist-Revised (PCL-R): 2nd edition.* Canada, Toronto: Multi-Health Systems Inc.

Hart, S. D., Douglas, K. S., & Guy, L.S. (2016). The structured professional judgement approach to violence risk assessment: Origins, nature, and advances. *The Wiley-Blackwell Handbook on the Assessment, Treatment and Theories of Sexual Offending.*

Harper, C. A., Bartels, R. M. & Hogue, T. E. (2016). Reducing stigma and punitive attitudes toward pedophiles through narrative humanization. *Sexual Abuse: A Journal of Research and Treatment, 30*(5), 533–555. DOI: 10.1177/1079063216681561

Hogue, T., Wesson, C. & Perkins, D. (2016). Eye tracking and assessing sexual interests in forensic context'. In D. P. Boer (Ed.). *The Wiley Handbook on the Theories, Assessment and Treatment of Sexual Offending, Volume 1.* Wiley.

Hogue, T. E. , Wesson, C. , & Perkins, D. (2018).Eye-tracking and assessing sexual interest in forensic contexts.*The Wiley Handbook on the Theories, Assessment and Treatment of Sexual Offending,* 995–1013.

Houston, R. J., Stanford, M. S., Villemarette Pittman, N. R., Conklin, S. M., & Helfritz, L. E. (2003). Neurobiological correlates and clinical implications of aggressive subtypes. *Journal of Forensic Neuropsychology, 3*(4), 67–8710.1300/j151v03n04_05.

James, J., Higgs, T., & Langevin, S. (2020). Reactive and proactive aggression in sexual homicide offenders. *Journal of Criminal Justice, 71,* 101728.

Johnson, M., & Bennett, E. (2015). *Everyday sexism: Australian women's experiences of street harassment.* Australia Institute.

Johnstone and Dallos, 2014 Johnstone, L., & Dallos, R. (Eds.). (2014). *Formulation in psychology and psychotherapy: Making sense of people's problems* (2nd Ed.). London, England: Routledge.

Krasowska, A., Jakubczyk, A., Czernikiewicz, W., Wojnar, M., & Nasierowski, T. (2013). Impulsivity in sexual offenders. New ideas or back to basics? *Psychiatria Polska, 47*(4), 727–740. 10.12740/pp/17648

Kamarajan, C., Porjesz, B., Jones, K. A., Choi, K., Chorlian, D. B., Padmanabhapillai, A., Rangaswamy, M., Stimus, A. T., & Begleiter, H. (2005). Alcoholism is a disinhibitory disorder: neurophysiological evidence from a Go/No-Go task. *Biological Psychology, 69*(3), 353–373. 10.1016/j.biopsycho.2004.08.004.

Lejuez, C. W., Read, J. P., Kahler, C. W., Richards, J. B., Ramsey, S. E., Strong, D. R., & Brown, R. A. (2002).Evaluation of a behavioral measure of risk taking: the Balloon Analogue Risk Task (BART). *Journal of Experimental Psychology: Applied, 8*(2), 75–84.

Lee, C. A., Derefinko, K. J., Milich, R., Lynam, D. R., & DeWall, C. N. (2017). Longitudinal and reciprocal relations between delay discounting and crime. *Personality and Individual Differences, 111,* 193–198.10.1016/j.paid.2017.02.023

Logan, G. D. (1994). On the ability to inhibit thought and action: A users' guide to the stop signal paradigm. In D. Dagenbach & T. H. Carr(Eds.), *Inhibitory processes in attention, memory, and language* (pp. 189–239). San Diego, CA: Academic Press.

Logan, C.   (2016). Risk formulation: The new frontier in risk assessment and management. In Treatment of sex offenders. (pp. 83–105). Cham: Springer.

Longshore, D. (1998). Self-control and criminal opportunity: A prospective test of the general theory of crime. *Social Problems*, 45(1), 102–113. 10.2307/3097145.

McGrath, R. J., Cumming, G. F., Burchard, B. L., Zeoli, S., & Ellerby, L. (2010). Current practices and emerging trends in sexual abuser management. The Safer Society 2009 North American Survey.

Millon, T., Grossman, S., & Millon, C.   (2015). Millon clinical multiaxial inventory-IV (MCMI-IV). Pearson Assessments.

Mishra, S., & Lalumière, M. L. (2016). Associations between delay discounting and risk-related behaviors, traits, attitudes, and outcomes. *Journal of Behavioral Decision Making*, 30(3), 769–781.10.1002/bdm.2000

Meyer, D., Cohn, A., Robinson, B., Muse, F., & Hughes, R. (2017). Persistent complications of child sexual abuse: Sexually compulsive behaviors, attachment, and emotions. *Journal of Child Sexual Abuse*, 26(2), 140–157. 10.1080/10538712.2016.1269144

Murphy, L., Gottfried, E., Dimario, K., Perkins, D., & Fedoroff, P. (2020). Use of penile plethysmography in the court: a review of practices in Canada, the United Kingdom and the United States. *Behavioral Sciences & the Law*, 38(2), 79–99. 10.1002/bsl.2453

Parsons, T., Gaggioli, A., & Riva, G. (2017). Virtual reality for research in social neuroscience. *Brain Sciences*, 7, 42. 10.3390/brainsci7040042

Pacific Psychological Assessment Cooperation. (2004). *The Not-Real People stimulus set for assessment of sexual interest*. Victoria, BC: Author.

Paulhus, D. L. (1999). *Paulhus Deception Scales (PDS): The Balanced Inventory of Desirable Responding-7 (User's manual)*. Toronto, Ontario, Canada: Multi-Health Systems.

Paulhus, D. L. (2002). Socially desirable responding: the evolution of a construct. In Braun, H., Jackson, D., & Wiley, D. (Eds.). *The role of constructs in psychological and educational measurement* (pp. 39–69). Mahwah, NJ: Lawrence Erlbaum.

Perry, J. L., & Carroll, M. E. (2008). The role of impulsive behavior in drug abuse. *Psychopharmacology*, 200(1), 1–2610.1007/s00213-008-1173-0

Pratt, T. C., & Cullen, F.T. (2000). The empirical status of Gottfredson and Hirschi's general theory of crime: A meta-analysis. *Criminology*, 38(3), 931–96410.1111/j.1745-9125.2000.tb00911.x

Renaud, P., Chartier, S., Rouleau, J.-L., Proulx, J., Goyette, M., Trottier, D., Fedoroff, P., Bradford, J.-P., Dassylva, B., & Bouchard, S. (2013). Using immersive virtual reality and ecological psychology to probe into child molesters' phenomenology. *Journal of Sexual Aggression*, 19(1), 102–120. 10.1080/13552600.2011.617014

Renaud, P., Trottier, D., Rouleau, J.-L., Goyette, M., Saumur, C., Boukhalfi, T., & Bouchard, S. (2014). Using immersive virtual reality and anatomically correct computer-generated characters in the forensic assessment of deviant sexual preferences. *Virtual Reality*, 18(1), 37–47.10.1007/s10055-013-0235-8

Reynolds, C. R. & Suzuki, L. A. (2012). Bias in psychological assessment: an empirical review and recommendations. In *Assessment Psychology*, 10. 10.1002/9781118133880.hop210004

Riener, R., & Harders, M.   (2012). *Introduction to virtual reality in medicine. In virtual reality in medicine*. (pp. 1–12). London: Springer.

Santtila, P., Mokros, A., Viljanen, K., Koivisto, M., Sandnabba, N. K., Zappalà, A., & Osterheider, M. (2009). Assessment of sexual interest using a choice reaction time task and priming: a feasibility study. *Archives of Sexual Behavior*, *39*(5), 1081–1090. DOI: 10. 1007/s10508-009-9530-6

Schmidt, A. F. & Perkins, D. E. (2020). Using the Explicit and Implicit Sexual Interest Profile (EISIP) in applied forensic or clinical contexts. In G. Akerman, D. Perkins & R. Bartels (Eds.). *Assessing and Managing Problematic Sexual Interests* (). NY: Routledge.

Shapiro, F. (1995). *EMDR: Basic principles, protocols, and procedures*. New York: Guilford Press.

Shapiro, F. (2001). *Eye Movement Desensitization and Reprocessing: Basic Principles, Protocols and Procedures*. 2nd edition. New York: Guilford Press.

Simmonds, D. J., Pekar, J. J., & Mostofsky, S. H. (2008). Meta-analysis of Go/No-go tasks demonstrating that fMRI activation associated with response inhibition is task-dependent. *Neuropsychologia*, 46(1), 224–232. 10.1016/j.neuropsychologia.2007.07.015.

Snowden, R. J., Wichter, J. & Gray, N. S. (2008). Implicit and explicit measurements of sexual preference in gay and heterosexual men: a comparison of priming techniques and the Implicit Association Task. *Archives of Sexual Behaviour*, *37*(4), 558–565. DOI: 10. 1007/s10508-006-9138-z

Stefanska, E. B., Carter, A.J., Higgs, T., Bishopp, D., & Beech, A. R. (2015). Offense Pathways of Non-Serial Sexual Killers. *Journal of Criminal Justice*, 43, 99–107. 10.1016/ j.jcrimjus.2015.01.001

Stephens, S., Seto, M. C., Cantor, J. M., & Lalumière, M. L. (2019). The revised Screening Scale for Pedophilic Interests (SSPI-2) may be a measure of Pedohebephilia. *The Journal of Sexual Medicine*, 16, 1655–166310.1016/j.jsxm.2019.07.015

Stahl, C., Voss, A., Schmitz, F., Nuszbaum, M., Tüscher, O., Lieb, K., & Klauer, K. C. (2014). Behavioral components of impulsivity. *Journal of Experimental Psychology: General*, 143(2), 850–88610.1037/a0033981

Stein, J. S., & Madden, G. J. (2013). Delay discounting and drug abuse: Empirical, conceptual, and methodological considerations. In J. MacKillop & H. de Wit (Eds), *The Wiley-Blackwell handbook of addiction psychopharmacology* (pp. 165–208). Wiley Blackwell. https://doi.org/10.1002/9781118384404

Turner, D., Laier, C., Brand, M., Bockshammer, T., Welsch, R., & Rettenberger, M. (2018). Response inhibition and impulsive decision-making in sexual offenders against children. *Journal of Abnormal Psychology*, *127*, 471–481. 10.1037/abn0000359

Turner, D., & Rettenberger, M. (2020). Neuropsychological functioning in child sexual abusers: a systematic review. *Aggression and violent behaviour*, *54*, 101405.

Verbruggen, F., & Logan, G. D. (2008). Response inhibition in the stop-signal paradigm. *Trends in Cognitive Sciences*, 12(11), 418–42410.1016/j.tics.2008.07.005

Ward, T, & Beech, A. (2006). An integrated theory of sexual offending. *Aggression and Violent Behavior*, 11, 44–63. 10.1016/j.avb.2005.05.002

Ward, T., & Beech, A. (2016). The integrated theory of sexual offending - revised. A multifield perspective, In D. P. Boer (Ed.), *The Wiley handbook on the theories, assessment and treatment of sexual offending* (pp. 123-137). Hoboken, NJ: John Wiley & Sons.

Walker, J. S. (2005). The Maudsley Violence Questionnaire: initial validation and reliability. Personality and Individual Differences, 38, 187–201. 10.1016/j.paid.2004.04.001

Walker, J. S., & Gudjonsson, G. H. (2006). The Maudsley Violence Questionnaire: Relationship to personality and self-reported offending. *Personality and Individual Differences*, 40, 795–806. 10.1016/j.paid.2005.09.009

Woerner, J., Abbey, A., Helmers, B. R., Pegram, S. E., & Jilani, Z. (2018). Predicting men's immediate reactions to a simulated date's sexual rejection: the effects of hostile masculinity, impersonal sex, and hostile perceptions of the woman. *Psychology of violence*, *8*(3), 349.

Webster, C. D., Douglas, K. S., Eaves, D. & Hart, S. D., 1997. *HCR-20: Assessing risk for violence (version 2)*. Burnaby, British Columbia: Mental Health, Law and Policy Institute, Simon Fraser University.

Wright, L. & Warner, A. (2019). EMDR treatment of childhood sexual abuse for a child molester: self-reported changes in sexual arousal. *Journal of EMDR Practice and Research*. DOI: 10.1891/EMDR-D-19-00060

27 Challenging Bias in Cross-Cultural Forensic Psychology Assessment and Testing: A Summary Perspective

Yilma Woldgabreal

Introduction

I accepted the invitation to write the summary perspective chapter with some degree of trepidation. First, I am a clinician and do not have a track record of academic acumen. Second, despite my background as a person of colour, I am acutely aware that ethnic minorities in forensic psychology field are heterogenous and represent culturally diverse groups in a society, and, therefore, my perspective on racial bias may not be fully generalisable. Third, I am equally mindful that many of the chapters in this book explore and discuss racial bias from different angles and with reference to diverse forensic populations, making the task of summarising and accounting for all perspectives in this chapter even more challenging. Caveats aside, however, I enjoyed reading all the chapters and found them intellectually stimulating and practically informative. Most importantly, the various conceptual and pragmatic approaches taken throughout the book gave me hope that issues of racial bias in forensic psychology practice can indeed be challenged and addressed meaningfully.

My reflection and summary perspective focuses on three broad themes. The first is about challenges involving the construct validity of forensic psychology assessment and testing, a common theme that seems to cut across many of the topics covered in this book. This relates to the broader argument that bias in forensic psychology assessment and testing can arise in part from, and maintained by, an assumption of culture neutrality or universality. I highlight this conceptual argument from the outset to provide a context as to why challenging and addressing racial bias in forensic psychology assessment and testing is a focal point in this book. I also note that improvement in the construct validity of forensic psychology assessment and testing requires a paradigm shift that seeks to incorporate data from both qualitative and quantitative traditions, and that this demands epistemic reform through ongoing research.

In the second part of this chapter, I focus on the integral role of ethical practice in forensic psychology assessment and testing. There are ethical and legal responsibilities requiring forensic psychologists to use assessment tools that are not biased culturally and across diverse populations. But how strong and enforceable are ethical obligations to ensure cross-cultural competence and for

DOI: 10.4324/9781003230977-30

working with diverse populations? In this regard, taking into account the diverse perspectives presented in this book, I reflect on the extent to which current ethical practices are effective in challenging racial bias more broadly and provide some practical suggestions for improvement. In the final section, I consider the role of cross-cultural competence in challenging bias in forensic psychology assessment and testing. I specifically stress on the importance of cross-cultural case formulation, evidence-based professional supervision, and reflective practice.

Rethinking the Cultural Context of Construct Validity

A subtle, but common theme in this book is bias involving the construct validity of forensic psychology assessment and testing practices. Construct validity refers to the extent to which a psychological assessment or test represents a theoretical construct. Cook and Campbell (1979) described construct validity within the context of three broad categories: a statistical conclusion on the relationship between variables and the magnitude of this relationship; internal validity (whether a hypothesised cause and effect relationship between variables is free from other alternative explanations), and external validity (whether examined relationship between variables can be generalised across samples, settings, and occasions). These assumptions underpin the development of many of the contemporary forensic psychology assessments and tests, which have predominantly been tested and normed using samples from mainstream populations and then applied across other diverse demographic groups. That is, the mainstream approach is deeply rooted in the positivism paradigm that assumes the universality of psychological instruments that can be explained through scientific (quantitative) methods (Shepherd & Lewis-Fernandez, 2016).

However, cross-cultural equivalence of forensic psychology instruments has been contested and challenged by a growing number of both mainstream and minority scholars and researchers (e.g., Day et al., 2018; Hart, 2016; Ugwudike, 2020; Woldgabreal et al., 2020). The central argument here is that forensic psychology instruments have historically been influenced by values, worldviews, beliefs, and perceptions of the dominant culture in western societies. This means that contemporary forensic psychology assessment and testing practices have largely been non-inclusive in their epistemic values and have neglected the specific historical contexts and concerns of disadvantaged populations such as indigenous peoples and other people of colour living across western societies. This argument infers that forensic mental health and correctional practitioners who use forensic psychology instruments based on this hegemonistic perspective operate from the assumption that assessment instruments can be applied to all populations, preserving claims of culture neutrality and colour blindness in their practice (see Day and colleagues in this book). As such, a cross-cultural perspective calls for a paradigm shift and takes a constructivism stance, asserting that psychological assessment and testing should also be operationalised and interpreted qualitatively in light of individual and cultural circumstances.

Indeed, many of the contributions in this book illuminate the extent to which our assessment and testing practices have been intimately connected to homogenisation and institutionalisation of different experiences, and often ignoring the inherent power differentials. It is, thus, encouraging to see the consistency with which the monopoly and dominance of the epistemic tradition has been challenged and suggestions have been put forward for the integration of diverse worldviews such as culture-specific or gender-specific information in our assessment and testing practices. For example, Stephanie Schmidt and colleagues' chapter on dynamic risk factors highlights the limitations of generalising construct validity and measurement equivalence across cultures. Christopher Dean and Monica Lloyd's chapter demonstrates how an assessment strategy that relies on dominant perspective that assumes universality of behaviour may not be effective for assessing extremist offending. Jo Ramsden and Kerry Beckley have also shown us how the Power Threat Meaning Framework can be sensitively utilised to assess and treat persons involved in extremist offending. Yet again, Vivienne de Vogel highlights the limitations of risk assessment instruments when used with offenders who identify as females and how bias may play a role in misinterpretation of risks and needs, especially in minority groups. Taken together, many of the contributions in this book show how bias is introduced through the "one size fits all" approach can lead to either the introduction or omission of information that may be detrimental for the assessment process, and thereby leading, for example, to inflated risk scores among people of colour who have committed violent offences (e.g., Woldgabreal et. al., in press) and misdiagnosis in forensic mental health settings (e.g., Neighbors et al., 2003; Schwartz & Feisthamel, 2009). The overall message is that there is a need for substantive and sustainable paradigm shift or epistemic reform if we are to keep up with the principles of evolving evidence-based practice.

Moving Forward with Epistemic Reform in Construct Validity

A good starting point to improve construct validity is to work on the integration of the mainstream and culturally specific perspectives as demonstrated throughout this book. There is an increasing recognition that although the mainstream and cross-cultural perspectives tend to pull each other in divergent positions and become fertile grounds for bias, the split is not irreconcilable, and that both perspectives are mutually relevant for the advancement of our assessment and testing practices. Many of the chapters in this book reflect the need for a pragmatic stance, and highlight that knowledge is constantly renegotiated, debated, interpreted, and therefore the best method in forensic psychology assessment and testing is the one that seeks to understand and resolve a specific problem at hand in a fairer and equitable manner. This means that some situations might warrant quantification or objective approaches, while others may demand culturally sensitive qualitative responses, and yet others may be better served by combining the two.

Therefore, discussions in this book appear to lend themselves to two inter-related propositions that are likely to improve the construct validity of forensic psychology assessment and testing. The first is to incorporate nomothetic and idiographic information that I have alluded to so far (Barlow & Nock, 2009). Contemporary forensic psychology assessments are dominantly nomothetic and standardised because of their focus on making generalisations about an in-dividual's experiences, beliefs, values, thoughts, feelings, and behaviours based on the broader normative data. By contrast, the idiographic approach is concerned with specific information that is unique to an individual being assessed or tested. This approach is person-specific and considers qualitative aspects of an individual's circumstance and experiences, including environmental and cultural influences. Kelly's (1963) Personal Construct Theory (PCT) as discussed by Nick Blagden and Adrian Needs's in this book provides useful guidance on how to incorporate more idiographic information in forensic psychology assessments. PCT posits that each individual has the capacity to construct their own reality depending on their own unique circumstance. From this perspective, cross-cultural forensic psychology assessment can be enhanced by focusing on individual experiences, views, and interpretation. This is very much in line with a single case study design (Hayes et al., 1999), which seeks to explore and gain deeper understanding of individual circumstances during an assessment or testing. In comparison to standardised approaches, assessments that rely on single-case designs enable "the generation of alternative interpretations of collected data and quite possibly, causal explanations of behaviors" (Sexton-Radek, 2014, p. 98).

There have also been suggestions that integration of nomothetic-idiographic information through the use of structured professional judgment (SPJ) can increase construct validity in cross-cultural forensic psychology assessment and testing, primarily because of the opportunity SPJ presents for combining standardised approaches that cover common mental health symptoms and/or risk factors with individual accounts of presenting problems (Douglas et al., 2003); however, it should be born in mind that SPJ "require a great deal of clinical acumen to op-erationalize properly" (Zink et al., 2015, p. 27). Indeed, it is important to reiterate here that clinicians or psychologists generally tend to score people of colour higher on a violence risk scale that relies on SPJ (Woldgabreal et. al., in press), and make overdiagnosis of mental illness in patients from minority ethnic backgrounds (e.g., Neighbors et al., 2003; Strakowski et al., 2003). This is due in part to questions and formats that guide the SPJ relying on a prior theory, which does not take into account individual differences. Thus, the need for research to develop cross-culturally tailored SPJ guide remains of paramount and practical importance. This would require careful translation of concepts and use of culturally meaningful questions to increase the validity of the assessment.

The second proposition, perhaps the most important, is to develop conceptual models that can guide cross-cultural forensic psychology assessment and testing practices (Day et al., 2018). This proposition is based on the argument high-lighted earlier that assessment instruments have historically been influenced by values, worldviews, beliefs, and perceptions of the dominant culture in western societies, and therefore, there is a need to "decolonise" westernised ideas of knowledge and knowledge production by reconceptualising knowledge as fluid, contextual, dynamic, and organic (e.g., Gillies, 2013; Gray et al., 2007; Tauri, 2017; Teo, 2015). It has been, for example, suggested in the context of Australia that research methodologies that identify and recognise Aboriginal knowledge as a legitimate epistemic resource should be part of the evidence-based correctional policies and programs (e.g., Butcher et al., 2021; Keikelame & Swartz, 2019). For this, genuine partnerships among key stakeholders, including scholars with cultural authority, relevant government and non-government institutions, and researchers are considered critical. In my view, partnerships will diversify forensic psychology assessment and testing practices and bridge the gap in equity and fairness. This means that a successful "decolonisation" of knowledge can pave the way for epistemic reform that has been well overdue.

It is, nonetheless, important to recognise the significance of the challenge here. Even a cursory review of the extant literature in the field of corrections, for example, would highlight a chequered history of resistance in paradigm shift, with proponents of established assessments or tests defending their approaches vigorously even in the face of obvious limitations and opportunities for improvement (Looman & Abracen, 2013). This is because that once standardised assessments and testing practices are implemented based on certain theoretical and empirical orientation, there is a risk of emotional attachment, which tends to cloud objectively. However, as Popper (1995) argued, scientific knowledge should be open for modification. This is a good reminder for us to remain pragmatic, open to paradigm shift, and sensitive to emerging social, cultural, and ecological contexts in which forensic psychology assessment and testing practices are embedded. It is, thus, imperative for all of us with vested interest in the field of forensic psychology to not fall into the trap of maintaining the status quo for a universal approach or engage in temporary or minor fixes in the hope that assessment or test validity problem discussed so far would simply go away.

Rethinking Ethical Practice

Psychology is a regulated profession in western societies. Codes of ethics, and guidelines exist to protect users of psychological services from both potentially foreseeable and unforeseeable practice-related harms. Whilst the depth and breadth of these ethical codes and guidelines differ across countries and legislatures, psychologists are generally expected to practice within the scope of certain universal ethical principles. These include, among others, respect for the dignity of persons and peoples, competent caring for the well-being of persons and peoples, integrity, and professional and scientific responsibilities to society (International Union of Psychological Science, 2008).

So, what do these four universal declarations of ethical principles entail? Well, the first, respect for the dignity of persons and peoples, is the most fundamental principle that recognises the universal rights and inherent worth of human beings irrespective of their race, gender, age, religion, status, and so on. A summary of the extant literature also indicates that when people are exposed to disrespectful behaviour, they tend to experience a range of dysfunctional life events such as poor mental health, emotional distress, reduced productivity, avoidant and un-cooperative behaviour, loss of trust, and even engagement in antisocial conducts (Allan & Davidson, 2013). Thus, it is not surprising that respect embodies both morally codified ethical principles and legally enforceable responsibility from the perspective of human rights and anti-discrimination legislative provisions that protect the welfare of disadvantaged and vulnerable members of a society.

The second principle, competent caring for the well-being of persons and peoples, is about doing no harm. It seeks to maximise benefits and minimise po-tential harm that can arise from bias in forensic psychology assessment and testing. In the context of cross-cultural practice, competent caring requires the application of knowledge and skills that are appropriate for clients of diverse ethnic back-grounds. It is incumbent on psychologists to ensure that their knowledge of cross-cultural practice is adequate. This involves openness to engaging in critical self-reflection and preparedness to assess their own values, experiences, social contexts, and how these might influence their actions and interpretations. Therefore, from the perspective of universal ethical principles, psychologists have moral obligations and responsibilities to do no harm by ensuring that forensic psychology assessment and testing practices are less susceptible to bias through the development and maintenance of cross-cultural competence.

The third broad principle, integrity, concerns the extent to which forensic psychology assessment and testing is underpinned by an honest, open, and cross-culturally accurate information. This principle again reminds psychologists about their responsibility to engender public confidence through the choice and ap-plication of ethically, conceptually, and practically defensible assessment and testing instruments that can minimise biases. The last, but a related ethical principle, is professional and scientific responsibility to society. This is about psychologists' obligation to work cooperatively with their colleagues and other professionals in the best interests of clients. This includes advocacy roles, chal-lenging unethical practices or behaviours of others, and preventing or avoiding their own unethical conduct.

Moving Forward with Ethical Practice

The aforementioned broad ethical principles are difficult to assess in practice, and their application to real-world settings depends on an individual psycholo-gist's commitment. In his famous book, *Nicomachean Ethics*, Aristotle noted that doing what we should and not doing what we should not is simply not enough in ethical practice. For Aristotle, ethical practice is about practicing virtues (e.g., courage, passion, justice, fortitude, and so on), showing practical wisdom, and taking actions (McKeon, 1971). This is exactly what we have collectively done in this book, taking practical actions to challenge and address bias through our scholarly contributions. However, much remains to be done. My own personal experience, observation, and insight into the forensic psychology field indicate that the goalposts for theoretical and empirical basis of assessment tools hardly move, which I think is the antithesis to the scientific basis of our profession and ethical principles. What is even more concerning is that substantive changes in the context of cross-cultural psychology have continued to lag behind, and there have been "many critical moments of silence and inaction at times when proactive acts or speaking out were warranted" (American Psychological Association, APA, 2021, para. 14).

Indeed, recent "Black Lives Matter" movement across many western countries has put a spotlight on this issue, culminating to the publication of position statements by peak and authoritative psychological associations across many countries. For example, the Australian Psychological Society (APS) in conjunction with the Australian Indigenous Psychologists Association, Association of Counselling Psychologists, Australian Clinical Psychology Association, Australian Psychology Accreditation Council, Heads of Departments and Schools of Psychology Association, Institute of Clinical Psychologists, and Institute of Private Practising Psychologists issued a joint position statement to take a stand against racism, systematic discrimination, and inequalities in the delivery of psychological services more broadly (Australian Psychological Society, 2020). Prior to this the APS made a formal apology to Aboriginal and Torres Strait Islander people, acknowledging psychology's contribution to historical injustices and failure to "respect their skills, expertise, worldviews, and unique wisdom developed over thousands of years" (APS, 2017, para. 4). It has also been noted that the root causes of ethical problems in psychological practice, including forensic psychology assessment and testing, reside in part due to explicit and implicit racial biases arising from socio-economic and political disadvantages experienced by Aboriginal and Torres Strait Islander people in Australia. The APS went on to affirm its commitment to pursue a different way of working with Aboriginal and Torres Strait Islander people by "listening more and talking less, following more and steering less, advocating more and complying less, including more and ignoring less and collaborating more and commanding less" (Australian Psychological Society, 2017, para. 6).

Comparable position statements were made in the United Kingdom, United States, Canada, and New Zealand in recent years, making explicit commitments to ensure that psychologists uphold their ethical responsibilities and provide equitable, non-discriminatory, and unbiased psychological services to people of colour. However, the APA (2021) warns that even with the explicit acknowledgement and encouragement of our peak professional bodies, taking action against racially biased psychological practices has been either slow or absent in many applied settings. In my own area of practice in corrections, psychologists rarely speak up or engage in advocacy roles to inform policies and practices that are non-discriminatory to people of colour who have offended. Silence seems to be the common code, which must be broken in the spirit of virtuous ethical principles to challenge racial bias. The collective ideas presented in this book echo this message. However, it is important to note that ethical principles on their own are ill-equipped to handle issues of racial bias in forensic assessment and testing. As detailed in the preceding section, more work is needed around epistemic reform as well as commitment to cross-cultural competence, which I am about to cover in the next section.

Strengthening Cross-Cultural Competence

Advancing cross-cultural competence may not seem an obvious message of this book; however, in my view, it is one of the subtle concepts discussed throughout the book. Even what brought us all together to contribute to this book, the very recognition of bias in forensic psychology assessment and testing, and our commitment to challenge bias through knowledge building are the most critical elements of cross-cultural practice. Before I comment and reflect on how ongoing improvement can be made in this space, it may be helpful to present a brief scan of the literature on cross-cultural competence. The literature provides no single definition of cross-cultural competence. However, most definitions refer to knowledge, perspective taking, and problem-solving skills needed to effectively work or interact with people from ethnically/racially diverse backgrounds (Whaley & Davis, 2007). A number of conceptual models have been proposed over the years, including Cross et al.'s (1989) six-stage model, which explains cross-cultural competence as sequentially developing knowledge and skills along a continuum (see Figure 27.1).

Cross et al. (1989) referred the Cultural Destructiveness stage as the early stage of the colonial period in western countries where institutions and professionals actively reinforced policies and practices of segregation, discrimination, exclusion, and maltreatment of racial minorities. The Cultural Incapacity stage on the continuum was where institutions and professionals began to understand the plight of racial minorities, but unable to help because of deeply held beliefs in racial superiority and paternalistic attitudes of the dominant group. The Cultural Blindness stage refers to denial of bias by either institutions or individual professionals, who assert that all human beings are inherently similar, and therefore, the dominant culture should be universally applicable. Cross and colleagues (1989) linked this stage of cultural competence to policies of assimilation, where institutions or individual practitioners failed to recognise power differentials, privileges of the dominant group, the specific needs of people of colour, and blaming them for their inability to succeed even in the face of considerable socio-economic disadvantages.

The Cultural Pre-Competence stage, according to Cross and colleagues (1989), refers to recognition of racial inequalities. This is a stage where institutions or individuals of the dominant culture have begun to improve some aspects of services, including hiring people of colour and implementing diversity policies such as mandating cultural awareness training for staff. However, Cross and colleagues (1989) warned about two potential dangers at this level of cross-cultural competence. The first is the possibility of developing a sense of accomplishment and the risk of failing to move forward along the continuum, and the second being tokenism or tendency to hire few assimilated people of colour and assume that that an organisation or institution is well-equipped to handle

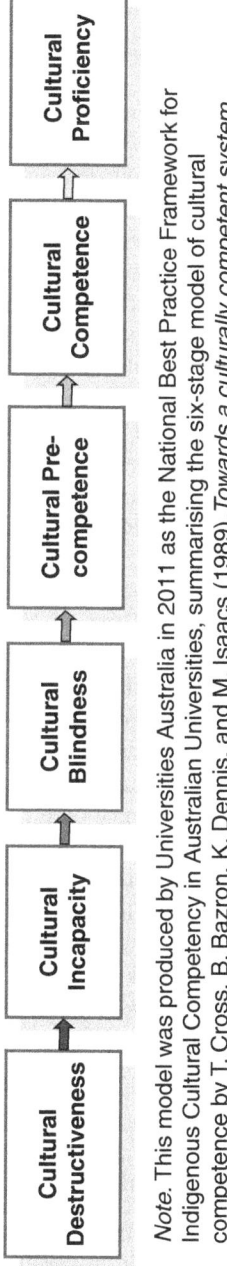

Note. This model was produced by Universities Australia in 2011 as the National Best Practice Framework for Indigenous Cultural Competency in Australian Universities, summarising the six-stage model of cultural competence by T. Cross, B. Bazron, K. Dennis, and M. Isaacs (1989). *Towards a culturally competent system*

Figure 27.1 Model of cross-cultural competence.

service needs of people of colour. In the context of individual practitioners, it would mean equating cross-cultural competence with having some friends who are from certain minority or disadvantaged backgrounds. The next stage, Cultural Competence, is where either an individual practitioner or institution accepts and respects cultural differences and engages in ongoing critical self-reflection to improve relationships or service needs of people of colour. The last stage on the continuum, Cultural Proficiency, is what Cross and colleagues (1989) referred to as "the most positive end of the scale" (p. 32). Individual practitioners or institutions at this stage are said to engage in knowledge building by conducting research, disseminating results, developing new assessment tools and intervention approaches based on culture.

Campinha-Bacote (1994) proposed a slightly different cultural competence model, involving a four-stage process in the development of cultural competence as depicted in Figure 27.2. This model posits that proficiency would be required at each stage for individuals or organisations to progress along the continuum. That is, cultural awareness leads to cultural knowledge which in turn results in skilfulness, and this translating into an ability to deal with cultural encounters. This model also assumes that cultural competence is an ongoing process and is not something that can be accomplished with a one-off lesson.

Another most commonly recognised model is Bennett and Bennett's (2004) developmental model of intercultural competence depicted in Figure 27.3, which is mainly similar to Cross et al.'s (1989) model. The denial, defense, and minimisation stages are considered to be "ethnocentric". That is, in the denial stage individuals or institutions do not recognise the presence of cultural differences; in the mini-misation stage, they acknowledge the difference but feel threatened and respond defensively; in the minimisation stage, they downplay the seriousness of cultural differences to preserve the dominance of the dominant culture. The last three stages of Bennett and Bennett's (2004) model are known as "ethno-relative". Specifically, the acceptance stage is said to occur when individuals or institutions recognise cultural differences without prejudice or judgement; the adaptation stage refers to adaptation of the cultural difference both cognitively and behaviourally; the integration stage reflects a state of comfort in everyday race-related discourses, humility, and celebration of cultural difference or diversity.

Overall, these conceptual models highlight the various stages of cross-cultural competence, and indicate the extent to which cross-cultural competence is embedded progressively. It is reassuring to know that racial bias can be challenged through ongoing knowledge building and acquisition of skills. Indeed, our collective effort in this book is part and parcel of this knowledge-building process to make forensic psychology assessments and tests fairer and unharmful when used with people of colour.

Moving Forward with Cross-Cultural Competence

As highlighted above, cross-cultural competence can be enhanced when we engage in knowledge building through research and development of new

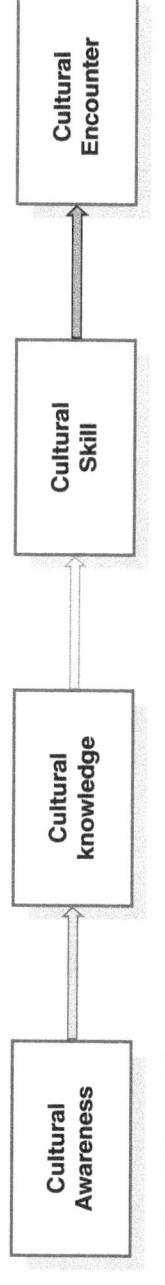

Note. This model was produced by Universities Australia in 2011 as the National Best Practice Framework for Indigenous Cultural Competency in Australian Universities, summarising the four-stage process model of cultural competence by J. Campinha-Bacote. 1994. Cultural Competence in Psychiatric Mental Health

Figure 27.2 Model of development of cultural competence.

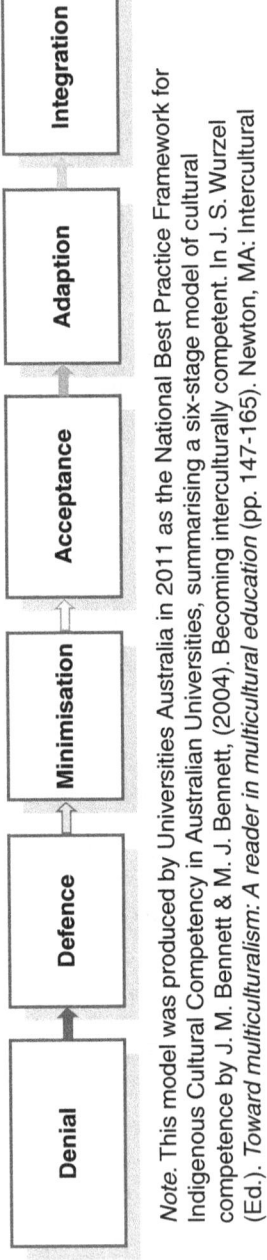

Note. This model was produced by Universities Australia in 2011 as the National Best Practice Framework for Indigenous Cultural Competency in Australian Universities, summarising a six-stage model of cultural competence by J. M. Bennett & M. J. Bennett, (2004). Becoming interculturally competent. In J. S. Wurzel (Ed.). *Toward multiculturalism: A reader in multicultural education* (pp. 147–165). Newton, MA: Intercultural

Figure 27.3 Developmental model of intercultural competence.

assessment and intervention strategies based on culture. Cultural difference is something that we can adapt through cognitively flexibility, perspective taking, and humility. This goes in tandem with ongoing acquisition of practical skills, including cross-cultural case formulation, seeking evidence-based professional supervision, and reflective practice, which I consider next.

Cross-Cultural Case Formulation

Forensic psychology assessment or testing practices are not ends in and of themselves, but they inform key decisions in forensic mental health care and provision of correctional services. For example, instruments that are designed for the assessment of risk of recidivism still disproportionality classify people of colour who have committed offences and contribute to their overrepresentation in the criminal justice system (Woldgabreal et al., 2020). Addressing the differential impacts of such tools remains a long-term goal and research priority. Meanwhile, we have responsibility to minimise the differential impact of assessment tools on people of colour through other readily available options. Cross-cultural case formulation is one of such options. For this, Heffernan and Ward's chapter in this book provides important suggestions and reminds us of potential challenges to overcome when completing cross-culturally informed case formulation. They note that,

> "… it is important not to jump to conclusions about the causes of behaviour, or to rely solely on identified risk factors to guide case formulations. Rather, practitioners can use these ratings as one source of information (i.e., as potential barriers to prosocial agency or red flags to explore), and later check whether they are likely to be linked with or addressed within their case formulation. The most important source of information for constructing the formulation will be the individual's account of their behaviour, including the motivations and values underpinning it and the context in which it occurred" (p. xx).

Kilcullen and Day (2017) proposed a similar approach to case conceptualisation in the context of Aboriginal and Torres Strait Islander people in Australia. They argued that case conceptualisation with clients of Aboriginal and Torres Strait Islander background cannot be objectively completed without considering historical experiences of injustice and systemic factors that continue to impact on their psychosocial mechanisms still today (e.g., integrational trauma, racism, and economic inequality). The authors emphasised the importance considering and integrating culturally relevant strength factors into case conceptualisation, and that this could involve recognising communal values, interdependence, cultural connectedness, family involvement, spirituality, knowledge transmission of myth and ritual practices that engender resilience.

Day (2017) noted that practitioner opinion matters in cross-cultural case conceptualisation, stating that the opinion section is the most important as "it seeks to offer an explanation of why a person acted as he or she did, rather than simply describing a person's level of risk or psychological functioning" (p. 56). This further provides practitioners with opportunities to consider some of the ethical issues that impact on people of colour (e.g., inequality and disadvantages), which are not commonly covered by standardised forensic psychology assessments (Delle-Vergine & Day, 2016). All of these propositions are clearly consistent with the integration of nomothetic-idiographic information discussed earlier in this chapter, and further emphasise the importance of eclectic approach in cross-cultural case formulation.

Evidence-Based Supervision

Evidence-based professional supervision is another important mechanism by which cross-cultural competence can be strengthened. Whilst a review of the types and forms of evidence-based supervision is beyond the scope of this chapter, it is important to highlight that Jason Davies's chapter in this book provides useful theoretical, empirical, and practical applications of evidence-based professional supervision. The message here is to stress on the role of professional supervision in driving cross-cultural competence. As noted in Jason Davies's chapter, professional supervision is key for maintaining, developing, and evaluating forensic psychologists' practical skills. It also offers opportunities for attending to ethical dilemmas and challenges, and thereby enhancing forensic psychologists' objectivity and impartiality in cross-cultural practice.

   However, the assumption that supervisors educating, guiding, mentoring, and supporting supervisees can be a complex idea. Supervisors can be equally susceptible to prejudice and may not be able to buffer the effects of racial bias through the supervision process. What is even more challenging, based on my own personal experience in correctional settings, is that a significant number of supervisors tend to have less training and limited insight into cross-cultural practices compared to supervisees. There have been, however, practical approaches to address this limitation through peer supervision and consultation with more experienced forensic psychologists in the context of cross-cultural practice. In my view, this can be further strengthened by holding regular reflective practice forums, involving practitioners and their supervisors.

Reflective Practice

The lived experiences chapter (Chapter 2) in this book by Palwinder Athwal-Kooner, Martine Ratcliffe, and Ana Da Silva is an excellent point of departure for the discussion of reflective practice. The authors have eloquently told their personal experience of bias both as forensic psychologists and members of the Black and Minority Ethnic communities in the United Kingdom. I have been particularly drawn to their stories of hope, optimism, and resilience. As an African immigrant and a person of colour living in Australia, their experience resonates with me very well. At the same time, however, I am mindful of the challenges associated with sharing a personal experience of bias as part of a reflective practice setting or discussion of bias involving people of colour who have offended. In my experience, scholarly reflections of lived experience rarely reach direct practice settings. When they do, they often end up in emotional turmoils and bad feelings on all sides, and consequently tend to be avoided or never to be repeated in a while. This then results in a self-perpetuating cycle of negative experience in forums, meetings, and even professional supervision sessions that seek to challenge instances of racial bias in applied work settings. As a result, we often seem to fall back to default paradigms or uncritical adoption of race-neutral approaches, which then tend to dominate topics of reflective practice. Forensic psychology assessment and testing is no exception in this regard.

So, why is race-related reflective practice or discussion of racial bias sensitive and emotionally charged? Well, in my view and personal experience, two fundamental challenges are readily apparent. First, discourses that involve racial bias or prejudice are inherently anxiety-provoking and uncomfortable because of the ways in which these issues have been conceptualised, interpreted, and discussed in practice settings. There is a general inclination to view issues of racial bias or prejudice as binary or categorical events, which tend to position people within "victims vs perpetrators" or "us vs them" dichotomy. This in turn seems to leave no room for constructive and critical reflection. It often discourages openness and leads to denial of personal responsibility as reflected in Pally, Martine, and Ana's chapter (Chapter 2). However, if we take a pragmatic approach to see race-related discourses along a continuum line, we are likely to appreciate the complexity and diversity of race-related issues, and acknowledge that bias can sometimes be a normal mental process and an inevitable human tendency. Indeed, some of the classical studies on racial bias (e.g., Gaertner & Bickman, 1971; Piliavin et al., 1969) and recent memory and neuroimaging experiments (e.g., Brown et al., 2017; Rubien-Thomas et al., 2021) suggest that we have a natural tendency to favour and pay attention to our own race. And none of us are immune to this possibility. Whilst my view here is not purported to legitimise and minimise the effects of racial bias, seeing bias along a continuum line is likely to help us challenge and tackle racial bias realistically.

The second challenge relates to our tendency to primarily focus on human deficits or negative events during reflective practice forums or meetings. We simply focus on encouraging practitioners to examine stereotypical beliefs and worldviews held about certain ethnic minorities or other disadvantaged sections of a society. This approach is very much in line with the idea of detecting deficits and weakness, and changing or correcting errors. However, we know that psychology has been challenged within for its preoccupation in trying to repair the worst things in human life, whilst paying limited attention to identify and build such character strengths as open-mindedness, gratitude, optimism, kindness, fairness, compassion, and so on (Seligman & Csikszentmihalyi, 2000). Indeed, research over the past two decades has shown the link between positive psychology interventions that seek to promote character strengths and a range of desirable life events such as healthy relationships, resilience, perspective taking, and more broadly optimal well-being

(Ellardus Van Zyl & Rothmann, 2019). Therefore, reflective practice that draws on strengths is likely to offer a different lens and buffer the effects racial bias, whether this is to do with seeing the positives in specific client populations or simply our daily conversations with practitioners of diverse backgrounds. With positive approaches we are likely to build bridges. With deficit-based approaches we are likely to encounter defensive responses and widen the gap and make issues of racial bias more subtle and insidious.

Concluding Thoughts

In closing, I would like to reiterate the three broad themes that I have identified in trying to understand and challenge bias in a cross-cultural forensic psychology assessment and testing context. The first relates to construct validity issues involving standardised instruments, which have historically been influenced by values, worldviews, beliefs, and perceptions of the dominant culture in western societies. This book offers scholarly, practical, and experiential suggestions on how to challenge some of the biases that can arise from the limitations of standardised forensic psychology instruments. Some of these recommendations include attention to the integration of nomothetic-idiographic information in the assessment and testing process. Nonetheless, the need for a paradigm shift or epistemic reform to recognise and legitimatise cultural knowledge remains to be a research priority if we are to bring about substantive and sustainable improvements in this area.

My second observation relates to the role of ethical practice in challenging bias in the context of cross-cultural assessment and testing. Whilst psychological practice is a regulated profession and guided by ethical codes and guidelines to protect users of psychological services from both potentially foreseeable and unforeseeable practice-related harms, enforcing these expectations remains a challenge. In many ways, the responsibility falls back on the individual psychologist to show practical wisdom and take actions to prevent bias and advocate for a fair and equitable psychological practice. This is what brought us together from all corners to contribute to the edition of this book, which is an exemplary effort and must continue in many different contexts to challenge racial bias that exists in our practice.

The third important theme, from my perspective, is the subtle overarching aim of this book to contribute to the knowledge base and help the development of skills that can lend themselves to cross-cultural competence in forensic psychology assessment and testing. The book consists of specific areas of forensic psychology practice (e.g., risk assessments) and strategies on how to challenge racial bias in all of those contexts, contributing to our knowledge base in cross-cultural competence. Indeed, cross-cultural competence is an area of continuous improvement in terms of challenging racial bias in forensic psychology practice more broadly. For these, the role of ongoing skills development in the context of cross-cultural case formulation, evidence-based professional supervision, and reflective practice cannot be stressed enough.

References

Allan, A., & Davidson, G. (2013). Respect for the dignity of people: What does this principle mean in practice? *Australian Psychologist, 48*(5), 345–352. 10.1111/ap.12012

American Psychological Association. (2021). *Historical chronology: Examining psychology's contributions to the belief in racial hierarchy and perpetuation of inequality for people of color in U.S.* https://www.apa.org/about/apa/addressing-racism/historical-chronology

Australian Psychological Society. (2020). *Black Lives Matter: Psychologists take a stand against racism.* https://psychology.org.au/getmedia/dece6e26-f3a9-4b1a-bc55-3abdab03293d/aps-black-lives-matter-position-statement-psychologists-take-a-stand-against-racism_1.pdf

Australian Psychological Society. (2017). Apology to Aboriginal and Torres Strait Islander People from the Australian Psychological Society. https://psychology.org.au/getmedia/dc5eb83c-9be9-4dce-95ec-232ac89e1d14/aps-apology-atsi.pdf

Barlow, D. H., & Nock, M. K. (2009). Why can't we be more idiographic in our research? *Perspectives on Psychological Science, 4*(1), 19–21. 10.1111/j.1745-6924.2009.01088.x

Bennett, J. M., & Bennett, M. J. (2004). Developing intercultural sensitivity: An integrative approach to global and domestic diversity. In D. Landis, J. M. Bennett & M. Bennett (Eds.), *Handbook of intercultural training* (pp. 147–165). Thousand Oaks, CA: Sage.

Brown, T. L., Vinson, E. S., & Abdullah, T. (2017). Cross-cultural considerations with African American clients: A perspective on psychological assessment. In L. T. Benuto & B. D. Leany (Eds.), *Guide to psychological assessment with African Americans* (pp. 9–18). Springer. doi: 10.1007/978-1-4939-1004-5

Butcher, L., Day, A., Miles, D., Kidd, G., & Stanton, S. (2021). Developing youth justice policy and programme design in Australia. *Australian Journal of Public Administration, 53*, 369–386. doi: 10.1111/1467-8500.12524

Campinha-Bacote, J. (1994). *The process of cultural competence: A culturally competent model of care* (2nd Ed). Wyoming, Ohio: Transcultural C.A.R.E. Associates.

Cook, T. D., & Campbell, D. T. (1979). *Quasi-experimentation: Design and analysis issues for fields settings.* Boston: Houghton Mifflin Company.

Cross, T., Bazron, B., Dennis, K., & Isaacs, M. (1989). *Towards a culturally competent system of care* (Vol. 1). Washington, DC: Georgetown University Child Development Center, CASSP Technical Assistance Center. https://files.eric.ed.gov/fulltext/ED330171.pdf

Day, A. (2017). Reporting case formulation and opinion. In: S. Brown, E. Bowen, & D. Prescott, (Eds.) *The forensic psychologist's report writing guide* (pp. 56–65). Abingdon, UK: Routledge.

Day, A., Tamatea, A. J., Casey, S., & Geia, L. (2018). Assessing violence risk with Aboriginal and Torres Strait Islander offenders: Considerations for forensic practice. *Psychiatry, Psychology and Law, 25*(3), 452–464. 10.1080/13218719.2018.1467804

Delle-Vergine, V., & Day, A. (2016). Case formulation in forensic practice: Challenges and opportunities. *Journal of Forensic Practice, 18*(3), 240–250. doi: 10.1108/JFP-01-2016-0005.

Douglas, K. S., Ogloff, J. R. P., & Hart, S. D. (2003). Evaluation of a model of violence risk assessment among forensic psychiatric patients. *Psychiatric Services, 54*(10), 1372–1379. doi: 10.1176/appi.ps.54.10.1372

Ellardus Van Zyl, L. & Rothmann Sr, S. (2019). *Evidence-based positive psychological interventions in multi-cultural contexts.* Springer. 10.1007/978-3-030-20311-5

Gaertner, S., & Bickman, L. (1971). Effects of race on the elicitation of helping behavior: The wrong number technique. *Journal of Personality and Social Psychology, 20*(2), 218–222. 10.1037/h0031681

Gillies, C. (2013). Establishing the United Nations' Declaration on the Rights of Indigenous Peoples as the Minimum Standard for All Forensic Practice with Australian Indigenous Peoples. *Australian Psychologist*, *48*, 14–27. doi:10.1111/ap.12003

Gray, M., Coates, J., & Hetherington, T. (2007). Hearing indigenous voices in mainstream social work. *Journal of Contemporary Human Services*, *88*(1), 55–66. doi: 10.1606/1044-3894.3592

Hart, S. D. (2016). Culture and violence risk assessment: The case of Ewert v. Canada. *Journal of Threat Assessment and Management*, *3*(2), 76–96. 10.1037/tam0000068

Hayes, S. C., Barlow, D. H., & Nelson-Gray, R. O. (1999). *The scientist practitioner: Research and accountability in the age of managed care* (2nd ed.). Allyn & Bacon.

International Union of Psychological Science (2008). Universal declaration of ethical principles for psychologists. Available at https://www.iupsys.net/about/declarations/universal-declaration-of-ethical-principles-for-psychologists/

Keikelame, M. J., & Swartz, L. (2019). Decolonising research methodologies: Lessons from a qualitative research project, Cape Town, South Africa. *Global Health Action*, *12*(1). 10.1080/16549716.2018.1561175

Kelly, G. (1963). *A theory of personality: The psychology of personal constructs*. New York: W. W. Norton & Company.

Kilcullen, M., & Day, A. (2017). Culturally informed case conceptualisation: Developing a clinical psychology approach to treatment planning for non-Indigenous psychologists working with Aboriginal and Torres Strait Islander clients. *Clinical Psychologist*, *22*(1), 280–289. doi: 10.1111/cp.12141

Looman, J., & Abracen, J. (2013). The risk need responsivity model of offender rehabilitation: Is there really a need for a paradigm shift? *International Journal of Behavioral Consultation and Therapy*, *8*(3–4), 30–36. 10.1037/h0100980

López, S. R. (1997). Cultural competence in psychotherapy: A guide for clinicians and their supervisors. In C. E. Watkins, Jr. (Eds.), *Handbook of psychotherapy supervision* (pp. 570–588). John Wiley & Sons, Inc.

McKeon, R. (1971). *The basic work of Aristotle*. New York: Random, House.

Neighbors, H. W., Trierweiler, S. J., Ford, B. C., & Muroff, J. R. (2003). Racial differences in DSM diagnoses using a semi-structured instrument: The importance of clinical judgment in the diagnosis of African Americans. *Journal of Health and Social Behavior*, *44*, 237–256. doi: 10.2307/1519777

Piliavin, I. M., Rodin, J., & Piliavin, J. A. (1969). Good Samaritanism: An underground phenomenon? *Journal of Personality and Social Psychology*, *13*(4), 289–299. 10.1037/h0028433

Popper, K. (1995). Knowledge and the shaping of reality. In K. Popper (Ed), In search of a better world: Lectures and essays from thirty years (pp. 3–29). Routledge.

Rubien-Thomas, E., Berrian, N., Cervera, A., Nardos, B., Cohen, A. O., Lowrey, A., Daumeyer, N. M., Camp, N. P., Hughes, B. L., Eberhardt, J. L., Taylor-Thompson, K. A., Fair, D. A., Richeson, J. A., & Casey, B. J. (2021). Processing of task-irrelevant race information is associated with diminished cognitive control in black and white individuals. *Cognitive, Affective, & Behavioral Neuroscience*, *21*, 625–638. 10.3758/s13415-021-00896-8

Schwartz, R. C., & Feisthamel, K. P. (2009). Disproportionate diagnosis of mental disorders among African American versus European American clients: Implications for counseling theory, research, and practice. *Journal of Counseling and Development*, *87*, 295–301. 10.1002/j.1556-6678.2009.tb00110.x

Seligman, M. E. P., & Csikszentmihalyi, M. (2000). Positive psychology: An introduction. *American Psychologist*, *55*(1), 5–14. 10.1037/0003-066X.55.1.5

Sexton-Radek, K. (2014). Single case designs in psychology practice. *Health Psychology Research*, *2*(3), 98–99. doi: 10.4081/hpr.2014.1551

Shepherd, S. M., & Lewis-Fernandez, R. (2016). Forensic risk assessment and cultural diversity: Contemporary challenges and future directions. *Psychology, Public Policy, and Law*, *22*(4), 427–438. 10.1037/law0000102

Strakowski, S. M., Keck Jr., P. E., Arnold, L. M., Collins, J., Wilson, R. M., Fleck, D. E., Corey, K. B., Amicone, J., Victor R. & Adebimpe, V. R. (2003). Ethnicity and diagnosis in patients with affective disorders. *Journal of Clinical Psychiatry*, *64*(7), 747–754. doi: 10.4088/jcp.v64n0702

Sue, D. W., & Torino, G. C. (2005). Racial-cultural competence: Awareness, knowledge, and skills. In R. T. Carter (Ed.), *Handbook of racial-cultural psychology and counseling, Vol. 2. Training and practice* (pp. 3–18). John Wiley & Sons, Inc.

Tauri, J. (2017). Imagining an indigenous criminological future. In A. Deckert & R. Sarre (Eds.), *The Palgrave handbook of Australian and New Zealand criminology, crime and justice* (pp. 769–786). Springer. doi: 10.1007/978-3-319-55747-2

Teo, T. (2015). Are psychological "ethics codes" morally oblique? *Journal of Theoretical and Philosophical Psychology*, *35*(2), 78–89. doi: 10.1037/a0038944

Ugwudike, P. (2020). Digital prediction technologies in the justice system: The implications of a 'race-neutral' agenda. *Theoretical Criminology*, *24*(3), 482–501. doi: 10.1177/1362480619896006

Universities Australia. (2011). *National best practice framework for indigenous cultural competency in Australian universities.* Canberra, ACT: Australian Government Department of Education, Employment and Workplace Relations. https://www.universitiesaustralia.edu.au/uni-participation-quality/Indigenous-HigherEducation/Indigenous-Cultural-Compet#.VCylEL6QcyE

Whaley, A. L., & Davis, K. E. (2007). Cultural competence and evidence-based practice in mental health services: A complementary perspective. *American Psychologist*, *62*(6), 563–574. 10.1037/0003-066X.62.6.563

Woldgabreal, Y., Day, A., & Tamatea, A. (2020). Do risk assessments play a role in the enduring 'color line'? *Advancing Corrections: Journal of the International Corrections and Prisons Association*, *10*, 18–28.

Woldgabreal, Y., Day, A., Daffern, M., Lloyd, C., & Graffam, J. (in press). An empirical test of the factor structure of the violence risk scale and its measurement invariance across time and cultural groups. *Criminal Justice and Behavior*. Advance online publication. https://doi.org/10.1097/PHM.0000000000001435

Zink, D., Lee, B., & Allen, D. (2015). Structured and semistructured clinical interviews available for use among African American clients: Cultural considerations in the diagnostic interview process. In L. T. Benuto & B. D. Leany (Eds.), *Guide to psychological assessment with African Americans* (pp. 19–42). Springer. doi: 10.1007/978-1-4939-1004-5

Index

Please note that page references to Figures will be in **bold**, while references to Tables are in *italics*.

Equality, Diversity and Inclusion (EDI) 20,
27–30, 31
Equality Act (2010), UK 339
equivalence: construct 54–55; cross-
cultural 54, 476; full score 56–57;
functional 55; importance in forensic
psychology 53–54; measurement 56;
structural 55; taxonomies 54
ERG22+ SPJ framework 429
Esposito, L. 316
ethical blindness 199
ethics: ethical issues fallacy, in forensic
practice 233; ethical practice 475–476,
479–480; moving forward with ethical
practice 480–482; rethinking ethical
practice 479–480
ethnicity: and criminal versatility 412;
double discrimination of minoritized
ethnic groups 364; psychopathy
assessment 447–448; *see also* BAME
(Black Asian Ethnic Minority)
community; culture(s); racism
Euclidean distances 267
European Federation of Psychologists
Association 190
EuroPsy 190
Evaluator Specific Factor Scale (ESF) 238
evangelical Christianity 377–378
Ewert v Canada (2015) 245–246, 250
Expanded Levenson Self-report
Psychopathy Scale (ELSRP) 442
expert immunity fallacy, in forensic
practice 234
Explicit and Implicit Sexual Interest Profile
(EISIP) 460, 462, 469
exploratory factor analysis 55
extremist offending 16, 423–438; assessing
potential risk before crime committed
427; assessment frameworks 429–430;
assessor bias 430–434; assessor
victimisation 430; contextual issues in
assessing 424–427; Far-Right extremist
narrative 426; Islamist extremist
narrative 425–426; London attacks
(2005) 424; low rate of offending and
recidivism 428–429; methodological
issues in assessing 428–430; race, power
and privilege 425–427; radicalisation
425; scene setting 424; terminology
424–425; terrorists 424, 425
Eye-Movement Sensitisation Reprocessing
(EMDR) 415

Facebook 278, 280, 282
Fadus, M. C. 376, 380
fake news 278
fallacies, bias in forensic practice 228,
233–237, 375; bad apples (second
fallacy) 233–234; blind spot (fifth fallacy)
234; ethical issues (first fallacy) 233;
expert immunity (third fallacy) 234;
illusion of control (sixth fallacy)
235–237; technological protection
(fourth fallacy) 234
FAM (*Female Additional Manual*) 305,
306, 307
Fausto-Sterling, A. 315
fire setting 409–410
First Nations groups 7, 246
Fischer, G. H. 117
Fitness to Plead 400
5-Level System (Justice Center, US
Council of State Governments) 10–11,
95, 96–98; benefits 99, 102; challenges
105; construct validity 97; core
assumptions 98–99; developing 102;
future research 106; recommendations
101; risk assessment bias 104–105; risk-
level placements, increasing consistency
in 99–100
Five-Factor Model (FFM) 443
Floyd, G., killing of 28–29
FMHA *see* Forensic Mental Health
Assessments (FMHA)
FMHS *see* Forensic Mental Health Services
(FMHS)
Forensic Clinical Risk Assessment 111
forensic context assessment *see* assessment,
forensic practice
Forensic Mental Health Assessments
(FMHA) 178; pretrial 180; remote
see remote FMHA; social media data,
use of 285, *288*, 289–292;
see also assessment, forensic practice
Forensic Mental Health Services (FMHS):
causes and consequences of service
disparities 178–180; in rural and
economically disadvantaged regions
178–180; social media evidence
281–285, *286–287*; technology, role in
closing the gap 180; *see also* e-mental
health; juvenile justice, e-mental
health for
forensic practice: bias in *see* bias in forensic
practice; fallacies, bias in forensic